Pudner's
Nursing the Surgical Patient

Editors

Ian Peate OBE, FRCN, EN(G) RGN, DipN(Lond), RNT B.Ed (Hons), MA, LLM

Ian began his nursing a career at Central Middlesex Hospital, becoming an Enrolled Nurse practicing in an intensive care unit. He later undertook three years of student nurse training at Central Middlesex and Northwick Park Hospitals, becoming a Staff Nurse then a Charge Nurse. He has worked in nurse education since 1989. His key areas of interest are nursing practice and theory. Ian has published widely. Ian was awarded an OBE in the Queen's 90th Birthday Honours List for his services to Nursing and Nurse Education and was granted a Fellowship from the Royal College of Nursing in 2017.

Jay Macleod BSc (Hons), DipHE ODP, PCTHE, Postgraduate Certificate in Coaching and Mentoring, Fellow of The Higher Education Academy

After years in various other industries, Jay trained in Operating Department Practice (ODP) with Oxford Brookes University as a mature student. He worked at the Royal United Hospital, Bath, as an ODP before being employed with Oxford Brookes University, firstly as a part-time Teaching Fellow and then as a full-time lecturer and international project lead. Jay's passion is to advance the ODP profession and help students reach their full potential; empowering them to become the theatre leaders of the future.

Pudner's Nursing the Surgical Patient

Fourth Edition

Edited by

Ian Peate
OBE, FRCN, EN(G) RGN, DipN(Lond), RNT B.Ed (Hons), MA, LLM
Head of School, School of Health Studies, Gibraltar Health Authority, Gibraltar;
Editor in Chief, British Journal of Nursing;
Visiting Professor, St George's University of London and Kingston University London;
Visiting Professor, Northumbria University;
Visiting Senior Clinical Fellow, University of Hertfordshire, UK

Jay Macleod
BSc (Hons), DipHE ODP, PCTHE, Postgraduate Certificate in Coaching and Mentoring,
Fellow of The Higher Education Academy
Lecturer and Placement Lead of Operating Department Practice Oxford Brookes University, Oxford, UK

Elsevier Ltd
London   New York   Oxford   Philadelphia   St Louis   Sydney   2021

ELSEVIER

First edition © Harcourt Publishers 2000
Second edition © Elsevier Science Ltd 2005
Third edition 2010
Fourth edition 2021

Notices

Practitioners and researchers must always rely on their own experience and knowledge in evaluating and using any information, methods, compounds or experiments described herein. Because of rapid advances in the medical sciences, in particular, independent verification of diagnoses and drug dosages should be made. To the fullest extent of the law, no responsibility is assumed by Elsevier, authors, editors or contributors for any injury and/or damage to persons or property as a matter of products liability, negligence or otherwise, or from any use or operation of any methods, products, instructions, or ideas contained in the material herein.

ISBN: 978-0-7020-7865-1

Printed in Scotland
Last digit is the print number: 9 8 7 6 5 4 3 2 1

Content Strategist: Robert Edwards
Content Development Specialist: Fiona Conn
Project Managers: Anne Collett and Julie Taylor
Design: Amy Buxton

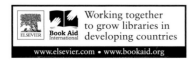

Contents

v

Preface

We were delighted to have been approached by Elsevier to undertake a review and revision of the third edition of the immensely popular and well-respected *Nursing the Surgical Patient*. Previous editions of the book have received many accolades and readers from varied backgrounds have found it to be a key text in their studies and in clinical practice.

In this, the fourth edition of the newly titled *Pudner's Nursing the Surgical Patient*, we have endeavoured to remain true to the book's original aim — to enable readers to link the theoretical concepts of surgical nursing to the application of clinical practice (wherever this may be). We have retained the user-friendly approach that Rosie Pudner successfully used over the years, ensuring that the reader is able to gain insight and understanding of the everchanging field of surgical care.

Each of the twenty-four chapters in the book has been fully reviewed and updated by either the original authors or new contributors. The chapters take into account the latest surgical procedures and technological advances, developments in clinical practice, an ageing population, complexity of care needs, the increasing challenges of long-term conditions and an epidemic of lifestyle-related morbidity.

Since the last edition, the Nursing and Midwifery Council's (NMC) *Future nurse: Standards of Proficiency for Registered Nurses* (NMC, 2018a) and the NMC's *Standards of Proficiency for Nursing Associates* (NMC, 2018b) have been published and implemented, along with the revision of *The Code* (NMC, 2018c). These have been given due consideration in this fourth edition, acknowledging that the new nursing standards are creating opportunity to redefine the essence of registered nursing practice.

Within the last decade, ambulatory (outpatient) care has developed considerably, with many procedures now being undertaken safely as a day case or with a single overnight stay, transforming the way surgical care is delivered. Transformation of service delivery supported by the British Association of Day Surgery and by patients recognizes the good and potential good for patients and service providers, enabling patients to return to normal life as quickly as possible. As the period of postoperative observation is brief and monitoring is not as intensive, ambulatory surgery is only appropriate for low-risk procedures and in those without serious comorbidities, where the possibility of major perioperative events is low.

Regardless of the developments and advances discussed, what is key to the role and function of those providing care to people undergoing surgery is that the patient remains at the centre of all that is done. As was the case with previous editions, this fourth edition uses a contemporary evidence base on which to inform practice and to offer care to people who are very often at a vulnerable juncture in their lives as they prepare for surgery, undergo surgery and recover from surgery.

The book is primarily written for those nurses who offer care and support to surgical patients, acknowledging that it is not possible to separate the care that is required by a surgical patient from other associated medical aspects of their care. The reader is directed to other sources of information, as well as to other specialist nursing texts and appropriate websites within the book.

The book will continue to be of value for undergraduate nursing students and trainee nursing associates with a focus on the adult patient. The hallmark clear, user-friendly and easy-to-understand approach has been retained for this fourth edition, providing a useful resource for revision and in clinical practice.

Preface

In Section I of the book, chapters relate to aspects of surgical nursing care that are applicable to all of those who are undergoing a surgical procedure. Section II focuses on specific areas of surgical nursing. These chapters provide a detailed discussion related to surgical procedures and the requisite nursing care, helping the reader to understand the complexities of surgical interventions.

The approach adopted in this book is patient-centred, using a problem-solving, evidence-based approach to care. The care required by people undergoing surgery is discussed and aligned to national guidelines and standards. Case studies and care plans have been included to demonstrate the use of a problem-solving approach to patient care. This new edition encourages the reader to reflect on their practice, to utilize critical thinking and to ensure that care is safe and compassionate.

Reference to relevant, best available evidence and research findings continues to be a key aspect in this new edition, as those who provide care are required to do so using a sound evidence base. As well as a reference list at the end of each chapter, the reader is offered a further reading list, and details of relevant websites are also provided to encourage the reader to delve deeper, extending their knowledge base beyond this text and to engender a sense of curiosity.

It is envisaged that the book will provide a guide to the theoretical and practical aspects required to offer safe and effective surgical care. It is not intended that the book is read from cover to cover; more so, the reader dips in and out of the relevant sections and chapters related to the care of surgical patients they have the privilege to support and care for.

The chapters have been written by a range of authors practising in the surgical field and academics who are actively engaged in clinical practice, further cementing the aspiration to relate theory and practice.

We hope you find this revised and updated edition a valuable resource as you strive to offer people care that is appropriate and, above all, safe. We have enjoyed editing the book and we hope you will enjoy using it. We anticipate that by using the book this will encourage you to delve deeper into the exciting and developing field of surgical care. Taking over as editors from Rosie Pudner has been a privilege and a worthwhile experience, providing us with the opportunity to continue her legacy and her passion to promote surgical care.

Ian Peate
Jay Macleod

References

Nursing and Midwifery Council (NMC). (2018a). *Future nurse: Standards of proficiency for registered nurses*. Available at: <www.nmc.org.uk/globalassets/sitedocuments/education-standards/future-nurse-proficiencies.pdf>

Nursing and Midwifery Council (NMC). (2018b). *Standards of proficiency for nursing associates*. Available at: <www.nmc.org.uk/globalassets/sitedocuments/education-standards/nursing-associates-proficiency-standards.pdf>

Nursing and Midwifery Council (NMC). (2018c). *The code. Professional standards of practice and behaviour for nurses, midwives and nursing associates*. Available at: <www.nmc.org.uk/standards/code>

Acknowledgements

Ian would like to acknowledge the ongoing support offered to him by his partner, Jussi Lahtinen, and the support offered to him by Mrs Frances Cohen. He would also like to thank the staff in the library at the School of Health Studies, Gibraltar, and the RCN Library, London.

Jay would like to thank his wife, Jo, his children, Connor and Mia, and his family for their continuous support, advice and encouragement in all of his endeavours.

We would like to thank those authors who have contributed chapters to earlier editions and the founding Editor, Rosie Pudner.

List of Contributors

The editor(s) would like to acknowledge and offer grateful thanks for the input of all previous editions' contributors, without whom this new edition would not have been possible.

Katie Adams FRCS
Consultant Colorectal & General
Surgeon
Department of Colorectal Surgery
Guy's & St Thomas' NHS Foundation
Trust
London, UK

Adèle Atkinson MEd, BA(Hons),
RN, RNT, ENB 264, SFHEA
Formerly Associate Professor
School of Nursing, Faculty of Health,
Social Care & Education, Kingston
University & St. George's, University of
London, Kingston Hill Campus,
Kingston upon Thames, UK

Claire Badger BN (Hons) Nursing,
**Post Grad Dip Perioperative Specialist
Practice, MSc Advancing Practice, MSc
by Research in Clinical Practice**
Consultant Nurse Lead Pre-Operative
Assessment Service
University Hospitals Coventry and
Warwickshire
Coventry, UK

Melanie Baker RD, BSc (Hons), MSc
Clinical & Speciality Lead, Nutrition
Support Team
Nutrition & Dietetic Service
University Hospitals of Leicester NHS Trust,
Leicester, UK

Kevin Barrett RN BSc(Hons) MRes
PgCHSCE SFHEA
Senior Lecturer
School of Health Sciences, University of
Brighton
Brighton, UK

Louise Best PGdip, BSc (Acute
Clinical Care), NMP
Advanced Nurse Practitioner in Cardiac
Surgery
Royal Sussex County Hospital, Brighton
& Sussex University Hospitals
Brighton, UK

Chris Brunker MRes, RGN
Clinical Nurse Specialist
Neuro-ICU, St George's University
Hospitals NHS Foundation Trust

Nigel Conway MSc, BA(Hons),
PGCert, RODP
Programme Leader, Faculty of Health &
Life Sciences,
Department of Psychology, Health &
Professional Development,
Oxford Brookes University,
Oxford, UK

Ali Curtis RN DipN, Bsc (Hons)
Matron and Clinical Operations Manager
Benenden Hospital, Cranbrook
Kent, UK

Nuala Davison B.Nurs (Hons) in
Adult Nursing
Clinical Nurse Specialist in Obesity Surgery
Department of General Surgery, Chelsea
and Westminster Healthcare NHS
Foundation Trust
London, UK

Marie Digner
Deputy Divisional Director of Operations/
Clinical Manager
Diagnostics and Support Services Division
Bolton Hospitals NHS Foundation
Trust
Greater Manchester, UK

Giles Farrington RODP MAcadMED
Senior Operating Department
Practitioner
Operating Department, York Teaching
Hospital NHS Foundation Trust
York, North Yorkshire, UK

Helen Gibbons MSc, PGCert
Medical Education , BA Hons
Clinical Lead Nurse Education
Course Director MSc Clinical Ophthalmic
Practice
Moorfields Eye Hospital NHS Trust
London, UK

Efua Hagan DipHE Operating
**Department Practice, Esc Health
Studies**
Practice Development Operating
Department Practitioner
King's College Hospital, NHS Foundation
Trust
London, UK

Fiona Hibberts BSc Hons) RN, MSc,
PGCert, FHEA
Head of the Nightingale Academy /
Consultant Nurse
Guy's and St. Thomas' NHS Foundation
Trust
London, UK

Barry Hill MSc. PGCAP. BSc (Hons), DipHE. O.A. Dip. SFHEA); NMC: TCH, RN
Director of Employability for Nursing, Midwifery and Health
Programme Leader BSc (Hons) Adult Nursing
Northumbria University, Faculty of Health and Life Sciences (HLS), Department of Nursing, Midwifery and Health, Newcastle upon Tyne, UK

Jane Holden RN ENB 264; BA Hons; PGC; MSc
Lead Clinical Nurse in Plastic Surgery
Department of Plastic Surgery, St. George's University Hospital's NHS Foundation Trust
London, UK

Bhuvaneswari Krishnamoorthy BSc (Hons), DNDM, DRCS, NMP, MPhil, PhD, SFHEA, PFHEA, FFPCEd
Postdoctoral NIHR fellow and Senior Lecturer for MSc Surgical Practice
Edge Hill University and Manchester Foundation Trust.
Manchester, UK

Georgina Lewis BSc MSc
Surgical Care Practitioner (Gynaecology)
Gloucestershire Hospitals NHS Foundation Trust
Gloucestershire, UK

Joseph Mahaffey RODP, DipHE
Divisional Clinical Educator
Surgery, Women's and Oncology Division
Oxford University Hospitals NHS Foundation Trust
Oxford, UK

Jo Mahoney BSc (Hons), RN, V300
National Clinical Specialist Pre-Operative Assessment
Spire Healthcare
London, UK

Sarah McKenna DipHE ODP
Associate Lecturer for Oxford Brookes University
and Resuscitation Officer (Operating Department Practitioner)
Great Western Hospital Foundation Trust
Swindon, UK

Julie McLaren RN, BN, BSc Hons, AFHEA
Lecturer
School of Health and Life Science
University of West of Scotland
Lanarkshire, UK

Janice Minter BSC Adult Nursing
Lead Cancer Nurse
St Georges University Hospitals NHS Foundation Trust
London, UK

Helen Ord
Senior Specialist Dietitian, Training and Education,
Nutrition and Dietetic Service, University Hospitals of Leicester NHS Trust
Leicester, UK.

Chloe Rich RODP, FHEA, PCTHE, BSc (Hons), DipHe
Programme Lead; Senior Lecturer, Operating Department Practice
University of Bolton
Bolton, UK

Deborah Robinson MSc Ed, ODP
Faculty Director of Professional External Engagement
Faculty of Health Sciences
University of Hull
Hull, UK

Madhini Sivasubramanian RN, RSCN, RNT, Paediatric ICU Nursing, FHEA, MSc, PGdip, PGCE (Mphil/PhD)
Senior Lecturer Adult Nursing.
Simulation Lead
University of East London
Stratford, London, UK

Lee Wadsworth RGN MSc Clinical Nursing V300
Nurse Clinician/Clinical Trainer
A & L Healthcare Consultancy & Training
Macclesfield, Cheshire, UK

Ashleigh Ward MSc PgDip BScHons RN
Lecturer
Faculty of Health Sciences and Sport, University of Stirling
Stirling, UK

Kate Woodhead RGN, DMS
Director, KMW (Healthcare Consultants) Ltd,
Leeds, UK

Anne Wright BSc (Hons)Nursing, Post Grad Dip Advanced Clinical Practice
Senior Sister Preassessment Services
Hywel Dda University Health Board, Withybush General Hospital
Haverfordwest, Pembrokeshire, UK

Glossary

Abduction Movement of a limb away from the midline of the body.

Absorption The passing of substances into the surrounding tissue.

Accommodation A process by which the refractive power of the lens is increased by contraction of the ciliary muscle, causing an increased thickness and curvature of the lens, allowing near objects to be focused on the retina.

Achlorhydria An abnormal condition where there is absence of hydrochloric acid in the stomach.

Adduction Movement of a limb towards the midline of the body.

Adhesions Following an inflammatory process, two surfaces, not normally joined, unite together.

Adjuvant A substance or treatment that can be used to enhance the action of an analgesic.

Agnosia Inability to recognize objects because of damage to the sensory pathways.

Alignment The state of being arranged in the correct anatomical position.

Amblyopia Subnormal vision associated with squints due to a lack of retinal stimulation in the first years of life.

Amenorrhoea Absence of periods (menses).

Anaesthetic Administration of a regimen of drugs and/or gases and/or volatile agents to abolish the sensation of feeling.

Anastomosis The joining of two hollow structures, usually by suturing together during a surgical procedure, e.g. two sections of the colon, or stomach to small intestine, or blood vessels.

Aneurysm Local dilatation of a blood vessel, usually an artery, caused by a fault in the wall due to defect, disease or injury, producing a pulsating swelling over which a murmur may be heard.

Angina Pain emanating from the heart, due to inadequate blood supply to the myocardium, which radiates into the chest, jaw and down the left arm.

Angiogenesis The process of new blood vessel formation.

Angiography X-ray of the arterial system by means of injecting a radio-opaque contrast medium.

Ankle brachial pressure index (ABPI) A non-invasive test to assess arterial blood supply to a lower limb by measuring the ankle–brachial systolic pressure ratio using a hand-held Doppler ultrasonic probe.

Anorexia Lack or complete loss of appetite, which may result in malnutrition and/or starvation.

Antacid A substance which buffers, neutralizes or absorbs the effects of hydrochloric acid in the contents of the stomach.

Antiseptics Solutions which are intended to inhibit the proliferation of pathogens.

Aperient Mild laxative medication which stimulates a bowel action.

Aphakia Absence of a lens in the eye, following cataract surgery or trauma.

Apposition Bringing together two opposing structures.

Arrhythmia An abnormal heart rhythm that may be regular or irregular.

Arterial occlusive disease Obstruction of the arteries by embolus, thrombus or atherosclerosis.

Arteriosclerosis/atherosclerosis Degeneration of the artery, with thickening and loss of elasticity of the arterial walls.

Arteriotomy Cutting or opening into an artery.

Arthrodesis An operation to produce bony fusion across a joint.

Arthroplasty Surgical reconstruction of a joint.

Arthroscopy Examination of a joint using an arthroscope.

Asepsis Prevention of wound contamination by using only sterile instruments and solutions.

Astigmatism Irregularity of the cornea in one or more planes.

Asymmetrical Not identical on both sides of a central line.

Atherectomy Removal of obstructing atheroma using high-speed cutters.

Atheroma Deposits of hard yellow plaques of lipoid material in the intimal layer of arteries.

Athetosis Involuntary, slow writhing movements.

Atrophy Degeneration of cells, resulting in wasting of any part of the body.

Bacteraemia Presence of bacteria in the blood.

Bioptome catheter An intravascular catheter device with a small opening and closing capsular mouth that can take tiny tissue samples from the heart.

Bitemporal hemianopia Tunnel vision.

Blepharo Conditions related to the eyelids.

Glossary

Blom–Singer valve A voice prosthesis for a laryngectomy patient; it allows air to enter the oesophagus, and the vibrating tissue, together with oral articulation, enables the patient to produce speech.

Body ideal The picture in our heads of how we would like our body to look and perform.

Body image A psychological experience focusing on conscious and unconscious attitudes and feelings. It is dependent on body ideal, body reality and body presentation.

Body presentation The body as it is presented to the world.

Body reality The physical body as it exists.

Bougie A flexible instrument which is used to dilate a tubular organ such as the oesophagus.

Brace A support used in orthopaedics to hold parts of the body in their correct position.

Bradyarrhythmia Abnormal regular or irregular heart rhythm with a rate that is less than 60 beats per minute, which may cause hypotension and hypoperfusion.

Bronchoscopy Endoscopic examination of the main bronchi.

Bunion Prominence of the head of the metatarsal bone at its junction with the great toe.

Buphthalmos Congenital glaucoma, also referred to as 'ox eye'.

Capillary refill The time taken for capillaries to refill – usually tested by pressing on area with a finger (to occlude the capillary) and then releasing the pressure.

Carpopedal spasm Cramp in the hands and feet due to a deficiency of ionized calcium in the blood.

Cataract Opacity of the lens.

Chalazion/meibomian cyst/internal hordeolum Enlargement and blockage of the meibomian gland.

Chemosis Oedema of the conjunctiva.

Chemotherapy A systemic cytotoxic drug treatment.

Cheyne–Stokes respiratory pattern A pattern of breathing which includes stertorous breathing with periods of apnoea.

Chorea Involuntary sudden movements which are both flexor and extensor.

Chvostek's sign Spasm of the facial muscles produced by tapping the facial nerve.

Circumcision Surgical removal of the foreskin.

Colic Severe spasmodic episodes of pain caused by involuntary muscular contraction.

Compartment syndrome Swelling within the muscle compartments of a limb due to haemorrhage or oedema, resulting in muscle necrosis and nerve damage.

Conjunctivitis Inflammation of the conjunctiva, usually caused by a bacterial or viral infection.

Contraction Drawing together of wound edges.

Contralateral Pertaining to the opposite side.

Cortical blindness Blindness caused by damage to the occipital lobe.

Counter-traction A force applied to oppose traction.

Cyanosis Bluish discoloration of the skin caused by a relative decrease in oxygen saturation levels within the capillaries.

Cycloplegia Paralysis of the ciliary muscle.

Cystectomy Surgical removal of the bladder.

Cystocele Herniation and descent of the bladder through the anterior vaginal wall.

Cystoscopy Endoscopic visualization of the urethra and bladder using a fibreoptic light source.

Cytology Study of cells used in diagnosis of pre-malignant disease.

Dacryocystorhinostomy Formation of an opening between the lacrimal sac and the nasal cavity.

Decortication Surgery to remove the thick cortex that is formed as a result of empyema within the pleural cavity.

Dehiscence Breakdown of a surgically closed wound.

Denervated Lacking nerve endings.

Depolarization A surge of charged particles that bring about muscle contraction.

Dermatome An area of the body corresponding to a particular nerve root.

Digital subtraction angiography (DSA) A computerized method of angiography without background information (e.g. bones, bowel).

Dilatation and curettage Gentle dilatation of the cervix and scraping (curetting) of the endometrium for diagnostic purposes.

Diplopia Double vision.

Dislocation Displacement of a bone from its anatomical position.

Dissection Tearing or splitting, e.g. the inner lining of the coronary artery wall.

Distension Enlargement of the abdomen with a collection of gas or fluid from the intestines.

Donor site Area from which a skin graft or flap has been taken.

Dorsiflexion Bending the ankle upwards.

Duct ectasia A benign condition affecting the breast.

Ductal carcinoma *in situ* A pre-invasive ductal carcinoma of the breast.

Duplex scan A non-invasive ultrasonic scan providing accurate diagnosis of arterial stenosis/occlusion or deep vein thrombosis.

Dysarthria Difficulty with articulating speech.

Dyscalculia Difficulty with calculating.

Dysgraphia Difficulty with writing, caused by brain damage.

Dyslexia Difficulty with reading and abstract thinking.

Dysmenorrhoea Painful periods.

Dyspareunia Painful sexual intercourse.

Dyspepsia Symptoms associated with indigestion, nausea, vomiting, discomfort of the abdomen and flatulence.

Dysphagia Difficulty in swallowing.

Dysphasia Difficulty with the processing of language. It can be (a) receptive, in which the individual experiences difficulty understanding language, or (b) expressive, in which the individual has a difficulty in expressing himself in words.

Dyspnoea Difficulty in breathing.

Dyspraxia Difficulty in performing a pattern of movements, e.g. locating and picking up a cup.

Dysuria Painful micturition.

Ectopic pregnancy Pregnancy which implants outside the uterus, most commonly in the fallopian tubes.

Ectropion Turning out of the lid margin, usually the bottom lid.

Electrosurgery The surgical application of heat to coagulate blood vessels to prevent excessive bleeding, and also to cut tissue.

Embolectomy Surgical removal of an embolism.

Embolism Obstruction of blood vessels by impaction of a solid body (e.g. thrombi, fat or tumour cells).

Empyema Collection of purulent fluid within the pleural space.

Endarterectomy Surgical removal of an atheromatous plug in an artery.

Endometriosis A condition where the endometrium grows in other parts of the body outside the uterus.

Enteral nutrition May refer to food or fluids taken orally or via a tube placed within the gastrointestinal tract.

Entropion Turning in of the lid margin, usually the bottom lid.

Enucleation Removal of the eye.

Epiphora Overflow of tears onto the cheek due to a defective or inadequate drainage system.

Euthyroid A normally functioning thyroid gland.

Evisceration Removal of the internal structures of the eye.

Excoriation Superficial breakdown of skin, usually surrounding a wound and caused by wound exudate.

Exenteration Removal of an organ.

Exostosis A bony outgrowth from the surface of the bone.

Exudate Fluid produced in wounds, which consists of serum, leucocytes and wound debris.

Fasciotomy Incision of a fascia to relieve damaging tension in a muscle compartment or prevent compression of arteries or nerves.

Fat necrosis Death of fat tissue, creating a hard craggy lump that often mimics cancer, and often occurs following trauma.

Fibroadenoma A benign tumour of fibrous or glandular tissue.

Fibroids Benign fibrous tumour found in the muscle of the uterus or cervix.

Fistula An abnormal track which may connect one epithelial surface to another, organ to organ, or organ to epithelial surface.

Flap Tissue which is moved from one part of the body to another and takes its own blood supply with it.

Flatus The presence of gas in the stomach or intestines.

Fluoroscope X-ray equipment that allows direct viewing of images without taking or developing X-ray pictures.

Foreign body Material found in the body which does not normally belong, e.g. prosthetic material, sutures, staples.

Gastrectomy Surgical removal of part or the whole of the stomach

Gastrostomy Incision into the stomach. A tube is placed within the incision; often used for feeding.

Glaucoma Raised intraocular pressure.

Glucose intolerance The inability to metabolize glucose efficiently as a result of the presence of large quantities of cortisol during the stress response.

Goitre An enlargement of the thyroid gland, which presents as a pronounced swelling in the neck.

Graft bed The wound site on which skin grafting will take place.

Growth factors Proteins which act as cell messengers and are vital for cell proliferation.

Guttae Eyedrops.

Haematoma A localized collection of blood within the tissues.

Haematuria Blood in the urine.

Haemostasis The cessation of bleeding.

Haemothorax The abnormal presence of blood in the pleural space.

Halitosis Unpleasant or foul-smelling breath which often results from systemic disease.

Haemolysis The rupture or destruction red blood cells.

Heimlich valve A small, portable, one-way valve device for draining air from a pneumothorax, but unsuitable if fluid is draining as well.

Hemiballismus Violent involuntary movements of the limbs.

Homonymous hemianopia Loss of vision in the right or left visual fields.

Hydatidiform mole A condition in pregnancy in which the chorionic villi degenerate into clusters of cysts.

Hydrocele Collection of fluid in the tunica vaginalis.

Hydrocephalus Excessive accumulation of cerebrospinal fluid in the ventricles or around the brain.

Hydrophilic A substance that attracts water.

Hypercholesterolaemia Excessive cholesterol in the blood.

Hyperlipidaemia Excessive fat in the blood.

Hyperthyroidism Excessive secretions of thyroid hormones.

Hypertrophic scar An increase in the volume of tissue produced by enlargement of existing cells.

Hyphaema Presence of red blood cells in the anterior chamber of the eye.

Hypocalcaemia Diminished amount of blood calcium.

Hypoparathyroidism Diminished function of the parathyroid glands.

Hypopyon Presence of white blood cells in the anterior chamber of the eye.

Hypothyroidism Insufficiency of thyroid hormone secretion.

Hypoxaemia Low levels of oxygen in the blood.

Hypoxia Lack of oxygen to the tissues and body organs.

Hysterosalpingogram Diagnostic X-ray examination of the uterus and fallopian tubes following the injection of a radio-opaque dye.

Hysteroscopy A diagnostic procedure examining the uterine cavity via an endoscope.

Induction The process of causing unconsciousness by the use of anaesthetic agents.

Infection The presence of microorganisms in sufficient numbers to cause a host reaction.

Infertility Inability to conceive.

Intermittent claudication Sudden, severe pain in the calves, thigh or buttock muscles, occurring after walking a certain distance; caused by an inadequate blood supply to the muscles.

Intra-abdominal pressure Increased pressure within the abdominal cavity.

Intraduct papilloma A wart-like growth in the duct of a breast.

Intramedullary Within the medullary cavity of long bone.

Intraoperative The phase which starts when the patient is transferred to the operating table and ends when the patient is transferred to the recovery room.

Intrathecal antibiotics Antibiotics introduced into the cerebrospinal fluid in the theca of the spinal canal.

Invasive ductal carcinoma An invasive cancer arising from the ducts of the breast.

Invasive lobular carcinoma An invasive cancer arising from the lobules in the breast.

Ipsilateral Pertains to the same side.

Ischaemia Lack of blood supply to a part of the body.

Jaundice The mucous membranes and sclera become yellow due to bile bilirubin in the blood.

Jejunostomy A surgically made fistula between the jejunum and abdominal wall. A fine tube is placed within the fistula, usually for feeding.

Keloid scar A type of scar which results from the formation of large amounts of scar tissue around the wound.

Keratitis Inflammation of the cornea.

Keratoconus Abnormality of the cornea, resulting in apical thinning and bulging.

Keratoplasty Corneal graft.

Ketosis An abnormal amount of ketones in the blood and urine as a result of inefficient metabolism of carbohydrates.

Kirschner wire A thin wire which may be passed through a bone.

Lacrimation Production of tears.

Laminectomy Excision of the posterior arch of the vertebra.

Laparoscopy A surgical procedure to internally examine the abdomen using minimally invasive techniques (keyhole surgery).

Laparotomy A surgical procedure where the abdominal wall is incised either for exploratory procedures or surgery.

Laryngeal mask airway A single use supraglottic airway device

Laryngoscopy Examination of the larynx using a laryngoscope.

Laryngospasm Spasm of the larynx.

Latissimus dorsi flap A flap of muscle and skin taken from the latissimus dorsi muscle in the back for reconstructive surgery of the breast, or head and neck.

Lipoma A fatty lump.

Lobectomy Surgical resection of one or more lobes of a lung.

Lymphadenitis Inflammation of the lymphatic glands.

Lymphoedema Oedema due to the obstruction of lymph vessels.

Malnutrition A condition that arises when the body's nutrition becomes depleted.

Mammogram A radiographic investigation of the breast.

Mastectomy Removal of the breast.

Mastitis An infection of the breast.

Meatotomy Incision of the urethral meatus.

Meatoplasty Surgical reconstruction of the urethral meatus.

Mediastinoscopy Invasive surgical procedure to visualize and biopsy the lymph glands of the mediastinum.

Mediastinotomy Opening of the mediastinum, allowing insertion of an endoscope.

Melaena Faeces are coloured black with altered blood, as a result of bleeding into the lower part of the digestive system.

Meningitis Inflammation of the meninges.

Menopause The normal cessation of menstruation, commonly occurring at around the age of 50 years.

Menorrhagia Heavy menstrual bleeding.

Mesothelioma A pleural tumour, often associated with contact with asbestos.

Metastases Spread of cancer from a primary tumour, via the blood and lymphatic systems, to other tissue/organs.

Microcalcification Minute chalky deposits in the breast.

Microdochectomy An operation performed to disconnect a duct in the breast.

Miotic An agent that constricts the pupil.

Morcellated Broken up into small pieces.

Motility The action of spontaneous movement.

Multimodal analgesia The use of different types of analgesics to provide enhanced analgesia while reducing side-effects.

Mydriatic An agent that dilates the pupil.

Myelography A radiological investigation of the spinal cord and subarachnoid space. A contrast medium is introduced through a lumbar puncture in order to identify spinal pathology.

Myomectomy Removal of fibroids, either through laparotomy or laparoscopy.

Myxoedema A syndrome due to hypothyroidism.

Necrotic tissue Localized dead tissue which has a leathery texture and is black/brown in colour.

Neo-bladder Reconstruction of the whole bladder using bowel.

Nephrectomy Surgical removal of the kidney.

Nephrostomy tube Temporary method of draining the renal pelvis.

Nociception The processing of damaging or potentially damaging stimuli.

Oesophagostomy The surgical creation of an opening from the surface of the body into the oesophagus.

Oesophagectomy The surgical removal of all or part of the oesophagus.

Oculentum An eye ointment.

Occult bloods The faecal occult blood test (FOBT) is a laboratory test that is used to check stool samples for hidden (occult) blood.

Olfaction The sense of smell.

Oncology The study and treatment of tumours.

Oophorectomy Surgical removal of one or both ovaries.

Orchidectomy Surgical procedure to remove testes.

Orthoptics Special eye exercises to develop binocular vision.

Ossification The process by which bone is developed.

Osteotomy An operation to cut across bone.

Ototoxicity The degree to which a substance is harmful to the structures of the ear.

Oxygen saturation (SaO$_2$) Measurement of the percentage of oxygen bound to haemoglobin; normal range is 95–99%.

Palmar Relating to the palm of the hand; also called volar.

Paralytic ileus Reduced peristalsis (motility) in a portion of the bowel, causing the ileum to become obstructed.

Paraphimosis Condition arising from inability to replace foreskin over glans penis.

Perception The way something is regarded or understood.

Percutaneous An invasive approach through the skin.

Percutaneous transluminal angioplasty (PTA) A balloon catheter is passed into the lumen of the artery at the site of stricture, usually under local anaesthetic, and the balloon inflated, dilating the stricture.

Pericardiocentesis Removal of excess fluid from the pericardial space by needle aspiration.

Perioperative The total surgical journey incorporating pre-, intra- and postoperative phases.

Peripheral vascular disease Impaired circulation to the limbs.

Peristalsis Movement along the wall of a tubular structure.

Pernicious anaemia Anaemia caused by the lack of absorption of vitamin B$_{12}$.

Peyronie's disease Fibrotic process of unknown aetiology, resulting in erectile deformity.

Phacoemulsification A form of cataract removal that uses high-frequency sound waves to emulsify the lens matter, which can then be aspirated more easily.

Phagocytosis The process by which foreign matter is engulfed by phagocytes, e.g. macrophages.

Phasing Regular and frequent measurements of intraocular pressure.

Phimosis Term given to the inability to retract the foreskin over the glans penis.

Phlebitis Inflammation of a vein, which is often associated with clot formation (thrombophlebitis).

Photophobia Sensitivity to light.

Photopsia The presence or perceived flashing of lights.

Pleural effusion (hydrothorax) Collection of fluid within the pleural space.

Pleurectomy Surgical removal of the parietal pleura, in the treatment of pneumothorax.

Pleurodesis Surgical procedure to introduce an irritant substance into the pleural space to cause an inflammatory reaction to adhere the pleural surfaces together.

Pneumonectomy Surgical resection of one lung.

Pneumothorax Abnormal presence of air in the pleural space, causing collapse of the underlying lung.

Postcoital bleeding Bleeding after sexual intercourse.

Postoperative This phase starts when the patient is transferred from the operating theatre to the recovery room.

Potency The dose of a drug required to produce 50% of the maximum response of that drug.

Preoperative Commences either when the patient decides to have surgery and includes the

preoperative assessment, or from the moment the patient arrives in the operating theatre. The phase concludes when the patient is transferred onto the operating table.

Presbycusis Progressive deafness that occurs with age.

Priapism A persistent painful erection.

Primary dressing A dressing which is applied directly to the wound surface.

Procidentia Complete prolapse of the uterus so that it extrudes through the vagina.

Proliferation Reproduction of cells.

Proprioception Sensory function which monitors and interprets spatial position and muscle activity.

Proptosis Abnormal protrusion of the eye.

Prosthesis Any artificial device attached to the body as a substitute for a missing or non-functional part.

Prosthetic tube An artificial tube fitted into the oesophagus to provide patency to the oesophagus and allow semi-fluid nutritional substances to be taken into the body.

Ptosis Drooping of the upper eyelid.

Pulmonary oedema Accumulation of fluid in the lung tissue, causing prolongation of oxygen transport.

Pulse oximeter An instrument that uses arterial pulsation to detect the level of oxygen saturated on haemoglobin.

Purulent Producing pus.

Pus Fluid containing exudate, bacteria and phagocytes which have completed their work. Is usually seen in infected wounds.

Pyeloplasty Operation to relieve obstruction at the pelviureteric junction in the kidney.

Quadrantectomy Excision of a quadrant of the breast.

Radiotherapy The treatment of disease with penetrating radiation.

Raised intracranial pressure Pressure within the cranium, resulting from a space-occupying lesion.

Rectocele Hernia and prolapse of the rectum through the posterior vaginal wall.

Reduction Putting a fracture or dislocation in its correct position.

Refraction The convergence of light rays so they focus on the macula.

Regurgitation Backward flow of blood against the normal direction of flow, i.e. blood flows backwards through regurgitant heart valves instead of forwards.

Resection Removal of part of the body by surgery.

Resident flora Microorganisms which reside on the skin and exist in harmony with their host.

Rest pain Severe pain in the leg or foot occurring while the patient is resting, which can prevent the patient from sleeping.

Salpingectomy Surgical removal of one of both fallopian tubes.

Salpingitis Inflammation and infection of the fallopian tubes.

Salpingo-oophorectomy Surgical excision of one or both fallopian tubes and ovaries.

Sclerotherapy A treatment for varicose veins in which the affected veins are injected with a solution that causes inflammation of the vein lining, clotting of the contained blood and adherence and closure of the vein.

Secondary dressing A dressing which holds a primary dressing in place.

Segmentectomy Surgical resection of an anatomical segment of a lobe of lung.

Self-concept An individual's percepts, concepts and evaluations about themselves, including the image they feel others have of them and of the person they would like to be.

Self-esteem The outcome of the process of self-evaluation and self-worth, i.e. thinking favourably of oneself; evaluation of one's self-worth.

Sensory inattention The inability to detect touch or pain in both limbs when the stimulus is applied to both the limbs simultaneously, caused by a lesion in the parietal lobe.

Sentinel node The first lymph node draining the site of a cancer.

Septicaemia Presence of bacteria in the bloodstream, accompanied by symptoms of infection and illness.

Sepsis A potentially life-threatening condition caused by the body's response to an infection.

Seroma A fluid collection.

Serosanguinous Composed of serum and blood.

Sinus A wound where one end is open to the skin, with a track leading to a blind cavity.

Skin graft A piece of skin that has been totally separated from its blood supply, to be used on another area.

Skin graft take The adherence and healing of a skin graft.

Sloughy tissue Devitalized tissue which contains some exudate, and is yellow, white or grey in colour.

Speculum A metal instrument used to dilate an orifice or canal in the body to allow inspection.

Staging Investigations to detect metastatic disease.

Stenosis An abnormal narrowing of an orifice or opening of a vessel.

Stent A small tubular mesh structure that prevents an artery or other hollow structure from collapsing.

Stoma An artificial opening of a tube that has been brought to the surface.

Strabismus Squint.

Stress A response to a difficult situation, or a set of circumstances which require an unusual response.

Stress incontinence Incontinence caused by increased abdominal pressure, e.g. in coughing.

Subarachnoid haemorrhage A haemorrhage from the vessels of the circle of Willis into the subarachnoid space.

Subcuticular Within the subcutaneous tissues.

Subluxation A partial dislocation.

Surgical emphysema Air in the subcutaneous tissue that can result from thoracic surgery and pneumothorax.

Sympathectomy Surgical excision to remove part of the sympathetic nervous system supply to an area in order to limit constriction of the

blood vessels and therefore increase blood flow.

Sympathetic ophthalmitis Severe uveitis in one eye following trauma involving the uvea of the other eye.

Synovectomy Excision of diseased synovial membrane.

Tachyarrhythmia Abnormal heart rhythm that may be regular or irregular at a rate greater than 100 beats per minute, e.g. ventricular tachycardia, which may cause hypotension and hypoperfusion.

Tachypnoea Rapid respiratory rate greater than 20 breaths per minute.

Tamponade The abnormal presence of blood or fluid in the pericardial space, which can prevent the heart chambers from filling adequately with blood, and may lead to shock and death.

Tenesmus A painful condition when the faeces will not be expelled from the rectum despite the effort of straining.

Tension pneumothorax Like a pneumothorax, but a flap of tissue allows air to enter but not leave the pleural space, causing increased intrathoracic pressure and is potentially fatal.

Tentorial herniation The herniation of the uncus of the temporal lobe between the brainstem and the tentorium cerebelli when the intracranial pressure is greater above the tentorium cerebelli than below it.

Tertiary centre A hospital that provides tertiary care, including highly specialized treatment such as neurosurgery, transplants, burns and plastics.

Tetany A condition marked by spasms of the hands and feet, due to a diminished blood calcium level.

Thiersch graft The name given to split skin grafts.

Thoracentesis Aspiration of fluid from the pleural cavity.

Thoracoscopy Endoscopic examination of the pleural surfaces.

Thoracotomy Surgical opening of the chest.

Thrombectomy Surgical removal of a thrombus from within a blood vessel.

Thrombosis Formation of blood clot within a blood vessel.

Thymectomy Resection of the thymus gland.

Thyroidectomy Surgical removal of the thyroid gland.

Thyrotoxicosis A condition produced by overactivity of the thyroid gland.

Tie-over pack A type of pressure dressing used on Wolfe grafts.

Tinnitus Noise in the ear, ringing, rushing or buzzing sound.

Tissue expander An inflatable device which is inserted under the skin and slowly expanded in order to provide enough skin to cover an adjacent defect without the need to use additional donor skin.

Total abdominal hysterectomy Surgical removal of the uterus and cervix, via an incision in the abdomen.

Total parenteral nutrition The provision of full nutritional support via routes (intravenous or subcutaneous) other than the mouth or rectum.

Tracheostomy An opening through the neck into the trachea with an indwelling tube inserted.

Traction A pulling or drawing force.

Transducer A device that converts a physical variable, e.g. pressure, into an electrical waveform, e.g. blood pressure is recorded directly from an artery, and the waveform and pressures are displayed on a monitor.

Transient flora Microorganisms that are transferred onto the skin through contact with other people or objects.

Transluminal Through the space/lumen of a blood vessel.

Transvaginal Through or across the vagina.

Transverse rectus abdominis myocutaneous flap A flap of muscle and skin taken from the abdominal muscle to reconstruct the breast.

Trousseau's sign A spasm of the muscles, occurring in tetany, if pressure is applied over large arteries or nerves.

Tru-cut biopsy An incisional biopsy taking a small core of tissue for histological diagnosis.

T-tube A tube placed into the common bile duct following exploration or surgery to keep the common bile duct patent, allowing bile to be passed freely until any oedema subsides.

Ultrasound A radiological investigation using sound waves.

Urethroplasty Open operation to reconstruct the urethra.

Urethrotomy Endoscopic cutting of urethral stricture.

Urgency Overwhelming desire to pass urine immediately.

Urinary flow rate The rate and volume of urine voided (in mL).

Urinary frequency Voiding frequency, e.g. up to 10–12 times per day.

Urinary incontinence Absence of voluntary control over the passing of urine.

Vacuum-assisted closure Application of topical negative pressure to a wound, to assist closure in wounds healing by secondary intention and after the application of skin grafts.

Valgus Displacement outwards.

Varicocele Varicose condition of the veins of the spermatic cord.

Varus Displacement inwards.

Vasectomy Surgical procedure for sterilization of the male.

Vasoconstriction Contraction of blood vessels.

Vasodilatation Dilatation of blood vessels.

Vasovasostomy Surgical procedure for reversal of vasectomy.

Venography X-ray examination of venous system by injecting a radio-opaque contrast medium.

Ventricular aneurysm Bulging, thinning and enlargement of part of the ventricle wall due to myocardial infarction.

Vertigo Hallucination of movement; dizziness.

Viscera The internal organs of the body cavities.

Vulvectomy Total or partial excision of the vulva.

Wedge resection Surgical excision of part of a lung without reference to anatomical divisions.

Wide local excision Removal of a lump plus a good margin of healthy tissue surrounding it.

Wolfe graft The name given to full-thickness skin grafts.

Wound An injury which causes tissue damage and may result in the loss of continuity of the skin or tissue.

Xenograft An animal graft.

Section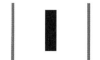

The basis of surgical care

Chapter | 1 |

Preoperative assessment

*Claire Badger, Marie Digner, Jo Mahoney, Ali Curtis, Lee Wadsworth and Anne Wright
(Preoperative Association Council Members)*

CHAPTER CONTENTS

KEY OBJECTIVES OF THE CHAPTER

By the end of the chapter the reader should be able to:
- be aware of the background to the development of preoperative assessment clinic
- have an understanding of the types, purpose and detail of preoperative assessments available
- identify rationale and guidance for preoperative investigations and how these guide patient management and optimization
- appreciate a legal and ethical approach to consent for anaesthesia
- understand how lifestyle and co-morbidities can affect health globally and how optimization of patients can improve patient outcomes
- determine how to care for and manage people considered high-risk patients
- outline the principles of protocol, audit, policy and guidance development in POA and the application of policy to practice
- and provide an overview of key national POA guidance.

Areas to think about before reading the chapter

- What do you understand by the terms prehabilitation and rehabilitation?
- What are the key skills required by the nurse to undertake a physical examination?
- When is the ideal time to carry out an initial preoperative assessment for elective surgery and why?

Introduction

Traditionally patients were admitted the day before elective surgery for a junior doctor-led clerking to identify health status and any co-morbidities, and for routine tests and specific preoperative preparation, e.g. bowel preparation, to be undertaken. This resulted in an unnecessary and often inconvenient overnight stay for the patient and financial implications for the healthcare organization. Late identification of patient co-morbidities often led to cancellation on day of surgery. Preoperative assessment (POA) services for elective surgical patients were developed as early as the mid 1980s to address some of these issues (Sabin, 1985; Pring et al., 1987).

Whilst not a new concept, the implement of POA clinics has been slow. Momentum increased from the late 1990s with the recommendations of the 'National Booked Admissions

Programme' (1998; McLeod et al., 2003), of which POA was seen as an essential part of the patient pathway to facilitate booking and effective theatre scheduling and utilization. The publication of the Association of Anaesthetists of Great Britain and Ireland (AAGBI) document 'Preoperative Assessment and the Role of the Anaesthetist' (AAGBI, 2001) was closely followed by recommendations for best practice from the Modernisation Agency (Janke et al, 2002). POA as a distinct speciality within the perioperative pathway had evolved.

In 2010, the AAGBI further cemented the concept when it stated that preoperative anaesthetic assessment services can decrease elective cancellations, reduce complications and mortality resulting in improved outcomes and an enhanced experience for the patient. It is now also a recommendation by the Royal College of Anaesthetists (RCoA, 2019) that most patients should attend a preoperative preparation clinic.

Aim of a preoperative assessment

The aim of the assessment process is to check it is safe to proceed with anaesthesia and elective surgery. The focus is to identify risk, optimize health issues, provide information and reduce anxiety. The assessment has a particular emphasis on the cardiovascular/respiratory systems and potential airway difficulties. Sociological considerations should also be included in the assessment as some patients may have little or no support at home resulting in delayed discharge or cancellation on the day of surgery.

The POA team should aim to get the patient as psychologically and physically fit as possible for surgery and anaesthesia. This process is known as optimization and the time from the POA to procedure date should be utilized to achieve this.

Shared decision-making should be evident throughout the patient journey. Evidence has shown that patients who are active participants in their care have better outcomes than those who are passive recipients of care. This is also reflected in Enhanced Recovery Programmes (RCoA, 2019).

When to undertake a preoperative assessment

The ideal time to carry out an initial POA for elective surgery is immediately following the decision to operate. However, it must be recognized that for some patients this is not convenient or appropriate – for example, for a patient receiving an unexpected or distressing diagnosis – and whilst guidance is useful it should not detract from an individual patient's needs.

In this case the assessment should be carried out as soon as possible following the decision to operate to ensure the patient is fully prepared, informed and safe for surgery.

Early POA can identify if the patient's medical condition requires further investigations or treatment, and early action can be taken to prevent cancellations and maximize theatre productivity. In addition, discharge planning can commence and any nursing needs can be identified.

Types of assessment

The American Society of Anesthesiologists (ASA) Classification is a system for assessing the fitness of patients before surgery. Grade one surgery, e.g. day surgery, can be a one-stop service (see Table 1.1). Alongside guidance, the basis for arranging tests such as blood tests may be on the grounds of professional judgement, individual patient clinical needs and evidence-based speciality-specific requirements. If this is not possible or convenient to the patient, then an appointment should be agreed with the patient to return within an appropriate timeframe. It may be appropriate for ASA 1 patients undergoing minor day case surgery to have telephone- or electronic-based assessments. Review of the information gained will then determine if further assessment is required (RCoA, 2019). This helps to direct resources appropriately, with a greater amount of time being made available for those requiring a more complex assessment and preoperative management plan.

ASA 2, 3 or 4 (see Table 1.1) patients requiring more complex surgery with an inpatient stay and preoperative investigations are usually seen in a face-to-face setting in POA. Although resource intensive in terms of the time required to undertake a comprehensive assessment in this way, it gives the clinical team the opportunity to ensure that all appropriate tests are undertaken preoperatively. Additionally, co-morbidities are identified and flagged to the appropriate teams and any specific requirements, such as medication or blood management, critical care level 2 or level 3 (Intensive Care Society, 2009) admission or discharge planning, can be planned for in advance of admission.

Preoperative assessment is carried out in National Health Service (NHS) or private hospitals, or in private clinics. However, assessments are increasingly being carried out in the primary care setting to enable prehabilitation activity to begin much sooner in the patient's pathway. In these cases, the POA should follow the same guidelines and processes as in secondary care ensuring a consistent approach and avoiding unnecessary cancellations. Patients assessed in secondary care may require referral back to their general practitioners (GPs) for specialist opinion and/or optimization.

Types of preoperative assessment clinics

Preoperative assessment clinics can be delivered in a variety of ways by different practitioners. These include by telephone, face-to-face, one-stop clinics, and, more recently and increasingly, via digital assessments online. Nurse

Table 1.1 ASA Classification

ASA Classification	Definition	Examples, including, but not limited to:
ASA 1	A healthy patient	Healthy, non-smoking, no or minimal alcohol use
ASA 2	A patient with mild systemic disease	Mild diseases only without substantive functional limitations. Examples include (but are not limited to): current smoker, social alcohol drinker, pregnancy, obesity (BMI >30 but <40 kg/m^2), well-controlled DM and/or hypertension, mild lung disease
ASA 3	A patient with severe systemic disease	Substantive functional limitations. One or more moderate to severe diseases. Examples include (but are not limited to): poorly controlled DM or hypertension, chronic obstructive pulmonary disease, morbid obesity (BMI $\geq$ 40 kg/m^2), active hepatitis, alcohol dependence or abuse, implanted pacemaker, moderate reduction of ejection fraction, ESRD, undergoing regularly scheduled dialysis, percutaneous coronary intervention <60 weeks, history (>3 months) of MI, CVA, TIA, or CAD/stents.
ASA 4	A patient with severe systemic disease that is a constant threat to life	Examples include (but are not limited to): recent (<3 months) MI, CVA, TIA, or CAD/stents, ongoing cardiac ischaemia or severe valve dysfunction, severe reduction of ejection fraction, sepsis, disseminated intravascular coagulation, acute renal disease or ESRD not undergoing regularly scheduled dialysis

BMI, body mass index; CAD, coronary artery disease; CVA, cerebrovascular vascular accident; DM, diabetes mellitus; ESRD, end-stage renal disease; MI, myocardial infarction; TIA, transient ischaemic attack.
(Adapted from *ASA Physical Status Classification System* [ASA, 2014].)

specialists often lead POA services comprising a team of nurses who have responsibility for assessing a patient's fitness for anaesthesia and surgery and organizing any necessary investigations or referrals. However, the sessions may also be delivered by junior doctors, anaesthetists, pharmacists or physiotherapists. Within the UK, the most common approach is still a mixture of face-to-face and telephone assessments, nurse-led with anaesthetic, physiotherapist and pharmacist support and anaesthetist-led clinics for patients with more complex needs.

Whichever method is used, POA as a speciality is clearly an integral part of the perioperative patient pathway that is best delivered by a multiprofessional team.

Core elements of a preoperative assessment

History taking

A medical history should start with the history of the presenting complaint. The aim of the history is to obtain a complete picture of the patient's present condition; why the patient first attended and what procedure they are scheduled for. This will include confirming their understanding of the complaint. The medical history, alongside the physical examination, will determine which tests, if any, are required or if the patient requires referral to primary care for additional investigations before surgery can proceed. The urgency of the procedure will determine if there is time to achieve the required improvement to health or if surgery proceeds with the patient accepting the risks involved (Walsgrove, 2011).

The past medical history should include all medical problems the patient has experienced including any chronic or acute illnesses, e.g. thyroid disease, diabetes mellitus (DM) and hypertension. Details of hospital visits, admissions and any reasons the patient is regularly attending their GP should be recorded. More detailed assessment of the following areas should be explored (Esland, 2018).

Cardiovascular history

The risk of an acute cardiac event is increased during anaesthesia. It is important to determine what cardiovascular risk factors the patient may have (if any), how symptomatic they are and how they are managed. Cardiac function, arrhythmias, valvular and peripheral vascular disease all require detailed assessment (Janke et al, 2002).

Respiratory history

There are significant risks associated with general anaesthetic and respiratory function. The aim is to determine which, if any, respiratory risk factors are present and how symptomatic the patient is.

The presence of dyspnoea, cough or sputum production will need to be explored further and, depending on the urgency and the severity of the surgery, may require referral to a respiratory physiotherapist preoperatively.

Gastrointestinal/liver/endocrine history

Gastric problems such as reflux, dyspepsia, regurgitation or hiatus hernia can increase the risk of pulmonary aspiration. Management of these conditions using preoperative medicines and/or alteration to lifestyle, e.g. weight loss and alcohol reduction, can prevent further complications.

Liver disease can lead to impaired metabolism of anaesthetic drugs. It can also have an effect on coagulation leading to increased bleeding and potential spinal haematoma after regional block.

Alcohol intake should be explored as this can also have an effect on clotting mechanisms. Patients with a high alcohol intake may also experience alcohol withdrawal so early intervention by alcohol dependence services may be required.

Renal history

The main risk perioperatively from renal disease is causing further deterioration of renal function or development of acute kidney injury which, if left untreated, can lead to renal failure (Doyle & Forni, 2017). A detailed history of renal disease should be gained, details of the cause and if the disease is newly diagnosed, stable or progressing. Drug history should include indications for treatment, e.g. hypertension, diabetes.

Surgical/anaesthetic history

Previous surgery, however minor, and dates of surgery should be recorded. Scar tissue from previous surgery can have an impact on the procedure to be performed. Early identification of this can help to reduce/avoid surgical complications.

Identification of complications with anaesthesia, e.g. difficult airway, postoperative nausea and vomiting, should be explored further. Previous anaesthetic notes/charts should be obtained to determine if further tests are required. Referral of notes for the anaesthetist's advice should occur to ensure potential airway problems are planned for.

Drug history

A detailed drug history is essential to ensure that correct advice regarding management of medicines is given prior to surgery. Patients should be advised to bring an up-to-date copy of their prescription medicines. Non-prescription medicines (e.g. herbal remedies, complementary therapies), recreational drugs, drugs of addiction and abuse should also be documented.

This section should also include questioning about any drug allergies, sensitivities, interactions or contraindications. Details of each allergy/interaction should be clearly documented describing the reaction and any other adverse effect.

Most medicines can be continued in the perioperative period and by doing this can help avoid complications of surgery and anaesthesia. For more complex cases specialist advice may be required.

The Handbook of Peri-operative Medicines (2017), alongside locally agreed guidelines on medicines management, should be used to determine if the patient is required to make any adjustments to their medication before surgery (UKCPA, 2017).

The pharmacological effects of some herbal remedies/complementary therapies are unknown. Adverse effects of these medicines include an increased tendency to bleed; in view of this, advice is to stop for two to three weeks before surgery (ASA, 2003).

The patient should be given clear written guidance or as appropriate to their needs (e.g. braille, large print, culturally applicable) on when to stop any medication and advice on recommencement should surgery be postponed.

Family history

It is important to determine if the patient has any familial illnesses, e.g. hypertension, coronary artery disease, stroke, diabetes, or an adverse reaction during surgery or anaesthesia. An important condition to include is malignant hyperpyrexia. This is an autosomal dominant condition that characteristically leads initially to muscle rigidity followed by a rise in temperature. This requires further tests and anaesthetic input preoperatively (Dougherty & Lister, 2015).

Social history/functional assessment

A good social history is essential to identify any issues that may delay discharge. Checking home circumstances and distance to travel to hospital can help in determining if a patient is suitable for day surgery or day of surgery admission.

Regardless of whether the patient is undergoing surgery as a day case or an inpatient, early discharge planning is essential. Establishing that the patient has support for discharge or if there is a need for input from other services is imperative for safety and to help prevent readmissions (Edward & Fitzgerald, 2012).

Establishing how the patient manages their daily activities including diet and fluid intake, elimination, mobility sleep pattern, communication, mood and coping strategies will give a picture of functional capacity. This will also help to determine how the patient will cope postoperatively.

A full smoking history should be taken and advice, support and encouragement to quit should be given or advice to temporarily abstain (NICE, 2013). Smoking has been highlighted as the single biggest cause of premature and preventable death in the UK (Action on Smoking and Health [ASH], 2015). Patients who smoke have been shown to be more likely to suffer a range of complications before, during and after surgery (Theadom & Cropley, 2006).

Venous thromboembolism assessment

Hospital admission increases the risk of blood clots (thrombosis) due to immobility. National Institute for Health and Care Excellence (NICE) guidance (NG89) suggests that the risk of blood clots can be prevented by following simple steps. Risk assessment should be completed as part of routine preoperative assessment (NICE, 2018).

In 2014 the All-Party Parliamentary Thrombosis Group (APPTG) identified venous thromboembolism (VTE) as an international patient safety issue (APPTG, 2014). It is firmly embedded in the post-Francis review patient safety agenda.

It is important that each nurse or allied health professional has access to locally agreed guidelines regarding VTE risk assessment and prophylaxis. Patients should be given verbal and written information regarding risks and of prophylaxis (Blann, 2011). Evidence of risk assessment and management of VTE prophylaxis should be documented in the patient record.

Special considerations

Elderly

Increasingly, patients aged over 65 years, who often have multiple co-morbidities, are frail or have cognitive impairment, are being scheduled for surgery and can be at increased risk of adverse postoperative outcomes. POA and preparation of these patients can take longer and should involve a greater range of healthcare professionals. There should be assessment for risk of postoperative delirium, postoperative functional decline, consideration of complex discharge issues and review of medications where there is polypharmacy (Key & Swart,

2019). Despite the identification of frailty as a considerable predictor of poor postoperative outcome, there is lack of consensus of how best to assess and diagnose it (Partridge et al, 2012). An example of a frailty assessment tool which can be used in the POA setting is the Edmonton Frail Scale or Reported Edmonton Frail Scale (Rolfson et al, 2006).

Vulnerable adults

If patients lack capacity to make decisions regarding surgery, clinicians involved in their care need to follow the Mental Capacity Act Code of Practice 2005 (Crown Copyright, 2007) and ensure they adhere to local policy and procedure.

Morbidly obese

The Society for Obesity and Bariatric Anaesthesia (SOBA) recommends that patients with a body mass index equal to or greater than 35 kg/m^2 are screened using the STOP-Bang Questionnaire (Nightingale & Redman, 2016). This tool suggests preoperative testing and advises on peri- and postoperative management as well as being the best validated tool for screening of obstructive sleep apnoea (OSA) (Chung et al, 2016).

Clinical examination

Clinical examination in POA is completed to build upon the information gained and to confirm a diagnosis suggested by the clinical history, plan treatment and prevent complications whilst the patient is under anaesthetic (Pickard, 2011). It is undertaken in the traditional systematic approach that is central to clinical medicine – with evaluation of anatomical findings by appropriately educated and competent practitioners, and through the use of observation, palpation, percussion, and auscultation. In POA following a general examination there is a focus on three body systems which are of key importance to clinicians working in this specialty: the respiratory system, the cardiovascular system and the abdominal system. The same principles are then applied to other systems if necessary (Pickard, 2011).

Accurate documentation of examination findings is essential to ensure effective communication to the surgical team and the anaesthetist on the day of surgery (Key & Swart, 2019). Traditionally this is via a paper document inserted into the patient's notes but digital records are the future with POA being part of IT solutions for Electronic Patient Records. A number of POA computerized software packages are now available that advise on preoperative investigations and optimization plan and stratify risk following completion of a patient health questionnaire. This is either completed at the POA appointment or remotely in the patient's home (Kenny, 2011).

General examination

A physical examination starts as soon as the clinician sees the patient. In POA this is often during the walk from the waiting area to the consultation room — noting of general demeanour, appearance and how the patient stands and walks. Height, weight, blood pressure, pulse and oxygen saturation are essential observations to document a baseline, ensure fitness to proceed to surgery and plan care (Innes et al, 2018).

Respiratory examination

A thorough respiratory examination is fundamental and should include airway examination to identify which patients with anatomical or pathological features may indicate difficult airway management, such as those with facial abnormalities, receding mandible, difficulty with mouth opening or neck flexion and extension, or poor or absent dentition (Pickard, 2011). There are several bedside tests that can be used, of which the Mallampati classification (Fig. 1.1) is the most common but can be subjective.

Cardiovascular examination

Cardiovascular signs should be noted as per a standard cardiovascular examination. Patients with internal cardiac devices, such as pacemakers, defibrillators and loop recorders, must be identified at POA so that any techniques used in surgery, particularly diathermy, do not cause harm to the patient or device (Higgins & Hill, 2017).

Preoperative tests for elective surgery

The purpose of preoperative investigations is to provide additional diagnostic and prognostic information to supplement the clinical history of a patient. Each hospital is likely to have local guidelines and these, in addition to NICE (2016a) guidance, advise which tests to offer patients before minor, intermediate and major or complex surgery, taking into account specific co-morbidities assessed by ASA Physical Status Classification (ASA, 2014). Unnecessary testing can promote patient anxiety, is labour intensive and expensive, and causes delays without influencing the outcome or changing perioperative management. The use of tests as part of POA and health optimization remains a high-volume activity and total expenditure remains significant (Czoski-Murray et al, 2012). Adherence to testing guidelines promotes efficiency by streamlining clinical decision-making and minimizing costly investigations. Test results should be included in the referral from primary care to avoid duplicate testing.

Blood tests

Full blood count

Full blood count (FBC; haemoglobin, white blood cell count and platelet count) is offered or considered predominantly to assess for undiagnosed anaemia or thrombocytopaenia, as these conditions require correction prior to surgical interventions to reduce the risk of perioperative cardiovascular events.

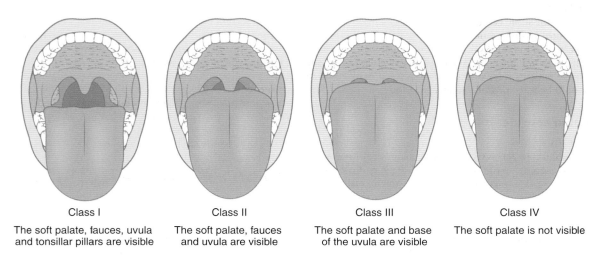

Class I	Class II	Class III	Class IV
The soft palate, fauces, uvula and tonsillar pillars are visible	The soft palate, fauces and uvula are visible	The soft palate and base of the uvula are visible	The soft palate is not visible

Figure 1.1 The Mallampati classification. (From Pardo, M., Miller, R. (2018). *Basics of anesthesia*, 7th edition. Philadelphia: Elsevier.)

Kidney function

Kidney function tests (estimated glomerular filtration rate (eGFR), electrolytes, creatinine and sometimes urea levels) are offered or considered to identify renal disease or patients at risk of acute kidney injury (AKI), such as those undergoing intraperitoneal surgery, with diabetes, heart failure, liver disease, eGFR <60 mL/min/1.73 m^2, over 65 years, or with use of drugs with nephrotoxic potential preoperatively.

Haemostasis

This should be considered in patients with chronic liver disease and/or those taking anticoagulants. Point-of-care testing (sometimes called bedside testing), which gives immediate results, should be used wherever possible (according to local guidance).

Group and save

This should be dictated by local policy to prevent unnecessary ordering of blood.

HbA1c

This reflects diabetic control over the previous three months and likely stability of glycaemic control at the time of surgery. This should not be offered in patients without diagnosed diabetes and in diagnosed diabetics where HbA1c result is available within the past three months. Diabetes can lead to increased length of stay, postoperative infections, myocardial infarction, acute kidney injury, inpatient costs and mortality (Barker, 2015). However, the impact of optimizing HbA1c levels preoperatively has not been assessed in a randomized clinical trial.

Sickle cell screening

Testing for sickle cell disease or sickle cell trait should not be routinely offered preoperatively. By adulthood the disease will be clinically evident and finding an unknown trait will not alter the patient's management and care. Where patients receive sickle cell specialist input, the team should be informed of intended surgery.

Other tests

Electrocardiogram (ECG) (resting)

This should be offered or considered in patients with known cardiovascular, renal or diabetic co-morbidities or in patients aged over 65 years where no ECG is available within the past 12 months, to detect underlying cardiac disease and provide a baseline to compare any perioperative changes.

Echocardiogram (resting)

Echocardiogram (resting) should be considered if the patient has a heart murmur and any cardiac symptoms including breathlessness, pre-syncope, syncope, chest pain or signs or symptoms of heart failure. Before this is completed, a resting electrocardiogram should be performed and the findings discussed with an anaesthetist.

Cardiopulmonary exercise testing (CPET)

In POA, this is used to assess how high-risk patients may respond to physiological stress during surgery. However, there is uncertainty about the predictive value of CPET on perioperative morbidity and mortality, and the use of results to inform preoperative optimization and perioperative management.

Lung function tests

Lung function tests (spirometry, including peak expiratory flow rate, forced vital capacity and forced expiratory volume) and arterial blood gas analysis are considered for patients with known or suspected respiratory disease and to predict perioperative pulmonary complications that contribute significantly to morbidity and mortality.

Polysomnography

This is used to diagnose and monitor treatment responsiveness in obstructive sleep apnoea (OSA) and other sleep disorders. OSA affects 9–24% of the population (Singh et al, 2013), especially those who are obese, and it is frequently undiagnosed before surgery. It is an independent risk factor for cardiovascular, neurological, endocrine morbidity and all-cause mortality. However, there is currently no robust evidence for whether POA and diagnosis of OSA leads to improved perioperative outcomes.

Methicillin-resistant Staphylococcus aureus (MRSA) screening

This status is important for avoiding cross-infection in hospital. A decolonization regimen can be initiated if indicated by hospital policy.

Pregnancy test

This should be offered on admission to women of child-bearing potential as elective surgery is generally avoided unless urgent due to the risk presented to the woman and fetus by the anaesthetic and the procedure.

Consent for anaesthesia

Information regarding anaesthesia and associated risks, benefits and possible consequences should be provided to patients ideally in written form as early as possible before admission for surgery. Consent is a process involving the surgeon and other members of the multidisciplinary team and may require more than one discussion. A separate signed form is not required for anaesthetic procedures that are performed in order to carry out another treatment. Consent can be delegated from a doctor to a suitably trained and qualified health professional who is sufficiently familiar with the procedure. The nature and amount of information provided should be tailored to the individual patient in order for them to make a decision regarding undergoing an anaesthetic. There should be a check for patient understanding, an opportunity for questions and clear documentation of discussions by nurse and anaesthetist in the patient record (Yentis et al, 2017).

Optimization in preoperative assessment

Lifestyle measures

There is a good evidence that cessation of alcohol prior to surgery can reduce infectious outcomes so therefore improve wound healing, lower incidence of cardiac arrythmias and reduce bleeding risk. The optimum timeframe identified is three to eight weeks (Tønnesen et al, 2009). Alcohol is also a risk factor for the development of hypertension and atrial fibrillation. We should therefore encourage patients to stop alcohol or seek help from the primary healthcare team if we suspect alcohol dependence. Assessment tools such as the Alcohol Use Disorders Identification Test can be used to identify those patients who may exhibit signs of alcohol dependence (WHO, 2001).

Improving aerobic fitness increases the body's ability to withstand the physiological stress of major surgery and decreases the risk of adverse perioperative outcomes. Nurses and other healthcare practitioners should encourage patients to increase activity both prior to surgery as part of a prehabilitation strategy and also after surgery. The World Health Organization (WHO) recommends 150 minutes of 'moderate' intensity exercise or 75 minutes of vigorous intensity per week. Exercise should include muscle strength and resistance in addition to an aerobic element (Ayyash et al., 2017).

All patients should be encouraged to stop smoking prior to surgery (Tønnesen et al, 2009). Patients should be given the appropriate help and resources to do this, i.e. patient information leaflet, help from the primary care team, smoking cessation service, mobile device apps or a pharmacist.

Patients should be encouraged to reduce weight if indicated prior to anaesthesia and surgery (AAGBI, 2010) as this is likely to improve wound healing, reduce blood pressure, reduce the risk of respiratory complications and lower the risk of OSA.

Preoperative assessment is an ideal and timely opportunity to promote health both for short-term and long-term benefit. The RCoA (2018) resource, *Fitter Better Sooner*, provides patient information, both written and digital, to encourage patients to prepare for surgery. Preoperative practitioners should provide brief interventions to address lifestyle issues as part of the *Making Every Contact Count* initiative (NHS Health Education England, 2019). Primary care can help with optimization by offering advice on lifestyle measures. This may help to increase survival, decrease perioperative morbidity and shorten the duration of hospital stay (AAGBI, 2010).

Co-morbidities

The American Society of Anesthesiologists recognizes the increased co-morbidities associated with increasing weight in patient populations and now classifies patients with a BMI of 40 or above as ASA category 3 (ASA, 2014). Patients with a STOP-Bang score of five or above will require sleep studies and treatment with continuous positive airway pressure (CPAP) (Danjoux & Habgood, 2017). Screening for OSA is now included in the updated NICE Guidelines on Preoperative Investigations (NICE, 2016a).

Anaemia should be viewed as a treatable medical condition rather than just an abnormal laboratory value. Optimization strategies incorporate iron therapies including intravenous iron, B_{12}, folic acid and erythropoietin. All possible measures to avoid blood transfusion due to the increased risk associated with these should be taken by the perioperative team (Lavies & Kotze, 2017). Simple clinical assessment measures such as an increased pulse and respiratory rate are effective tools to identify anaemic patients.

Diabetes UK (2018) has identified that there are 3.8 million diabetic patients in the UK. Management of diabetic patients in POA focuses on thorough evaluation and optimization; defined by a HbA1C of 69 mmol/mol or less. The AAGBI Guidelines for the Pre-Operative Management of the Surgical Patient with Diabetes (Hartle et al, 2016) provides detailed guidance of how to manage all the groups of diabetic drugs at POA including insulin. Patients who are unfit for surgery based on their HbA1C or comply poorly to lifestyle measures or their medicines should be referred back to their GP for optimization (Diabetes UK, 2016).

People who are hypertensive are at risk of damage to organs, i.e. the heart and kidneys. Therefore, their management and care should involve testing urea and electrolytes, eGFR and recording of a 12-lead ECG, primarily to identify atrial fibrillation (AF), left bundle branch block and left ventricular hypertrophy. The evidence supports that if a patient's blood pressure is less than 180/110 mmHg without target organ damage, then surgery should still proceed (Sear, 2017). Regarding medicines management, there is evidence to support the continuation of most anti-hypertensive drugs other than angiotensin converting enzymes (ACE 1) or angiotensin II receptor blockers (ARBs), which should be stopped for one dose, and diuretics, which may be discontinued, for both the risk of intraoperative hypotension and patient comfort (Sear, 2017).

Atrial fibrillation (AF) increases the risk of thromboembolism (Enga et al, 2014). Nurses should attempt to identify undiagnosed patients by simply palpating the pulse. An irregularly irregular pulse is a strong clinical sign that the patient has AF. This can be confirmed by an ECG. These patients may require deferral of surgery until cardiac imaging can be performed to exclude structural heart disease (Gallagher & Gonna, 2018). In practice, patients are referred by back to the GP service for investigation. Patients who have established and therefore treated AF should be assessed to establish the ventricular response, as a bradycardia may indicate too much beta-blockade or tachycardia suboptimal treatment. Either of these circumstances would require referral back to the GP for optimization or, in the case of a symptomatic, tachycardic AF, referred to the Emergency Department.

Medicines management

Anticoagulants such as warfarin or the novel oral anticoagulant (NOAC) drugs such as apixaban require stopping prior to most types of surgery. The general consensus is that warfarin should be stopped five days prior to surgery and patients who have an increased $CHADS_2$ or more recently CHA_2DS_2-VASc score (above 4) may require bridging with low-molecular-weight heparin (Keeling et al, 2016). Stopping a NOAC is a little more complicated as it requires the practitioner to consider the particular agent, bleeding risk from surgery and the patient's eGFR (UKCPA, 2017). The British Society for Haematology (2016) states that the operating surgeon 'has to assess the risk of bleeding for the individual patient and discuss both this and the plan for peri-operative anticoagulation with them. The plan must be recorded clearly in the notes, including a plan for when the patient is discharged.'

In practice, the operating surgeon may refer to the opinion of the haematologist, cardiologist or anaesthetist in perioperative anticoagulation management planning as the expert. Aspirin, which is one of the most commonly used antiplatelet drugs, is generally continued unless there is risk of bleeding into an enclosed space. Clopidogrel given as a monotherapy exerts a much stronger antiplatelet effect. In many circumstances it is continued, though should be stopped for procedures that may cause bleeding into an enclosed space and for spinal anaesthesia.

Patients who have drug-eluting coronary stents that have been inserted for acute coronary syndrome/myocardial infarction receive dual antiplatelet therapy for a minimum of 12 months. This regimen should not be interrupted for elective procedures as this can result in an increased risk of stent thrombosis. The commonest regimen used is a combination of aspirin and clopidogrel, though other antiplatelet drugs are used. If the procedure is urgent or an emergency, the practitioner should seek the advice of an anaesthetist, who may well want to discuss this with a cardiologist (UKCPA, 2017).

Other groups of drugs that require review are oestrogen-containing products such as the combined oral contraceptive pill and hormone replacement therapy. The consensus advice is that both of these products should be stopped four to six weeks prior to major surgery, especially if there is the possibility of a lengthy immobilization, and all surgery of the lower limbs (UKCPA, 2017), although the recent NICE guidance stipulates a cessation period of 4 weeks (NICE, 2018). However, in many circumstances these patients attend for their POA in a very short timeframe before their operation date and there simply is not the recommended time to stop oestrogen-containing products. The importance of a VTE assessment for this group of patients is even more important. This group of patients may be advised to continue but be treated as higher risk and require more intense interventions.

Protocols, policies and guidelines

The Care Quality Commission (CQC) inspection framework in England for the NHS and independent acute hospitals mandates that risk-based POAs are completed in line with guidelines (CQC, 2017). To maintain safe and effective practice in POA, practice must be underpinned by evidence-based ratified protocols, policy and guidelines, education and competency assessment. Agreed service measures and audit should be adopted to provide assurance of safety, quality, efficiency and parity of service provision in POA.

The Royal College of Anaesthetists (RCoA) (2019) guidance states that each hospital should have approved written policies, protocols or guidelines following national guidelines where published, covering key areas of POA practice (Box 1.1), to set standards, and reduce variation. Staff must, however, be mindful of the distinction between protocols and guidelines (Knight & Kenny, 2011), noting that guidance offers best practice recommendations.

Box 1.1 Policies, Protocols and Guidelines

Each hospital should have approved written policies, protocols or guidelines following national guidelines where published, covering:
- the time allocated for the anaesthetist to undertake preoperative care in both outpatient clinic and ward settings. Job plans should recognize an adequate number of programmed activities
- preoperative tests and investigations
- preoperative blood ordering for potential transfusion
- management of anaemia including parenteral iron therapy to reduce the risk of allogenic blood transfusion
- management of diabetes and anticoagulant therapy, including newer anticoagulant drugs
- preoperative fasting schedules and the administration of preoperative carbohydrate drinks
- antacid prophylaxis
- latex and chlorhexidine allergies
- escalation of care in the event of perioperative complications to the intensive care unit
- continuation of regular medication
- locally agreed protocol for the administration of thromboprophylactic agents to patients undergoing surgery, including VTE risk assessment, for identification of patients at low, moderate and high risk, and a recommended prophylactic method for each group (including timing of administration to patients undergoing regional anaesthesia)
- referral of patients from a nurse-led clinic to medical staff for further review
- pregnancy testing before surgery
- use of the WHO *Surgical Safety Checklist*
- management of acute pain in complex patients, e.g. opioid-tolerant patients
- perioperative management of pacemakers including implantable cardioverter defibrillators

(Reproduced here with permission from the Royal College of Anaesthetists. Taken from Chapter 2: Guidelines for the Provision of Anaesthesia Services for Preoperative Assessment and Preparation 2019).

The POA service is part of the responsibility of the anaesthetist (RCoA, 2019) and as such anaesthetists should be involved in the development of protocols, policy and guidelines for the POA clinic (NCEPOD, 2002a). To ensure a multidisciplinary approach, this should include the lead registered nurse in POA and clinicians from other disciplines, as appropriate. Guidelines should be drafted in consideration of the local circumstance, using key sources of evidence, and should be subject to frequent review (Knight & Kenny, 2011). Such documents should be easily accessible in the POA clinical setting, and viewed as working tools. Local variance from national guidelines may be adopted in policy following consultation with key stakeholders, and ratified through the hospital Clinical Governance Committee.

POA may identify a new clinical finding or a change in the patient's health status that may not previously have been noted. Clinical staff should have knowledge of key guidance that extends beyond POA, for example that from NICE and Scottish Intercollegiate Guidelines Network (SIGN) with local referral pathways, enabling patients to make long-term health gains. Such guidance could include the management of hypertension in both secondary and primary care (Hartle et al, 2016; NICE, 2016b).

POA and planning improves efficiency (NHS Modernisation Agency, 2003) and protocols, policy and guidelines should include administrative processes that will increase effectiveness of the POA service covering:
- clinic booking to ensure effective capacity and demand management
- patient tracking system to maintain flow and ensure the patient is not lost in the POA process (Hill & Jackson, 2018)
- receipt of medical records in preparation for the POA consultation
- POA documentation, such as integrated pathways, risk assessments, and patient information in preparation for the POA consultation.

Protocols and policy to ensure compliance with administration of Patient Reported Outcome Measures (PROMs) (NHS England, 2017) and National Joint Registry (NJR, 2017) consent should further be adopted.

National guidelines

The early work of the University of Southampton (Janke et al, 2002) and the NHS Modernisation Agency (2003) was fundamental in establishing guidance in POA. There is now a plethora of national guidance and research accessible to support preoperative and perioperative practice from the NHS, medical societies, the Royal Colleges and medical foundations, some of which is offered as further reading.

The *Guidelines for the Provision of Anaesthesia Services for Preoperative Assessment and Preparation* from the RCoA (2019) have provided a clear national framework for patients requiring anaesthesia or sedation, providing annual updated recommendations. Since its establishment in 2004, the Preoperative Association has been pivotal in the development of POA nationally, establishing best practice in the field of preoperative medicine through consensus, published guidance, research and audit. The Association of Anaesthetists (AoA, formerly Association of Anaesthetists of Great Britain & Ireland [AAGBI]) has published guidance on the role of the anaesthetist in POA (AAGBI, 2010), obesity (AAGBI & SOBA, 2015), diabetes (AAGBI, 2015) and dementia (AoA, 2019) to name but a few.

Primarily, registered nurses must maintain the knowledge and skills needed for safe and effective practice according to the Nursing and Midwifery Council (NMC) Code of Conduct (NMC, 2018) and be accountable, which includes having the authority to perform the task, through delegation and the organizational policies and protocols (Royal College of Nursing, 2019). In addition to robust protocols, policy and guidance, clinical curiosity should be fostered in the practice setting with resources and access to research databases to maintain knowledge.

Research and audit

All staff completing POA should undertake comprehensive training in preoperative clinical assessment skills (NCEPOD, 2002b). Training and competency will ensure staff have the knowledge and skills to relate policy to practice (Hill & Jackson, 2018).

'We can only improve what we can measure' (Darzi, 2008). The cornerstone of clinical governance is audit and it is strengthened by critical and objective examination (RCoA, 2012). To this end, the POA service should have a dashboard of agreed service measures and programme of audit, with established pathways for reporting, and service improvements.

The RCoA (2012) *Compendium of audit recipes for continuous improvement in anaesthesia* includes the audit of POA clinics with suggested indicators and targets, and more recently the RCoA (2019) guidelines include a list of regular audits that can be undertaken in POA (Box 1.2). Objective examination through audit may highlight the potential for further training and, if appropriate, may result in policy changes, updated and communicated through the interprofessional team at clinical governance meetings (Hill & Jackson, 2018).

The Francis Report (2013) is clear: 'Audit of protocols, policy and guidance should not be considered the sole method of assurance of safety and quality. In policing compliance with standards, direct observation of practice, direct interaction with patients, carers and staff, and audit of records should take priority over monitoring and audit of policies and protocols' (Francis, 2013:88).

POA service improvement will not be achieved solely by implementation of ratified protocol, policy and guidelines, knowledge and skills in the application of policy to practice is required, underpinned with a robust clinical governance framework to provide assurance of safety and quality.

Box 1.2 **Undertaking Audit**

Regular audits of the following aspects of preoperative care may include:
- the effectiveness of preoperative information provided to patients
- preoperative documentation of consultation by anaesthetists
- consent to anaesthesia
- the effectiveness of POA services
- preoperative visiting (patient waiting time, proportion of one-stop visits)
- preoperative airway assessment
- preoperative fasting in adults and children
- appropriate preoperative medication
- thromboprophylaxis
- choice of technique: general, local or regional anaesthesia
- cancellation on day of surgery due to a failure in the preoperative assessment process

(Reproduced here with permission from the Royal College of Anaesthetists. Taken from Chapter 2: Guidelines for the Provision of Anaesthesia Services for Preoperative Assessment and Preparation 2019).

SUMMARY OF KEY POINTS

With the need to manage finite resources within healthcare, nurse-led POA is recognized and valued as a service. It has reduced day-of-surgery cancellations, improved patient experience and assisted with workforce issues following the reduction in junior doctors' hours. Moving forward, POA supports workforce and recruitment pressures by utilizing appropriately skilled and registered nurses, which frees up pharmacists and medical staff to undertake other tasks whilst ensuring a patient is informed, and is safe for their anaesthesia and surgery.

REFLECTIVE LEARNING POINTS

Having read this chapter, think about what you now know and what you still need to find out about. These questions may help:

- Describe the ASA classification and critically discuss the advantages and disadvantages of its use.
- How can the nurse ensure that POA is patient-centred with a focus on the unique needs of the individual?
- In clinical practice, how is audit of policies and protocols undertaken?

References

Action on Smoking and Health (ASH). (2015). *Fact sheet: Smoking statistics, illness and death*. Available from: < http://ash.org.uk/category/information-and-resources/fact-sheets/ > .

All-Party Parliamentary Thrombosis Group (APPTG). (2014). *Healthcare commissioners' guide to VTE prevention. VTE: What does it mean to me as a commissioner?* London: NHS England.

American Society of Anesthesiologists (ASA). (2003). *What you should know about herbal and dietary supplement use and anesthesia. Patient Information Leaflet*, cited in Wong, A., & Townley, S.A. (2010). Herbal medicines and anaesthesia. *Continuing Education in Anaesthesia Critical Care and Pain* 11 (1):14–17.

American Society of Anesthesiologists (ASA). (2014). *ASA physical status classification system*. Available from: < https://www.asahq.org/standards-and-guidelines/asa-physical-status-classification-system > .

Association of Anaesthetists (AoA). (2019). *Guidelines: Perioperative care of people with dementia*. Available from: < https://anaesthetists.org/Home/Resources-publications/Guidelines/Peri-operative-care-of-people-with-dementia-2019 > .

Association of Anaesthetists of Great Britain & Ireland (AAGBI). (2001). *Preoperative assessment the role of the anaesthetist*. London: AAGBI.

Association of Anaesthetists of Great Britain & Ireland (AAGBI). (2010). *Preoperative assessment and patient preparation. The Role of the Anaesthetist 2*. London: AAGBI.

Association of Anaesthetists of Great Britain & Ireland (AAGBI) & Specialists in Obesity and Bariatric Anaesthesia (SOBA). (2015). *Peri-operative management of the obese surgical patient*. Available from: < https://www.aagbi.org/sites/default/files/Peri_operative_management_obese_patientWEB.pdf > .

Ayyash, R., Durrand, J., & Danjoux, G. (2017). Peri-operative exercise: an evidence-based review and guidelines for peri-operative teams. In N. Lavies, & R. Hill (Eds.), *Evidence-based guidelines for preoperative assessment units. A practical guide, 2017 edition* (pp. 2–13). London: The Preoperative Association.

Barker, P. (2015). Peri-operative management of the surgical patient with diabetes 2015. Association of Anaesthetists of Great Britain and Ireland. *Anaesthesia, 70*, 1427–1440.

Blann, A. (2011). The role of haematology in preoperative assessment. In M. Radford, A. Williamson, & C. Evans (Eds.), *Preoperative assessment and peri-operative management* (pp. 187–217). Keswick, Cumbria: M and K Publishing.

British Society for Haematology. (2016). *Peri-operative management of anticoagulation and antiplatelet therapy*. Available from: < https://b-s-h.org.uk/guidelines/guidelines/peri-operative-management-of-anticoagulation-and-antiplatelet-therapy/ > .

Care Quality Commission (CQC). (2017). *Inspection framework: NHS and independent acute hospitals*. Available from: < https://www.cqc.org.uk/sites/default/files/20190122_Surgical_Core_Services_framework_NHS_and_IH_providers_v9.pdf > .

Chung, F., Abdullah, H. R., & Liao, P. (2016). STOP-Bang questionnaire: a practical approach to screen for obstructive sleep apnoea. *Chest, 149* (3), 631–638.

Crown Copyright. (2007). *Mental capacity act 2005 (Code of Practice)*. Norwich: The Stationary Office.

Czoski-Murray, C., Lloyd Jones, M., McCabe, C., Claxton, K., Oluboyede, Y., Roberts, J., et al. (2012). What is the value of routinely testing full blood count, electrolytes and urea, and pulmonary function tests before elective surgery in patients with no apparent clinical indication and in subgroups of patients with common co-morbidities: a systematic review of the clinical and cost-effective literature. *Health Technol Assess, 16*(50), i–xvi.

Danjoux, G., & Habgood, A. (2017). Guidelines for the pre-operative assessment and management of patients with obstructive sleep apnoea. In N. Lavies, & R. Hill (Eds.), *Evidence-based guidelines for preoperative assessment units. A practical guide, 2017 Edition* (pp. 14–25). London: The Preoperative Association.

Darzi, A. (2008). *High quality care for all: NHS next stage review final report*. Available from: < https://www.gov.uk/government/publications/high-quality-care-for-all-nhs-next-stage-review-final-report > .

Diabetes UK. (2016). *Management of adults with diabetes undergoing surgery and elective procedures; improving standards (2016)*. Joint British Diabetes Societies for inpatient care. Available from: < https://www.diabetes.org.uk/resources-s3/2017-09/Surgical%20guidelines%202015%20-%20full%20FINAL%20amended%20Mar%202016_0.pdf > .

Diabetes UK. (2018). *Diabetes prevalence 2018*. Available from: < https://www.diabetes.org.uk/professionals/position-statements-reports/statistics/diabetes-prevalence-2018 > .

Dougherty, L., & Lister, S. (Eds.), (2015). *The royal marsden manual of clinical nursing procedures* (9th ed.). West Sussex: Wiley and Sons.

Doyle, J., & Forni, L. (2017). Guidelines for the pre-operative assessment and peri-operative management of the patient with renal impairment. In N. Lavies, & R. Hill (Eds.), *Evidence-based guidelines for preoperative assessment units. A practical guide, 2017 edition* (pp. 31–37). London: The Preoperative Association.

Edward, J., & Fitzgerald, F. (2012). Surgical preoperative assessment. What to do and why. *Student BMJ, 20,* 29–31.

Enga, K. F., Rye-Holmboe, I., Hald, E. M., Lochen, M. L., Mathieson, E. B., Njolstad, I., et al. (2014). Atrial fibrillation and future risk of venous thromboembolism: The Tromso study. *Journal of Thrombosis and Haemostasis, 13,* 1–16.

Esland, J. (2018). *The preoperative assessment*. Available from: < https://teachmesurgery.com/perioperative/preoperative/assessment/ > .

Francis, R. (2013). *Report of the mid staffordshire NHS foundation trust public inquiry executive summary*. Available from: < https://webarchive.nationalarchives.gov.uk/20150407084231/http://www.midstaffspublicinquiry.com/report > .

Gallagher, M. M., & Gonna, H. (2018). Cardiac arrhythmias. In A. Crerar-Gilbert, & MacGregor (Eds.), *Core topics in preoperative anaesthetic assessment and management* (p. 27). Cambridge: Cambridge University Press.

Hartle, A., McCormack, T., Carlisle, J., Anderson, S., Pichel, A., Beckett, T., et al. (2016). The measurement of adult blood pressure and management of hypertension before elective surgery: Joint guidelines from the AAGBI and the British Hypertension Society. *Anaesthesia, 71,* 326–337.

Higgins, N., & Hill, R. (2017). Guidelines for perioperative management of cardiac pacemakers and implanted defibrillators. In N. Lavies, & R. Hill (Eds.), Evidence-based guidelines for preoperative assessment units. A practical guide, 2017 edition (pp. 64–68). London: The Preoperative Association.

Hill, R., & Jackson, J. (2018). Challenges of setting up preoperative service. In A. Crerar-Gilbert, & M. Macgregor (Eds.), *Core topics in preoperative anaesthetic assessment and management* (pp. 290–299). Cambridge: Cambridge University Press.

Innes, J. A., Dover, A. R., & Fairhurst, K. (Eds.), (2018). *Macleod's clinical examination*. Edinburgh: Elsevier.

Intensive Care Society. (2009). *Levels of critical care for adult patients*. Available from: < https://www.ics.ac.uk/AsiCommon/Controls/BSA/Downloader.aspx?iDocumentStorageKey = 74ca75c6-67c4-4400-96a2-4e7e14b8d9a3&iFileTypeCode = PD-F&iFileName = Levels%20of%20Critical%20Care%20for%20Adult%20Patients > critical care levels.

Janke, E., Chalk, V., Kinley, H., & NHS Modernisation Agency, Southampton University. (2002). *Preoperative assessment: Setting a standard through learning*. Southampton: University of Southampton.

Keeling, D., Tait, R. C., & Watson, H. (2016). Peri-operative management of anticoagulation and antiplatelet therapy. *British Journal of Haematology, 175,* 602–618.

Kenny, L. (2011). Clinical examination. In M. Radford, A. Williamson, & C. Evans (Eds.), *Preoperative assessment and perioperative management* (pp. 1–13). Keswick, Cumbria: M and K Publishing.

Key, W., & Swart, M. (2019). *Guidelines for the Provision of Anaesthesia Services (GPAS) Guidelines for the provision of anaesthesia services for preoperative assessment and preparation 2019*. London: Royal College of Anaesthetists (RCoA).

Knight, P., & Kenny, L. (2011). Developing protocol and guidance to support assessment service. In M. Radford, A. Williamson, & C. Evans (Eds.), *Preoperative assessment and perioperative management* (pp. 379–393). Keswick, Cumbria: M and K Publishing.

Lavies, N., & Kotze, A. (2017). Guidelines for pre-operative management of anaemia in patients having major orthopaedic surgery. In N. Lavies, & R. Hill (Eds.), *Evidence-based guidelines for preoperative assessment units. A practical guide, 2017 edition* (pp. 26–27). London: The Preoperative Association.

McLeod, H., Ham, C., & Kipping, R. (2003). Booking patients for hospital admissions: evaluation of a pilot programme for day cases. *British Medical Journal, 15,* 327.

National Confidential Enquiry into Patient Outcome and Death (NCEPOD). (2002a). *The NCEPOD classification of intervention*. Available from: < https://www.ncepod.org.uk/ > .

National Confidential Enquiry into Patient Outcome and Death (NCEPOD). (2002b). *Functioning as a team? The 2002 report of the national confidential enquiry into peri-operative deaths*. Available from: < https://www.ncepod.org.uk/2002report/02_s3.pdf > .

National Institute for Health and Care Excellence (NICE). (2013). *PH48 Smoking: acute, maternity and mental health services 2013*. Available from: < https://www.nice.org.uk/guidance/ph48 > .

National Institute for Health and Care Excellence (NICE). (2016a). *NG45 Routine preoperative tests for elective surgery*. Available from: < https://www.nice.org.uk/guidance/ng45 > .

National Institute for Health and Care Excellence (NICE). (2016b). *Hypertension in adults: diagnosis and management. CG127*. Available from: < https://www.nice.org.uk/guidance/cg127 > .

National Institute for Health and Care Excellence (NICE). (2018). *NG89 Venous thromboembolism in over 16s: reducing the risk of hospital-acquired deep vein thrombosis or pulmonary embolism*. Available from: < https://www.nice.org.uk/guidance/ng89 > .

National Joint Registry (NJR). (2017). *Information for healthcare providers*. Available from: < http://www.njrcentre.org.uk/njrcentre/Healthcare-providers > .

NHS England. (2017). *National patient reported outcome measures (PROMs) programme guidance*. Available from: < https://www.england.nhs.uk/wp-content/uploads/2017/09/proms-programme-guidance.pdf > .

NHS Health Education England. (2019). *Make every contact count*. Available from: < https://www.makingeverycontactcount.co.uk/ > .

NHS Modernisation Agency. (2003). *National good practice on preoperative assessment for inpatient surgery*. Available from: < http://www.hello.nhs.uk/documents/Preoperative%20assessment%20guidance%20for%20inpatient.pdf > .

Nightingale, C. & Redman, J. (2016). *The SOBA single sheet guideline*. Available from: < https://www.sobauk.co.uk/downloads/single-sheet-guideline > .

Nursing and Midwifery Council. (2018). *The code: Professional standards of practice and behaviour for nurses, midwives and nursing associates.* London: Nursing and Midwifery Council.

Partridge, J. S. L., Harari, D., & Dhesi, J. K. (2012). Frailty in the older surgical patient: a review. *Age and Ageing, 41,* 142—147.

Pickard, H. (2011). Clinical examination. In M. Radford, A. Williamson, & C. Evans (Eds.), *Preoperative assessment and perioperative management* (pp. 55—87). Keswick, Cumbria: M and K Publishing.

Pring, D. J., Naidu, A., Burdette-Smith, P., & England, J. P. (1987). An assessment of orthopaedic preadmission clinic. *Journal of the Royal College of Surgeons Edinburgh, 32*(4), 221—222.

Rolfson, D. B., Majumdar, S. R., Tsuyuki, R. T., Tahir, A., & Rockwood, K. (2006). Validity and reliability of the Edmonton Frail Scale. *Age and Ageing, 35,* 526—529.

Royal College of Anaesthetists (RCoA). (2012). *Raising the standard: A compendium of audit recipes for continuous quality improvement in anaesthesia,* 3rd ed. Available from: < https://www.rcoa.ac.uk/system/files/CSQ-ARB-2012.pdf > .

Royal College of Anaesthetists (RCoA). (2018). *Fitter better sooner.* Available from: < https://www.rcoa.ac.uk/ patient-information/preparing-surgery-fitter-better-sooner > .

Royal College of Anaesthetists (RCoA). (2019). *Guidelines for the provision of anaesthesia services (GPAS).* Available from: < https://www.rcoa.ac.uk/ gpas2019 > .

Royal College of Nursing. (2019). *Accountability and delegation.* Available from: < https://www.rcn.org.uk/professional-development/accountability-and-delegation > .

Sabin, N. (1985). Dedicated preadmission testing centre cuts costs. *LOS Hospitals, 59*(6), 66 & 70.

Sear, J. (2017). Peri-operative control of hypertension: When and how does it adversely affect peri-operative outcome? In N. Lavies, & R. Hill (Eds.), *Evidence-based guidelines for preoperative assessment units. A practical guide, 2017 edition* (pp. 43—51). London: The Preoperative Association.

Singh, M., Liao, P., Kobah, S., Wijeysundera, D. N., Shapiro, C., & Chung, F. (2013). Proportion of surgical patients with undiagnosed obstructive sleep apnoea. *British Journal of Anaesthesia, 110*(4), 629—636.

Theadom, A., & Cropley, M. (2006). Effects of preoperative smoking cessation on the incidence and risk intraoperative and postoperative complications in adult smokers: a systematic review. *Tobacco Control, 15,* 352—358.

Tønnesen, H., Neilson, P. R., Lauritzen, J. B., & Møller, A. M. (2009). Smoking and alcohol intervention before surgery: evidence for best practice. *British Journal of Anaesthesia, 102*(3), 297—306.

United Kingdom Clinical Pharmacy Association (UKCPA). (2017). *The handbook of peri-operative medicines.* 2nd ed.. Available from: < http://ukclinicalpharmacy.org > .

Walsgrove, H. (2011). History taking. In M. Radford, A. Williamson, & C. Evans (Eds.), *Preoperative assessment and perioperative management* (pp. 33—54). Keswick, Cumbria: M and K Publishing.

World Health Organization (WHO). (2001). *The alcohol use disorders identification test — guidelines for use in primary care,* 2nd ed. Available from: < https://apps.who.int/iris/bitstream/handle/10665/67205/WHO_MSD_MSB_01.6a.pdf?sequence = 1 > .

Yentis, S. M., Hartle, A. J., Barker, I. R., Barker, P., Bogod, D. G., Clutton-Brock, T. H., et al. (2017). Association of Anaesthetists of Great Britain and Ireland (AAGBI) Consent for Anaesthesia 2017. *Anaesthesia, 72,* 93—105.

Further reading

NHS Modernisation Agency. (2002). *National good practice guidance on preoperative assessment for day surgery 2002: Operating Theatre and pre-operative assessment programme.* London: NHS Modernisation Agency.

Chapter | 2 |

Perioperative care

Kate Woodhead

KEY OBJECTIVES OF THE CHAPTER

The aim of this chapter is to provide a broad introduction to the holistic care given by nurses within the perioperative environment during the patient's immediate preoperative, intraoperative and postoperative phases of their surgical experience.

This chapter will:

- give a definition of the perioperative period
- explore in depth the needs of patients during the phases of their surgical journey, and how care for the individual physical and psychological needs can be adapted
- identify some of the hazards of the perioperative environment for patients and how their effects can be minimized proactively.

Areas to think about before reading the chapter

- What do you understand by the 'perioperative period'?
- Describe the Safe Surgery Saves Lives surgical checklist.
- How is anaesthesia defined?

Introduction

For patients, student nurses and other hospital staff, the perioperative or theatre area has been seen as one of high drama and action, as portrayed regularly by the media, with many having preconceived ideas about the roles and contribution made by those within the environment. Yet, for many individuals, it is a time when they are most vulnerable or scared. For patients, they are asleep, unsure if they will wake up and what will happen to them; for student nurses, it is a strange experience, which to begin with they feel unable to relate to other environments; and for other hospital staff, they feel as if they are entering an environment where everything is mysterious. Ensuring that the highest standard of patient care is delivered to each individual patient throughout their surgical journey is fundamental to the perioperative nurse's role. Patient interaction and communication is essential, although covert if the patient is asleep, as perioperative nurses assess, prepare, plan and implement care. This chapter will demonstrate that perioperative nursing care is patient orientated and that nurses must have a thorough knowledge and understanding of the environment. This will enable them to deliver patient care safely, effectively and without harm to any patient.

Perioperative period

'Perioperative' refers to the three phases of a patient's surgical journey – preoperative, intraoperative and postoperative. For the purposes of this chapter the perioperative period is from the minute the patient arrives in through the operating theatre doors to the moment they leave through those same doors after surgery.

Elective or emergency surgery

Surgical procedures can be broadly categorized as either elective (that which is planned) or emergency (that which is unplanned). Elective surgery aims to be performed when the patient is in optimal health but before the surgery affects the quality and threatens their life: e.g. an inguinal hernia can become life-threatening if the bowel becomes obstructed within the sac. Clinicians decide if a planned procedure is 'urgent' due to clinical deterioration or can be arranged at a time convenient for the surgeon, hospital and patient (NCEPOD, 2004).

The majority of patients for elective surgery now arrive at the hospital on the day of surgery already pre-assessed, starved according to local policy for the individual and optimized prior to their admission (Radford & Palmer, 2012).

Immediate surgery may be as a result of trauma or an accident, gastrointestinal obstruction, or from perforated viscera. The injury may be immediately life-threatening, and therefore the procedure will be carried out within minutes of the decision to operate. Other emergencies may require procedures within 24−48 hours following the injury, but in both instances the preoperative time for preparing the patient is significantly reduced and changes in the patient's condition occur rapidly. A diversity of skills is required by the perioperative team in a number of challenging clinical scenarios from day case assessment to the transfer of unstable surgical patients to the operating theatres. Patient safety must be a continuing aspect of all care delivered to patients throughout their perioperative journey; good communication is an essential feature of this care delivery (Radford & Palmer, 2012).

For this chapter the emphasis will be on the care of the patient for elective surgery, as many of the principles discussed apply to any patient undergoing any surgical procedure.

Preoperative care

Patient preparation

The perioperative environment is dynamic and ever changing with developments in anaesthesia and surgical technologies, but underpinned by practitioners promoting and maintaining a safe environment for each individual patient. Preparing the perioperative environment starts before the patient arrives and the only information that may be available for the staff is retrieved from the operating theatre list, which is written daily and produced 16−24 hours before the scheduled surgery (AfPP, 2016).

At a minimum, this should detail the patient's name, age, gender and procedure. This will enable the perioperative nurse to prepare their own area to ensure a safe working environment. For example, knowing the patient's age allows the anaesthetist and recovery nurses to prepare the correct equipment for the management of that patient's airway; the procedure will identify the patient's tolerance to the planned position and potentially the length of surgery (AfPP, 2016). However, liaison with the pre-assessment clinic may also have highlighted specific needs for the individual, such as immobility problems, hearing impairment or medical history requiring additional interventions from the clinicians (Oakley, 2010). In addition, the patient has an opportunity to gather more information about anaesthetic technique, postoperative pain relief, and risks, all within a calm environment (AAGBI, 2010).

Meeting and greeting the patient

The patient is escorted to the operating theatre by either a porter or ward nurse, or both. Ward staff must check the patient's identity, surgical consent form, patient notes and appropriate marking and ensure that all documentation is completed before the patient is transferred to theatre (AfPP, 2016). The patient may be transported on a wheelchair or their bed, or if they wish and are fit enough, they can walk to theatre with their escort. Depending on the facilities within each unit, the patient is either admitted to the holding area or waits in reception. The patient at this time may be stressed and anxious due to the impending event and unfamiliar staff and environment. It is therefore essential that the perioperative nurse communicates effectively with patients, to ensure that they reassure them (and their relatives) as well as focusing on the handover of information (Radford & Palmer, 2012). An accurate assessment at this time by the perioperative nurse will identify any clinical changes which may affect the plan for care.

An adult or parent may accompany a child to the operating department, thus including the family in the plan for perioperative care. Parents will be anxious as they relinquish care of their child for surgery and consideration of their needs, as well as the child's, has to be undertaken.

Adolescents have different needs to children and adults. They may have concerns about their surgery and confidentiality must be able to be ensured together with providing information to parents, which can be a delicate balance (McArthur, 2012). An elderly patient may be confused and require additional explanations and reassurance. The nurse with experience will assess the older patient's skin condition, mobility and general appearance as an indication of the patient's health and well-being (Hehir, 2012).

The patient should be greeted by name and the nurse should introduce themselves to the patient. A preoperative checklist should be completed in accordance with local policy.

Patient safety in surgery

In 2009, the National Patient Safety Agency implemented the World Health Organization's Safe Surgery Saves Lives surgical checklist. It may be amended locally to suit conditions and is often used with Five Steps to Safer Surgery (AfPP, 2016). The development of the checklist was designed to improve teamwork and minimize the most common and avoidable patient safety risks which can occur during surgery (Wicker, 2015). It is a simple tool, to help all of the team to focus on key safety checks at three points during vital phases of perioperative care: prior to the induction of anaesthesia, prior to skin incision and before the team leaves the operating room (WHO, 2008).

All those professionals working in the perioperative team have a duty of care to ensure that the patient is not harmed by their care (WHO, 2008). There are a core set of standards devised by the World Health Organization (WHO) that provide that the team will:

1. Operate on the correct patient at the correct site.
2. Use methods known to prevent harm from anaesthetic administration, while protecting the patient from pain.
3. Recognize and effectively prepare for life-threatening loss of airway or respiratory function.
4. Recognize and effectively prepare for risk of high blood loss.
5. Avoid inducing any allergic or adverse drug reaction known to be a significant risk for the patient.
6. Consistently use methods known to minimize risk of surgical site infection.
7. Prevent inadvertent retention of instruments or swabs in surgical wounds.
8. Secure and accurately identify all surgical specimens.
9. Effectively communicate and exchange critical patient information for the safe conduct of the operation.

The Five Steps to Safer Surgery (Vickers, 2011) added a further two elements to the safe surgery checklist: briefing, which involves all the team members discussing the surgical schedule, patient by patient at the beginning of the day, undertaken to anticipate and resolve issues proactively; and debriefing at the end of the list to ensure any 'lessons learned' can be discussed by all the team.

Safe Surgery Saves Lives Patient Safety Challenge acknowledged the complexity of modern surgery and identified the checklist as a means to reduce possible errors (WHO, 2008).

As the patient arrives in the operating theatre department, additional checks need to be undertaken, which are identified in Table 2.1.

Perioperative nurses also need to provide equitable and appropriate care with respect to cultural, religious, ethnic and racial beliefs. This will involve a knowledge and understanding of religious practices, family role and cultural orientation.

Care during anaesthesia

The anaesthetic nurse will, based on the information known or relayed by the anaesthetist, prepare the anaesthetic room, anaesthetic machines and all other equipment to ensure the maintenance of a safe environment for the delivery of care during anaesthesia. This includes preparing the anaesthetic equipment and also applying knowledge and skills of anaesthesia related to age, medical history and surgical procedure to ensure that the patient's individual needs are met: e.g. if the patient is elderly, then additional precautions are needed when caring for their skin; if the patient has language difficulties, an interpreter may be required.

Anaesthetic assistance may be provided by a specialized nurse or an operating department practitioner. The safe administration of anaesthesia cannot be carried out by the anaesthetist alone; competent assistance is necessary at all times (AAGBI, 2018).

The role of an anaesthetic nurse has many dimensions and involves technical, communication, clinical and supervisory skills. Barriers, such as the wearing of a mask when greeting the patient, undue background noise such as talking and telephones, and lack of explanations when performing tasks, must be avoided. A clear function of the anaesthetic practitioner is to promote the well-being of the patient, to act as advocate, and provide a professional approach to their duties (Chilton & Thompson, 2012). Communication is not always verbal and the use of touch, holding the patient's hand and just being a physical presence can offer additional support for the patient. The anaesthetic nurse may also need to remove dentures, glasses, prostheses or wigs in preparation for surgery. Reassurance, comfort and sensitivity about the patient's potential loss of dignity are essential in reducing the patient's anxiety further (AfPP, 2016).

The first of the Safe Surgery Saves Lives checks is undertaken as the patient arrives in the anaesthetic room, and before induction of anaesthesia. It is known as the 'Sign In' and includes the patient in the final safety checks to confirm their identity, site of surgery, skin marking and any possible risks which may become important, such as a difficult airway or anticipated blood loss.

Anaesthesia is defined as the loss of the sensations of pain, pressure, temperature and touch in a part or the whole of the body (Bryant & Knights, 2015). When

Table 2.1 Preoperative checklist

To check	Rationale
Name/date of birth of patient	To ensure that this is the correct patient with the correct notes. The date of birth acts as an additional check, as patients with the same name may be on the same ward.
Consent	Written consent is preferred as it provides documentary evidence (AfPP, 2016). The consent form should clearly state without abbreviations the operative procedure and should be signed by the patient (exceptions apply such as minors, life-threatening situations, legally or mentally incompetent) (Royal College of Surgeons, no date) and by a qualified practitioner competent to carry out the procedure. For consent to be valid, the patient must be informed of the procedure, its expected outcomes, benefits, potential risks and alternatives (AfPP, 2016). The perioperative nurse must check the patient's understanding of the procedure to safeguard their autonomy (Reid, 2005).
Procedure site is marked	Side or site is clearly marked with an indelible marker to avoid confusion. This should then be confirmed with the patient's notes, X-rays and the operating list. It is the responsibility of the person performing the procedure to ensure that the correct side/site is marked (AfPP, 2016).
Last ate or drank	Patients must fast preoperatively to minimize the risk of inhaling gastric contents whilst undergoing general anaesthetic, which could prove fatal (AfPP, 2016; RCN, 2013). The Royal College of Nursing recommends the oral intake for adults be restricted — clear fluids (water, tea and coffee without milk) may be taken up to 2 hours before surgery — and a fasting time of 6 hours for solid foods or drinks with milk. Chewing gum and sweets are not recommended on the day of surgery (RCN, 2013). Patients must be given enough information to understand and realize the importance of preoperative fasting and the consequences if these instructions are not followed, i.e. the operation will be delayed or cancelled (AfPP, 2016). Liddle (2014) identified that prolonged fasting preoperatively can result in dehydration, anxiety, electrolyte imbalances and glycaemic disturbances. Certain groups of patients are particularly susceptible to such complications, including the elderly, pregnant women, children and the critically ill. Reducing fasting times will reduce postoperative nausea and vomiting (PONV) and improve wound healing, comfort and postoperative outcomes.
Allergies	Identify allergies to minimize risk for the patient during surgery. These should include Elastoplast, specific drugs (antibiotics, suxamethonium, or any that contain eggs or nuts), fluids such as iodine, and latex, and also note patient's adverse reactions to anaesthetic or blood transfusions (AfPP, 2016).
State of teeth	Caps, crowns, dentures or loose teeth can become dislodged or damaged during intubation and may compromise the airway. Dentures, if tight fitting, and if the patient does not normally remove them routinely, may be left in place throughout the procedure at the anaesthetist's discretion.
Jewellery	Some items of jewellery are worn for religious or cultural reasons and may cause offence if removed, so perioperative nurses must respect patient needs. Muslim and Sikh women may wear gold or glass bangles or nasal stones and a wedding ring to signify marriage and the AfPP recommends that these remain in place if they do not compromise venous or surgical access (AfPP, 2016). Some body piercings may interfere with the surgery or compromise the airway and may be removed if required. Secure all rings and other jewellery to ensure that they are not lost during positioning or moving of the patient (AfPP, 2016).
Wearing of any prosthesis	Hearing aids are essential for the patient to communicate with theatre staff, so can be left in until the patient reaches the anaesthetic room and is about to be anaesthetized. The hearing aid should then be removed and given to recovery staff so that they can insert it once the patient regains consciousness. Glasses can also be worn to theatre for the same reason.
	Contact lenses should not be worn, because during the procedure there is a risk that they can become dry and may scratch the cornea.
	Other prostheses such as wigs, false eyes and artificial limbs should be removed prior to surgery and retained on the ward for safe-keeping. However, patients may express anxiety and every effort should be made to preserve a patient's dignity and respect during the perioperative period (AfPP, 2016).
Medical and nursing records	All medical and nursing records should accompany the patient to the operating theatre so that an accurate assessment of the patient's history can be made for the delivery of safe perioperative care. Documentation includes results from investigations completed at preoperative assessment, blood tests, X-rays and baseline observations (AfPP, 2016).

Source: AfPP (2016); RCN (2013); Liddle (2014).

making a decision about the type of anaesthesia to be administered – i.e. general, regional or local – the anaesthetist will be influenced by the type and technique of the planned surgery, the patient's risk factors, their personal skills and the patient's preference.

A general anaesthetic can be divided into three components, called the triad of anaesthesia. These three elements are hypnosis (loss of consciousness), analgesia and akinesia (prevention of movement). Different surgical procedures require differing degrees of each. Surgical stimulation and pain can cause a series of physiological responses such as tachycardia, hypertension, sweating and vomiting. Analgesics reduce the body's response to such stimulation, which may prevent or reduce postoperative complications (Bonnet & Marret, 2005). Anaesthetic techniques and drug therapy have evolved, allowing the anaesthetist to adjust the proportions of each part of the triad of anaesthesia to suit individual requirements. For procedures requiring little or no muscle relaxation, the anaesthetist may induce anaesthesia using an intravenous agent (although a gas induction can be used with patients with a needle phobia), and maintain anaesthesia with an intravenous agent, or a volatile agent; allowing the patient to breathe the gases spontaneously via a mask or a laryngeal mask airway attached to the appropriate breathing system. Where muscle relaxation is required after anaesthesia is induced, a muscle relaxant is given and the patient's airway maintained via an endotracheal tube or a laryngeal mask airway, and the patient is connected to a ventilator. The third part of the triad of anaesthesia is analgesia. This is achieved using differing categories of drugs, which block the stimulation of pain at the nerve impulses. Opioid analgesics such as fentanyl are used intraoperatively because of their short duration of action and can be titrated to meet the patient's needs (Stanley, 2014).

Regional and local anaesthesia provide the patient with a reversible regional loss of sensation leading to a reduction of pain, thereby facilitating surgical procedures (Wicker, 2015). Techniques include peripheral nerve blocks (injection of a local anaesthetic agent into a plexus of nerves); central neuroaxial blocks (injection of local anaesthetic into the subarachnoid space or epidural space for surgery on lower abdomen or lower limbs and postoperative analgesia); and infiltration anaesthesia (injection of local anaesthetic around the surgical incision site or prior to cannulation) (Chilton & Thompson, 2012).

During regional anaesthesia the patient is awake or sedated, therefore requiring additional reassurance and support from all perioperative staff. Diligence by clinical staff is essential in maintaining confidentiality of other patients and ensuring that minimal noise and interference occurs during the procedure, which may distract the patient and so cause them to move. Conversely, if the procedure is long, it may be difficult for the patient to stay still on an uncomfortable table/bed and therefore sedation may be administered or a combination of general and regional anaesthesia to produce a state of drug-induced tolerance. Patients are likely to be rousable in this state and should also be able to respond to commands or physical stimuli (Williams, 2014).

The Association of Anaesthetists recommends minimum standards of monitoring during anaesthesia and recovery. During induction of anaesthesia, this will include pulse oximetry, non-invasive blood pressure monitoring, electrocardiogram and capnography (measurement of CO_2 in expired air at end of respiration) (AfPP, 2016). For those patients undergoing complex procedures, or who are high risk due to co-morbidities, monitoring of urine output, body temperature and invasive monitoring such as central venous pressure and arterial pressure are essential.

During the induction of anaesthesia, it is important that all personnel are calm, and that noise, disruption and disturbance are minimal, as hearing is the last sense to go when the patient loses consciousness.

During the maintenance phase, the anaesthetic nurse will observe and monitor the patient's well-being. Eye pads may be applied over the eyes to prevent corneal abrasions and to maintain closure of the eyelids to prevent drying of the corneas due to a reduced eye reflex.

Intraoperative care

Patient and staff safety is paramount throughout the perioperative environment and a proactive clinical risk management strategy involves identifying and adopting strategies to reduce the risk (Vincent, 2016). Throughout the intraoperative phase, the patient is vulnerable and totally reliant on the perioperative team to ensure that they come to no harm. Some of these risks have already been addressed with patient identification, informed consent and patient monitoring in the anaesthetic room. Intraoperatively, such clinical risks are associated with patient positioning, the risks of infection, deep vein thrombosis, and hypothermia. This list is not exhaustive but identifies some of the potential risks to each patient undergoing surgery. The perioperative care team addresses the risks to minimize harm whilst the patient is having surgery.

Prior to the first incision being made, the team will stop to review whether they are sure that they are about to start surgery on the right patient at the correct site and side. Other critical aspects of safe surgery, such as whether there are any anticipated critical events, are also addressed at this time. This is known as the 'Time Out'.

Surgical access and positioning

Positioning the patient correctly to enable easy surgical access requires coordination and cooperation from the whole team (Table 2.2). Manual handling regulations recommend that the team involved undertake a risk assessment prior to moving and positioning of each individual patient. An assessment will include the physical condition of the patient, nature of the intervention and individual patient needs. When positioning patients, consideration should be given to avoiding nerve and joint injury, avoiding mechanical trauma such as shearing, friction burns and damage to soft tissue, and ensuring that at all times the anaesthetized patient is physically well supported, with particular emphasis on natural body alignment and protection of skin, nerves and bony prominences (AfPP, 2016).

Nerve injuries are an outcome of poor positioning, with direct pressure resulting in ischaemia to that area,

e.g. radial nerve injury if the arm is left hanging over the edge of the operating table; ulna nerve injury due to compression by an inappropriately placed arm support; and fibular nerve injury due to compression when using the lithotomy poles. Perioperative nurses must therefore ensure that mechanical aids and supports are padded and used appropriately together with other commonly used devices, such as gel pads, head rests, head rings and shoulder support (Wicker, 2015).

Shearing forces can occur when moving the patient on the operating table, resulting in tissue damage, which may go undetected. Skin risk assessment should be undertaken at the beginning and end of surgery and documented, using specially designed tools according to local policy. The use of gel mattresses or similar pressure-relieving adjuncts can redistribute the pressure across a wider area (Pirie, 2012).

Common sites for skin pressure injury during surgery are the elbows, heels, buttocks and sacrum. National Institute

Table 2.2 Common surgical positions

Surgical position	Description and potential risks	Procedures performed
Supine	Patient lies on their back, with their arms folded and secured across their chest, or on an arm board at less than 90 degrees to the body to prevent brachial plexus injury, or at their side. A lumbar support should be used to prevent postoperative backache. Pressure-relieving devices for the ankles should not hyperextend the knee as this may result in injury.	Administration of general anaesthesia Patient transfer to and from the operating table Abdominal, breast and lower limb surgery
Lateral	Patient is turned onto their side and the head, rear of chest and pelvis is supported with padded table attachments. Arms are secured to allow venous access. A pillow should be placed between the knees to prevent pressure on bony contact.	Hip surgery Some kidney procedures Thoracic surgery
Prone	Patient lies on their stomach with their head supported on a ring or turned to one side, and their arms positioned to prevent extension and abduction at the shoulder, either above their head or by their side. The chest must be supported to allow movement of the abdomen for respiration.	Spinal surgery Neurosurgery
Trendelenburg	Patient is in a supine position with a head-down tilt. Abdominal organs fall towards diaphragm due to gravity, allowing greater surgical access. Legs may be bent at the knee to add stability.	Lower abdominal surgery, e.g. abdominal hysterectomy Lower limb surgery, e.g. varicose veins
Lithotomy	Patient lies supine with their legs raised in supporting poles. These may support the calf to ankle or just the ankles are secured. The patient's arms are secured across their chest while the end of the table is removed. The legs are elevated, lowered and positioned simultaneously to prevent lower back injury, sacroiliac ligament damage and pelvic asymmetry. Nerve damage may occur from pressure applied directly from lithotomy poles, which are inadequately padded, to the medial or lateral side of the leg. A lumbar support will prevent postoperative backache.	Gynaecological procedures Urological surgery Rectal surgery Obstetric procedures

Source: Wicker (2015).

for Health and Care Excellence (NICE) guidance advises that risk assessment and preventative measures should be taken for those who are going to be immobile for some time, thus including surgical time (NICE, 2014). The risk to the patient increases as the surgery time increases but all patients undergoing surgery are at risk of intraoperative ulceration.

Prevention of deep vein thrombosis

Deep vein thrombosis (DVT) is a serious postoperative complication and one where the actions of perioperative nurses can influence the outcome for the patient. DVT occurs as a result of venous haemostasis, tissue or vessel wall trauma and increased coagulant activity. NICE guidance specifies risk assessments on each patient to enable the perioperative team to make decisions about the mechanical or pharmacological regimen for thromboembolic prophylaxis (NICE, 2018).

Maintenance of normothermia

The impact of patients losing heat during their surgery leads to many postoperative complications including an increased likelihood of surgical site infection, as well as cardiac and metabolic difficulties. Perioperative nurses can adopt a variety of measures to control and maintain the patient's temperature above 36°C throughout a surgical procedure which includes the control of the environmental temperature (21−24°C), use of forced air warming blankets, warming intravenous fluids, irrigation and skin preparation fluids, and the monitoring of a patient's core temperature (NICE, 2016).

Infection control in the perioperative environment

Much of the practice around every surgical procedure, such as the patient bathing before their operation and surgical skin antisepsis, are indicated to reduce the potential for surgical site infection. Infection prevention comprises various vital components, all of which are aimed at reducing the risk of infection to the patient (Table 2.3). Setting of the sterile field and using flawless aseptic technique is an essential skill for the scrub practitioner and the rest of the team to have heightened awareness of at all times.

Technology and advances in surgical practice

Minimally invasive surgical procedures, drug therapy (particularly in anaesthesia) and the development of electrical

Table 2.3 Infection control practices	
Area	**Infection control**
Theatre design	Location of operating theatre department within the hospital Ventilation system with minimum 20 air changes per hour Scheduled preventative maintenance Controlled access to the department by visitors
Cleaning	Cleaning between patients Cleaning at the end of a list Policies for using correct cleaning fluid depending on purpose Correct disposal of waste and linen
Staff	Wearing of protective clothing: scrub suits, hats and footwear Appropriate use of personal protective equipment and use of standard precautions Appropriate use of masks Hand hygiene Safe handling and disposal of sharps Scrubbing and gowning techniques based on evidence and best practice Maintenance of aseptic technique Correct sterilization and disinfection procedures
Patient preparation	Hair removal if absolutely necessary, with a clipper not a razor immediately prior to the procedure Use of alcohol-based skin preparation fluids Identification of risk factors such as old age, obesity, malnutrition, other co-morbidities Surgical intervention such as operative site, duration of surgery, wound contamination (such as bowel contents, pus)
Source: AfPP (2016); Wilson (2019).	

equipment (lasers, robotic assistance) have revolutionized the patient's surgical pathway, altering the length of stay, reducing recovery time and increasing the potential for an early return to normal activity (Esmail & Wrona, 2013). As new technology is introduced, perioperative nurses must understand the principles and specifics of each new piece of equipment, drug or procedure and ensure that risk assessments have been undertaken and all staff have received appropriate training on the equipment and its potential dangers. Nurses are accountable for their own practice and should ensure that they and their colleagues do not harm the patient (Nursing and Midwifery Council, 2018). Technology that is not new, but remains hazardous, is in regular use to reduce bleeding during surgery. Details are provided in Table 2.4.

Swab and instrument counting

Managing risks to patients from the sterile field includes the use and handling of instrumentation; care and handling of specimens; and the swab, needle and instrument count. Negligently using defective equipment during

Table 2.4 Electrosurgery risks

Electrosurgery hazard	Prevention
Insulation on equipment not intact	Ensure that all equipment, including cables, surgical instrumentation and patient plates, are fully insulated and that any faulty equipment is removed immediately and reported as per hospital policy Always ensure that surgical electrosurgery equipment is kept within an insulated container throughout the procedure Do not coil the return electrode cable while in use
Using alcohol-based fluids Alcohol-based fluids are used to prepare the surgical site prior to surgery. However, if the fluid pools in the patient's skin or drapes, then it may be ignited by a spark from the electrosurgery, resulting in a burn	Ensure that if alcohol-based preparation fluid is used, it is allowed to dry or is removed with a sterile swab Ensure that surgical drapes are free from contact with alcohol Avoid any fluid contact with the electrosurgery unit
Alternative pathways Unintended routes for the electrical pathway due to the patient being in contact with other conductors, or if the patient is wearing a pacemaker	Patient plate should be as close to the surgical site as possible to reduce length of pathway through patient Ensure no exposed metal, e.g. from armrests, mayo table stands or metal infusion poles, are touching the patient For patients with a pacemaker, diathermy should be avoided, or if it cannot, then precautions should be taken to minimize the interference from the electrical current
Smoke inhalation Research has shown that surgical smoke is hazardous to the perioperative team who are exposed on a daily basis. The risks are from biological and chemical hazards found in the particulate matter of the smoke (AfPP, 2016)	Utilization of dedicated smoke evacuators Wearing of compliant respiratory masks Regular changing of filters and maintenance of theatre departments
Patient preparation Incorrect preparation of the patient could mean an increase in current density to one area and result in a burn	Ensure that the patient plate/return electrode is clean and, if single-use, is never reused Ensure good contact with the plate and the skin by placing the plate over a muscular area, away from bony prominences or scar tissue, and remove hair from directly below the plate prior to positioning if the patient is hirsute. If the patient is moved during surgery, ensure that the plate remains intact or replace with another Record the position of the plate on the patient and the skin condition before and after

Source: AfPP (2016); Wicker (2015).

invasive procedures and leaving foreign objects within patient cavities is against the law, as all clinical staff have a duty of care to the patient (AfPP, 2016). All swabs, instruments, needles and other sharps must be accounted for at all times throughout the surgical procedure, and are recorded on a 'swab board' for all invasive procedures according to local policy. A count is performed by the scrub nurse and a circulating practitioner, who may be unqualified. The surgeon is informed at the end of the procedure that the count is correct, and it is documented in the patient's care plan (AfPP, 2017).

Preparation for transfer of the patient to recovery

Prior to the staff and patient leaving the theatre, the 'Sign Out' element of the safe surgery checklist should be completed, to confirm satisfactory completion of the surgery and for team members to reflect what might be improved for the next time. The debriefing is completed at the end of the surgical operating list.

At the end of the operation, the patient's perioperative care plan is completed, which details the procedure; patient position; position of diathermy plate and other equipment used; skin condition due to position and site of diathermy plate; signatures confirming that the needle, swab and instrument count are correct; skin closure used; and indication of presence of any drains or catheters (AfPP, 2016). The patient is prepared for transfer to the recovery or post-anaesthetic care unit, which may involve moving the patient to a bed. Preservation of the patient's dignity and maintaining their safety is paramount. Once the patient has been transferred, the theatre can be cleaned and prepared for the next patient in accordance with local hospital policy.

Immediate postoperative care

For this chapter, the author will use the term 'recovery room' indicating the area within the operating theatre department where patients recover from anaesthesia and surgery. The area is also known as the post-anaesthetic care unit or PACU. Emergence from anaesthesia is potentially hazardous, with patients requiring close observation until recovery is complete. Appropriately staffed recovery facilities must be available during whatever hours of the day elective and emergency surgery is undertaken (RCoA, 2019).

The recovery nurse is a skilled and knowledgeable practitioner, able to deal quickly and efficiently with any changes in the patient's condition. Within the perioperative environment, recovery nurses have the greatest autonomy, as they manage a patient's care in the recovery

area from arrival through to discharge, only requesting medical assistance when needed. Recovery room nurses must also have knowledge of both anaesthetic and operating theatre techniques.

The postoperative phase of a patient's journey starts when the patient is transferred from the theatre to the recovery room. However, preparation for each individual patient commences well before the patient arrives. All equipment, such as resuscitation, oxygen and monitoring, is checked and additional resources acquired if necessary, e.g. patient warming apparatus, provision of analgesic pumps, or pillows if the patient needs to be nursed sitting up. The patient's age will also influence the size of the equipment needed, particularly for children.

The anaesthetist and a nurse from the perioperative team accompany the patient to the recovery area. The recovery nurse immediately assesses and establishes a patent patient airway before monitoring vital signs and undertaking a more detailed assessment. The Association of Anaesthetists of Great Britain and Ireland states that patients must be observed on a one-to-one nurse:patient ratio until the patient has regained airway control, respiratory and cardiovascular stability and can communicate (AAGBI, 2013).

Airway

- The patient's airway must be patent, clear of blood or mucus.
- Adequate ventilation must be achieved and this may require assistance with the position of the head/neck or an airway adjunct, e.g. Guedel or laryngeal mask airway.
- The patient's position may also affect ventilation, and therefore the patient may need to be moved to a different position.
- Oxygen therapy is commenced immediately via an oxygen mask or nasal cannulae. Usually, this is at 40%. Contraindications include chronic obstructive airway disease or where a prescribed percentage of oxygen is required.
- A pulse oximeter is attached to monitor oxygen saturation levels.

Breathing

- Observe the movements of the chest to ensure bilateral even movement and feel the air flowing in and out of the mouth.
- Noisy breathing is obstructed breathing and action must be taken to relieve the obstruction. The nurse may support the patient's airway. However, obstructed breathing is not always noisy, as complete obstruction is characterized by silence.
- Skin colour (lips, nail beds) may indicate cyanosis.

- Respiratory rate is taken to include depth and pattern. Changes could be an early indication of future respiratory or cardiac arrest.

Circulation

- Once the airway has been established, blood pressure and pulse can be monitored.
- Assessment of perfusion status includes conscious state, skin temperature, and pulse and blood pressure, as an indication of perfusion to all vital organs.
- Wounds and drains should be observed for evidence of haemorrhage.

It should be remembered that monitors alert staff to changes in condition, but ongoing physical visual assessment and observation allow the detection of subtle changes in condition without relying on monitors.

Once the initial assessment has been completed, the nurse can gather information through an extensive handover from the anaesthetist and theatre/anaesthetic nurse. This should include past medical history, surgical procedure, vital signs, pharmacology given (particularly analgesics), blood loss, intravenous infusions, catheters and drains. It will detail any untoward events that occurred during the surgery and highlight any potential problems for the postoperative period. The anaesthetist will outline any specific postoperative instructions for each patient: e.g. analgesic regimen, oxygen therapy and any additional monitoring requirements.

The nurse can then carry out a more thorough patient assessment to include:

- checking of consciousness levels and signs of protective reflexes returning
- intravenous infusions – type, rate and patency of site
- drains – types, amount draining and rate
- urinary catheters – patency, colour of drainage and amount.

Monitoring will include:

- temperature (hypothermia remains a potential risk)
- pulses and sensation following arterial or limb surgery
- wound site
- plaster of Paris casts
- pressure areas (AfPP, 2016; Wicker, 2015).

All postoperative assessment and observations must be recorded in the patient's documentation. The immediate postoperative period is fraught with potential complications for each patient, and the recovery room nurse plays a vital role in detecting, preventing and managing dangerous life-threatening conditions by continuous, ongoing assessment of the patient visually and with the aid of monitors.

Waking up from an anaesthetic can be a frightening experience for the patient. Constant communication with the patient during this phase and throughout their recovery is vital to reduce the patient's anxiety. The nurse should communicate any procedures being undertaken even before the patient regains consciousness, as hearing is the first sense to return.

Recovery rooms are often large areas with bays segregated by curtains or screens. Maintaining confidentiality, privacy, dignity and respect is a challenge to all recovery room nurses, as they must juggle the individual needs with those of patient safety.

Managing a patient's pain

A pain assessment tool should be used to quantify a patient's postoperative pain, whilst recognizing that it is a subjective and highly individual experience. The American Society of PeriAnesthesia Nurses recommends that this assessment should occur preoperatively (ASPAN, 2003) because in the postoperative period an accurate assessment is difficult if the patient is drowsy, confused or crying. The recovery nurse can observe non-verbal clues such as restlessness, grimacing and hyperventilation (Cox, 2012). Hypoxia, hypothermia, anxiety, nausea, fatigue and pain are all symptoms of the body's stress response to surgery. Pain postoperatively can magnify these responses and delay a return to normal function, as well as impair wound healing and predispose the patient to infection.

Analgesics can be administered through a variety of techniques and routes, i.e. intramuscular injection, intravenous bolus, intravenous patient-controlled analgesia (PCA), epidural, or rectally. Recovery nurses must have the knowledge and skills to understand and administer the different methods and analgesics available and monitor the incidence and severity of side-effects. PCA is popular with both patients and clinicians, as it avoids injections, eliminates the delay to the patient in receiving analgesia and allows the patient to feel more in control of their own pain. A PCA is a much more efficient way of giving opioids, as it avoids the peaks and troughs in blood concentration associated with intramuscular injections (Chumbley, 2009). Assessment of the patient is ongoing, in order to monitor the efficacy of the pain relief. If the pain is controlled, then the patient should be able to move easily on the trolley/bed, take deep breaths and generally feel more comfortable and less anxious. Documentation of the assessment and actions taken must be made in the patient's care plan. See Chapter 8 for more detailed information on pain management in the surgical patient.

Managing postoperative nausea and vomiting

Postoperative nausea and vomiting (PONV) is a significant postoperative complication and causes the patient stress, discomfort and additional pain. Literature widely recognizes that 25–30% of patients experience nausea and vomiting following general anaesthesia, which is highly unpleasant for the patient (Pierre & Whelan, 2013). It can range from feeling nauseated to active vomiting which may lead to dehydration and delay recovery time (Smedley & Quine, 2012).

Pierre and Whelan identified the patient risk factors for PONV as non-smoker, female, and previous history of travel sickness or PONV. The risk increases dependent on the type of surgery – oral, ENT or laparoscopic – and if opioids are used during surgery. The risk score then identifies the management and treatment for the patient, including general measures such as reduced fasting times, use of non-opioid analgesics preoperatively, and pharmacology prophylaxis such as ondansetron or dexamethasone.

PONV is self-limiting but can be debilitating for the patient if prolonged. Patients may become pale and experience excessive swallowing or salivation and tachycardia prior to vomiting. Complications may arise, such as aspiration and regurgitation of stomach contents, wound dehiscence due to muscular contractions damaging sutures within the wound, postoperative bleeding, hypotension and shock, which can result in delayed postoperative recovery and discharge (ASPAN, 2003). Electrolyte imbalance and dehydration can occur if the episode of PONV is prolonged, particularly in children. The recovery nurse must prevent hypovolaemia, ensure adequate hydration, and may need to administer alternative anti-emetics.

Other postoperative complications include:
- pulmonary complications (upper airway obstruction, pneumothorax, aspiration of gastric contents)
- shock
- neurological complications (loss of sensation to affected limb)
- cardiovascular complications (hypotension, arrhythmias, myocardial ischaemia)
- postoperative bleeding
- and for diabetic patients, hypo- or hyperglycaemia (AAGBI, 2013).

Enhanced recovery

Enhanced recovery is the outcome of applying a range of multimodal strategies, originally devised for day surgery, to prepare and optimize patients before, during and after surgery, ensuring prompt recovery and discharge from hospital. It has good outcomes for patients, enabling them to return home sooner and frees surgical beds, saving hospitals money (ERPP, 2010).

Discharge of the patient to the ward

The patient's stay in the recovery room varies considerably, depending on the patient, type of anaesthetic, surgical procedure and postoperative recovery. The AAGBI identify that the anaesthetist is responsible for discharging the patient from the recovery room although this is often delegated to a competent practitioner (AAGBI, 2013). Discharge criteria are usually set locally but should be mutually agreed with the department for anaesthesia. The recovery room nurse must provide detailed information to a competent nurse who will take on the responsibility for that patient's care (AAGBI, 2013).

General postoperative care on the ward

The ward nurse then escorts the patient back to the ward, monitoring the patient's condition throughout the transition. Having settled the patient on the ward, regular recording of vital signs and systemic observation can reveal early indicators of postoperative complications. Close monitoring of the patient will allow immediate action to be taken in the event of a complication. Observations should be recorded initially every 30 minutes and compared to the baseline assessment, and observations in recovery, to provide an overall view of the patient's condition. Observations and their frequency can be reduced as the patient's condition improves (Table 2.5).

The aim of the care is to allow the patient to move along the patient dependence–independence continuum.

Conclusion

Entering the perioperative environment is a daunting prospect both for student nurses and for the patient. Yet it is an essential part of the surgical patient's journey.

Perioperative nursing is perceived as technical, assisting the surgeon or anaesthetist – 'handmaidens' – and as such not real nursing. The author hopes that through providing a rationale for nurses' actions, those who visit the operating theatre department can gain an understanding of the high standard of nursing care that is required and delivered to the individual patient undergoing a surgical procedure.

Each perioperative nurse, no matter what their role is, is personally accountable for their practice and the author has demonstrated that the concept of perioperative nursing is centred on individual risk assessment and prevention of harm.

Table 2.5 General postoperative nursing care

Observation	Action and rationale	Complication
Level of consciousness	Patient can be roused easily Patient becomes gradually aware of surroundings Patient can explain where they are and what has happened to them	Patient not rousable or confused: • check baseline admission nursing and medical notes • review medication in theatres or recovery • inform medical staff immediately
Respirations	Monitor rate, depth and chest movement Breathing should be unhindered Skin colour is pink or based on baseline assessment of the individual patient Be alert for signs of cyanosis and poor oxygenation Sitting patient upright as soon as possible will encourage lung expansion and oxygenation	Reduced respiratory rate may indicate early respiratory arrest Reduced respiratory rate may be due to analgesics or other drugs administered, and nurses should be aware of what the patient has received and their potential side-effects Nurses must be aware of patient's medical history when administering oxygen
Pulse	Monitor and assess against baseline recording Monitor rate, volume and irregularities Nurses need to be aware of drugs given in theatre and recovery as they can affect pulse rate	Rising pulse rate may indicate reduced circulating volume due to haemorrhage Arrhythmias may indicate cardiac problems and therefore an ECG may be required Bradycardia may indicate reaction to drugs or cardiac arrest. Inform medical staff immediately
Blood pressure	Monitor and assess against baseline recording Nurses need to be aware of drugs given in theatre and recovery as they can affect blood pressure Blood pressure should return to within patient's normal limits	Hypotension may indicate haemorrhage or lack of fluid replacement Hypotension may also be indicative of pain or nausea
Temperature	Body temperature can alter significantly in surgery and should be monitored on the ward	A reduction in body temperature may indicate hypothermia, a reaction to surgical assault or anaesthetic drugs. Warmed blankets, increasing the room temperature and forced air warming systems may be used Increase in body temperature may indicate postoperative infection; inform medical staff so that appropriate action can be taken
Pain and nausea	Monitoring of patient's pain and nausea by scoring or dependency Type and rate of analgesics must reflect patient's needs Nurses need to be aware of patient's allergies and any drugs administered in theatre and recovery	Restlessness, agitation, confusion and non-verbal clues indicate increasing pain levels Restlessness, hypotension and excessive salivation can indicate nausea
Fluid intake	Encourage fluid intake as soon as possible, dependent on the surgery performed Accurately record fluid intake if intravenous infusion sited Monitor infusion site, rate of infusion and type of fluid being administered	Oral intake should be gradual and should be halted if the patient is nauseous, until more comfortable If intravenous site becomes blocked or damaged, it may need to be re-sited, depending on patient's condition and needs postoperatively Administration of a blood transfusion requires careful observations and patient monitoring
Fluid output	Every postoperative patient should have noted on their records when they pass urine	Restlessness and agitation may indicate a full bladder. The patient must be assisted and encouraged to pass urine

(Continued)

Table 2.5 General postoperative nursing care—cont'd

Observation	Action and rationale	Complication
	Urinary catheters must be checked for patency and flow of urine The colour, smell and amount of urine must be recorded	If catheterized, ensure patency, no blockages; if no flow, a bladder washout may be performed on medical instructions
Neurovascular status	Monitor colour, warmth, sensation and movement, and circulation return to the affected limb	Report any change in condition as this may reflect constriction of blood supply or nerve damage Dressings and plaster casts may also restrict blood supply and may need to be loosened or reapplied
Wounds and drains	Observe for excess blood loss or haemorrhage Ensure patency of drain	Excessive blood loss may indicate further haemorrhage. Further pressure wound dressings may be applied and the patient's overall physical status observed closely

Source: AfPP (2016); Hamlin et al. (2016).

SUMMARY OF KEY POINTS

This chapter has:

- provided a broad introduction to the holistic care given by practitioners within the perioperative environment during the patient's immediate preoperative, intraoperative and postoperative phases of their surgical experience.
- defined the patient's perioperative journey and the nurse's role in delivering individualized patient care.
- discussed the importance of good communication skills.
- explored in depth the needs of patients during the phases of their surgical experience, and how care for the individual physical and psychological needs can be adapted.
- identified potential risks for each patient in all three areas in the operating theatre department and the actions taken to prevent these occurring.

REFLECTIVE LEARNING POINTS

Having read this chapter, think about what you now know and what you still need to find out about. These questions may help:

- Why must all swabs, instruments, needles and other sharps be accounted for throughout the surgical procedure?
- What is the role and function of the recovery room nurse?
- What might be the impact of patients losing heat during their surgery?

References

American Society of PeriAnesthesia Nurses (ASPAN). (2003). ASPAN pain and comfort clinical guideline. *Journal of Perianesthesia Nursing, 18*(4), 232–236. Available at: <http://www.aspan.org/Portals/6/docs/ClinicalPractice/Guidelines/ASPAN_ClinicalGuideline_PainComfort.pdf>.

Association of Anaesthetists of Great Britain & Ireland (AAGBI). (2010). *Preoperative assessment and patient preparation. The role of the anaesthetist.* London: AAGBI. Available at: <https://anaesthetists.org/Home/Resources-publications/Guidelines/Pre-operative-assessment-and-patient-preparation-the-role-of-the-anaesthetist-2>.

Association of Anaesthetists of Great Britain & Ireland (AAGBI). (2013). *Immediate post-anaesthetic recovery 2013.* London: AAGBI. Available at: <https://anaesthetists.org/Home/Resources-publications/Guidelines/Immediate-post-anaesthesia-recovery>.

Association of Anaesthetists of Great Britain & Ireland (AAGBI). (2018). *The anaesthesia team 2018.* London: Association of Anaesthetists. Available at: <https://anaesthetists.org/Home/Resources-publications/Guidelines/The-Anaesthesia-Team-2018>.

Association for Perioperative Practice (AfPP). (2016). *Standards and recommendations for safe perioperative practice.* Harrogate: AfPP.

Association for Perioperative Practice (AfPP). (2017). Accountable items, swab, instruments and sharps count 2017 *(Poster).* Harrogate: AfPP. Available at: <https://www.afpp.org.uk/filegrab/1accountable-items-final.pdf?ref = 2138>.

Bonnet, F., & Marret, E. (2005). Influence of anaesthetic and analgesic techniques on outcome after surgery. *British Journal of Anaesthesia, 9*(1), 52–58.

Bryant, B., & Knights, K. (2015). *Pharmacology for health professions* (4th ed.). Sydney: Elsevier.

Chilton, R., & Thompson, R. (2012). Anaesthetic care. In K. Woodhead, & L. Fudge (Eds.), *Manual of perioperative care: an essential guide*. Chichester: John Wiley & Sons Ltd.

Chumbley, G. (2009). Patient-controlled analgesia. In F. Cox (Ed.), *Perioperative pain management* (pp. 161–185). Chichester: Wiley-Blackwell.

Cox, F. (2012). Pain management. In K. Woodhead, & L. Fudge (Eds.), *Manual of perioperative care: an essential guide*. Chichester: John Wiley & Sons Ltd.

Enhanced Recovery Partnership Programme (ERPP). (2010). *Delivering enhanced recovery. Helping patients to get better sooner after surgery*. London: ERPP. Available at: <https://ebpom. org/download.php/?fn=NHS +Delivering+Enhanced+Recovery. pdf&mime=application/ pdf&pureFn=NHS+Delivering +Enhanced+Recovery.pdf>.

Esmail, N., & Wrona, D. (2013). Improved medical technology leads to better overall health. In C. Ullmann, & L. M. Zott (Eds.), *Medical technology*. Detroit: Greenhaven Press. Available at <https://pdfs.semanticscholar.org/ cd97/7d7c02ebc52758795388477a 8149091914ca.pdf>.

Hamlin, L., Davies, M., Richardson-Tench, M., & Sutherland-Fraser, S. (2016). *Perioperative nursing: an introduction*. Sydney: Elsevier.

Hehir, R. (2012). Care of the elderly patient. In K. Woodhead, & L. Fudge (Eds.), *Manual of perioperative care: an essential guide*. Chichester: John Wiley & Sons Ltd.

Liddle, C. (2014). Nil by mouth best practice and patient education. *Nursing Times, 110*(26), 12–14. Available at: <https://www.nursingtimes.net/ Journals/2014/06/20/r/m/t/250614- Nil-by-mouth-best-practice-and- patient-education.pdf>.

McArthur, E. (2012). Care of the adolescent in surgery. In K. Woodhead, & L. Fudge (Eds.), *Manual of perioperative care: an essential guide*. Chichester: John Wiley & Sons Ltd.

National Confidential Enquiry into Patient Outcome and Death (NCEPOD). (2004). *The NCEPOD classification of intervention*. Available at: <www.ncepod.org.uk/classification. html>

National Institute for Health & Care Excellence (NICE). (2014). *Pressure ulcers: prevention and management*. Clinical guideline [CG179]. Available at: <https://www.nice.org.uk/guid- ance/cg179>

National Institute for Health & Care Excellence (NICE). (2016). *Hypothermia: prevention and management in adults having surgery*. Clinical guide- line [CG65]. Available at: <https:// www.nice.org.uk/guidance/cg65>

National Institute for Health & Care Excellence (NICE). (2018). *NICE Guideline [NG89] Venous thromboembo- lism in over 16s: reducing the risk of hospital-acquired deep vein thrombosis or pulmonary embolism*. NICE guideline [NG89]. Available at: <https://www. nice.org.uk/guidance/ng89/chapter/ Recommendations>

Nursing and Midwifery Council (NMC). (2018). *The Code: standards of conduct, performance and ethics for nurses and midwives*. London: NMC.

Oakley, M. (2010). Preoperative assess- ment. In R. Pudner (Ed.), *Nursing the surgical patient* (3rd ed.). Edinburgh: Elsevier.

Pierre, S., & Whelan, R. (2013). Nausea and vomiting after surgery. *Continuing Education in Anaesthesia Critical Care & Pain, 13*(1), 28–32. Available at <https://academic.oup.com/bjaed/arti- cle/13/1/28/281153>.

Pirie, S. (2012). Safer moving and han- dling and patient positioning. In K. Woodhead, & L. Fudge (Eds.), *Manual of perioperative care: an essential guide*. Chichester: John Wiley & Sons Ltd.

Radford, M., & Palmer, R. (2012). Pre- operative care. In K. Woodhead, & L. Fudge (Eds.), *Manual of perioperative care: an essential guide*. Chichester: John Wiley & Sons Ltd.

Reid, J. (2005). Ethical dimensions of peri- operative practice. In K. Woodhead, & P. Wicker (Eds.), *A textbook of periopera- tive care* (2nd ed.). Edinburgh: Churchill Livingstone.

Royal College of Anaesthetists. (2019). *Guidelines for the provision of anaesthesia services for postoperative care*. Available at <https://www.rcoa.ac.uk/gpas/chap- ter-4>

Royal College of Nursing (RCN). (2013). *Perioperative fasting in adults and chil- dren. An RCN guideline for the multidis- ciplinary team*. Available at: <https:// www.rcn.org.uk/professional-develop- ment/publications/pub-002779>

Royal College of Surgeons. (no date). *Consent*. Available at: <https://www. rcseng.ac.uk/standards-and-research/ gsp/domain-3/3-5-1-consent/>

Smedley, P., & Quine, N. (2012). Postoperative care. In K. Woodhead, & L. Fudge (Eds.), *Manual of perioperative care: an essential guide*. Chichester: John Wiley & Sons Ltd.

Stanley, T. (2014). The fentanyl story. *The Journal of Pain, 15*(12), 1215–1226. Available at: <https://www.jpain.org/ article/S1526-5900(14)00905-5/pdf>.

Vickers, R. (2011). Five steps to safer sur- gery. *Annals of the Royal College of Surgeons of England, 93*(7), 501–503. Available at: <https://www.ncbi.nlm. nih.gov/pmc/articles/PMC3604917/>.

Vincent, C. (2016). *Safety strategies in hospi- tals. Safer healthcare: Strategies for the real world*. Cham (CH): Springer. (Chapter 7) Available at: <https:// www.ncbi.nlm.nih.gov/books/ NBK481877/>.

Wicker, P. (2015). *Perioperative practice at a glance*. Chichester: John Wiley & Sons Ltd.

Williams, A. (2014). Anaesthesia for thera- peutic and diagnostic procedures. In J. Nagelhout, & K. Plaus (Eds.), *Nurse anaesthesia*. St Louis: Elsevier Saunders.

Wilson, J. (2019). *Infection control in clini- cal practice* (3rd ed.). London: Elsevier.

World Health Organization (WHO). (2008). *Patient safety*. Available at: <https://www.who.int/patientsafety/ en/>

Further reading

Rothrock, J. (2018). *Alexander's care of the patient in surgery* (16th ed.). St Louis: Mosby.

Chapter | 3 |

Day surgery

Efua Hagan

KEY OBJECTIVES OF THE CHAPTER

At the end of the chapter the reader should be able to:

- give a definition of day surgery and an explanation of what it involves
- discuss the history and development of day surgery
- state the advantages and possible disadvantages of day surgery
- discuss the surgical and anaesthetic techniques employed in day surgery
- describe the recovery of the patient following surgery
- discuss the discharge criteria for the day surgery patient.

Areas to think about before reading the chapter

- What criteria must be satisfied prior to a patient being considered for day surgery?
- List three types of anaesthesia used in the day surgery setting.
- What do you understand by second stage recovery in day surgery?

Introduction

What is day surgery?

Day surgery is also known as ambulatory care, day case surgery and outpatient surgery. In the UK and Ireland this is defined by a patient who is admitted into hospital for a planned procedure, whether an investigation or a procedure, and is discharged home on the same day. This differs from patients who are admitted in inpatient theatres and are discharged on the same day and will be noted as a patient who has had a zero-hour length of stay (Quemby & Stocker, 2014). Patients who come in for a day surgery procedure will also need recovering in a ward area before being discharged and this will take place in a specially adapted unit that has been designed for this purpose. According to the British Association of Day Surgery (BADS), day surgery is not a procedure but a process (BADS, 2016).

History and development of day surgery

Professor James H. Nicoll is known as the father who created the foundations for day surgery. In a paper that was published in 1901 in the *British Medical Journal*, the Glaswegian was reported to have performed approximately 9000 paediatric operations. The motivation behind the day cases was due to Professor Nicoll's concerns over infection rates and also lack of beds (Quemby & Stocker, 2014). The principles Professor Nicoll incorporated into his care of patients, follow-up by a nurse and early mobilization, went against the established medics' advice of bed rest after surgery. No progress with the provision of day surgery units was made until the first units opened in 1951 in Michigan and then in Los Angeles the following year in the United States. The

31

United Kingdom did not open its first unit until 1969 in Hammersmith by James Calnan. The Royal College of Surgeons (RCS) then suggested that a target of 50% of surgeries should be performed as day cases after it was noted in the 1980s that less than 15% were day cases. This was due to junior doctors performing surgeries, which meant surgical times were slow; part of the RCS's recommendation was that senior clinicians would perform the surgeries to increase the turnaround time. An association was created in 1989, named the British Association of Day Surgery (BADS), and in 1995 BADS, along with eleven other organizations, went on to create the International Association for Ambulatory Surgery (IAAS).

Advantages of day surgery

The reduction of waiting lists and the increased availability and use of the inpatient service for patients who are in need are seen as some of the economic benefits of day surgery. Patients who are accepted on the day surgery pathway will expect to receive a high-quality, efficient and economical service. The high flow of patients coming through day surgery has also led to a reduction to surgical waiting lists. It also has a low incidence of major morbidity, reduced cross-infection risks, and lends itself to audit (Jackson, 2012).

Many patients prefer to have their aftercare at home rather than in hospital, and patient surveys indicate high levels of satisfaction with day case treatment (Darwin, 2015). Patients can avoid an unnecessary hospital stay, have minimal disruption of daily routine, and can return home to recover in familiar surroundings. Day surgery is not a new concept of care; it has been used throughout the last century. However, now that the benefits of day case procedures are evident, it has become increasingly popular.

Day case surgery is good news for the health service; it now accounts for approximately 80% of elective procedures each year, with space to increase (Appleby, 2015). Appleby (2015) states that, in 2013−2014, 22% of cases were inpatient vs 78% day case; with the spending on elective care during this period and developments in surgery, by 2023−2024 this would mean 13% inpatient cases vs 87% day case, a 22% increase for day cases. This data demonstrates that day cases are a popular option for patients.

The majority of surgical specialties can utilize a day surgery unit. In 1990, the Audit Commission produced a 'basket of procedures', which numbered 20; however, this 'basket' was updated in 2001 (Darwin, 2015; Anderson et al, 2016) (Box 3.1). The British Association of Day Surgery put forward a further list of major procedures that can also be performed as day surgery in 50%

Box 3.1 The Audit Commission 'basket of 25'

- Orchidopexy
- Circumcision
- Inguinal hernia repair
- Excision of breast lump
- Anal fissure dilatation and excision
- Haemorrhoidectomy
- Laparoscopic cholecystectomy
- Varicose vein stripping and ligation
- Transurethral resection of bladder tumour
- Excision of Dupuytren's contracture
- Carpal tunnel decompression
- Excision of ganglion
- Arthroscopy
- Bunion operations
- Removal of metal ware
- Extraction of cataract with/without implant
- Correction of squint
- Myringotomy
- Tonsillectomy
- Submucous resection
- Reduction of nasal fracture
- Operation for bat ears
- Dilatation and curettage/hysteroscopy
- Laparoscopy
- Termination of pregnancy

Box 3.2 British Association of Day Surgery 'trolley' of procedures suitable for day surgery in some cases

- Laparoscopic hernia repair
- Thoracoscopic sympathectomy
- Submandibular gland excision
- Partial thyroidectomy
- Superficial parotidectomy
- Wide excision of breast lump with axillary clearance
- Urethrotomy
- Bladder neck incision
- Laser prostatectomy
- Transcervical resection of endometrium (TCRE)
- Eyelid surgery
- Arthroscopic meniscectomy
- Arthroscopic shoulder decompression
- Subcutaneous mastectomy
- Rhinoplasty
- Dentoalveolar surgery
- Tympanoplasty

---

of cases, which is based upon the complexity, length and anaesthesia involved in the surgery (Quemby & Stocker, 2014) (Box 3.2). This was extended with the Directory of Procedures (British Association of Day

Table 3.1 British Association of Day Surgery (BADS) Directory of Procedures (2016)

Treatment option	Definition of length of stay in Directory
Procedure room	Operation that may be performed in a suitable clean environment outside of theatres, e.g. GP surgery
Day surgery	Traditional day surgery
23-hour stay	Patient is admitted and discharged within 24 hours
Under 72-hour stay	Patient is admitted and discharged within 72 hours

Surgery, 2016), where each procedure is listed against four possible treatment options (Table 3.1). There are procedures that may require a patient to have a longer recovery time. This means that the patient will need to have their surgery during a morning session. Procedures such as ophthalmology may also require specialist equipment and training for clinicians to reach their full potential.

Disadvantages of day surgery

Training and educational programmes have been developed to increase interest in their care pathway and have changed some negative attitudes that have been associated with day surgery. As anaesthesia has and continues to develop alongside the increase in standards of preoperative assessment, this has meant practitioners and doctors have needed to receive further education in this area. There may be some patients who might feel they will be a burden to their relatives due to their home circumstances. This can be combated with patients receiving a comprehensive preoperative assessment, which needs to include discharge planning in advance with a high input of quality patient education. Patient anxieties can be reduced, which can enable the patient to understand that day surgery care could be the best option for them. Patients selected for day surgery are usually physically fit for surgery and need a responsible adult to take care of them for at least the first 24 hours after surgery and a suitable home environment. However, healthcare professionals may be unable to assess this, which could mean the environment may not be suitable (Jackson, 2012).

Day surgery nursing

Day surgery nursing differs from ward or theatre nursing as there is the potential for nurses to work in and across all areas of the day surgery unit. Most planned day surgery units have areas identified for preoperative assessment, anaesthetics, operating theatre, recovery and ward facilities. All nurses working in day surgery should ideally be trained to be multi-skilled and able to work in each area, perhaps on a rotation system. Staff can expand their practice by becoming competent anaesthetic, operating theatre and recovery nurses, as well as being skilful in patient assessment before and after surgery (Bailey et al, 2019).

The benefits of staff rotation are greater job satisfaction, more effective and efficient staffing and good staff morale. Patients also benefit from a more knowledgeable nursing staff, and it highlights the specialized role of the day surgery nurse. The rotation system prevents work becoming too routine and allows staff to become competent in nursing patients from a variety of specialities (Bailey et al, 2019).

In order to facilitate nurse rotation throughout a day surgery unit, nurses should be intensively trained so that they achieve a variety of skills. They will need theatre nursing skills, knowledge of anaesthetic techniques and the ability to deliver immediate postoperative care to patients. This is in addition to demonstrating good communication skills and a caring attitude towards patients and their relatives (Bailey et al, 2019).

Day surgery nursing – patient care

Day surgery is now being touted as the 'norm' in the NHS but it is important to ensure the unit is run in a safe and effective way. The patients that are admitted into day surgery need to be carefully selected. The surgery must match the correct patient profile (medically and practically safe) so that the patient is able to return home the same day. If the length of time of recovery takes 1 day or longer, the impact on the patient may be great. Hospitalization and subsequent recovery at home will impinge on the patient's social circumstances. It will have implications for work commitments, and the necessary help and arrangements will be needed to achieve a satisfactory and uneventful recovery. It should not be forgotten that fears and anxieties regarding treatment may be just as real in the day surgery patient (Anderson et al, 2016).

Preoperative assessment in day surgery

The role of the preoperative assessment for surgical patients has been discussed in depth in Chapter 1. However, it is worth noting at this point that preoperative assessment in day surgery is a fundamental part of the patient's journey to surgery. The Nursing and Midwifery Council (2018) note that the nurse must put the interests of people who require nursing services first. The nurse has to make the care and safety of the patient their main concern and ensure that the patient's needs are recognized, assessed and responded to.

Day surgery has led the way in preoperative assessment because, particularly at the inception of widespread day surgery, there were very strict criteria laid down as to which patients were suitable for day surgery and which patients were not. It is important that the patient is fully informed so that this can reduce stress levels and also help with the postoperative care at home. It is important that those who are involved in preoperative assessments are trained in the area. It is common for nurses who are trained in the area to also ask for input from anaesthetists, usually consultants, who have an interest in the same area. This also allows for patients who are found to be complex to be reviewed so as not to delay their surgery.

Preoperative assessments usually take place in a designated area within a day surgery unit. This enables not just the patient but also relatives to have some familiarity with the environment and to meet staff who may be involved in their care when admitted (Anderson et al, 2016; Bailey et al, 2019).

Admission to the day surgery unit

When patients are admitted to the day surgery unit, there is only a short amount of time available for the nursing staff to assess, plan, implement and evaluate the care required to ensure that the needs of the patient are met. However, the opportunity to practise excellent nursing care should not be dependent on the length of a patient's hospital stay, and effective communication skills should be used to convey information and understand the patient's fears and anxieties. Communicating with the patient, putting them at ease and giving clear understandable information forms the basis of good day surgery care. The nurse in the day surgery unit should recognize that, to each patient, their operation is a major source of anxiety and will be a stressful event. However, minor the surgical condition may seem, there is no such thing as a 'minor' general anaesthetic.

On admission to the day surgery unit, the nurse should explain to the patient the routine they should expect and offer adequate preoperative instructions and information. It should be remembered that the patient may be very anxious and nervous, and the nurse should ascertain that the patient understands the information given and allow time for any questions. The patient's preoperative assessment questionnaire will be checked by the nurse to identify any change in the patient's health status since their first assessment. The patient's baseline observations will also be measured and recorded. It is important that all patients should have a responsible adult to take them home after the operation and to stay with them for the first 24 hours. This will ensure patient safety, as their coordination and memory may be impaired following general anaesthesia. Therefore, the patient's discharge arrangements should be carefully checked during the admission procedure.

Anaesthesia in day surgery

As stated previously, there is no such thing as a 'minor' general anaesthetic. The anaesthetic technique for day surgery must ensure adequate anaesthesia and analgesia without compromising the recovery and subsequent discharge of the patient. Thus, the technique is tailored specifically to minimize the pain the patient will experience postoperatively, without the use of drugs that will hinder discharge from the day surgery unit. Added to this, an antiemetic anaesthetic technique will be employed to reduce the incidence of postoperative nausea and vomiting. It is obvious from this that the anaesthetic service in a day surgery unit should be consultant-led.

The ideal anaesthetic for the day surgery patient should produce very little cardiorespiratory depression, and the induction should be smooth and rapid. The anaesthetic must facilitate the fast turnover of day surgery without pain and postoperative nausea and vomiting, and a rapid return of psychomotor state with minimal hangover effects, allowing for a prompt discharge.

Patients may walk into the operating theatre from the ward to undergo induction of anaesthesia on the operating table or trolley. A nurse or operating department practitioner (ODP) will escort the patient into theatre and is, therefore, responsible for collecting the correct patient for the correct procedure. The nurse or ODP stays beside the patient until anaesthesia has been induced.

The Association of Anaesthetists of Great Britain and Ireland (AAGBI) recommended that day case surgery should be a consultant-led speciality. However, it is important that trainee anaesthetists are also educated in the speciality so they are competent to manage patients within this pathway (Anderson et al, 2016).

Anaesthetic technique

It is important that anaesthesia given to the patient needs to be tailored to them. This is to reduce the amount of discomfort and encourage the quickest recovery possible.

The most commonly used induction agent is propofol, as it has a rapid onset and facilitates airway management easily, particularly the insertion of the laryngeal mask airway (LMA). There are two methods to maintain a patient's anaesthesia — either with inhalation gases such as sevoflurane and desflurane or the 'total intravenous anaesthetic technique' (TIVA), which has reduced the need for inhalation agents and also reduces the incidence of postoperative vomiting and nausea. This drug also allows a patient to return to full cognitive function (Quemby & Stocker, 2014; Darwin, 2015; Anderson et al, 2016).

Prophylactic oral analgesia such as paracetamol has been recommended as the drug of choice. In a high-turnover day surgery department, the use of these drugs can assist as a time-saving measure, as patients are more likely to mobilize earlier. However, it is important to take renal function into consideration, so drug doses need to be tailored (Darwin, 2015).

Analgesia could also be given during the procedure to ensure the patient is as pain-free as possible; examples of drugs used are fentanyl and alfentanil, which are given in relation to the patient's need. Infiltration of the wound with local anaesthesia and non-steroidal anti-inflammatory drugs (NSAIDs) are the other forms of analgesia used in day surgery.

If a patient is to be ventilated, a muscle relaxant will be given; there are two categories — depolarizing and non-depolarizing. Depolarizing muscle relaxants act by mimicking the action of acetylcholine, a neurotransmitter, which is broken down naturally in the body by plasma cholinesterase. The only depolarizing muscle relaxant in clinical use in the United Kingdom is suxamethonium, which is used when a rapid endotracheal intubation is required.

Non-depolarizing muscle relaxants work by blocking the receptor sites at the motor end plate at the neuromuscular junction. The action of non-depolarizing muscle relaxants has to be reversed, and this is done by the administration of an anticholinesterase such as sugammadex, neostigmine and glycopyrronium bromide. Rocuronium is increasingly being used as an alternative to suxamethonium, as it has fewer negative side effects and allows the patient to breathe spontaneously quicker (Dean & Chapman, 2018).

If a patient is to have a laryngeal mask airway (LMA) inserted, the preferred choice is the i-gel as it is quicker to insert and gives a better fibreoptic view when the equipment is needed. The disadvantage of the LMA is that it cannot be used in patients who have a full stomach or a history of reflux, as it does not protect the airway from vomit and the patient is at risk of aspiration. However, this category of patient is highly unlikely to fit the day surgery criteria (Dean & Chapman, 2018).

Recovery in day surgery

Recovery in day surgery can be divided into two distinct phases: first stage recovery, where the patient comes to straight from theatre, and second stage recovery, which is usually where they are discharged. In first stage recovery, the care of the patient is the same as that given to any post-anaesthesia patient — i.e. airway and pain management and, where necessary, management of postoperative nausea and vomiting. Where day surgery recovery is at variance with inpatient recovery is that the patient will not be allowed to 'sleep it off', as the main aim is one of discharge. Although all care will be given to the patient and analgesics administered as appropriate, this will be with a view to getting the patient into second stage recovery and discharge.

First stage recovery

The majority of patients will arrive in first stage recovery with an LMA in place and this will maintain the airway until the patient wakes up. Depending on the type of LMA, this is removed fully inflated to allow secretions to be removed with it and usually the patient is encouraged to take it out themselves. Note that the i-gel is a type of LMA that does not need to be inflated.

The two most important areas in first stage recovery are management of the patient's pain and prevention of postoperative nausea and vomiting. These are the main reasons why patients cannot be discharged home from the day surgery unit and have to be admitted as inpatients (Rae, 2016).

Pain management

The prevention of pain is managed from pre-assessment of the patient, where patients are told what to expect and how the pain will be treated. The anaesthetic technique will incorporate strategies that will enable the patient to be pain-free in the recovery period, and each unit will have protocols in place as to the analgesics the patient will take home following surgery. Obviously, the use of opioids postoperatively is avoided in favour of other forms of analgesics, but opioids should not be withheld if the patient really needs them; the implications of this can be dealt with as they occur and the patient may have to be admitted, but this is preferable to the patient experiencing pain.

Management of postoperative nausea and vomiting (PONV)

It is important for PONV to be risk-assessed before a procedure so that intraoperatively it can be managed appropriately. It is important for fluids to be administered as needed to lessen the incidence of PONV. The use of regional blocks or non-steroidal anti-inflammatory drugs also reduces the incidence of PONV (Apfel et al, 2012; Quemby & Stocker, 2014; Darwin, 2015).

Second stage recovery

Once the patient is conscious, pain is managed to an appropriate level, the patient is not suffering from post-operative nausea and vomiting, and all observations are within normal limits, they will be moved to second stage recovery. This will vary from unit to unit. Some units have their patients on beds/trolleys, whereas others have recliner chairs. When appropriate, the nursing staff will start encouraging the patient to mobilize and start taking oral fluids and food. Once the patient has reached the pre-set criteria for discharge, arrangements will be made to send the patient home.

Discharge of the patient from the day surgery unit

In the day surgery setting, patients are usually discharged home by nurses, following protocols laid down by the medical staff. The nursing staff are responsible for assessing the patient's fitness for discharge from the day surgery unit once the anaesthetist and surgeon have seen the patient postoperatively. All patients have to fulfil a series of discharge criteria designed by the medical staff (Box 3.3). If the nurse is concerned about the patient's condition, the anaesthetist or the surgeon should return to the unit to reassess the patient.

Failure to fulfil all these criteria will mean either a delay in the patient's discharge or their transfer to an inpatient bed. No compromises can be made, as the safety of the patient is paramount and only patients who fulfil the criteria for discharge can be discharged home. Various studies summarized by Rae (2016) conclude the following reasons for readmission: PONV, urinary retention, pain, bleeding, chest pain and adverse drug events, amongst others.

Patients attending a day surgery unit require a great deal of education and support if they are to go home and care for themselves competently within a few hours of having received a general anaesthetic. Working in an area where nurses care for patients from their admission to discharge home, within a compressed time span, imposes a responsibility for nurses to educate their patients prior to their discharge from the day unit.

Postoperative information

It is important to give clear written and verbal instructions outlining essential postoperative information, because a patient's ability to understand and remember information may be impaired following a general anaesthetic (Quemby & Stocker, 2014; Bailey et al, 2019). It is therefore important for all nursing staff to develop and maintain a high standard of interpersonal and teaching skills. Many patients have unrealistic expectations and believe that, because they are only staying in hospital for a short time, they will be completely well before going home. Therefore, the importance of educating and informing patients cannot be overstressed. Prior to discharge, the nurse must check the patient understands their aftercare at home. Information should be given about whom to contact if a problem arises and how to cope in an emergency situation, and advice should be given on pain management and wound management, if appropriate. Details of further appointments, suture/staple removal and specific aftercare instructions should also be given (Box 3.4).

If appropriate, the patient may be seen by a physiotherapist prior to discharge, when postoperative exercises and the correct use of crutches can be explained, and further written information can be provided.

The nurse discharging the patient should ensure that the patient fully understands the effects of the anaesthesia, and the importance of not driving or drinking alcohol for 24

Box 3.3 Criteria for discharge

- The patient should be alert and orientated
- The patient should have tolerated diet and fluids, i.e. not vomiting
- The patient should have voided urine, although anecdotally many units do not insist on this
- The patient should be comfortable and mobile, i.e. should be pain-free
- Baseline observations must be satisfactory
- Wound checks must be satisfactory, i.e. the dressing is dry, there is no fresh bleeding
- Any follow-up appointments (if required) should be arranged
- Any mobility aids such as crutches (if required) should be supplied
- The patient must have a discharge letter for their general practitioner
- Verbal and written discharge information should be given
- Any medication to take home (if required) must be given

Box 3.4 **Summary of patient advice**

- How and when to take medication, if any is required
- How to manage wound care, e.g. when to remove any dressings
- When to bathe/shower while any sutures/staples are in place
- When and what exercises can be taken
- When to return to work
- When to start driving following surgery
- Advice about diet and fluids, e.g. to avoid alcohol for 24 hours postoperatively
- Whether a follow-up appointment is necessary in the outpatient clinic
- When any sutures/staples will be removed
- Warnings about nausea and light-headedness that may occur
- What activities may and may not be carried out in the immediate postoperative period, e.g. not to drive a car or operate machinery for 24 hours following discharge

hours. A responsible escort should collect the patient from the day surgery unit, as the patient will not be allowed to travel home alone by car or on public transport. It is the nurse's responsibility to ensure the safety of the patient at all times in the unit, and this is also carried beyond the hospital stay to the post-discharge period. Adequate arrangements for the patient's aftercare must be ensured, with back-up facilities arranged as necessary. Arrangements for informing the general practitioner must be adhered to. Failure to abide by strict criteria could result in unpleasant and perhaps dangerous consequences for the patient, and this is unacceptable.

Conclusion

In this chapter, the principles of caring for the patient as a day surgery case have been discussed. Where possible, this chapter has followed the patient journey through the day surgery unit. Day surgery is a team effort and nurses working within the unit have to be skilled in more than one area. The scope for nurses to develop their professional portfolio is inexhaustible as new surgical techniques are developed and the role of the day surgery nurse is enhanced.

Day surgery is preferable for patients, as most patients prefer to come to hospital for one day and in many cases half a day, and then go home to their own environment to recover.

SUMMARY OF KEY POINTS

- Day case surgery has proved to be universally popular with carefully selected patients.
- The economic benefits of day case surgery may be observed in terms of reduced waiting lists and cost savings.
- Anaesthetic and surgical technique must be tailored to patient discharge.
- Discharge planning and patient education play major roles in the duties of nurses in day surgery units.

REFLECTIVE LEARNING POINTS

Having read this chapter, think about what you now know and what you still need to find out about. These questions may help:

- How is pain managed in the day surgery setting and what advice is given to the patient on discharge?
- If no responsible adult is available to escort a patient home after day surgery, how might this be managed?
- In a day care unit where you have been placed, describe the various roles and responsibilities of those healthcare staff working in the unit.

References

Anderson, T., Walls, M., & Canelo, R. (2016). Day case surgery guidelines. *Surgery, 35*(2), 85–91.

Apfel, C. C., Meyer, A., Orhan-Sungur, M., Jalot, L., Whelan, R. P., & Jukar-Rao, S. (2012). Supplemental intravenous crystalloids for the prevention of postoperative nausea and vomiting quantitative review. *British Journal of Anaesthesia, 108*, 893–902.

Appleby, J. (2015). Day case surgery: a good news story for the NHS. *BMJ, 351*, h4060.

Bailey, C. R., Ahuja, M., Bartholomew, K., Bew, S., Forbes, L., Lipp, A., et al. (2019). Guidelines for day-case surgery 2019. *Anaesthesia, 2019* 1–15.

British Association of Day Surgery (BADS). (2016). *BADS directory of procedures* (5th ed.). London: BADS.

Darwin, L. (2015). Patient selection for day surgery. *Anaesthesia and Intensive Care Medicine, 17*(3), 151–154.

Dean, C., & Chapman, E. (2018). Induction of anaesthesia. *Anaesthesia and Intensive Care Medicine*, *19*(8), 383–388.

Jackson, I. (Ed.) (2012). Section 5: Day surgery services. In J.R. Colvin & C.J. Peden (Eds.), *Raising the standard: a compendium of audit recipes* (3rd ed.) (pp. 155–169). London: Royal College of Anaesthetists.

Nursing and Midwifery Council. (2018). *The Code. Professional standards of practice and behaviour for nurses, midwives and nursing associates*. London: NMC. Available at https://www.nmc.org.uk/globalassets/sitedocuments/nmc-publications/nmc-code.pdf.

Quemby, D. J., & Stocker, M. E. (2014). Day surgery development and practice: key factors for a successful pathway. *Continuing Education in Anaesthesia, Critical Care and Pain*, *14*(6), 256–261.

Rae, A. (2016). Reasons for delayed patient discharge following day surgery: a literature review. *Nursing Standard*, *31*(11), 42–51.

Further reading

Patient information for preparing for surgery

Royal College of Anaesthetists (RCoA). (2018). *Fitter Better Sooner*. Available from: https://www.rcoa.ac.uk/patient-information/preparing-surgery-fitter-better-sooner.

Relevant websites

British Association for Day Surgery — https://daysurgeryuk.net/en/home/
Royal College of Anaesthetists — www.rcoa.ac.uk

The Association of Surgeons in Training — www.asit.org
The Royal College of General Practitioners — www.rcgp.org.uk

Chapter | 4 |

Perioperative stress and anxiety in the surgical patient

Chloe Rich

KEY OBJECTIVES OF THE CHAPTER

At the end of the chapter the reader should be able to:

- discuss the concepts of perioperative stress and anxiety in the adult patient
- evaluate key factors that can attribute to surgical patients' stress and anxiety
- appreciate the benefits of reducing stress and anxiety in the surgical patient
- utilize various methods of reducing stress and anxiety in the surgical patient.

Areas to think about before reading the chapter

- How can stress manifest in an individual undergoing surgery?
- Describe the role of the nurse in helping those people undergoing surgery to reduce their stress levels and anxiety.
- Make a list of factors that people undergoing surgery may find stressful and describe how these can be removed or reduced

Introduction

In this chapter, the concepts of perioperative stress and anxiety will be examined, including current influencing factors and methods that can be used to reduce levels in the surgical patient. It has long been argued that surgery is a form of psychological stress. Stress can be defined as a response to external demands upon the body that requires a physical, mental or emotional adjustment or response (Kumar & Bhukar, 2013). A 'stressor' is any physical or psychological threat that evokes a physiological stress response, such as a threat to safety and well-being, or pain (Hannibal & Bishop, 2014).

Surgical trauma is a known body stress, causing psychophysiological stress responses from the endocrine system, central nervous system and immunological system (Ramos et al, 2008). The stress response begins in the brain, within the amygdala, responsible for processing emotional data. The amygdala transmits a message of threat to the hypothalamus, which in turn rouses a response from the sympathetic nervous system.

The hypothalamus first activates the secretion of adrenaline and noradrenaline from the adrenal medulla (glands) into the blood circulation, increasing heart rate, respiratory rate and blood pressure. Further effects include bronchodilation, vasoconstriction of arterioles, stimulation of sweat secretion, pupillary dilation and reduction of gastrointestinal activity to allow the circulating blood volume to fuel vital organs and muscles. Adrenaline triggers the release of glucose and fat from temporary storage into the blood circulation to balance the increased energy consumption. This short-term response is an inflammatory process, functioning to destroy invading microorganisms (Hannibal & Bishop, 2014).

The hypothalamus then releases the peptide hormone corticotrophin, stimulating the pituitary gland to synthesize and secrete adrenocorticotropic hormone (ACTH) into the blood circulation. ACTH acts within the cortical area of the adrenal glands, triggering a systematic and sustained release of glucocorticoid (cortisol) approximately 15 minutes after the onset of stress (Dedovic et al, 2009). Cortisol effects include further glucose and fat metabolism, suppression of non-vital organ systems and decrease in inflammation to allow for the management of stress.

The perception of stimuli as threatening or frightening is subjective to each individual. The internal anticipation of this future threat is anxiety. The amygdala responds to fear or danger by initiating a sympathetic and neuroendocrine stress response in an attempt to restore homeostasis (Mora et al, 2012). Stress and anxiety are interconnected, and the perioperative practitioner can be directly involved in their recognition and management.

Anxiety in the surgical patient

Anxiety is an 'alarm' reaction of the human body to a perceived physical or psychological threat (Ahmetovic-Djug et al, 2017). Experts believe that some individuals by nature are more prone to fear and discomfort, but it is also possible for past events to serve as a trigger for a particular anxiety (Alanazi, 2014). Patients who are anxious typically exhibit nervous behaviours and are more reactive and alert to an increased number of stimuli (Muglatti & Komarik, 2008).

Kindler et al (2000) propose that perioperative anxiety can be categorized into three areas: fear of the unknown, fear of feeling unwell, and fear for one's life. Suggested common triggers for perioperative anxiety include waiting for surgery, fear of disability, anticipation of postoperative pain, loss of independence, the fear of the unknown, separation from family members and death (Ay et al, 2014; Yilmaz et al, 2012). Other authors suggest triggers that include the anticipation of nausea and vomiting, having a mask placed over their face, cannulation, the unease of trusting a stranger, and the fear of waking up during surgery (Mitchell, 2010; Pierre & Whelan, 2012; Gilmartin & Wright, 2008).

Certain patient factors have been associated with preoperative anxiety, including a low level of education (Chan et al, 2004; Wang et al, 2008), female gender (Ayral et al, 2002; Jawaid et al, 2007; Perks et al, 2009), age (Chan et al, 2004), extent and type of surgery (Jawaid et al, 2007), marital status (Karanci & Dirik, 2003) and levels of social support (Lincoln et al, 2005). Females, those who are literate, patients living alone and those with lower levels of social support are all believed to have significantly higher perioperative anxiety levels (Yilmaz et al, 2012).

With the increased use of regional and local anaesthesia for surgical procedures, practitioners must also consider different concerns with these techniques. Patients experiencing surgery under local or regional anaesthesia are thought to be less anxious overall (Mitchell, 2012a); nonetheless, they are concerned about the procedure being painful, seeing their body being 'cut open', numbness wearing off too quickly and being able to feel what the surgeon is doing (Mitchell, 2008).

The increased use of laparoscopic surgical techniques and advancements in anaesthetic practice, in conjunction with pressure on the NHS to reduce costs and increase patient satisfaction, has resulted in a drastic reduction in the need for inpatient surgical stays. The evolution of day case surgery has drastically increased the range of procedures for patients that do not require an overnight stay in hospital, which overall increases patient satisfaction with their surgical journey (McWhinnie, 2018). However, this modern approach limits the ability for perioperative staff to interact with patients, alleviate possible anxieties and provide information on the day of surgery (Jlala et al, 2010). This is most apparent in postoperative care units, where the increasing complexity of day case procedures requires the practitioner to give the patient detailed information for their recovery in a short amount of time.

A final consideration must be the reduction of anaesthetic inductions being performed in an anaesthetic room within the UK. There are strong opinions from anaesthetists that the most important reasons to anaesthetize patients in anaesthetic rooms are that the environment is quieter, there are fewer interruptions and it has a positive impact on patient experience (Velzen et al, 2015). The NAP5 report by the Royal College of Anaesthetists and Association of Anaesthetists of Great Britain and Ireland (AAGBI) (2014) commented in particular on the lack of evidence published so far with regards to the measurable difference in anxiety levels between patients anaesthetized in theatres versus anaesthetic rooms. Some patients surveyed preferred being induced in the anaesthetic room as it felt warmer, smaller and cosier, less technical looking, less intimidating and more familiar. In contrast, others preferred being anaesthetized in the operating theatre itself as it felt more spacious, brighter and airy, a nicer colour and they did not want to be moved after an anaesthetic. This variation further supports the discussions that anxiety is subjective and should be managed on an individual patient basis. The NAP5 report concluded that departments should rule out patient anxiety as the dominant reason to continue the use of anaesthetic rooms for induction.

Benefits of reducing anxiety in the surgical patient

Perioperative anxiety is considered to be a normal part of a patient's surgical experience, although extremely harmful because of its negative impact upon patient outcomes (Mitchell, 2012b). Physiological responses to anxiety include tachycardia, hypertension, elevated temperature, sweating, muscle tension, nausea and a heightened sense of touch, smell or hearing (Alanazi, 2014; Pritchard, 2009). Patients can also present with shaking hands, dry mouth, headaches, back pain and 'blotchy' skin from the stress response (Keegan, 2003), all of which can help the practitioner identify an anxious individual. Psychological effects include feelings of restlessness, impaired concentration, nervousness, unpredictability and expression of illogical thoughts (Robinson et al, 2013). These negative emotions increase the likelihood of behaviours which affect the immune system, such as poor sleep patterns, inadequate nutrition and reduced physical activity, associated with delayed wound healing and recovery (Vileikyte, 2007). The impact of perioperative anxiety may be prolonged, affecting the patient's capacity to carry on everyday activities, impacting quality of life (Wong et al, 2010).

Anxiety is known to aggravate reactive airway diseases such as chronic obstructive pulmonary disease (COPD) and asthma, and can increase the risk of bronchospasm during general anaesthesia (Kocaturk & Oguz, 2017). It has been directly linked to an overall increase in incidences of adverse events during anaesthetic induction and patient recovery from correlated effects, including increased postoperative pain, increased analgesic and anaesthetic consumption, and exposing the patient to greater physiological and haemodynamic changes, e.g. hypotension, bradycardia and respiratory depression (Caumo & Ferreira, 2013; Pritchard, 2009).

As part of the 'fight or flight' response, patients who are anxious will present with peripheral vasoconstriction and cool peripheries (Pritchard, 2009), making cannulation more difficult for the practitioner. As a result, anxiety can again rise due to the multiple attempts and associated pain and discomfort. Overall, perioperative anxiety is associated with prolonged hospital stays and a decrease in patient satisfaction (Caumo & Ferreira, 2013).

Methods of relieving anxiety in the surgical patient

It has been suggested that long waiting times with little information, inadequate respect, and insufficient empathy increase patient and family member anxiety, resulting in reduced confidence in the healthcare system (Jangland et al, 2009). Therefore, simple measures of reassurance and updates on changing situations can have a great impact in the patient's overall surgical experience. As a result of heightened senses and reactivity, anxious surgical patients are greater affected and responsive to the surgical environment. Factors such as the sound of alarms on machinery, the sight of unfamiliar medical equipment and the noise of surgical instruments being unpacked can have a significant effect on increasing anxiety (Haugen et al, 2009). With more patients now being anaesthetized within the operating theatre itself, this should always be considered, and reassurance and explanations given.

It is known that long periods of waiting can lead to boredom and increase anxiety, whilst a clean and efficient environment can evoke feelings of professionalism and safety (Mottram, 2011). For patients undergoing conscious surgery, additional fears and discomfort may be introduced when the patients are exposed to further sights, sounds and smells within the operating room. It is suggested that talking to patients immediately before anaesthesia, offering the option of some physical contact throughout surgery, limiting the impact of the environment and enabling someone to accompany the patient during or immediately after may all be beneficial (Mitchell, 2012b). Perioperative nurses and practitioners have expert knowledge of the surgical environment, procedures and experiences patients will encounter, so are in a privileged and vital position to begin to address patient anxiety with non-pharmacological interventions. Each nurse must ensure that they are acting in the patient's best interests and this will include helping patients to manage and cope with stress and anxiety prior to, during and after surgery (Nursing and Midwifery Council, 2018).

Information giving and effective communication

Creating and maintaining effective therapeutic communication with the surgical patient is the first recommended step for reducing perioperative anxiety. Therapeutic communication can be defined as demonstrating care, genuine concern and empathy, and interest in the patient as a unique individual by actively listening (hearing, understanding and believing the patient) (Levett-Jones, 2014). It is vital to remember that each surgical patient will bring with them their own previous experiences and anxieties and will have their own style of coping with stress and anxiety.

Patient education is widely used to reduce perioperative anxiety, with needs-based patient education delivery suggesting the most effective results (Wongkietkachorn et al, 2018; Ndiosi & Adebajo, 2015; Ndiosi et al, 2015). This involves a process of assessing the patient's individualized needs prior to providing education to ensure that the level of information and method of delivery support the patient's coping style. Grieve (2002) proposes a popular model of four major coping styles that individual patients use to manage anxiety: vigilant, avoidant, fluctuating and flexible. Patients with a vigilant coping style require extended information to reduce anxiety, whereas those with an avoidant style prefer a minimal amount of information. Patients with fluctuating coping mechanisms generally desire a small amount of information, but with greater detail in certain areas, and those who are flexible are able to adapt to whatever information is provided to them.

The patient's coping style must be identified to prevent inadvertent heightening of anxiety levels, e.g. giving extended information using a leaflet or video demonstration to an individual with an avoidant coping style. Thus, the nurse or practitioner can use shared decision-making with their patient to identify the extent of information they need to be given for safety purposes, and any further information they wish to receive. Using needs-based education techniques is said to decrease anxiety, increase overall satisfaction and require less time than conventional patient education (Wongkietkachorn et al, 2018). It is consistent with adult learning theory, which stresses the importance of learning being matched to individual backgrounds and needs.

Overall it is thought that providing simple explanations about the surgical environment and safety procedures, and dispelling common misconceptions, can reassure patients and help them feel more in control (Mitchell, 2010). Effective verbal communication, including the tone and rate of speech, can convey understanding, sympathy or empathy, and acknowledgement. However, using technical language may hinder the patient's ability to make informed decisions, and any speech that is rushed or perceived as disinterested by the patient may increase their anxiety (Pritchard, 2011). Actively listening and providing positive non-verbal communication and encouragement to the patient can in turn offer reassurance and build trust within a therapeutic relationship (Kornhaber et al, 2016). It is said that patients undergoing general anaesthesia are likely to want more information than those requiring local or general procedures (Mitchell, 2012a). It is important to note that it cannot be assumed that patients will remember all that they are told, as anxiety can interfere with comprehension and memory.

Nurses and practitioners can also promote other measures to help reduce patients' anxiety, including self-efficacy enhancement, self-control enhancement, and therapeutic use of self (Mitchell, 2012b). To enhance patients' perception of self-control, providing minor choices and involving patients in decision-making processes, where appropriate, are the most effective measures. This can be simply giving them the option of remaining dressed until they need to be escorted to theatre or asking which ear they would like their tympanic temperature measurement taken from. Self-efficacy enhancement centres around increasing the patient's perception of their ability to 'cope' with the surgical experience. Patients who experience a high degree of self-efficacy may recover more quickly from surgery (Brembo et al, 2017). Using positive statements to reassure them that support channels are available and alleviate concerns in key areas of anxiety, such as pain control and postoperative recovery, will ultimately boost their positive outlook of the experience. Therapeutic use of self aims to use supportive interventions including the physical and emotional presence of a healthcare professional or relative in close proximity. It can be considered in terms of social support, optimistic outlook and cognitive coping strategies. Using phrases such as 'you will be monitored continually whilst asleep' and 'the medications used are very safe and effective' can collectively give patients the 'tools' to promote fewer negative thoughts (Chan et al, 2012).

Alternative therapies

There is ongoing research into the following interventions to alleviate anxiety in surgical patients: virtual reality, smartphone apps, preoperative theatre visits, hypnotherapy, hand massage, aromatherapy and acupuncture. All techniques have some supporting evidence for positive results, but further research is needed to form grounded conclusions.

Music therapy

Music therapy is an intervention that has shown effectiveness in reducing stress and anxiety in surgical patients (Wu et al, 2017; Wakim et al, 2010; Arsian et al, 2008). The majority of studies reviewed demonstrated that being able to listen to music had a positive impact on both psychological and physiological patient outcomes. Patients who have access to music therapy may respond with lower blood pressures, lower respiratory rates and lower heart rates (Lee et al, 2014; Hu et al, 2013), as well as a reduction in feelings of fear, anxiety and postoperative pain (Lin et al, 2011). No differences were noted in the results obtained in different clinical settings or healthcare systems, and it is strongly suggested that more favourable results are witnessed when patients have control over the type of music they are exposed to. Allowing the patient to listen to their choice of music or bring in a portable music device from home to use during the pre-, during and postsurgical phases, where appropriate, could foster a feeling of familiarity and empower the patient's self-efficacy. It is thought that the rhythms of music not only distract the patient from their environment and promote positive thoughts, but can also reduce the secretion of neurotransmitters and the activity of the autonomic nervous system. Ultimately music therapy is a simple, safe and cost-effective intervention in assisting patients to perceive a lower level of anxiety.

Cognitive behavioural therapy

Cognitive behavioural therapy (CBT) is a form of psychotherapy that incorporates cognitive and behaviour interventions to reduce symptoms of stress and anxiety. The technique includes psychoeducation, cognitive restructuring, exposure therapy, and/or relaxation training. The interventions aim to change negative and irrational thought patterns associated with anxious feelings. Numerous trials have found CBT to be an effective treatment for specific anxiety disorders, including generalized anxiety disorder, panic disorder, social anxiety disorder, posttraumatic stress disorders, and obsessive–compulsive disorder (Heilmann et al, 2016; Aust et al, 2016; Dao et al, 2011). The authors suggest patients who are treated preoperatively with CBT, and continue techniques throughout their extended surgical journey, will have a significantly reduced perioperative anxiety level.

Relaxation techniques

Relaxation and meditation have been linked to great potential in reduction of anxiety (Appukuttan, 2016). It must be noted that further research is needed to provide recommendations on the most effective technique for perioperative anxiety, and this intervention relies upon patients first being taught and then performing these methods.

There is robust evidence that meditative therapies may be an effective treatment for reducing anxiety symptoms in surgical patients (Chen et al, 2012). Meditation has consistently been shown to reduce cortisol, adrenaline and noradrenaline levels that may trigger biologically based anxiety responses (Brand et al, 2012). It is believed to train the individual to condition and control the mind as a means to reduce anxiety, develop coping mechanisms and facilitate a calm response to stress. This method involves a whole package of biological, behaviour and cognitive changes, used to adjust the breathing, body and mind.

Deep relaxation or diaphragmatic breathing is believed to be a vital technique for helping patients to reduce tension and prevent hyperventilation (Appukuttan, 2016). Diaphragmatic breathing is achieved by contracting the diaphragm muscle in a conscious effort to take smooth, slow and regular breaths. It reduces tension in the chest, provides more oxygen for the body per breath and decreases the overall work of breathing (Ma et al, 2017).

Guided imagery relaxation is a mind–body intervention that uses the patient's own imagination and mental processing to form a mental representation of an object, place, event or situation perceived through the senses (Felix et al, 2018). An example of this could be asking the patient to imagine they are standing in the warm sunshine on a sandy beach, listening to the sound of waves crashing against the shore. This technique focuses on pleasing images to replace negative or stressful feelings, and has been shown to be effective in reducing anxiety levels in patients undergoing laparoscopic bariatric surgery (Felix et al, 2018). Further evidence now needs to be collected with larger, diverse samples to form grounded conclusions on its overall effectiveness.

Pharmacological interventions

The Royal College of Anaesthetists (RCOA, 2012) stance on preoperative sedation for alleviating patient anxiety is that premedication should not be the mainstay of achieving preoperative anxiolysis, or inhibiting anxiety, in adults. However, there is a strong argument for sedative premedication in cases of significant patient anxiety not alleviated by non-pharmacological means. The RCOA propose a standard for best practice of anaesthetists having the opportunity to order sedative premedication in these circumstances for 100% of surgical cases but recognize common barriers to this practice. These include patients being admitted after lists have started, change in list order or time, and same day facilities unable to accommodate patients requiring sedative medication. The choice of sedative drug depends on the individual, the nature of the procedure, the anaesthetic to be used and other factors such as recovery facilities. Premedication in this nature aims to not only inhibit anxiety, but also enhance the action of anaesthetics and provide some degree of preoperative amnesia.

The most common preoperative sedative drugs administered to patients belong to the benzodiazepine group, such as midazolam, lorazepam, temazepam and diazepam (BNF, 2019). These drugs can be administered orally, intranasally or intravenously, most commonly given by the anaesthetist once the patient reaches the operating theatre. Diazepam is used to produce mild sedation with amnesia and is long acting with second periods of drowsiness occurring several hours after its administration. Temazepam is given for a short duration of action and more rapid onset than diazepam, with anxiolytic and sedative effects lasting for approximately ninety minutes. Lorazepam produces more prolonged sedation than temazepam and has marked amnesic effects. Midazolam is often the preferred benzodiazepine of anaesthetists due to its rapid onset of sedative and anxiolytic effects and faster recovery. Caution is taken in the elderly, those with a low cardiac output or after repeated dosage, and profound sedation is associated with midazolam when given intravenously. Common side-effects of these drugs include confusion, dizziness, drowsiness, hypotension, nausea and vomiting, respiratory depression, fatigue, and sleep disorders. Therefore, the risks of administration must be weighed up against the negative impact of the patient's anxiety levels. Patients who regularly take benzodiazepines or are dependent on alcohol or drug misuse commonly require a higher dose than usual to account for any tolerance to the drug. Adverse effects of benzodiazepines can be treated and reversed with flumazenil, but due to its shorter half-life a second dose may need to be administered to prevent re-sedation. Clonidine and dexmedetomidine are alternative drugs used in sedative premedication, with their sedative properties being a secondary effect of administration.

Conclusion

Perioperative stress and anxiety remain a consistent threat to surgical patients, with the ability to negatively impact their physical and psychological health and well-being. Ultimately, more current research is needed in the field to bridge the existing knowledge gap. As discussed in this chapter, there are many interventions that can be adopted by the healthcare practitioner to reduce the anxiety levels of patients. Non-pharmacological techniques, including needs-based patient education and effective therapeutic communication, appear to be the most effective and safest interventions to reduce patients' anxiety levels.

Other alternative techniques, such as music therapy, have been shown to be effective, but are perhaps being underutilized due to the challenge of facilitating patients bringing in their own device or having one readily available for each patient. Further alternative therapies, such as relaxation techniques and CBT, have shown positive results in recent studies, but their use is currently limited due to staffing and resources required to teach patients and reinforce their use.

In cases of high levels of anxiety that cannot be alleviated through these techniques, preoperative sedation, most commonly a benzodiazepine, can be administered to the patient to provide sedative, anxiolytic and amnesic effects. When administering these medications, or caring for patients who have had preoperative sedation, the nurse or practitioner must be aware of potential side-effects and the reversal process.

SUMMARY OF KEY POINTS

- Creating and maintaining effective therapeutic communication with the surgical patient is the first recommended step for reducing perioperative anxiety.
- Patient education is widely used to reduce perioperative anxiety, with needs-based patient education delivery suggesting the most effective results.
- Music therapy is an intervention that has shown effectiveness in reducing stress and anxiety in surgical patients.
- Relaxation and meditation therapies have been linked to great potential in reduction of anxiety.
- There is a strong argument for sedative premedication in cases of significant patient anxiety not alleviated by non-pharmacological means.

REFLECTIVE LEARNING POINTS

Having read this chapter, think about what you now know and what you still need to find out about. These questions may help:

- What is meant by 'talking therapies'?
- What is mindfulness and how might it be practised?
- Describe the differences between complementary therapies and alternative therapies.

References

Ahmetovic-Djug, J., Hasukic, S., Djug, H., Hasukic, B., & Jahic, A. (2017). Impact of preoperative anxiety in patients on hemodynamic changes and a dose of anesthetic during induction of anesthesia. *Journal of the Academy of Medical Sciences in Bosnia and Herzegovina, 71* (5), 330–333.

Alanazi, A. (2014). Reducing anxiety in perioperative patients: a systematic review. *British Journal of Nursing, 23*(7), 387–393.

Appukuttan, D. (2016). Strategies to manage patients with dental anxiety and dental phobia: literature review. *Clinical, Cosmetic and Investigational Dentistry, 8,* 874.

Arsian, S., Ozer, N., & Ozyurt, F. (2008). Effect of music on preoperative anxiety in men undergoing urogenital surgery. *Australian Journal of Advanced Nursing, 26*(2), 46–54.

Aust, H., Rüsch, D., & Schuster, M. (2016). Coping strategies in anxious surgical patients. *BMC Health Services Research, 16,* 1492–1495.

Ay, A., Ulucanlar, H., & Ozden, M. (2014). Risk factors for perioperative anxiety in laparoscopic surgery. *Journal of the Society of Laparoendoscopic Surgeons, 18* (3), 1–13.

Ayral, X., Gicquere, C., Duhalde, A., Boucheny, D., & Dougados, M. (2002). Effects of video information on preoperative anxiety level and tolerability of joint lavage in knee osteoarthritis. *Arthritis & Rheumatology*, 47(4), 380–382.

BNF. (2019). *Pre-medication and peri-operative drugs*. London: National Institute for Health and Care Excellence.

Brand, S., Holsboer-Tracgsker, E., Naranjo, J., & Schmidt, S. (2012). Influence of mindfulness practice on cortisol and sleep in long-term and short-term meditators. *Neuropsychobiology*, 65(3), 109–118.

Brembo, E., Kapstad, H., Dulmen, S., & Eide, H. (2017). Role of self-efficacy and social support in short-term recovery after total hip replacement: a prospective cohort study. *Health Quality Life Outcomes*, 15, 68.

Caumo, W., & Ferreira, M. (2013). Perioperative anxiety: psychobiology and effects in postoperative recovery. *The Pain Clinic*, 15, 87–101.

Chan, C., Hon, H., Chien, W., & Lopez, V. (2004). Social support and coping in Chinese patients undergoing cancer surgery. *Cancer Nursing*, 27, 230–236.

Chan, Z., Kan, C., Lee, P., Chan, I., & Lam, J. (2012). A systematic review of qualitative studies: patients' experiences of preoperative communication. *Journal of Clinical Nursing*, 21(5-6), 812–824.

Chen, K., Berger, C., Macheimer, E., Forde, D., Magidson, J., Dachman, L., et al. (2012). Meditative therapies for reducing anxiety: a systematic review and meta-analysis of randomized controlled trials. *Depression and Anxiety*, 29, 545–562.

Dao, T., Youssef, N., & Armsworth, M. (2011). Randomized controlled trial of brief cognitive behavioural intervention for depression and anxiety symptoms preoperatively in patents undergoing coronary artery bypass graft surgery. *Journal of Thoracic Cardiovascular Surgery*, 142(3), 109–115.

Dedovic, K., Duchesne, A., Andrews, J., Engert, V., & Pruessner, J. (2009). The brain and the stress axis: the neural correlates of cortisol regulation in response to stress. *Neuroimage*, 47(3), 864–871.

Felix, M., Ferreira, M., Oliveria, L., Barichello, E., Pires, P., & Barbosa, M. (2018). Guided imagery relaxation therapy on perioperative anxiety: a

randomized clinical trial. *Revista Latino-Americana De Enfermagem*, 26, 1–10.

Gilmartin, J., & Wright, K. (2008). Day surgery: patients' felt abandoned during the preoperative wait. *Journal of Clinical Nursing*, 17(18), 2418–2425.

Grieve, R. (2002). Day surgery preoperative anxiety reduction and coping strategies. *British Journal of Nursing*, 11(10), 670–678.

Hannibal, K., & Bishop, M. (2014). Chronic stress, cortisol dysfunction, and pain: a psychoneuroendocrine rationale for stress management in pain rehabilitation. *Journal of the American Physical Therapy Association*, 94(12), 1816–1825.

Haugen, A., Eide, G., Olsen, M., Haukeland, B., Remme, A., & Wahl, A. (2009). Anxiety in the operating theatre: a study of frequency and environmental impact in patients having local, plexus or regional anaesthesia. *Journal of Clinical Nursing*, 18(16), 2301–2310.

Heilmann, C., Stotz, U., & Burbaum, C. (2016). Short-term intervention to reduce anxiety before coronary artery bypass surgery- a randomised controlled trial. *Journal of Clinical Nursing*, 25(3-4), 351–361.

Hu, C., Lin, Y., Lin, M., & Han, R. (2013). Effectiveness of music therapy on anxiety and physiological responses for patients with myocardial infarction. *Chang Gung Nursing*, 24(4), 357–365.

Jangland, E., Guinningberg, L., & Carsson, M. (2009). Patients' and relatives' complaints about encounters and communication in health care: evidence for quality improvement. *Patient Education and Counseling*, 75(2), 199–204.

Jawaid, M., Mushtaq, A., Mukhtar, S., & Khan, Z. (2007). Perioperative anxiety before elective surgery. *Neurosciences*, 12, 145–148.

Jlala, H., French, J., Foxall, G., Hardman, J., & Bedforth, N. (2010). Effect of preoperative multimedia information on perioperative anxiety in patients undergoing procedures under regional anaesthesia. *British Journal of Anaesthesia*, 104(3), 369–374.

Karanci, A., & Dirik, G. (2003). Predictors of pre and postoperative anxiety in emergency surgery patients. *Journal of Psychosomatic Research*, 55, 363–369.

Keegan, L. (2003). Alternative and Complementary Modalities for Managing Stress and Anxiety. *Critical Care Nurse*, 23(3), 55–58.

Kindler, C., Harms, C., Amsler, F., Ihde-Scholl, T., & Scheidegger, D. (2000). The visual analogue scale allows

effective measurement of preoperative anxiety and detection of patients' anesthetic concerns. *Anesthesia & Analgesia*, 90, 706–712.

Kocaturk, O., & Oguz, E. (2017). The effect of preoperative anxiety on the incidence of perioperative bronchospasm: a prospective observational study. *Medicine Science International Medical Journal*, 6(4), 746–749.

Kornhaber, R., Walsh, K., Duff, J., & Walker, K. (2016). Enhancing adult therapeutic interpersonal relationships in the acute health care setting: an integrative review. *Journal of Multidisciplinary Healthcare*, 9, 537–546.

Kumar, S., & Bhukar, J. (2013). Stress level and coping strategies of college students. *Journal of Physical Education and Sports Management*, 4(1), 5–11.

Lee, C., Yen, W., Lin, S., Hsu, T., & Lai, C. (2014). Effects of music intervention on preoperative anxiety in patients undergoing spinal surgery. *VGH Nursing*, 31(4), 343–350.

Levett-Jones, T. (2014). *Critical conversations for patient safety: An essential guide for health professionals*. Pearson Australia: Frenchs Forest NSW.

Lin, P., Lin, M., Huang, L., Hsu, H., & Lin, C. (2011). Music listening for patients receiving spine surgery. *Journal of Clinical Nursing*, 20(7–8), 960–968.

Lincoln, K., Chatters, L., & Taylor, R. (2005). Social support, traumatic events, and depressive symptoms among African Americans. *Journal of Marriage and Family*, 67, 754–766.

Ma, A., Yue, Z., Gong, Z., Zhang, H., Duan, N., Shi, N., et al. (2017). The effect of diaphragmatic breathing on attention, negative affect and stress in healthy adults. *Frontiers in Psychology*, 8, 874.

McWhinnie, D. (2018). *Evolution of day surgery in the UK: Lessons learnt along the way?* London: British Association of Day Surgery.

Mitchell, M. (2008). Conscious surgery: influence of the environment on patient anxiety. *Journal of Advanced Nursing*, 64(3), 261–271.

Mitchell, M. (2010). General anaesthesia and day-case patient anxiety. *Journal of Advanced Nursing*, 66(5), 1059–1071.

Mitchell, M. (2012a). Influence of gender and anaesthesia type on day surgery anxiety. *Journal of Advanced Nursing*, 68(5), 1014–1025.

Mitchell, M. (2012b). Anxiety management in minimal stay surgery. *Nursing Times*, 108(48), 14–16.

Mora, F., Segovia, G., Del Arco, A., de Blas, M., & Garrido, P. (2012). Stress, neurotransmitters, corticosterone and body-brain integration. *Brain Research, 1476*, 71–85.

Mottram, A. (2011). Patients' experiences of day surgery: a Parsonian analysis. *Journal of Advanced Nursing, 67*(1), 140–148.

Muglatti, M., & Komarik, N. (2008). Factors related to patients' anxiety before and after oral surgery. *Journal of Oral and Maxillofacial Surgery, 66*(5), 870–877.

Ndiosi, M., & Adebajo, A. (2015). Patient education in rheumatoid arthritis: is the needs-based approach the way forward? *Clinical Rheumatology, 34*(11), 1827–1829.

Ndiosi, M., Johnson, D., Young, T., Hardware, B., Hill, J., & Hale, C. (2015). Effects of needs-based patient education on self-efficacy and health outcomes in people with rheumatoid arthritis: a multicentre, single blind, randomised controlled trial. *Annals of the Rheumatic Diseases, 75*(6), 1126–1132.

Nursing and Midwifery Council. (2018). *The code. professional standards of practice and behaviour for nurses, midwives and nursing associates.* Available from: <https://www.nmc.org.uk/standards/code/>

Perks, A., Chakravarti, S., & Manninen, P. (2009). Preoperative anxiety in neurosurgical patients. *Journal of Neurosurgical Anesthesiology, 21*, 127–130.

Pierre, S., & Whelan, R. (2012). Nausea and vomiting after surgery. *British Journal of Anaesthesia, 13*(1), 28–32.

Pritchard, M. (2009). Identifying and assessing anxiety in pre-operative patients. *Nursing Standard, 23*(51), 35–40.

Pritchard, M. (2011). Reducing anxiety in elective surgical patients. *Nursing Times, 107*(3), 22–23.

Ramos, M., Cardoso, M., Vaz, F., Torres, M., García, F., Blanco, G., et al. (2008). Influence of the grade of anxiety and level of cortisol on post-surgical recovery. *Actas Españolas de Psiquiatria, 36*, 133–137.

Robinson, O., Vytal, K., Cornwell, B., & Grillon, C. (2013). The impact of anxiety upon cognition: perspectives from human threat of shock studies. *Frontiers in Human Neuroscience, 7*, 203.

Royal College of Anaesthetists (RCOA). (2012). *Raising the standard: a compendium of audit recipes* (3rd edn). London: RCOA.

Royal College of Anaesthetists and Association of Anaesthetists of Great Britain and Ireland. (2014). 5th national audit project: Accidental awareness during general anaesthesia in the United Kingdom and Ireland. London: RCOA and AAGBI.

Velzen, J., Atkinson, S., Rowley, E., & Martin, J. (2015). The tradition of anaesthetic rooms: Best practice or patient risk? *6th International conference on applied human factors and ergonomics and the affiliated conferences, AHFE 2015, 3*, 59–66.

Vileikyte, L. (2007). Stress and wound healing. *Clinics in Dermatology, 25*, 49–55.

Wakim, J., Smith, S., & Guinn, C. (2010). The efficacy of music therapy. *Journal of PeriAnesthesia Nursing, 25*(4), 226–232.

Wang, Y., Shen, J., Lu, J., & Yang, X. (2008). Preoperative anxiety and depression in patients undergoing cardiac surgery and related influencing factors. *Zhonghua Yi Xue Za Zhi, 88*, 2759–2762.

Wong, E., Chan, S., & Chair, S. (2010). Effectiveness of an educational intervention on levels of pain, anxiety and self-efficacy for patients with musculoskeletal trauma. *Journal of Advanced Nursing, 66*(5), 1120–1131.

Wongkietkachorn, A., Wongkietkachorn, N., & Rhunsiri, P. (2018). Preoperative needs-based education to reduce anxiety, increase satisfaction, and decrease time spent in day surgery: a randomized controlled trial. *World Journal of Surgery, 42*(3), 666–674.

Wu, P., Huang, M., Lee, W., Wang, C., & Shih, W. (2017). Effects of music listening on anxiety and physiological responses in patients undergoing awake craniotomy. *Complementary Therapies in Medicine, 32*, 56–60.

Yilmaz, M., Sezer, H., Gürler, H., & Bekar, M. (2012). Predictors of preoperative anxiety in surgical inpatients. *Journal of Clinical Nursing, 21*, 956–964.

Chapter | 5 |

Wound healing in the surgical patient

Nigel Conway

KEY OBJECTIVES OF THE CHAPTER

At the end of this chapter the reader should be able to:

- describe the structure and function of the skin
- discuss the different mechanisms of wound closure
- discuss the normal physiology of wound healing and factors which may affect this
- list the various methods used in wound healing
- discuss the use and care of surgical wound drains
- discuss the principles of caring for the surgical patient's wound
- discuss the potential postoperative complications of wound healing.

Areas to think about before reading the chapter

- What are the characteristics of acute and chronic wounds?
- Describe the stages of wound healing and the role of the nurse in optimizing wound healing.
- What is the tumour necrosis factor?

Introduction

Wounds can be divided into two main types:
- Acute wounds, which include surgical and trauma wounds.
- Chronic wounds, which include venous and arterial ulcers, diabetic ulcers and pressure ulcers.

This chapter explores acute wound healing.

The integumentary system is an organ system made up of the skin, hair, nails, and exocrine glands. Surgical wounds are formed from an incision in the skin and underlying structures, as informed by the patient's surgical treatment intervention. The surgical intervention is usually performed in a clean, specially designed operating theatre environment where asepsis and infection prevention is a key focus.

Examples of common general surgical sites for incisions and wounds can be seen in Fig. 5.1.

The majority of surgical wounds heal by primary (first) intention, with minimal intervention from healthcare professionals. The type of surgical incision, surgical approach,

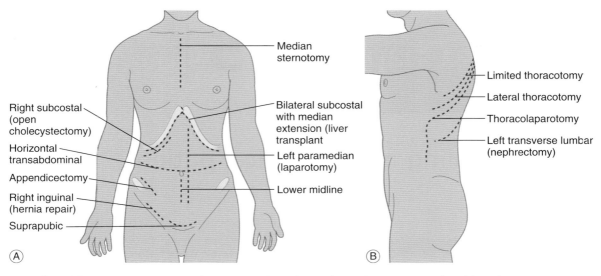

Figure 5.1 Adult torso — common surgical incision sites. (From https://thoracickey.com/surgery-for-adults-2/.)

manner and type of material used in wound closure, and length of time spent in an acute hospital setting have changed over the years, which has, in turn, influenced contemporary approaches to wound management.

The main principles of surgical wound management are to:

- Achieve healing of the wound
- Avoid complications (e.g. infection)
- Achieve optimal patient comfort and pain control
- Consider patient body image and ensure cosmetically acceptable scar
- Facilitate the individual to return to normal or as close to normal lifestyle as soon as possible.

Perioperative and postoperative complications of the surgical wound can be minimized by preoperative assessment, planning, implementation of care, patient education and evaluation of recovery/healing of the wound. A sound knowledge and understanding of anatomical structures and functions of the skin, underlying structures and physiology of wound healing and factors which can interfere with this process are essential to optimize the standard of wound care.

This knowledge and understanding is fundamental to the assessment of an individual patient with a surgical wound and future management, with regard to cleansing and application of appropriate wound dressing.

Nearly every nurse at some point in their professional career will care for people with wounds; there are some nurses who will care for these patients on a daily basis. All nurses should know how to recognize, assess and effectively treat routine wounds, adhering to local policies and protocols. The nurse is required to provide care that is

evidence-based, ensuring the safety of the patient is paramount. The Nursing and Midwifery Council (2018) requires the nurse to assess needs and deliver or advise on treatment, or offer help (including preventative or rehabilitative care) without too much delay, to the best of their abilities, on the basis of best available evidence. These principles are applicable when promoting wound care.

Structure and function of the skin

The skin is the largest organ in the integumentary system in relation to surface area. It covers the body and gives protection to the underlying structures. It varies in thickness in different parts of the body and has variations in pigmentation (Tortora & Derrickson, 2017).

The skin performs five main functions:

1. Protection: acts as a physical barrier, protecting underlying structures from minor mechanical trauma, chemicals and gases, bacterial invasion, dehydration, cold, heat and ultraviolet (UV) radiation.
2. Sensation: acts as a sensory organ of the body as it contains numerous nerve endings which are sensitive to temperature, chemical changes, pain, touch, pressure and vibration. Facilitates the process of sensory perception of the external environment.
3. Temperature regulation: plays a vital role in maintaining a constant core temperature. Homeostasis is facilitated by conduction, convection or radiation of heat from the surface of the skin. Secretion and evaporation of sweat assist in cooling of the body. The

circulatory mechanism of vasodilation and vasoconstriction helps to control body temperature.

4. Excretion: water, salts and other organic materials are excreted through the skin.

5. Synthesis of vitamin D: the effect of ultraviolet rays on the skin stimulate the synthesis with skin cells of vitamin D from 7-dehydrocholesterol, which indirectly promotes the absorption of calcium from the intestine/gut.

The skin also has an absorptive capability. This physiological factor can be used clinically to administer therapeutic treatments/drugs such as:

- Oestrogen
- Glyceryl trinitrate (GTN)

These hormones/drugs can be applied as a slow-release skin patch, allowing the substance to be slowly absorbed through the skin (Montague & Watson, 2005).

Note: This absorptive physiology can also have negative outcomes if individuals accidently spill chemicals onto the skin, which may then be absorbed into the circulatory system (e.g. petrochemicals, volatile anaesthetic agents) and go on to have unwanted physiological effects on the body.

The skin is a complex and multilateral structure, comprising the epidermis, dermis and subcutaneous tissue shown in Fig. 5.2. These layers and structures within each layer will now be discussed.

The epidermis

The epidermis is the most superficial layer and is connected to the dermis. It is avascular, receiving nutrients from the dermis layer below. The epidermis is composed of keratinized stratified squamous epithelial cells.

Four types of cells are found in this layer:
- Keratinocytes
- Melanocytes
- Langerhans cells
- Merkel cells

The epithelial cells are produced in the basal layer and gradually migrate upwards over a period of 40–56 days.

The epidermis has variable thickness (four of five layers of cells) depending on the location of the body. The first layer, next to the dermis, is the stratum basale. Cell division occurs here, with the cells dipping down into the dermis to the surrounding sweat gland and hair follicles. Keratin is manufactured by the keratinocytes found in this layer. Keratin is an insoluble protein that is resistant to changes in temperature and pH, and helps waterproof and protect the skin. Merkel cells are also found in the

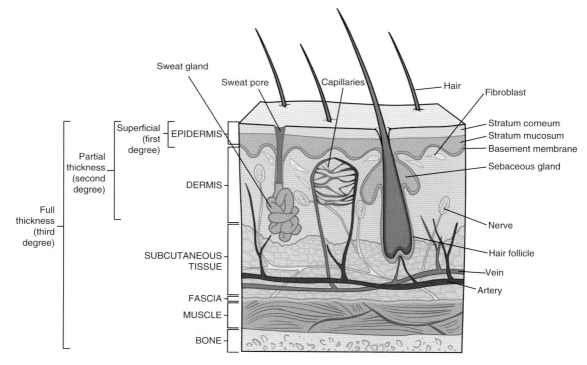

Figure 5.2 Anatomical structures of the skin. (From Klas K.S.A., (2013), Chapter 20, Burns. In Sole, M.L., Klen, D.G., & Mosely. M.J; Introduction to critical care nursing (6th edn.). Elsevier Inc.)

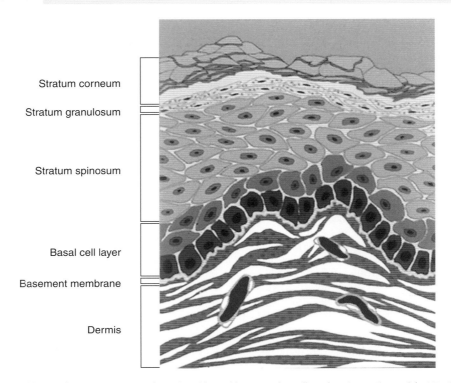

Stratum corneum

Stratum granulosum

Stratum spinosum

Basal cell layer

Basement membrane

Dermis

Figure 5.3 Epidermal layers. (From Bennon, S.D (2011). Epidermal layers and papillary dermis, In; Fitzpatrick, J.E., & Morelli, J.G., Dermatological Secrets Plus (4th edn.). Elsevier Inc.)

epidermis (Figs. 5.2 and 5.3). Merkel cells are in contact with the flattened end of sensory neurons and are involved in the sensation of touch. The second layer is the stratum spinosum which contains prickle cells or spinous cells and Langerhans cells (Fig. 5.4) (Tortora & Derrickson, 2017).

The prickle cells or spinous cells are keratin-producing epidermal cells; their name derives from their prickly appearance. These 'prickles' form numerous intracellular connections or bridges that prevent separation. They make up the stratum spinosum (prickly layer) of the epidermis and provide a continuous net-like layer of protection for underlying tissue. Langerhans cells participate in immune responses and are thought to have a role in allergic or immunological skin disorders (Beldon, 2010).

The third layer is the stratum granulosum (see Fig. 5.3), where the keratinocytes flatten and accumulate lamellar granules. Secretion from the lamellar granules slow the loss of body fluids and entry of foreign materials (Tortora & Derrickson, 2017).

The fourth layer is the stratum lucidum, this is found in the thick skin of the palm of the hands and soles of the feet (i.e. areas of excessive wear and tear). The cells in this layer start to undergo nuclear degeneration and contain large amounts of keratin.

The fifth and final layer is the stratum corneum, consisting of many layers of dead cells that are completely filled with keratin. These cells are constantly shed from the body surface (desquamation) as a result of friction and washing. They also have the ability to soak up extra moisture (Montague & Watson, 2005).

The dermis

The dermis lies beneath the epidermis (see Fig. 5.2) and forms the main part of the skin, providing strength and elasticity. It is formed of connective tissue containing collagen and elastic fibres, blood and lymph vessels, sensory nerve endings, hair follicles, sweat and sebaceous glands. In the dermal–epidermal junction, melanin is produced by melanocytes, under the influence of sunlight. Melanin gives colour to various body structures (e.g. hair, iris and skin). The main function of melanin is to protect the body from ultraviolet light (Tortora & Derrickson, 2017).

The upper region of the dermis is the papillary region, which consists of a series of undulations called dermal papillae (see Fig. 5.2). This structural undulation prevents the epidermis shearing off the dermis when shearing forces are applied to the skin. The reticular layer is the remaining portion of the dermis; it consists of dense,

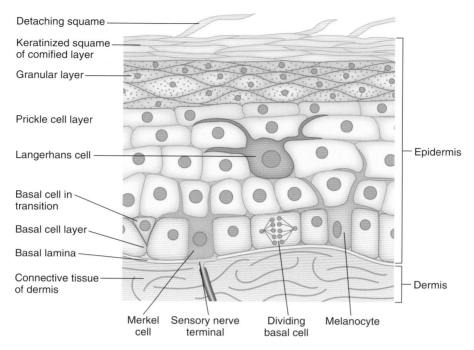

Detaching squame

Keratinized squame
of comified layer

Granular layer

Prickle cell layer

Langerhans cell

Basal cell in
transition

Basal cell layer

Basal lamina

Connective tissue
of dermis

Epidermis

Dermis

Merkel
cell

Sensory nerve
terminal

Dividing
basal cell

Melanocyte

Figure 5.4 Specialist cells within the epidermal layer.

irregularly arranged connective tissue containing interlacing bundles of collagenous reticular and course elastic fibres. It is within the spaces between these fibres that hair follicles, sensory nerves and sweat glands are located (Montague & Watson, 2005).

The dermis is constructed of ground substance or matrix, connective fibres and cells. Ground substance is an amorphous matrix, resembling a gel. This gel provides connective tissue with its bulk. Strands of collagen, elastin, fibronectin and other cells permeate through it. The gelatinous material is composed of water, electrolytes, glycoproteins and proteoglycans, and is synthesized by fibroblasts (Waugh & Grant, 2018).

Collagen, reticular fibres and elastin fibres are produced by mesodermal fibres, located in the dermis. Collagen is a category of connective tissue protein that has immense tensile strength. These fibres come together to form thick bundles in which numerous cross links form, increasing their overall combined strength. Collagens are important as structural support, but also control other cellular functions, including cell shape and differentiation. Ascorbic acid is necessary for the formation of collagen.

There are different types of collagen with types I and III found to be important in wound healing (Penelope et al, 2018; Rangara et al, 2011). Type I is usually physically allied with type III collagen. Type III collagen is dominant in the early stages of wound healing. Type I synthesis is more predominate in the later stages of healing. The reticular fibres form a framework in the dermis and envelop the collagen bundles. The yellow branching elastin fibres provide elasticity and resilience to the skin (Tortora & Derrickson, 2017).

Other cells found in the dermis include:

- Fibroblasts: found between collagen bundles linked with collagen and elastin syntheses.
- Tissue macrophages (histiocytes): wandering phagocytic cells.
- Tissue mast cells: produce histamine and heparin, found near blood vessels and hair follicles.
- White blood cells: neutrophils, lymphocytes and monocytes are transient cells constantly moving between blood vessels (Peate & Muralitharan, 2016).

The cutaneous blood vessels lie within the dermis and have a rich sympathetic nerve supply. This sympathetic nerve supply allows for vasoconstriction of vasodilation, depending on the environment and other factors (e.g. use of pharmaceutical agents). The lymphatic vessels are found within the dermis and are responsible for draining excess tissue fluid and plasma proteins that may have leaked from the tissues.

The dermis contains sensory nerves which have three types of nerve ending, each responding to specific

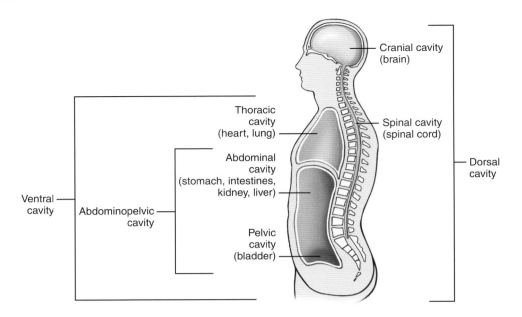

Figure 5.5 Dorsal and ventral body cavities, their subdivisions and anatomical contents. (From Brookes, D.L., & Brookes M.L., (2016). Basic medical Language (5th edn.). Elsevier Inc.)

stimulus. The hair follicles lie in the dermis, each surrounded by its own blood and nerve supply.

The basal layer of the epidermis dips down to surround the hair follicle, so the process of epithelialization can occur from this area. The sweat glands (eccrine and apocrine) are found as coiled tubular downgrowths from the epidermis. The sebaceous glands are formed as outgrowths of the developing hair follicles, producing sebum which waterproofs the skin and has some action against fungal and bacterial infection (Waugh & Grant, 2018; Peate & Muralitharan, 2016; Tortora et al, 2014).

The subcutaneous layer (fat)

Adipose tissue lies beneath the dermis and is a source of triglycerides, which provide a potential source of energy. The adipose tissue insulates the body preventing heat loss and acts as a shock absorber, helping to prevent trauma to the underlying structures.

This layer has very little ground substance and the tissue is divided into lobes by the septa which carry blood vessels and nerves. The cells which make up adipose tissue consist of a fat nucleus surrounded by large single fat globule (Waugh & Grant, 2018).

Beneath the adipose layer will be muscle structures and beneath the muscle layers organ structures, depending on the anatomic region. Figure 5.5 shows dorsal and ventral body cavity regions with an overview of the main body organs located within them.

The cavities can be further divided into regions for descriptive, diagnostic or surgical purposes in relation to anatomical features and organ location. This anatomical knowledge can help in the planning, assessment and care of wounds (Fig. 5.6).

Mechanisms of wound closure

There are three mechanisms of wound closure: primary intention, secondary intention and tertiary intention (delayed primary closure).

- **Primary intention**: the skin edges are pulled together and held in apposition by a mechanical means (e.g. surgical sutures, staples, adhesive strips of tissue adhesive). This closure method is adapted in most surgical incision wounds (see Fig. 5.1).
- **Secondary intention**: the wound is left open to allow granulation, contraction and epithelialization to occur. The method is adopted if there is extensive tissue loss, large superficial area, or presence of infection.
- **Tertiary intention** (delayed primary closure): the wound is initially left open to allow granulation to begin; after approximately 3−5 days, wound closure is

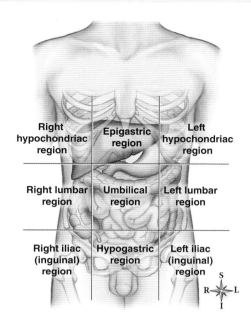

Figure 5.6 Common abdominal surgical regions in adults. (From Patton, K.T., (2014). Survival Guide for Anatomy & Physiology (2nd edn.) Elsevier Inc.)

achieved by either approximation of the skin edges or by the application of a skin graft. This method is adopted in wounds where there is high risk of contamination and possible infection, poor blood supply or excessive swelling in the area (e.g. orthopaedic trauma). The wound is managed in this way to reduce the risk of infection, help improve blood supply and reduced swelling before final skin closure is attempted (Wicker & Dalby, 2017).

Process of wound healing

This is a complex systematic process comprising interaction of cellular, chemical and physical events. The process can be divided into several phases of wound healing. Wound healing is a continuous process; there is, therefore, an overlap between phases.

The phases of wound healing are haemostasis (bleeding), early inflammatory phase, late inflammatory (destructive) phase (Fig. 5.7, stages 1 and 2), proliferative phase (including epithelialization and contraction) and maturation or remodelling phase (Fig. 5.7, stages 3 and 4). These phases are controlled by a variety of mediators such as growth factors. Growth factors are proteins which are secreted from a variety of cells acting as soluble mediators in cutaneous repair. Their effect is exerted locally via specific receptor sites or surface membranes of the target cells with the wound. They stimulate a physiological signalling network which helps regulate, coordinate and control cellular interactions during wound healing (Wicker & Dalby, 2017; Peate & Glencross, 2015).

Haemostasis and the early inflammatory phase

This phase occurs from the time of injury to approximately three days. The body's immediate response to a wound is to try to stop any bleeding and prevent the entry of microorganisms. Vasoconstriction occurs in the immediate area as a result of the release of serotonin and other chemical mediators from the platelets and damaged cells. Vasoconstriction helps to reduce the flow of blood in the wound.

Damage to the blood vessels in the wound causes the platelets to become sticky and clump together to form a platelet thrombus, further reducing the blood loss. The clotting cascade is also initiated by injury to the vascular endothelium resulting in the formation of a fibrin thrombus in the wound (Hussey & Bagg, 2011).

Inflammation also occurs as a natural response to trauma. Other biochemical mediators including prostaglandins are released into the wound causing vasodilation, increased capillary permeability and the stimulation of pain fibres. The effect of increased permeability is that mediators, plasm proteins, antibodies, neutrophils and monocytes migrate into the wound and surrounding tissue.

The neutrophils and macrophages phagocytose any microorganisms of dead tissue present in the wound space. The wound and surrounding area will appear red, swollen hot and painful with possible loss of function (Beitz, 2016; Wicker & Dalby, 2017).

Late inflammatory (destructive) phase

This phase occurs approximately 2–5 days after the injury. The polymorphonuclear leucocytes (polymorphs) and macrophages continue the process of phagocytosis, cleaning the wound of debris or microorganisms. The tissue macrophages also control wound healing through the production of growth factors such as platelet-derived growth factor (PDGF), transforming growth factor (TFGF), interleukin (IL) and tumour necrosis factor (TNF) (Department of Health, 2011; Nicks et al, 2010).

These growth factors stimulate the growth of blood vessels (angiogenesis). This process demands substantial resources and energy. Considerable heat and fluids can be lost, especially in open wounds.

WOUND HEALING

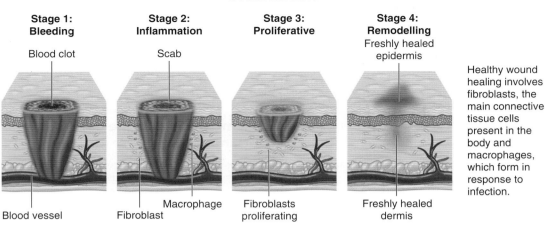

| Stage 1: Bleeding | Stage 2: Inflammation | Stage 3: Proliferative | Stage 4: Remodelling |

Freshly healed epidermis

Blood clot · Scab

Healthy wound healing involves fibroblasts, the main connective tissue cells present in the body and macrophages, which form in response to infection.

Blood vessel · Fibroblast · Macrophage · Fibroblasts proliferating · Freshly healed dermis

Figure 5.7 Stages of healing. (Adapted from Jain, S., & Tanwar, R (2018). Surgery for Medical Graduates. Elsevier India.)

Proliferative phase (including epithelialization and contraction)

This phase occurs from approximately 4–28 days but may be longer in some wounds. The macrophages continue phagocytosis of cell debris and microorganisms. Through monocyte-derived growth factor (MDGF) the macrophages attract fibroblasts to the damaged area. The fibroblast in the presence of vitamin C, ferrous iron, nutrients, oxygen and slightly acidic environment produce collagen fibrils, which are laid down in a haphazard fashion.

Vitamin C is vital in this phase of healing as it is involved in the hydroxylation of proline in collagen to hydroxyproline, which aids cross-linkage of the collagen fibres. Endothelial cells respond to the secretion of various growth factors and form new capillaries, which grow into the wound. This process is known as angiogenesis and is stimulated by the hypoxic environment. The matrix of the collagen fibres forms scaffolding for the new capillaries while the new capillaries provide nutrients and oxygen for the continued growth (Flannigan, 2013; Moores, 2013).

This process is often called granulation because in a wound healing by secondary intention the wound bed appears red and granular. As the wound defect is filled with the newly formed tissue the numbers of macrophages and fibroblasts reduce.

Contraction of the wound can also occur in wounds healing by secondary intention during this phase. This process of contraction is thought to be linked to the myofibroblasts in the wound. Myofibroblasts are cells containing the features of a fibroblast and a smooth muscle cell which appears to have contractile qualities so reducing the surface area of a wound (Flannigan, 2013).

Epithelialization is the last stage of this phase. Epithelial cells at the wound edges divide and migrate across the surface area of the wound until they meet other epithelial cells. When this occurs migration ceases, a process known as contact inhibition. If the remnants of hair follicles are still present in the wound bed, epithelial cells will migrate from the surface area and traverse the wound bed until they meet other epithelial cells. The rate of epithelialization is enhanced by maintaining a moist environment, as it allows epithelial cells to migrate across the surface of the wound more easily (Tortora & Derrickson, 2017; Hess, 2010). Figure 5.8 shows this process.

In surgical wounds it is important that the incisional wound is not allowed to become too wet as maceration can occur, so affecting the cosmetic results of the scar.

Maturation phase

This is the final phase of wound healing, occurring from 15 to 365 days approximately. The original type III collagen laid down in the wound bed is converted to type I collagen, which is laid down following the tension lines within the wound, it is cross-linked giving strength to the scar tissue. As this remodelling process continues, cellular activity reduces with a corresponding reduction and closure of the nutrient blood vessels within the wound. The scar may appear paler and flatter in appearance to the surrounding tissue. For some individuals this process may lead to hypertrophic scars (thickened appearance of scar), whereas keloid scarring is due to a local disturbance during the healing process where the scar tissue extends outside of the wound margins (Beitz, 2016).

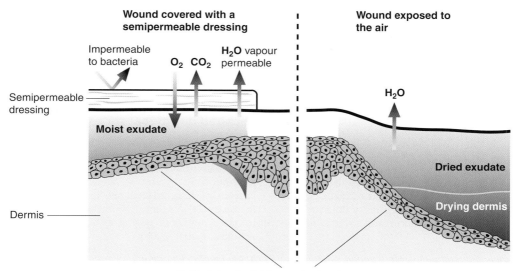

Figure 5.8 Epithelialization in wound healing in a moist and a dry environment.

Box 5.1 **Factors affecting wound healing**

Intrinsic

- Advancing age
- Dehydration
- Disease process
- Impaired blood supply
- Poor nutrition
- Reduced supply of oxygen

Extrinsic

- Drug therapy
- Infection
- Inappropriate wound management
- Obesity
- Poor surgical technique
- Smoking
- Stress
- Wound temperature

Social

- Poverty
- Poor housing
- Cultural/religious beliefs
- Patient's lifestyle

Psychological

- Motivation of patient
- Concordance with treatment
- Knowledge and understanding of patient/carer
- Altered body image

Factors affecting the healing process

A number of factors can affect the healing process, slow the rate of healing or impair healing altogether. These factors can be divided into intrinsic factors, extrinsic factors and social and psychological factors (Box 5.1).

Intrinsic factors

Advanced age

The inflammatory response is reduced, increasing the risk of invasion by microorganisms and infection. The ageing process reduces fibroblastic activity and migration. Collagen metabolism is reduced, resulting in weaker and thinner collagen less able to support the blood vessels in the dermis, allowing for these blood vessels to be more easily damaged. Angiogenesis and epithelialization are slower (Tortora & Derrickson, 2017; Mufti, 2016). Advancing age is also often associated with multiple medical problems which may affect wound healing and respiratory problems (affecting external and internal respiratory oxygenation).

Fluid intake/dehydration

This affects metabolism. The subsequent electrolyte imbalance can impair cellular function and repair. Guidelines on fluid intake suggest that 2−2.5 litres of fluid per day is required for efficient metabolism and cellular function (Dorner et al, 2016).

Disease process

Cancer, diabetes, inflammatory diseases, jaundice and diseases affecting the immune response can all affect wound healing (Mufti, 2016). Patients suffering from cancer may be on chemotherapy in order to destroy malignant cells or radiotherapy. Chemotherapy may be non-discriminatory and thus also destroy other non-malignant cells (e.g. newly forming epithelial cells within a wound). Radiotherapy has a fibrosing effect on local blood vessels, potentially impairing the blood vessel supply to wound areas. At the end stage of cancer a patient may suffer from cachexia, a chronic state of malnutrition resulting from the absorption of toxins.

Diabetes can delay healing due to the altered metabolism associated with it (Beitz, 2016). Hyperglycaemia has a detrimental effect on phagocytosis, therefore increasing the risk of infection. Diabetes is also linked to a decrease in collagen synthesis causing reduced tensile strength and retarded capillary growth.

Jaundice appears to affect the tensile strength of the wound and has been associated with abdominal wound dehiscence. Wound dehiscence is a surgical complication in which the surgical wound ruptures along the incision line (Brindle & Creehan, 2016).

Uraemia causes a delay in the proliferation stage in healing, i.e. delay in granulation of tissue (Maroz & Simman, 2014).

Impaired oxygen delivery to the wound

This can be caused by prolonged hypoxia due to shock, anaemia, impaired arterial blood supply or in patients with chronic obstructive airway disease. Inflammation is delayed as neutrophils are not able to reach the wound; collagen synthesis and epithelial growth are impaired.

Lack of oxygen will lead to ischaemia and the compromise of nearly formed tissue. Excessive caffeine intake, through drinking large quantities of coffee, caffeine or cola drinks, can lead to vasoconstriction, which then leads to impaired tissue perfusion (Waugh & Grant, 2018; Dorner et al, 2016).

Impaired nutritional status

Sufficient supplies of protein, calories, vitamin C and K, zinc and copper are necessary for wound healing. Inadequate supply of these due to poor intake, abnormal absorption or greatly increased demands can impair wound healing, reduce tensile strength of the scar, increase risk if wound dehiscence, and increase risk of infection and poor quality of scar (Dorner et al, 2016; Arnold & Barbal, 2006).

Extrinsic factors
Drug therapy

Steroids and non-steroidal anti-inflammatory drugs (NSAIDs) reduce the normal inflammatory response. Corticosteroids also suppress the syntheses of fibroblasts and collagen, with long-term usage leading to 'tissue paper' skin, which is easily damaged. Cytotoxic drugs delay the inflammatory response, suppress protein synthesis and inhibit the replication of cells. Immunosuppressive drugs reduce white blood cell activity, delaying the inflammatory response and increasing the risk of infection. Anticoagulant therapy, if not given in the correct dosage, can cause excessive bleeding and the potential formation of a haematoma within a wound. Wound haematoma is a common wound complication. Haematomas produce elevation and discoloration of the wound edges, discomfort, and swelling. Blood sometimes leaks through skin sutures (Bates-Jensen, 2016).

Infection

Healing is delayed as invading bacteria compete with macrophages and fibroblast for oxygen and nutrients. The inflammatory phase is prolonged, collagen synthesis is delayed and epithelialization may be prevented. Infection can lead to further local tissue destruction resulting from the inflammatory cytokines being produced, which can then lead to the formation of an abscess and breakdown of the wounds (Tortora & Derrickson, 2017; van Driessche, 2016).

Inappropriate wound management

The inaccurate assessment of the patient and their wound, or failure to evaluate care, can lead to inappropriate management of the patient's wound. Inappropriate application of a wound dressing can cause maceration of the surrounding skin, or from adherence of a dressing to the wound bed. Maceration is the softening and breakdown of skin resulting from prolonged exposure to moisture, delaying the healing process and increasing discomfort or pain (Bates-Jensen, 2016).

Obesity

Obesity can lead to an increased risk of infection in clean wounds, especially in abdominal surgical wounds. Obesity decreases perfusion to the wound tissue, which can result in wound infection, and dehiscence can occur. Contraction is reduced and the risk of dehiscence increased because of the amount of tension on the wound in an obese patient (Morello, 2016).

Smoking

Smoking has a vasoconstriction effect, inhibits epithelialization, can affect the immune response and can cause problems with scarring (Broughton et al, 2006). The width of a scar in smokers can be larger than in non-smokers, and the colour lighter in smokers compared to non-smokers. Smoking can also lead to a deficiency in vitamin C, an essential factor for tissue repair (Beitz, 2016; Wound Healing, 2017),

Poor surgical technique

If any type of tissue is handled roughly during surgery, it can become 'devitalized' (i.e. deprived of strength and vigour) and so provide a suitable site for infection. If haemostasis is not achieved or a drain is not inserted in a dead space, then a haematoma can form. This can also cause tissue damage through the pressure exerted at the wound edges and is also an ideal environment in which microorganisms can grow. The inappropriate use of diathermy can also cause problems with healing, and if sutures or staples are applied too tightly, this increases the risk of tissue trauma and tissue death, as well as poor cosmetic results (Charoenkwan et al, 2017; Brindle & Creehan, 2016; Kirk, 2010).

Stress

Psychological problems can affect a patient's health and wound healing through its effects on the endocrine, nervous and immune systems. The stress of surgery can also stimulate the sympathetic nervous system, continuing over into the postoperative period. Stress caused by hypoxia, hypothermia, pain and hypovolaemia stimulates the sympathetic nervous system whereby excess levels of noradrenaline (norepinephrine) cause vasoconstriction and altered peripheral perfusion, decreasing the oxygen

available for healing in these anatomical regions. The release of glucocorticoids may also impair the inflammatory response (Tortora & Derrickson, 2017; Bootun, 2013; Broadbent & Koschwanez, 2012).

Temperature

Frequency of dressing changes and use and temperature of wound cleansing solutions should be determined by the stage of healing (Jaszarowski & Murphee, 2016). Changes in room temperature ($21-22°C$) may also reduce intra-wound temperature. Cell division takes place at normal body temperature; a drop of $1°C$ may affect normal mitotic cell division and delay wound healing (Peate & Glencross, 2015).

Social and psychological factors
Social factors

Poverty can lead to poor nutritional intake. It can also affect a patient's ability to have sufficient heating during the cold weather leading to peripheral vasoconstriction and decreased blood supply to the wound. Poor housing can also lead to lower levels of cleanliness, increasing the potential risk to infection. Cultural and religious beliefs can have an influence on diet, hygiene and acceptance of medical interventions. Patient lifestyle can therefore influence healing, especially if the person smokes, drinks excessive amounts of alcohol or abuses drugs (Beitz, 2016).

Psychological factors

Poor motivation of a patient or their carers can affect concordance with treatments as they may lack the capability to continue with a recommended wound treatment regime. Known psychological effects on wound healing include stress, coping style, positive effect, environmental enrichment and social support (Beitz, 2016). Psychological factors exert physiological effects such as blood vessel size and leucocyte distribution via mediators such as oxytocin, vasopressin, epinephrine and cortisol (Broadbent & Koschwanez, 2012). It is also worth considering the impact on patients of the surgical postoperative period in terms of the resulting scar and possible altered patient body image (see Chapter 7 for information on altered body image).

Methods of skin closure

The purpose of wound closure is to achieve approximation of the wound edges to produce a strong scar, with minimal disturbance of the function and good cosmetic results. In wound healing by primary intention various types of suture material, staples, adhesive strips and tissue adhesives can be used to bring the skin edges together and hold them in apposition until healing has occurred.

The choice of wound closure and technique depend upon the:

- Best clinical evidence or guidance
- Type of tissue
- Position of the wound
- Surgeon's preference.

Sutures

Sutures are used to promote healing by eliminating dead space in a wound, realigning of tissue planes, and holding skin edges in apposition until healing has taken place and the wound no longer needs the support of the suture material. Sutures can be used to aid haemostasis. However, if applied too tightly they can cause tissue trauma or necrosis of the surrounding tissue. The type of suture technique, technique of knot tying, and the width of the tissue all affect wound strength and healing (Goodman & Spry, 2014; Kirk, 2010).

Suture materials are chosen for their strength, handling characteristics and absorptive properties. Different types of suture material are required in a variety of circumstances, and for different types of tissue, organs and parts of the body (Conway et al, 2019). The choice of suture material depends on the rate at which the tissue is likely to heal, the amount of strain or stress to which the wound site will be subjected, the likely growth of the wound and whether the suture is to give a temporary or permanent support (Ethicon, 2019a; Kirk, 2010). The surgeon will choose a suture material which loses its tensile strength relative to the gain of strength of the wound itself as it heals.

Types of suture material

These are either absorbable or non-absorbable (Table 5.1).

Absorbable sutures are made from materials which are digested either by proteolytic enzymes released from the polymorphonuclear cells, or by hydrolysis whereby the action of water on the suture causes the breakdown of material (Conway et al, 2019).

The action of hydrolysis is increased by the rise in temperature or a change in the percentage hydrogen (pH). Non-absorbable sutures are made out of materials which resist enzymatic digestion and therefore need removal when applied to the skin (e.g. Ethilon).

Non-absorbable skin sutures are left in place for different periods of time depending on the wound site and amount of tension the wound is under (Box 5.2).

Any non-absorbable suture material that is left in place for too long can cause excessive scarring and is a focus for infection, leading to the formation of a stitch abscess or sinus (Kirk, 2010).

Non-absorbent sutures can be left within hernia repairs in a form of mesh. Prolene can be used for suturing blood vessels and grafts in place.

Suture material is either monofilament or braided. Monofilament sutures are made from a single smooth strand of material. This smoothness makes them easy to handle and reduces tissue trauma. Braided sutures increase handling, manipulation and knotting features. However, these features may also increase infection risk as the braided nature of material can attract bacteria to it.

No one suture material is suitable for all purposes; the choice of material depends on the type and location of wound. Each suture material within a wound stimulates its own inflammatory response; this can last for approximately 7 days.

Suture techniques

The choice of suturing technique is informed by the type of tissue, site and size of wound (Alexander & Trott, 2012; Kirk, 2010). Three factors in suturing technique are:

- tightness of the tied suture
- size of tissue bite
- distance between the sutures.

If these factors are not addressed, then wound healing may be impaired as well as leading to poor cosmetic results. Sutures that are pulled too tight do not allow for swelling and may lead to vascular compromise at the wound edges resulting in tissue necrosis, delayed healing and poor cosmetic results. A poor cosmetic scar can also be the result of sutures inserted too loosely, allowing the wound to gape as the wound edges have not been brought together. Overlapping of the wound edges may also lead to dehiscence or cause a ridge effect within the scar. Sutures placed too near the edges of the wound can result in the suture pulling apart from the wound edges, causing further trauma to the wound.

Sutures can be inserted in a continuous or an interrupted pattern. The continuous method of insertion is used to close an incision with one running stitch, which is tied to the skin at each end ensuring tension is the same along the incision, e.g. subcuticular, continuous over-and-over stitch, blanket stitch and mattress stitch (Fig. 5.9). When a Prolene subcuticular suture is inserted, it is held in place by means of a bead at each end of the incision (see Fig. 5.9). A disadvantage of using a continuous suture is that if it breaks, the wound edges are not held together and so the suture has to be reinserted.

Interrupted sutures are where a suture is knotted and cut individually along the incision, e.g. interrupted over-and-under stitch, vertical or horizontal mattress stitch (Fig. 5.10). It produces a stronger incisional line and avoids devascularization of the skin edges. Abdominal incisions are generally closed using a layered approach, where each layer is closed separately with either

Table 5.1 Types of suture material

Suture	Type	Absorption	Area of use
Absorbable suture materials			
Coated VICRYL Rapid	Braided	42 days	Skin, perineum, scalp, oral
MONOCRYL	Monofilament	90–120 days	Subcuticular, muscle
Coated VICRYL	Braided Monofilament	56–70 days	Ligating, suture all tissue except where extended approximation is required. Ophthalmic: surgery only
Coated VICRYL Plus	Braided	56–70 days	Ligating, suture all tissue except where extended approximation is required
PDS II	Monofilament	180–210 days	All tissue except where approximation is required indefinitely
DEXON	Multifilament (can be coated)	60–90 days	
Non-absorbable suture materials			
PROLENE	Monofilament	Non-absorbable remains encapsulated in tissue	Cardiac, facia, skin, blood vessels
ETHILON	Monofilament		Fascia, skin, nerves, blood vessels
ETHIBOND *EXCEL*	Braided		Vascular, cardiac
NUROLON	Braided		Most body tissue, skin
MERSILENE	Monofilament		Most body tissue
MERSILK	Braided		Ligating, most tissue (buried), skin
Virgin silk	Twisted		Ophthalmic
Stainless steel	Monofilament/ multifilament		Cardiac, thoracic
PRONOVA	Monofilament		Cardiac, vascular

Source: Ethicon (2019b); Wicker & Dalby (2017); Brindle & Creehan (2016).

Box 5.2 **Indicative time for removal of non-absorbable sutures**

- Skin on head or neck: 205 days
- Upper limbs: 7 days
- Trunk or abdomen: 10 days
- Lower limbs: 14 days
- Retention sutures: 2–6 weeks

Source: Ethicon (2019b).

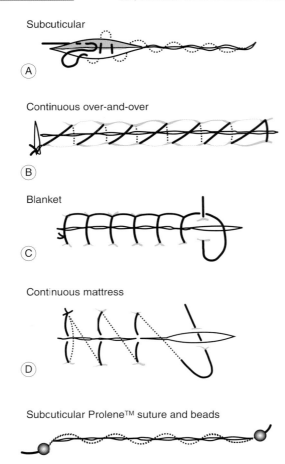

Subcuticular

(A)

Continuous over-and-over

(B)

Blanket

(C)

Continuous mattress

(D)

Subcuticular Prolene™ suture and beads

(E)

Figure 5.9 Types of continuous suture techniques.

continuous or interrupted sutures (Phillips, 2012; Kirk, 2010; Price & Sinclair, 2008).

Sometimes a purse-string suture is inserted around a drain. This is a continuous suture that is placed around an opening, so that once the drain is removed, the edges can be pulled together.

Retention or deep tension sutures are used when there is a risk of gross contamination of the wound, excessive tissue damage, recurrent suturing of a wound, or a patient is very obese; they are mainly used in abdominal surgery. By passing the retention sutures through all the layers of the wound and by approximating the skin edges with a large non-absorbent suture, as well as the smaller interrupted sutures, it reduces tension and holds the wound edges together until healing is completed. A bolster or plastic sleeve is placed over the retention sutures so as to prevent the sutures from cutting into the skin.

Removal of sutures

The time period for removal of sutures depends upon the position of the wound (see Box 5.2), condition of the skin and any underlying pathologies which could delay the healing process, e.g. steroid therapy. When removing sutures, it is important to ensure that the suture material that has been above the skin is not pulled through under the skin edges, as microorganisms may be dragged through into the underlying tissue and so cause infection.

In interrupted sutures, each suture layer is lifted by the knot and cut below the knot, as near the skin as is possible, at the point where it has been withdrawn from the skin. The suture is then pulled out towards the side on which it has been cut, to avoid the risk of dragging the skin edges apart. It is important to ensure that no portion of the suture has been left behind, as it will act as a foreign body and cause a local inflammatory response (Bogdanske et al, 2013).

In continuous subcuticular sutures, one end of the suture is cut, and the suture is then gently pulled away from the incision, ensuring the wound is supported during this procedure, as it can be very uncomfortable for the patient. In subcuticular Prolene suture with beads, one end of the suture is cut and the bead removed, while the opposing beaded end is pulled in order to remove the suture. In other types of continuous sutures, several cuts in the suture are required to ensure that all the suture material is removed without causing contamination to the underlying tissues.

Staples

The use of staples for skin closure can have an advantage in relation to cosmetic appearance of the scar. This closure method is time-saving and has the benefit of painless removal (Conway et al, 2019). As the stapler is squeezed, the open staple is forced against an anvil within the nose of the stapler. This action bends the staple legs, causing them to penetrate the everted skin edges and results in the staple's final rectangular shape (Fig. 5.11). They allow for haemostasis without causing necrosis to the tissue.

Removal of staples is achieved by inserting the lower jar of the staple remover under the staple and closing together the two edges of the staple remover. The staple needs to be placed in the V-shaped retaining slot situated in the bottom jar of the staple remover in order to ensure it is removed correctly. Squeezing the handles of the staple remover reforms the staple, so that it can be lifted from the skin.

Adhesive skin tapes

Adhesive skin tapes are used for some types of skin closure, especially if the cosmetic appearance of the scar is of

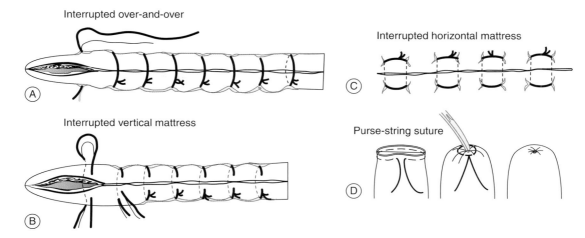

Figure 5.10 Types of interrupted suture techniques.

concern to the patients. This technique can also limit inflammation of skin edges (Broughton et al, 2006). The lax skin of the face and abdomen makes them amenable sites for wound closure by adhesive tape, whereas the skin over joints is subjected to frequent movement and so has limited adherence to tapes for successful wound closure (Alexander & Trott, 2012). It is important that skin edges are dry before the application of tape (Kirk, 2010).

Adhesive tapes can also be used in conjunction with subcuticular continuous sutures, to give extra support to the wound closure, e.g. reconstructive breast surgery. Adhesive skin tapes are usually left in place until they peel off by themselves. If there is leakage of exudate from the wound the adhesive skin tapes may need to be carefully removed and then reapplied until healing has occurred.

Tissue adhesives

This method can be used for minor lacerations, especially in children as it requires no anaesthesia. The wound edges are approximated and a small amount of glue is applied to the outside surface of the closed wound, and left for approximately 30 seconds (Conway et al, 2019). This approach to wound closure is a quick, efficient and relatively painless method of wound closure in some traumatic wounds with low overall complications (Hazalina et al, 2011).

Topical negative pressure

This is a non-invasive technique whereby negative pressure is applied in a uniform manner to promote wound healing (NICE, 2018). There are disposable pumps that use Hydrofiber Technology (gels) within a silicone

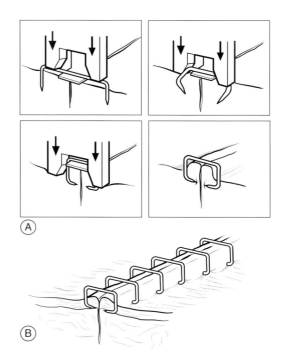

Figure 5.11 (A) Formation of skin staples. (B) Skin staples *in situ*.

adhesive border to absorb and lock in wound exudate and microorganisms, with a foam layer to aid distribution of negative pressure across the dressing. Once the treatment is completed or after a fixer period determined by the manufacturer of these single use devices (e.g. 30 days), the pumps are disposed of.

Another example of this technique is when a foam dressing is cut to the shape of the wound and applied over the wound itself, which is then covered with a vapour-permeable film. Suction tubing is attached and connected to a vacuum unit, which is set to the amount and type of pressure required. The negative pressure can be set at continuous or intermittent and can be administered between 50 mmHg (0.07 bar/6666 Pa) and 200 mmHg (0.27 bar/26664 Pa), depending on patient comfort, the type of wound and the system used (Yesuel & Kyong-Je, 2019; Bates-Jensen, 2016)

The foam dressing should be changed every 48 hours, unless the wound is infected, when it should be changed twice a day. If topical negative pressure therapy is used on meshed skin grafts, the foam should not be changed for 3−5 days. Older pumps also use a canister to collect exudate. This canister can act as a reservoir for bacteria and potentially increase the risk of infection. The canister should therefore be changed regularly, dependent on manufacturer and local guidelines.

The technique of using topical pressure creates a non-compression force to the tissue, which encourages the arterioles to dilate. This improves blood flow, promotes a moist environment and assists in the proliferation of granulation tissue. This approach also helps to reduce the amount of bacteria colonization within the wound and can remove excess fluid from the area, so reducing oedema (Bates-Jensen, 2016; Beitz, 2016). The use of topical negative pressure results in progressive wound closure in wounds healing by secondary intention, e.g. following dehiscence of a wound or application of a skin graft.

Negative pressure treatment is contraindicated in wounds with exposed organs, tendons or blood vessels, malignancy in wounds, or presence of fistula, it should be used with caution in patients with actively bleeding wounds, clotting disorders or patients taking anticoagulants (Netsch, 2016).

Tranexamic acid (TXA)

This is a medication used to treat or prevent excessive blood loss. It can be administered orally, topically or by intravenous injection. TXA can significantly reduce postoperative blood loss, accelerate removal of drainage tube and shorten duration of hospital stay (Mu et al, 2019; Ren et al, 2017).

Use of wound drains

Surgical drainage is undertaken for the following reasons:
- where an accumulation of fluid or cellular debris is expected within the wound

- to remove air, serum or fluid from a cavity or dead tissue space.

The insertion of a surgical drain provides a channel to the body surface for fluid which might otherwise be trapped or collect within the wound space. This can reduce the incidence of infection, allow closer apposition of the tissue, and facilitate the healing process (Findik et al, 2013). Drainage of fluid takes place along the surface of the drain and the flow of fluid is affected by the size, shape and number of holes in the drainage tube.

Surgical drains are a foreign body and can cause a local inflammatory response; causing pressure against vital structures (e.g. blood vessels, which can then lead to pressure necrosis; microorganisms on the skin can gain access to the wound and cause infection) (Durai & Ng, 2010; Durai et al, 2009).

The risk of infection due to the presence of a drain in a clean wound increases significantly after 304 days, as does the risk of mechanical damage to local tissue (Carlomango et al, 2013; Ikeanyi et al, 2013). Surgical drainage can be therapeutic or prophylactic (Wicker & Dalby, 2017). Therapeutic drainage is undertaken to remove bacteria, dead tissue and other infected material that has collected in the anatomical area (e.g. drainage of abscess or to remove excess inflammatory mediators so as to reduce further damage to healing tissue). This also reduces the amount of dead tissue space, alters the fluid environment of the wound and reduces the risk of bacterial contamination. Therapeutic drainage may be undertaken by needle aspiration or by insertion of a drain (Findik et al, 2013).

Prophylactic drainage is undertaken for a number of reasons, one being to prevent infection development within the wound (Wicker & Dalby, 2017). It is often used where physiological fluid is expected to collect after a surgical intervention, or when an anastomosis or closure of a viscus may leak. This method can also be used to redirect body fluids along an alternative route in order to rest an anastomosis, e.g. insertion of a T tube following exploration of the common bile duct, or insertion of a nephrostomy tube following urinary diversion. If haemostasis has been difficult to achieve, the insertion of a surgical drain allows early diagnosis of a secondary or reactive haemorrhage. It can prevent the formation of a haematoma and is used when a seroma or haematoma may affect the healing of a skin flap. It can also be used in mastectomy, amputations of a limb and plastic reconstructive surgery (Durai et al, 2009).

Types of wound drains

There are numerous types of drain available (Box 5.3), these adopt either a passive or active drainage approach.

Both active and passive drainage approaches should remove fluid efficiently, avoid damage to the surrounding

Box 5.3 **Types of surgical drain**

Passive drainage

- Gauze wick
- Penrose drain
- Corrugated drain
- Yeates drain
- T tube

Active drainage

- Redivac

Closed drain/underwater drain

- Chest drain

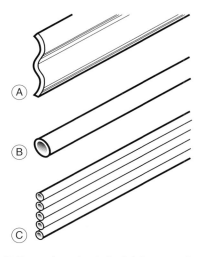

Figure 5.12 Types of passive drain. (A) Corrugated. (B) Penrose. (C) Yeates.

tissue, avoid the risk of infection and be easily removed (Durai et al, 2009).

In closed/underwater drains, the tube end is under water in a closed bottle so that atmospheric air is not able to access the drainage tube. It is essential to ensure that the bottle is always below the level of the wound. If the bottle is higher than the wound, the water within the bottle can drain back into the wound. Chest drains allow for the removal of air and fluid from the plural cavity (Wicker & Dalby, 2017; Wicker & O'Neil, 2010).

Passive drainage is achieved by two methods:

- Closed systems drain via a tube into a bag, which is under the force of gravity or capillary action.
- Open systems drain into a bag or dressing and are dependent on capillary action, gravity or changes in body cavity pressure (e.g. intra-abdominal pressure).

This type of drain must be inserted at an upward angle in order to facilitate drainage. Examples of this type of drain are Penrose drain, corrugated drain and Yeates drain (Fig. 5.12). An active drainage system uses vacuum pressure (Fig. 5.13) to encourage drainage.

These drains are inserted through a stab wound usually close to the main incision wound site. The drainage tubing is more rigid in order to prevent it collapsing under the negative pressure exerted by the vacuum. These drains are often held *in situ* by a loop suture to the skin.

Note: in orthopaedic surgery, a plaster cast may be used, in which case a loop suture to fix the drain would *not* be used to aid later removal. This type of drainage also facilitates more accurate record keeping of fluid volume loss (Zinn, 2012).

Care of surgical drains

Minimal handling and aseptic technique should be used to reduce the risk of infection. Sterile 'keyhole' dressings can be used around the drain/skin entry wound to absorb exudate.

A passive drain should have either a sterile absorbent dressing placed over the drain or a drainage bag applied over it, to collect the drained fluid (Durai et al, 2009; Simpson & Brooks, 2008).

Universal precautions should be adopted when dealing with body fluids (e.g. emptying a drainage bottle or removing a surgical drain). Patency of the drainage system should be checked regularly to ensure free drainage of fluid from the wound site. Wound exudate/fluid loss should be monitored and recorded. In the initial 24-hour period postoperatively there can be a high level of serous drainage from the surgical wound; this should reduce in the following 24-hour period. Excessive amounts of wound drainage should be reported, as this may indicate haemorrhage, which may need further investigation or may lead to fluid and electrolyte loss.

The drain, bag or drainage bottle should be well secured and easily observed. The drainage tubing should be protected from kinking, blockage or accidental removal (e.g. transfer of patient from bed to chair or bed to surgical trolley). The area around the drain should be inspected regularly in order to detect signs of infection; the immediate surrounding skin can be inflamed due to local trauma caused by movement of the drain. Pain levels should also be assessed in relation to any discomfort the drain or tubing may be causing to the patient.

Removal of surgical drains

The drain should be removed when drainage has stopped, the abscess cavity has closed, wound repair is complete, or if there is risk of drain-related complications (e.g. infection, tissue ingrowth or obstruction). Prior to removal of

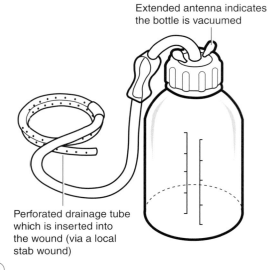

Extended antenna indicates the bottle is vacuumed

Perforated drainage tube which is inserted into the wound (via a local stab wound)

(A)

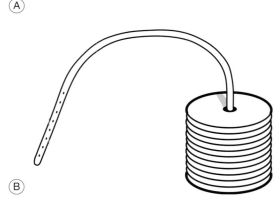

(B)

Figure 5.13 Types of active drain. (A) High vacuum wound drainage. (B) Concertina-type drain.

the drain, it is important to seek consent from the patient, inform the patient of what is going to happen to help reduce anxiety and fear. Analgesics may also be required by the patient, and these must be given in sufficient time before undertaking the removal procedure. Gloves should be worn by the healthcare professional removing the drain, as guided by universal precautions and local policy. If the drain has a retaining/securing suture in place, this suture should be cut and removed to facilitate full drain removal.

With active suction drainage systems, the suction vacuum created by the bottle should be released prior to removal of the drain in order to reduce trauma to tissue during the removal procedure (Wicker & Dalby, 2017). On removal of the drain a small absorbent dressing is required over the drain site, this dressing should also be observed for excessive amounts of leakage.

In the case of passive drains some surgeons will request the drain be shortened daily, to facilitate healing from the base of the wound. The retaining suture needs to be cut before the drain is shortened by 1–2 cm. In order to keep the drain in place or be drawn back into the wound, a sterile safety pin can be inserted into the drain. The drain is shortened by 1–2 cm every 24–48 hours until it falls out. A small absorbent dressing should then be applied to the drain site until healing has occurred and the amount of leakage closely monitored.

Principles of care for a patient with a surgical wound

A surgical wound is an intentional wound. The main focus for care is to monitor the progress of the wound healing, so that problems can be identified early, and appropriate interventions adopted to reduce the incidence of wound infection and improved postoperative outcomes.

Risk factors for surgical site infection

Two core factors in determining the development of a wound infection are:
- the virulence of bacteria within the wound
- the host's resistance.

A surgical classification of wounds is given in Box 5.4. These classifications have a strong link with the incidence of emergent wound infection. In elective surgery the degree of wound contamination relates to the type of operation (i.e. clean, clean contaminated, contaminated or dirty).

Other significant factors associated with the development of a wound infection are:
- Underlying medical conditions
- Age
- Length of hospital stay
- Surgical shaving
- Duration of the surgical intervention
- Perioperative interventions
- Use of wound drain
- Use of prophylactic antimicrobials/antibiotics
- Skin preparation of operative site
- Methods of wound closure
- Use of adherent dressing

It is worth noting that surgical site infections may not appear until up to 30 days after a surgical procedure, therefore vigilance and monitoring of patients postoperatively and on their return home is vitally important (Shiffman & Low, 2019; Tanner et al, 2009).

Box 5.4 **Surgical classification of wounds**

- Class I: Clean surgical wound — operation where there is no opening of the bronchi, genitourinary or gastrointestinal tracts.
- Class II: Clean contaminated wound — operation where the bronchi, genitourinary or gastrointestinal tract is opened.
- Class III: Contaminated wound — open fresh traumatic wound or incision where there is non-purulent inflammation.
- Class IV: Dirty wound — old traumatic wound and wound involving abscess or perforated viscera.

Source: Wicker & Dalby (2017); Zinn & Swofford (2014).

Underlying medical conditions

Chronic obstructive pulmonary disease (COPD), malnutrition, hypoalbuminaemia, excessive alcohol use, and hyperglycaemia can all increase the risk of surgical site infection (Dorner et al, 2016; Leaper, 2010).

Age of the patient

This is important to acknowledge. Paediatric patients will require smaller sutures than adults, the child's age will also inform the decisions around removal of sutures. Absorbable sutures may be preferred to negate manual removal. Infection risk will also increase with age. Older patients have decreased elasticity in their skin tissue alongside an increased incidence of bruising or other injury, the skin being thinner and more fragile as a result of the ageing process, medication or possible disease (Wicker & Dalby, 2017; Davis, 2009).

Length of hospital stay

Prolonged periods of stay within an acute area can allow for nosocomial acquisition of resistant orgasms, e.g. methicillin-resistant *Staphylococcus aureus* and other potentially infectious flora (Rosman et al, 2015). The longer the stay prior to surgery and postoperatively, the higher the risk to the patient of developing a wound infection.

Preoperative showering and bathing

Ideally the patient will have a shower or bath one day prior to surgery, or on the day of surgery, prior to putting on a clean operating gown. The use of soap is recommended rather than stronger skin disinfection (Wilson et al, 2015; National Institute for Health and Care Excellence (NICE), 2008, 2013a, 2013b).

Removal of body hair

Shaving, particularly with a razor, has been found to increase the risk of surgical site infection (NICE, 2008, 2013a, 2013b). However, for some body types (i.e.

extremely hairy patients), hair removal may be required to reduce interference and complications associated with wound closure and dressing (i.e. sinus formation, pain and discomfort on dressing removal). The use of electric clippers immediately prior to surgery is the preferred option (Wilson et al, 2015).

Surgical environment and duration of the surgical intervention

An effective air change ventilation system should be operational and regularly monitored. Doors to the operating theatre should remain closed, traffic movement should be kept to a minimum to facilitate the ventilation system. The number of staff in theatre should be kept to a minimum and all equipment should be cleaned prior to its admission into the operating theatre environment (Wilson et al, 2015; Department of Health, 2011). A correlation between wound infection rates and an increased length of the surgical procedure appears to exist (Haridas & Malangoni, 2008; Vilar-Compte et al, 2008).

Perioperative interventions

Perioperative hypothermia in surgery stimulates thermoregulatory vasoconstriction, leading to decreased subcutaneous oxygen tension. Alongside this drop in core body temperature, the risk of wound infection increases. NICE (2017) and Wilson et al (2015) recommend that all patients should be assessed within one hour prior to surgery for their risk of perioperative hypothermia. Ideally an anatomical site indicative of the body's core temperature should be used. Active warming should commence on the surgical ward or Accident and Emergency Department 30 minutes prior to induction of anaesthesia for all patients with a core temperature below 36°C unless there is a need for emergency surgery.

The patient's core temperature should continue to be measured and documented every 30 minutes until the end of the operation. This may be continued postoperatively.

Use of surgical drains

Wound drains can facilitate the removal of dead space and reduction of haematoma. It should also be noted that the drain can also act as a channel of microorganism entry. This risk should be reduced with good aseptic technique and wound management strategies.

Use of prophylactic antibiotics

Specific types of surgery (i.e. where prosthesis or prosthetic material are inserted) carry an increased risk of infection. Opportunistic microorganisms may infect the implanted material (Bratzler et al, 2013). Local guidelines to antibiotic prescribing including appropriate surgical prophylaxis should be referred to. Guidance on the use of the correct antibiotic for specific types of surgery and within a correct time frame is given by National Institute for Health and Care Excellence (2008).

Skin preparation of the operation site

Skin should be disinfected immediately prior to the incision with chlorhexidine (Hibiscrub) or povidone iodine (Betadine), alcohol or aqueous with the aim of removing transient and pathogenic organisms on the surface of the skin and reduce the number of resident flora (Kamel et al, 2012; NICE, 2008).

Surgical technique

Variance in surgical techniques from one surgeon or surgical team to another can be observed. Examples of this include the handling of tissue during surgery, excessive use of diathermy, and variations in approaches to wound closure from one clinician to another clinician.

Robust reporting and recording of surgical site infections are essential to audit surgical outcomes, inform hospital infection control teams, surgical teams and the perioperative and surgical ward teams.

Hospital infection control teams monitor practice and infection rates. The team is responsible for prevention, surveillance, investigation and control of infection. They also provide an advisory and education role to staff at all levels (Health Protection Scotland, 2014). The infection control team will normally consist of:

- Director of infection prevention and control
- Infection control medical doctor
- Antimicrobial pharmacist
- Infection control nurse or practitioner
- Infection control nursing service administrator.

The team works closely with staff from all areas to monitor and analyse infection rate data; this includes audits of operating theatres, surgical wards and surgical team outcomes in relation to incidence of infections (Wilson, 2012).

Potential postoperative wound complications

Some common complications that can occur following surgery include haemorrhage, haematoma, infection, wound dehiscence, sinus formation and fistula formation.

Haemorrhage

Haemorrhage commonly occurs at the time of surgery, in the immediate postoperative period and up to 10 days postoperatively (secondary haemorrhage). Failure to control bleeding during surgery or failure to tie blood vessels securely can result in haemorrhage in the early postoperative period. Secondary haemorrhage is commonly linked to infection.

Perioperative bleeding can affect fibroblast function particularly in relation to collagen production; on closure this can lead to a weakened suture line.

Haemorrhage can be visually detected by observation of blood loss in drains or on the wound dressing. In severe cases the patient may have to return to the operating theatre to have the bleeding point tied off or sealed using diathermy (Peate & Glencross, 2015).

Haematoma

A collection of blood within the tissue can exert an internal pressure, which can in turn restrict the blood supply and so lead to tissue ischaemia. The haematoma can have a toxic effect on tissue and harbour microorganisms potentiating the risk of infection. Haematomas can be detected by a raised hard area close to the incision wound or when it is released following the removal of sutures or staples. Release of the haematoma can be achieved by gentle aseptic probing of the wound to allow drainage of the collection of haemoserous fluid, i.e. a thin, watery, pink-coloured fluid composed of blood and serum (Brindle & Creehan, 2016).

Surgical site infection

The presence of a wound infection will delay healing and patient discharge increasing pressure on resources. Surgical site infection (SSI) can be defined as the infection of a wound by the invasion of microorganisms through tissue when patient defences, both local and systemic, break down (Jenks et al, 2012). It is worth noting that SSI at the site of surgical procedure can occur after discharge within 30 days of operation but may extend to 12 months, postoperative, if prosthetic or implant surgery is performed (Mangram et al, 1999).

Sources of SSI can be primary (acquired from a community or endogenous source, such as that following a perforated peptic ulcer) or secondary or exogenous (healthcare-

Table 5.2 American Society of Anesthesiologists (ASA) physiology score

ASA PS classification	Definition	Examples
ASA I	A normal healthy patient	Healthy, non-smoking, no or minimal alcohol use
ASA II	A patient with mild systemic disease	Mild diseases only without substantive functional limitations. Examples include (but not limited to): current smoker, social alcohol drinker, pregnancy, obesity (BMI 30–40), well-controlled diabetes mellitus (DM)/hypertension (HTN), mild lung disease
ASA III	A patient with severe systemic disease	Substantive functional limitations. One or more moderate to severe diseases. Examples include (but not limited to): poorly controlled DM or HTN, chronic obstructive pulmonary disease (COPD), morbid obesity (BMI ≥40), active hepatitis, alcohol dependence or abuse, implanted pacemaker, moderate reduction of ejection fraction, end stage renal disease (ESRD) undergoing regularly scheduled dialysis, premature infant post conceptional age (PCA) <60 weeks, history (>3 months) of myocardial infarction (MI), cardiovascular disease (CVA), transient ischaemic attacks (TIA), or coronary artery disease (CAD)/stents
ASA IV	A patient with severe systemic disease that is a constant threat to life	Examples include (but not limited to): recent (<3 months) MI, CVA, TIA, or CAD/stents, ongoing cardiac ischaemia or severe valve dysfunction, severe reduction of ejection fraction, sepsis, disseminated intravascular coagulation (DIC), ascites reinfusion dialysis (ARD) or ESRD not undergoing regularly scheduled dialysis
ASA V	A moribund patient who is not expected to survive without the operation	Examples include (but are not limited to): ruptured abdominal/thoracic aneurysm, massive trauma, intracranial bleed with mass effect, ischaemic bowel in the face of significant cardiac pathology or multiple organ/system dysfunction
ASA VI	A declared brain-dead patient whose organs are being removed for donor purposes	

associated infections (HCAIs) acquired from the operating theatre, i.e. due to poor or inadequate air filtration systems, or the surgical ward, e.g. poor hand-washing compliance, or from contamination at or after surgery, such as poor wound management or an anastomotic leak).

Secondary or HCAIs include respiratory infection (e.g. ventilator–associated pneumonia), urinary tract infections (urinary catheter–associated infections), bacteraemia (associated with vascular catheter) and surgical site infections (Jenks et al, 2012).

SSIs can be subcategorized into:
- Superficial surgical site infection (when infection involves skin and subcutaneous tissue of the incision within 30 days of operation)
- Deep surgical site infection (infection in the deeper musculofascial layers)
- Organ space infection (such as an abdominal abscess after an anastomotic leak)

The incidence of SSI risk can increase depending on other factors such as higher American Society of Anaesthetists (ASA) physiology score (Table 5.2), type of operation, length of surgery and wound classification.

The addition of 'E' to a category denotes emergency surgery – an emergency is defined as existing when delay in treatment of the patient would lead to a significant increase in the threat to life or body part.

Many SSIs occur after discharge. In light of the increasing use of ambulatory settings for minor operative procedures, developments of day surgery provision and emerging legislative accountability (i.e. delay in returning to work, loss of income to the patient) and development of broader monitoring of postoperative complications and infection rate is critical. Current hospital-based surveillance methods therefore need to be cognizant of these methods (Rhee et al, 2015).

The diagnosis of wound infection is based on clinical criteria (i.e. signs of inflammation, pyrexia, discharge of pus, pain in the area and possible breakdown of the wound). However, it is also possible that the early inflammatory stage could be mistaken for the beginning of a wound infection in ambulatory/day surgical patients. Surgical wounds which are healing by primary or secondary intention may present with different features (Box 5.5).

Wound infection is confirmed by the clinical symptoms and a positive result from a wound swab which should be taken prior to antibiotic therapy. It should be noted that the swab may also pick up other contaminants as well as the pathogenic organism that is causing the infection (Alavi et al, 2010). Clinical practitioners must therefore adopt wound swabbing methods advocated by appropriate microbiology departments relevant to their specific area of practice. It is important to obtain as much patient information as possible to inform laboratory investigations and best detect the infecting organism. Microbiology, culture and sensitivity of wound exudate will identify the pathogenic organism and best advise the antibiotic to be prescribed. If left untreated, wound infection can lead to deeper systemic infection such as lymphadenitis, bacteraemia, septicaemia and even death.

In primary care, a swab remains a common method used for obtaining a wound sample. An example of another method is biopsy of aspirate of pus. Wound swabs can provide acceptable samples for bacterial culture provided an appropriate technic is used. If a wound is not purulent it should be cleaned prior to swabbing (Siddiqui & Bernstein, 2010). With this technique the cleaning removes the organisms present on the surface material, which can be different from those bacteria responsible for the pathology. Wounds should be washed with sterile saline. Cotton, alginate or rayon-tipped swabs can be used to superficially debride the wound. Other literature suggests that cleaning the wound prior to taking a swab sample is unnecessary. However, if the wound is not cleaned, the sample taken may include multiple organisms which may not be relevant to the emergent infection and result in misleading data (i.e. mixed bacterial infection rather than an individual strain) (Rajan, 2012; Bowler et al, 2001).

Antibiotic prophylaxis is recommended to patients scheduled for surgery that may involve contaminated, clean contaminated or clean surgery but involving insertion of implants or prosthetics. Patients with a dirty or infected wound may need additional antibiotics (Borchardt & Rolston, 2012). Adverse effects of antibiotics need to be considered before administration. A single dose of antibiotic before commencing the anaesthetic may be necessary. It may also be necessary to give the antibiotic earlier if the patient is to have a tourniquet during the procedure. A repeat dose may be required if the operation is longer than the half-life of the antibiotic.

Note: the optimum dose of antibiotic should be in the tissue at the time of surgical incision and therefore needs to be administered 30 minutes prior to the surgical intervention or incision commences (Wicker & Dalby, 2017; NICE, 2017).

A number of scoring systems have been devised to assess patients with a suspected wound infection. Three commonly used methods are:

- Additional treatment, Serous discharge, Erythema, Purulent exudate, Separation of deep tissue, Isolation of bacteria and Stay as inpatient prolonged over 14 days (ASEPSIS method). This method was first developed for use in cardiothoracic surgery, allocating points for the appearance of the surgical wound in the first week and the emergent clinical consequences of infection (van Walraven & Musselman, 2013).
- Southampton Wound Assessment Scale. This method was initially designed for use on patients having had hernia surgery; it enables surgical wound healing to be graded according to specific criteria, usually giving a numerical value (JBI Library, 2011). This can then be placed into one of four categories:
  - Normal healing with mild bruising and erythema
  - Erythema plus other signs of inflammation (minor complication)
  - Clear or haemoserous discharge (wound infection)
  - Major haematoma
- Centres for Disease Control (CDC). This method is based on the principle that the risk of infection increases as the numerical score increases. It is calculated on a score of $0-1$ for each of the following four patient factors:
  - An abdominal operation
  - An operation lasting 2 hours or more
  - An operation that is contaminated
  - A patient who has three or more diagnoses at discharge, exclusive of wound infection

The use of scoring systems to assess possible wound infection provides clinical practitioners with a range of tools to audit surgical outcomes and inform further clinical interventions and best use of resources.

Dehiscence

This is the term used when there is partial or complete separation of a surgically closed wound. Dehiscence can occur within any surgical wound; however, more common examples have been associated in the past with abdominal

Box 5.5 Criteria for identifying wound infection in surgical wounds

Traditional criteria

- Abscess
- Cellulitis
- Discharge: serous exudate with inflammation, seropurulent, haemopurulent, pus

Additional criteria

- Delayed healing
- Discoloration
- Friable granulation tissue that bleeds easily
- Unexpected pain/tenderness
- Pocketing at the base of the wound
- Bridging of the epithelium/soft tissue
- Abnormal smell
- Wound breakdown

Surgical wounds healing by primary intention

- Cellulitis
- Pus/abscess
- Delayed healing
- Erythema +/− induration
- Haemopurulent exudate
- Malodour
- Seropurulent exudate
- Wound breakdown/enlargement
- Increase in local skin temperature
- Oedema
- Serous exudate with erythema
- Swelling with increase in exudate volume
- Unexpected pain/tenderness

Surgical wounds healing by secondary intention

- Cellulitis
- Pus/abscess
- Delayed healing
- Erythema +/− induration
- Haemopurulent exudate
- Increase in exudate volume
- Malodour
- Pocketing
- Seropurulent exudate
- Wound breakdown/enlargement
- Discoloration
- Friable granulation tissue that bleeds easily
- Increase in local skin temperature
- Oedema
- Unexpected pain/tenderness

Source: van Driessche (2016); Scales & Huffnagle (2013).

wounds following open abdominal surgery, resulting in a burst abdomen. Other examples of dehiscence have been associated with sternotomy, episiotomy and caesarean section (Brindle & Creehan, 2016).

Wound dehiscence can be categorized as early or late:

- Early wound dehiscence: occurs during the early stages of healing and linked more to the surgical closer technique used (i.e. type of suture or suturing technique).
- Late wound dehiscence: attributed to wound separation as a result of infection.

Wound dehiscence can also be due to other risk factors listed in Box 5.6.

A lack of development of a ridge of skin along either side of an incision line plus a discharge of serosanguinous fluid from the wound may indicate dehiscence. Patients may also report that 'something has given way' and that a 'warm wet' sensation is felt.

Total dehiscence will require further surgical intervention and exploration of the wound, removal of any devitalized tissue and closure of the wound.

Partial dehiscence can be lightly filled with an appropriate dressing such as alginate or Hydrofiber or topical negative pressures used.

Sinus formation

A sinus is a blind ending track which opens onto a body surface (Fig. 5.14). Often caused by the presence of an abscess or foreign material which is irritant and becomes infected, e.g. suture material or an ingrowing hair. It may be recognized by a point on the incision line or in other parts of the body (e.g. pilonidal sinus) which does not heal or repeatedly breaks down. The most effective way to manage a sinus is a surgical excision and removal of the foreign material or laying open the sinus to facilitate growth of healthy granulation tissue at the base of the wound.

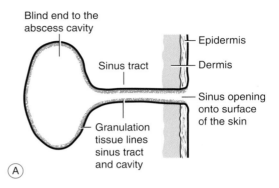

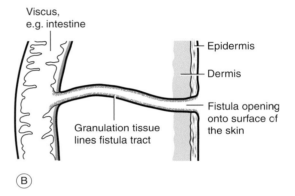

Figure 5.14 The difference between a sinus and a fistula. (A) Sinus. (B) Fistula.

Fistula formation

A fistula is an abnormal track connecting two viscera (see Fig. 5.14), such as between the rectum and vagina or between a viscera and the body surface. Fistula can occur following surgery where an anastomosis of the

---

Box 5.6 **Risk factors associated with wound dehiscence**

- Wound closure
- Tension of the wound
- Experience of surgeon, surgical practitioner or surgical team
- Obesity
- Renal failure
- Anaemia
- Wound infection
- Corticosteroids
- Radiotherapy

- Age of patient
- Emergency surgery
- Haematoma
- Diabetes
- Jaundice
- Malnutrition
- Increased abdominal pressure
- Cytotoxic therapy
- Chronic cough

Source: Wicker & Dalby (2017).

gastrointestinal tract has taken place (e.g. sigmoid colectomy). This type of wound will ooze large quantities of fluid and examination of the fluid will determine the source of the fistula (Nix & Bryant, 2016). Fistula can close spontaneously with minimal intervention and can therefore be managed conservatively, the aim being to maintain:

- integrity of the skin around the fistula
- fluid and electrolyte balance
- nutritional support
- use of appropriate ostomy or wound drainage systems.

Assessment of patient and the wound

Ongoing assessment of the patient's general condition is essential; factors that may influence healing should be identified and used to inform further treatment interventions, if required (Bates-Jensen, 2016; Netsch, 2016). Assessment of the wound should include the:

- method of closure
- presence of any drains
- indication of any complications.

If the wound is healing by primary intention, it should be observed for normal signs of inflammation, commonly seen in the first few days following surgery (Wicker & Dalby, 2017; Brindle & Creehan, 2016). If the wound appears inflamed and clinical infection is suspected, the patient should be treated in line with best practice and local guidelines.

A surgical wound that is healing by secondary intention should be observed in relation to the:

- appearance of the wound bed
- size of the wound
- shape of the wound
- depth of the wound
- amount and type of exudate
- presence of any complications (e.g. necrotic or sloughy tissue or infection).

Wound assessment should be conducted with a structured approach and clearly documented so that a baseline of information is recorded to inform the progress of wound healing, general monitoring and communication. Local guidelines and use of wound assessment tools should be reviewed in order to provide a framework to structure this process and documentation.

Wound management

Optimum conditions and environment for healing should be maintained both with the patient and for their specific wound type. Factors such as the nutritional state of the patient and their general health need to be taken into account. If any deficiencies exist, they should be corrected. This means that the patient should be in an optimal physical condition, if possible, and the optimum environment in relation to the patient/wound interface maintained.

The wound should be kept warm and moist, and measures to avoid causing pain and trauma to the wound during the changes of dressing should be taken. A wide range of wound dressing material and products are available. Some examples of these are identified in Table 5.3. When selecting the most suitable dressing product, the following factors should be taken into account:

- the patient (e.g. comfort/activities of living)
- their occupation
- how the wound occurred
- type of healing
- the site and type of wound
- the amount of exudate produced
- size and depth of wound
- patient allergies
- tissue perfusion
- type and state of skin around the wound
- actual dressings available to the clinician

(Wicker & Dalby, 2017; Bates-Jensen, 2016; Peate & Glencross, 2015).

Surgical wounds healing by primary intention

An initial dressing is applied to protect the wound and absorb excessive amounts of exudate. The dressing is removed later at 24–48 hours. The wound can then be left exposed if there is no leakage or exudate. Individual patients may prefer a small dressing over the wound for cosmetic reasons and comfort. The dressing should only be changed if there is leakage or exudate, or if clinical infection is suspected.

If haemostasis has been achieved and there is minimal exudate, a vapour-permeable dressing or a film dressing may be used over the incision wound and left in place until suture or staple removal. This approach allows for the wound healing to be monitored without having to remove the dressing, plus it also allows the patient to shower or bathe.

Incision wounds rarely require cleaning unless there is excessive leakage or exudate. If this is the case, the wound should be gently cleaned with normal saline at body temperature before the application of a new dressing (Weir & Schulz, 2016; Brindle & Creehan, 2016).

Surgical wounds healing by secondary intention

The wound is likely to be filled with an absorbent dressing material to facilitate haemostasis, absorb exudate and help with the formation of granular tissue at the base of the wound.

Table 5.3 Example range of wound dressing material and products (note: this is representative and by no means exhaustive)

Category of dressing	Trade names	Product information
Hydrogels	IntraSite Gel, Nu-Gel, Purilon Gel, GranuGel, Actiform Cool, Curagel, Geliperm, Hydrosorb	Non-adherent, non-absorbent, water and starch-based products. They aid autolytic debridement in dry, necrotic or sloughy wounds. The gel should be put into the wound about 5 mm thick, with caution so that it does NOT seep onto surrounding skin as this can cause maceration. If the dressing variant is used, it should be cut to the appropriate wound size. The wound should be gently covered, or the cavity loosely filled to prevent moisture loss. A semi-permeable dressing can be used and removed 3–5 days later depending on the exudate levels.
Hydrocolloid	Granuflex, DuoDerm, Comfeel, Tegasorb, Hydrocoll, Aquacel	On contact with the wound the hydrocolloid becomes a gel, creating a barrier to infection and microorganisms. This dressing can be used in exudation wounds across a range, e.g. pressure sores, surgical wounds, granulating, sloughy or necrotic wounds. The dressing aids rehydration and debridement of dry, sloughy and necrotic wounds. It is worth noting this dressing can encourage growth of anaerobic bacteria on infected wounds.
Semipermeable films	Opsite, C-View, Hydrofilm, Mepore Film	Can be used as primary or secondary dressing. Sterile, transparent films. Made from plastic sheets of polyurethane-coated adhesive. Some water and air vapour can pass through, but the film is impermeable to fluids and bacteria. Not indicated for use in wet wounds and do not absorb exudate. If there is poor moisture transmission through the film this can lead to moisture build-up, wrinkling, maceration of the skin and movement of the dressing. The dressing should be applied with no traction on it as this can lead to blistering of the skin.
Alginate	Aquacel, Kaltostat, Tegagen, Seasorb, Algosteril	These dressings can absorb many times their own weight in exudate, often changing either partially or fully into a gel (e.g. alginate can absorb up to 30 times its weight). These dressings are useful in moist wounds. Come in ribbon or square form which are either put onto or into the wound. These dressings promote granulation and comfort for patients.
Foam	Allevyn, Iyofoam, Mepilex, Tielle	Manufactured as either polyurethane or silicone. These transmit moisture vapour and oxygen. These dressings provide thermal insulation. Polyurethane is highly absorbent and designed to prevent exterior wound leakage. Silicone variant is used to contain exudate and protect the area surrounding the wound from additional damage.

(Continued)

Table 5.3 Example range of wound dressing material and products (note: this is representative and by no means exhaustive)—cont'd

Category of dressing	Trade names	Product information
Occlusive		Current thinking is that this dressing increases cell proliferation and activity by maintaining the level of wound exudate which in turn contains useful proteins and cytokines for wound healing.
Low-adherent (non-adherent and membrane)	NA ultra, Melonin, Tegapore, Tricotex, Release, Exu-Dry, Mepital, Mesorb	Used on lightly exudating wounds. Some have an absorbent layer. Membrane dressing can be used for variation of wound exudate (i.e. low to high) combined with a secondary absorbent dressing.
Deodorizing	Carboflex, Actisorb Silver 200, Clinsorb, Lyofoam C, Carbonet	Used for fungating and malodourous wounds. Dressing may contain charcoal cloth, which can absorb gas molecules. Other dressings in this group use materials such as foam, silver, absorbent pads and alginates.
Honey	Activon, Mesitran	Has antibacterial, anti-inflammatory and debridement properties.
Biologically based wound products	Hyaluronic acid	The dressing helps to improve phagocytic action. They simulate the healing process and inform good tissue repair. Used on neuropathic diabetic foot ulcers and venous leg ulcers.
Antimicrobial	Cadexomer Iodine (Iodoform, Lodosorb)	0.9% concentration of iodine which is slowly released as the wound fluid is absorbed into the lattice. A moisture-retentive dressing which provides an antimicrobial environment as it absorbs exudate. Note: caution to be used in patients with thyroid disease. Other variants of this dressing are impregnated with silver ions, which are effective against antibiotic-resistant organisms.

Source: Wicker & Dalby (2017); Adis Medical Writers (2014); Broussard & Powers (2013); Tickle (2013); Bennet-Marsden (2010).

Traditional surgical dressings for this purpose have been ribbon gauze soaked in antiseptic solution. Over time these dressings dry out, leading to dressing adherence to the wound bed. On removal, a dried-out dressing causes trauma to the wound bed, often seen as bleeding as well as pain and discomfort to the patient. Table 5.3 lists other more suitable dressings that can be used for this purpose (e.g. foam). These newer products should not adhere to the wound bed as much and be removable without causing as much trauma, pain or discomfort. Topical negative pressure may also be used to promote wound closure.

Cleansing of the wound in order to remove excessive amounts of exudate from the wound edge may be necessary. The patient can also facilitate this by showering and irrigating the wound with warm water. Using aseptic technique or using antiseptic solutions may have detrimental effects on normal healing (Weir & Schulz, 2016). Application of a new wound dressing will need to be guided by the specific dressing manufacturer's instruction and local guidelines.

As healing takes place, the amount of exudate will reduce and the cavity shape will change, becoming shallower and eventually showing signs of epithelialization. The wound dressing will need to be reviewed to protect the new epithelial tissue.

Infected wounds

If a wound is infected, the focus will be on removal of pus, devitalized tissue or accumulated fluids, as well as instigating an appropriate antibiotic therapy. The wound edges may also contain discharge that has collected within that needs to be released. The wound will need to be irrigated to remove any purulent material. Drainage bags may need to be used, which can help monitor future wound discharge and type of fluid, as well as helping to keep the patient clean and dry. Once the discharge has reduced, the wound dressing can be reviewed and an appropriate new dressing applied (see Table 5.3). Topical antiseptic dressing (i.e. contain ionic silver) may be of use here (van Driessche, 2016; Dumville et al, 2013).

Discharge advice

Robust guidance and information is essential to inform the patient on how best to manage their wound at home. The patient's carer or relative may also need to be informed.

If the patient is discharged prior to suture or staple removal, they will either need to return to hospital or visit their general practitioner to arrange for suture/staple removal.

Patient information should include the signs to look out for that may indicate wound infection and what to do if this happens. If a wound dressing is still required, the patient will need to be given instruction as to when, where and by whom it will need to be changed. This may need to take into account the patient's normal activities of living.

Patients will want to know if they have to continue wearing the wound dressing once healing has occurred and if they can shower or bathe. Once the wound has healed the patient does not need a dressing although if the scar is irritated by friction/rubbing from clothing, a light dressing may help to protect the scar. Some patients may also feel the scar is very sensitive to touch and therefore prefer to wear a light dressing. Such patients will also be able to shower and bathe normally although it may be helpful to pat the scar dry to avoid any discomfort.

If the wound is still exuding, the patient can still shower/bath but will need to apply a suitable dressing afterwards. Patient information should always include a contact number in case of concerns or problems relating to the wound.

Regenerative medicine

Human stem cell research offers a unique opportunity to provide both undifferentiated and differentiated cells for regenerative medicine or therapy, such as wound management and healing. Wound repair and healing is complex and influenced by numerous factors. The selection of a suitable stem cell progenitor remains a challenge for researchers and clinicians in terms of achieving the most desirable result specific to wound healing.

Clinical laboratory studies indicate improved healing in relation to texture, thickness and contours of the skin when used alongside other wound closure techniques (e.g. skin grafts).

Endogenous epidermal stem cells in the basal layer can regenerate skin but there is not normally a sufficient quantity of these endogenous stem cells in traumatic situations to facilitate full wound repair. Therefore, exogenous approaches to supply additional stem cells for wound healing are potential therapeutic strategies to aid wound healing in the future.

Embryonic stem cells could prove favourable over adult stem cells for the repair and regeneration of skin tissues due to their capacity for self-renewal and unlimited supply of differentiated keratinocytes or keratinocytes progenitors. However, embryonic stem cell–related research also raises difficult ethical issues. More recent research indicates adult stem cells could now have greater efficacy than previously thought (Nourian Dehkordi et al, 2019). Examples of potential sources of stem cells include:
- pluripotent stem cells
- mesenchymal stem cells
- adipose-derived stem cells
- hematopoietic stem cells

(Kanji & Das 2017).

Conclusion

This chapter has covered the structure of the skin, mechanisms of wound healing, methods of skin closure, principles of care for a patient with a surgical wound, wound management and healing, and regenerative medicine. This information is supported by peer-reviewed literature to help inform healthcare practitioners to apply theory to practice.

Surgical wounds are preconceived wounds. The perioperative surgical team will undertake to reduce the risk of complications, including infection. A key emergent theme is that postoperative complications can be minimized by the healthcare practitioner's approach to preoperative care and assessment, the information and education given to the patient, and evaluation of the healing process.

SUMMARY OF KEY POINTS

- Surgical wounds can heal by primary, secondary or tertiary intention.
- Many factors influence wound healing and increase the risk of infection.
- Surgical drains facilitate closer apposition of the tissue and can reduce the incidence of infection.
- Postoperative wound complications can often have a related link to infection.
- The patient and their wound should be assessed in order to best plan appropriate interventions.
- Wound cleansing is not required unless there is excessive exudate or presence of purulent material.
- Wound dressings should maintain an optimum environment for healing, and not cause pain or trauma on removal.
- Guidance on how to manage the wound should be given to the patient and/or carer prior to discharge.

REFLECTIVE LEARNING POINTS

Having read this chapter, think about what you now know and what you still need to find out about. These questions may help:

- What are the intrinsic and extrinsic factors that can affect the wound healing process?
- How can psychological problems affect a patient's health and wound healing, and what is the nurse's the role in helping to reduce psychological factors that can have a negative impact on wound healing?
- The choice of suturing technique is informed by what?

References

Adis Medical Writers. (2014). Selecting appropriate wound dressings by matching the properties of the dressing to the type of wound. *Drugs and Therapy Perspectives, 30*, 213—217.

Alavi, A., Niakosari, F., & Sibbald, R. (2010). When and how to perform a biopsy on a chronic wound. *Advanced Skin Wound Care, 23*, 132—140.

Alexander, T., & Trott, M. D. (2012). *Wounds and lacerations; emergency care and closure* (4th edn). Philadelphia: Elsevier Saunders.

Arnold, M., & Barbal, A. (2006). Nutrition and wound healing. *Plastic and Reconstructive Surgery, 117*(7s), 42S—58S.

Bates-Jensen, B. (2016). Assessment of the patient with a wound. In D. B. Doughty, & L. L. McNichol (Eds.), *Core curriculum: wound management*. Philadelphia: Wolters Kluwer.

Beitz, J. M. (2016). Wound healing. In D. B. Doughty, & L. L. McNichol (Eds.), *Core curriculum: wound management*. Philadelphia: Wolters Kluwer.

Beldon, P. (2010). Basic science of wound healing. *Surgery, 28*(9), 409—412.

Bennet-Marsden, M. (2010). How to select wound dressings. *Clinical Pharmacist, 2*, 363—366.

Bogdanske, J. J., Stelle, H.-V. S., Riley, M. R., & Schiffman, B. M. (2013). *Suturing principles and techniques in laboratory animal surgery*. Florida: CRC Press.

Bootun, R. (2013). Effects of immunosuppressive therapy on wound healing. *International Wound Journal, 10*, 98—104.

Borchardt, R. A., & Rolston, K. V. I. (2012). Surgical site infection: knowledge of likely pathogens is key. *Journal of American Academy of Physicians Assistants, 25*(5), 27—28.

Bowler, P., Duerden, B., & Armstrong, D. (2001). Wound microbiology and associated approaches to wound management. *Clin Microbiol Rev, 14*(2), 244—269.

Bratzler, D. W., Dellinger, E. P., Olsen, K. M., et al. (2013). Clinical practice guidelines for antimicrobial prophylaxis in surgery. *Am J Health-Syst Pharm, 70*, 195—283.

Brindle, C. T., & Creehan, S. (2016). Management of surgical wounds. In D. B. Doughty, & L. L. McNichol (Eds.), *Core curriculum: wound management*. Philadelphia: Wolters Kluwer.

Broadbent, E., & Koschwanez, H. E. (2012). The psychology of wound healing. *Current Opinion in Psychiatry, 25*(2), 135—140.

Broughton, G., Janis, J. E., & Attinger, C. (2006). Wound healing: an overview. *Plastic and Reconstructive Surgery, 117* (7s), 1e-S—32e-S.

Broussard, K. C., & Powers, J. G. (2013). Wound dressings: selecting the most appropriate type. *Journal of Clinical Dermatology, 14*(6), 449—459.

Carlomango, N. I., Santangelo, M., Grassia, S., La Tessa, C., & Renda, A. (2013). Intralumen migration of a surgical drain: report of rare complications and literature review. *Annali Italiani Di Chirugaria, 84*, 219—223.

Charoenkwan, K., Iheozar-Ejiofar, Z., Rerkasem, K., & Matovinovic, E. (2017). Scalpel versus electrosurgery for major abdominal incisions. *Cochrane Systematic Review, Cochrane Library, 6*.

Conway, N., Ong, P., White, N., & Rich C. (2019). Operating Department practice. Clinical Pocket Reference. 3rd Edition. Oxford.

Davis, N. B. (2009). Suturing materials and technique. In J. C. Rothrock, & P. C. Seifert (Eds.), *Assisting in surgery: patient-centered care* (pp. 195—242). Denver: Competency & Credentialing Institute.

Department of Health. (2011). *High impact intervention: care bundle to prevent surgical site infection*. Available from: < https://webarchive.nationalarchives.gov.uk/20120118171639/ http://hcai.dh.gov.uk/files/2011/03/2011-03-14-HII-Prevent-Surgical-Site-infection-FINAL.pdf >

Dorner, B., Posthauer, M. E., & Freidrich, E. (2016). Nutritional assessment and support in relation to wound healing. In D. Doughty, & L. L. McNichol (Eds.), *Wound management*. Philadelphia: Wolters Kluwer.

Dumville, J. C., McFarlane, E., Edwards, P., Lipp, A., & Holmes, A. (2013). Preoperative skin antiseptics for preventing surgical wound infections after clean surgery. *Cochrane Database of Systematic Reviews, 3*, CD003949.

Durai, R., Mowbah, A., & Ng, P. C. H. (2009). Use of drains in surgery: types, uses and complications. *AORN Journal, 91*, 266−271.

Durai, R., & Ng, P. C. (2010). Surgical vacuum draining; types, uses and complications. *AORN Journal, 91*, 266−271.

Ethicon. (2019a). *Sutures and wound closure.* Available from: < https://www.ethicon.com/na/epc/search/platform/wound%20closure?lang = en-default >

Ethicon. (2019b). *Wound closure.* Available from: < https://jnjinstitute.com/online-profed-resources/resources/wound-closure/suture-techniques-layer >

Findik, U. Y., Topcu. S. Y., & Vantansever, O. (2013). Effects of drains on pain, comfort and anxiety in patients undergone surgery. *International Journal of Caring Sciences, 6*(3), 412−419.

Flannigan, M. (2013). *Wound healing and skin integrity. Principles and practice.* Chichester: Wiley-Blackwell.

Goodman, T., & Spry, C. (2014). *Essentials of perioperative nursing* (5th ed.). Burlington MA: Jones and Bartlett Learning.

Haridas, M., & Malangoni, M. A. (2008). Predictive factors for surgical site infection in general surgery. *Surgery, 144*(4), 496−503.

Hazalina, N., Hussaine, N., Huda, N., Ali, M., & Ismail, G. (2011). *Tissue adhesives versus standard wound closure technique for laparoscopic procedure.* Lambert Academic Publishing.

Health Protection Scotland. (2014). *National infection prevention and control manual. Version 2.5.* Available from: < http://www.nhsdg.scot.nhs.uk/Departments_and_Services/Infection_Control/Infection_Control_Files/2.01_National_Infection_Control_Precautions.pdf >

Hess, C. (2010). Checklist for factors affecting wound healing. *Advances in Skin and Wound Care, 23*(4), 192.

Hussey, L., & Bagg, M. (2011). Principles of wound closure. *Operative Techniques in Sports Medicine, 19*, 206−211.

Ikeanyi, U. O., Chukwuka, C. N., & Chukwuanukwu, T. O. (2013). Risk factors for surgical site infections following clean orthopaedic operations.

Nigerian Journal of Clinical Practice, 16, 443−447.

Jaszarowski, K. A., & Murphee, R. W. (2016). Wound cleansing and dressing selection. In D. B. Doughty, & L. L. McNichol (Eds.), *Core curriculum: wound management.* Philadelphia: Wolters Kluwer.

JBI Library. (2011). A systemic review of surgical infection scoring system in surgical patients. *JBI Library of Systematic Reviews, 9*(60), 2627−2683.

Jenks, P. J., Laurant, M., McQuarry, C., & Watkins, R. (2012). Clinical and economical burden of surgical site infection (SSI) and predicted financial consequences of elimination of SSI from English hospital. *Journal of Medical Microbiology and Diagnosis, 1,* 111.

Kamel, C., McGrahan, L., Polisena, J., Mierzwinski-Urban, M., & Embil, J. M. (2012). Preoperative skin antiseptic preparations for preventing surgical site infections: a systematic review. *Infection Control & Hospital Epidemiology, 33,* 608−617.

Kanji, D., & Das, H. (2017). Advances of stem cell therapeutics in cutaneous wound healing and regeneration. *Mediators of Inflammation, 2017,* 5217967.

Kirk, R. M. (2010). *Basic surgical techniques* (6th ed.). Oxford: Elsevier Churchill Livingstone.

Leaper, D. J. (2010). Surgical site infection. *British Journal of Surgery, 97,* 1601−1602.

Mangram, A. J., Horan, T. C., Pearson, M. L., Silver, L. C., & Jarvis, W. R. (1999). Guideline for prevention of surgical site infection, 1999. Hospital Infection Control Practices Advisory Committee. *Infection Control and Hospital Epidemiology, 20,* 250−278.

Maroz, N., & Simman, R. (2014). Wound healing in patients with impaired kidney function. *Journal of American College of Clinical Wound Specialists, 5* (1), 2−7.

Montague, S. E., & Watson, R. (2005). *Physiology for nursing practice* (3rd ed). Oxford: Elsevier.

Moores, J. (2013). Vitamin C: a wound healing perspective. *British Journal of Community Nursing, Suppl*(Suppl12), S6, S8−11.

Morello, S. S. (2016). Skin and wound care for bariatric population. In D. B. Doughty, & L. L. McNichol (Eds.), *Core curriculum: wound management.* Philadelphia: Wolters Kluwer.

Mu, X., Wei, J., Wang, C., Ou, Y., Yin, D., Liang, B., et al. (2019). Intravenous administration of tranexamic acid significantly reduces visible and hidden blood loss compared with its topical administration for double-segment posterior lumbar interbody fusion: a single-center, placebo-controlled, randomized trial. *World Neurosurgery, 122,* e821−e827.

Mufti, A. (2016). Anatomy and physiology of the skin. In D. B. Doughty, & L. L. McNichol (Eds.), *Core curriculum: wound management.* Philadelphia: Wolters Kluwer.

National Institute for Health and Care Excellence. (2008). *Clinical guideline 74 − Surgical site infection: Prevention and treatment of surgical site infection.* London: National Collaborating Centre for Nursing and Supportive Care, NICE.

National Institute for Health and Care Excellence (NICE). (2013a). *Quality standard: Surgical site infection.* London: NICE.

National Institute for Health and Care Excellence (NICE). (2013b). *Surgical site infection: evidence update 43.* London: NICE, June 2013.

National Institute for Health and Care Excellence (NICE). (2017). *Surgical site infection: prevention and treatment.* Available from: < https://www.nice.org.uk/guidance/ng125 >

National Institute for Health and Care Excellence (NICE). (2018). *PICO negative pressure wound therapy for closed surgical incision wounds. Medtech innovation briefing (MIB 149).* London: NICE.

Netsch, D. S. (2016). Refractory wounds: assessment and management. In D. B. Doughty, & L. L. McNichol (Eds.), *Core curriculum: wound management.* Philadelphia: Wolters Kluwer.

Nicks, B., Ayello, E., Woo, K., Nitzia-George, D., & Sibbald, G. (2010). Acute wound management: revisiting the approach to assessment, irrigation, and closure considerations. *International Journal of Emergency Medicine, 3*(4), 399−407.

Nix, D., & Bryant, R. A. (2016). Fistula management. In D. B. Doughty, & L. L. McNichol (Eds.), *Core curriculum: wound management.* Philadelphia: Wolters Kluwer.

Nourian Dehkordi, A., Mirahmadi Babaheydari, F., Chehelgerdi, M., et al. (2019). Skin tissue engineering: Wound healing based on stem-cell-based therapeutic strategies. *Stem Cell Res Ther, 10,* 111.

Nursing and Midwifery Council. (2018). *The Code. Professional standards of practice and behaviour for nurses, midwives and nursing associates.* Available from: < https://www.nmc.org.uk/globalassets/sitedocuments/nmc-publications/nmc-code.pdf>

Peate, I., & Glencross, W. (2015). *Wound care at a glance.* Chichester: Wiley-Blackwell.

Peate, I., & Muralitharan, N. (2016). *Fundamentals of anatomy and physiology* (2nd ed). Chichester: Wiley Blackwell.

Penelope, J., Kallis, B. S., BA, & Friedman, A. J. (2018). Collagen powder in wound healing. *Journal of Drugs in Dermatology*, 17(4), 403–408.

Philips, N. (2012). *Berry and Kohn's operating room technique* (12th ed). St Louis: Elsevier.

Price, C. J., & Sinclair, R. (2008). *Fast facts: minor surgery* (2nd ed). Oxford: Health Press Limited.

Rajan, S. (2012). Skin and soft-tissue infections: classifying and treating a spectrum. *Cleveland Clinic Journal of Medicine*, 79(1), 57–66.

Rangara, A., Handy, K., & Leaper, D. (2011). Role of collagen in wound management. *Wounds UK*, 7(2), 54–63.

Ren, Z., Li, S., Sheng, L., Zhuang, Q., Li, Z., Xu, D., et al. (2017). Topical use of tranexamic acid can effectively decrease hidden blood loss during posterior lumbar spinal fusion surgery: A retrospective study. *Medicine*, 96(42), 1–4.

Rhee, C., Huang, S., Berrios-Torres, S., Kaganov, R., Bruce, C., Lankiewicz, J., et al. (2015). Surgical site infection surveillance following ambulatory surgery. *Infection Control and Hospital Epidemiology*, 36(2), 225–228.

Rosman, M., Rachminov, O., Segal, O., & Segal, G. (2015). Prolonged patients' in hospital waiting period after discharge eligibility is associated with increased risk of infection, morbidity and mortality: a retrospective cohort analysis. *BMC, Health Service Research*, 15, 246.

Scales, B., & Huffnagle, G. (2013). The microbiome in wound repair and tissue fibrosis. *The Journal of Pathology*, 229(2), 323–331.

Shiffman, M. A., & Low, M. (2019). *Burns, infections and wound management: recent clinical techniques, results and research in wounds.* Berlin: Springer.

Siddiqui, A., & Bernstein, J. (2010). Chronic wound infection: facts and controversies. *Clinics in Dermatology*, 28, 516–526.

Simpson, A., & Brooks, A. (2008). Surgical wounds. In A. Brooks, P. Mahoney, & B. Rowlands (Eds.), *ABC of tubes, drains, lines and frames.* Oxford: Blackwell.

Tanner, J., Khan, D., Aplin, C., Ball, J., Thomas, M., & Bankart, J. (2009). Post-discharge surveillance to identify colorectal surgical site infection rates and related costs. *Journal of Hospital Infection*, 72(3), 243–250.

Tickle, J. (2013). Wound care: quality dressing and assessment. *Nursing and Residential Care*, 16(9), 486–488.

Tortora, G., Berdell, R. F., & Case, C. L. (2014). Microbiology: an introduction ((12th ed). Pearson.

Tortora, G. J., & Derrickson, B. H. (2017). *Principles of anatomy and physiology* (15th ed). New Jersey: Wiley.

van Driessche, F. (2016). Wounds caused by infectious process. In D. B. Doughty, & L. L. McNichol (Eds.), *Core curriculum: wound management.* Philadelphia: Wolters Kluwer.

van Walraven, C., & Musselman, R. (2013). The Surgical Site Infection Risk Score (SSIRS): a model to predict the risk of surgical site infections. *PLoS One*, 8(6), e67167.

Vilar-Compte, D., Alvarez de Iturbe, I., Martin-Ornreat, A., et al. (2008). Hyperglycaemia as a risk factor for surgical site infection in patients undergoing mastectomy. *American Journal of Infection*, 36(3), 192–198.

Waugh, A., & Grant, A. (2018). *Ross & Wilson; Anatomy and physiology in health and illness* (13th ed.). Oxford: Elsevier.

Weir, D., & Schulz, G. (2016). Assessment and management of wound related infections. In D. B. Doughty, & L. L. McNichol (Eds.), *Core curriculum: wound management.* Philadelphia: Wolters Kluwer.

Wicker, P., & Dalby, S. (2017). *Rapid perioperative care.* Chichester: Wiley Blackwell.

Wicker, P., & O'Neil, J. (2010). *Caring for the perioperative patient* (2nd ed). London: Wiley-Blackwell.

Wilson, J. (2012). Surgical site infection: the principles and practice of surveillance. Part 1: Key concepts in the methodology of SSI surveillance. Surgical site infection: the principles and practice of surveillance. *Journal of Infection Prevention*, 14, 6–12.

Wilson, J., Topley, K., Stott, D., Neachell, J., & Gallagher, R. (2015). The OneTogether collaborative approach to reduce the risk of surgical site infection: identifying the challenges to assuring best practice. *Journal of Infection Prevention*, 16(3), 99–100.

Wound Healing. (2017). *Smoking negatively impacts on wound healing.* Available from: < https://advancedtissue.com/2017/03/smoking-negatively-impacts-wound-healing/>

Yesuel, E., & Kyong-Je, W. (2019). Negative pressure wound therapy for managing complicated wounds at extracorporeal membrane oxygenation sites. *Advances in Skin and Wound Care*, 32(4), 183–189.

Zinn, J. (2012). Surgical wound classification: communication is needed for accuracy. *AORN Journal*, 95(2), 274–278.

Zinn, J., & Swofford, V. (2014). Quality improvements initiative: classifying and documenting surgical wounds. *American Nurse Today*, 9(1). Available at: < https://www.americannurseto-day.com/quality-improvement-initiative-classifying-and-documenting-surgical-wounds/>.

Chapter | 6 |

Nutrition and the surgical patient

Helen Ord and Melanie Baker

KEY OBJECTIVES OF THE CHAPTER

The nurse will be able to promote recovery after surgery, and reduce the harmful effects of malnutrition, through understanding:

• the causes and consequences of malnutrition in the surgical patient
• identification of nutritional risk
• methods of preventing and treating malnutrition
• monitoring and evaluation of nutrition care.

Areas to think about before reading the chapter

• What do you understand by the term malnutrition?
• What factors can impact on the risk of malnutrition?
• Compare and contrast the role of the registered dietician and the registered nurse with regards to meeting the nutritional needs of the patient.

Introduction

The relationship between poor nutritional status and post-operative complications has been recognized for over 80 years (Studley, 1936). More recently, prospective studies have shown that malnutrition is negatively associated with surgical outcomes (Ho et al, 2015; Panis et al, 2011).

Of all healthcare professionals, nurses have the most constant contact with patients and play a pivotal role in identifying nutritional problems, and ensuring the delivery of adequate nutrition from a variety of routes. Communicating nursing observations and evaluation of care to doctors, dietitians, pharmacists and other professionals is equally important as direct nursing interaction with patients, in ensuring good nutrition.

This chapter aims to provide background information on the causes and consequences of malnutrition in surgical patients, highlighting the importance of assessing nutritional risk and providing adequate nutrition in the surgical patient. It will describe ways in which nurses can take a proactive role in the planning, delivery and evaluation of nutritional care.

Malnutrition

Malnutrition can be defined as a state of nutrition in which a deficiency or excess (or imbalance) of energy, protein and other nutrients causes measurable adverse effects on tissue/body form (body shape, size and composition) function and clinical outcome (Elia, 2003). It is under-nutrition (rather than over-nutrition) which is the key focus and concern within this chapter.

It is estimated that malnutrition affects more than three million people in the UK, the overall mean prevalence of 'malnutrition' in patients admitted to UK hospitals is reported as 29%, although it is higher in older people. More specifically, the prevalence on surgical wards is reported as 26% (Russell & Elia, 2014).

Malnutrition can be very difficult to recognize, particularly in patients who are overweight or obese to start with. Malnutrition can happen very gradually, which can make it very difficult to spot in the early stages. Key causes of malnutrition in the surgical patient include:

- Diagnosis or type of surgery may increase a patient's likelihood of developing malnutrition.
- Underlying disease process causing a reduction in food intake and/or increased nutrient losses.
- The metabolic response to trauma and surgery.
- Enforced periods of nil by mouth.
- Reduced appetite and nutritional intake, which may be further affected by pain, nausea anxiety and depression.
- Unfamiliar or unappetizing hospital food.

There are also many social factors, such as poverty and social isolation, that can increase the risk of malnutrition. High-risk groups include older people (over the age of 65 years), those with long-term conditions or chronic progressive conditions and when there is substance abuse (Bapen, 2018).

Malnutrition affects every system in the body and is a risk factor for postoperative complications. The adverse effects of malnutrition include impaired immune response, reduced muscle strength, impaired or prolonged wound healing, surgical wound dehiscence, anastomotic breakdown, development of post-surgical fistulae and increased risk of wound infection (Sanders et al, 2019; Verma et al, 2018; Llop et al, 2012). In addition, the undernourished patient is often apathetic, with little desire to eat and drink, or engage in other therapeutic activities. Malnutrition leads to greater healthcare use (including hospital (re)admissions, longer hospital stays, more GP visits, increased prescription costs). Expenditure associated with malnutrition in adults and children in England in 2011–2012 was estimated to be £19.6 billion, or about 15% of the total expenditure on health and social care, and with the ageing population this is set to increase (Elia, 2015).

Identifying patients at risk of malnutrition

Nutritional screening

Early identification of patients who are nutritionally depleted (or likely to become so) is vital. There is no one single objective test that can accurately define whether a patient is malnourished. This has led to the development of nutritional screening tools and there are a wide variety of tools available, with most considering current weight and height (body mass index, BMI, in kg/m^2), recent unintentional weight loss and likelihood of further future weight loss. This may be due to inadequate nutritional intake or those patients who have poor absorptive capacity, and/or high nutrient losses and/or have increased nutritional needs from causes such as catabolism.

NICE (2006) recommend using the *Malnutrition Universal Screening Tool (MUST)* (Elia, 2003), a validated tool designed to be used across all care settings (Fig. 6.1). The scores for BMI, unplanned weight loss and acute illness with current nutritional intake are added to provide a low-, medium- or high-risk grading for malnutrition, from which specific management guidelines can be instituted. All patients should be screened, and screening should occur on first contact with the patient and at regular intervals thereafter (NICE, 2006; NICE, 2012; Department of Health, 2014). Nutritional screening in the surgical patient will help ensure nutritional therapy is started early, and as soon as a nutritional risk becomes apparent.

Nutritional assessment

Nutritional screening will identify patients who require a more detailed, in-depth evaluation of nutritional status. This should be performed by an expert such as a dietitian. Clinical situation, physical state, diet, anthropometric measurements (such as measures of fat and muscle stores or muscle function) and biochemical markers should all be considered. A nutritional assessment determines to what extent an individual's nutritional needs have been or are being met and is followed by a plan of how the shortfall can be provided.

The nutritional needs of the surgical patient

When nutritional intake is inadequate to meet needs, the body breaks down its own tissues to provide the necessary energy/nutrients for the body's functions. In simple starvation, metabolic adaptations occur with the utilization of adipose tissue fat to meet energy requirements. As starvation continues, the metabolic rate falls as the body tries to conserve depleted tissues, but there is a breakdown of the body's protein stores, initially from skeletal muscle. Without food, death would occur within 40–60 days (Pichard & Jeejeebhoy, 1994).

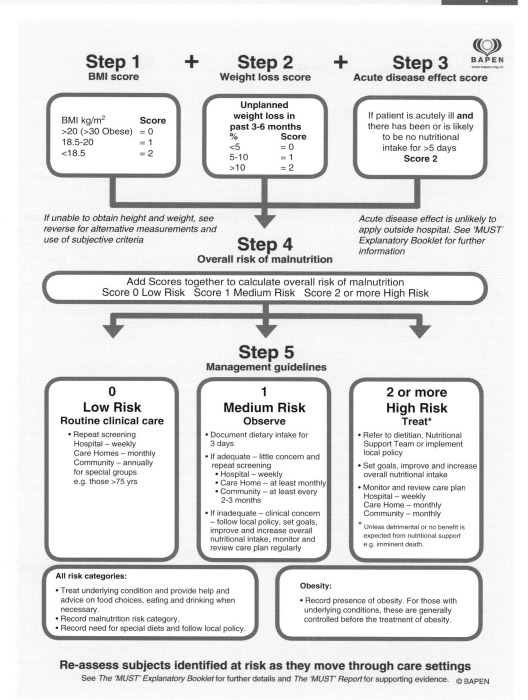

Figure 6.1 The 'MUST' flow chart summarizes the calculation of the 'MUST score'.
The 'Malnutrition Universal Screening Tool' ('MUST') is reproduced here with the kind permission of BAPEN (British Association for Parenteral and Enteral Nutrition). For further information on 'MUST', see www.bapen.org.uk. Copyright BAPEN (2012).

In contrast to simple starvation, trauma and surgery causes a metabolic stress response, causing catabolism of the body's stores of fat, protein and glycogen to release substrates used in the healing and immune response. This results in a loss of muscle tissue during a time when nutritional intake is often also impaired.

In elective surgery measures can be taken to reduce surgical stress, of which nutritional considerations are paramount. Enhanced Recovery After Surgery (ERAS) programmes are designed to help recovery and consider pre-surgical nutritional optimization, limiting preoperative fasting, carbohydrate loading and early reintroduction of nutrition post operation (Varadhan et al, 2010).

Nutritional requirements

Energy

During the catabolic phase of illness (following trauma, surgery or during sepsis/infection), metabolic rate is increased and energy requirements have been shown to be elevated (Barak et al, 2002). While the provision of nutritional support during this time is important, it cannot prevent the metabolic changes seen. The aim should be to provide balanced nutritional support to reduce the loss of lean body mass, while avoiding the negative effects of overfeeding.

Malnourished individuals who continue to have no/inadequate nutritional intake are at risk of metabolic complications when re-fed (commonly referred to as refeeding syndrome) (Friedli et al, 2017). Clinical and biochemical abnormalities — acute micronutrient deficiencies (especially B vitamins), fluid and electrolyte imbalance (hypophosphataemia, hypokalaemia, hypomagnesaemia) and disturbances of organ function (cardiac failure) — may occur when excessive, imbalanced nutritional support is given to malnourished patients. It is important to introduce nutritional support slowly (whether it is given via the oral, enteral or parenteral nutrition route) alongside biochemical monitoring (NICE, 2006).

After the catabolic phase of illness, the individual enters the recovery phase, when they are no longer hypermetabolic and can utilize additional nutrients. In this stage it is appropriate to increase intake to replenish the body's stores of lean and fat mass. More recently, interventions that combine both nutritional support and physical activity to promote a return to normal function have been investigated in surgical and cancer populations (Hall et al, 2018).

Protein

Protein is made up of chains of amino acids, and makes up the main structural and functional components of all cells in the body. Proteins within the body are continuously being broken down and resynthesized and this balance is altered by trauma or surgery. Attempts to restore lean body (muscle) mass and improve nitrogen balance by giving large amounts of protein and energy may result in complications such as hyperglycaemia, and have been shown to have no additional benefit over giving standard amounts (Ishibashi et al, 1998).

Levels of blood proteins such as albumin/pre-albumin were historically used as a marker of malnutrition. Albumin levels often fall post-surgery (Cuthbertson & Tompsett, 1935) or during trauma or infection when inflammatory markers (such as white cell count and C-reactive protein) are raised (Fleck et al, 1985). Malnourished patients due to starvation often maintain a normal albumin level (Lee et al, 2015); therefore, in catabolic surgical patients a low albumin level is more likely to indicate severity of illness than simply malnutrition.

Fluid and electrolytes

Water is an essential component of body tissues, constituting approximately 50%—70% of the total body weight, within cells or as extracellular fluid. Fluid is ingested as fluid drunk and in food eaten or provided by other routes such as in enteral tube feeds or intravenous fluids. It is excreted in urine, faeces, sweat from the skin and is exhaled from the lungs. Surgical patients may have increased losses of fluid and electrolytes from drains, stoma, fistulae which must be adequately recorded and replaced appropriately.

It is common after surgical intervention for a patient to be given intravenous (IV) fluids. Although large volumes may be required to restore blood volume during surgery, the excessive provision of IV fluids postoperatively (particularly those high in sodium, such as 0.9% sodium chloride (saline)) has been shown to increase complications (Brandstrup et al, 2003). Postoperative fluid overload can result in oedema and delay in the return of normal gastrointestinal function (gastric emptying and passing of bowel motions) (Lobo et al, 2002).

It is vital that a patient's fluid and electrolyte needs are assessed on an individual basis, and the nurse has a key role in ensuring that IV fluids are not used indiscriminately. Detailed fluid balance charts should be kept, although these do not take into account insensible losses (such as sweat). Regular (daily) measurements of body weight are the best clinical measure of fluid balance but are often not routinely undertaken in hospital patients.

Micronutrients

Adequate quantities of vitamins and minerals are essential for optimal functioning of the body. Micronutrient deficiencies are common, especially in certain populations such as the elderly (Finch et al, 1998). In the surgical patient, absorption of micronutrients may be reduced by malabsorption, poor gastrointestinal motility, or loss of intestinal mucosa. Some micronutrients such as vitamin C (ascorbic acid) and zinc are essential for wound healing.

Patients should be taking a minimum of 100% of daily recommended amounts of micronutrients, and, whenever possible, this should be met by intake of food and fluids. Where dietary intake is inadequate or requirements are raised, a multivitamin and mineral preparation may be necessary to ensure an adequate intake. The use of single nutrient supplements should be avoided where possible, due to potential problems with toxicity, drug nutrient interactions and competing bioavailability, but may be required to correct confirmed deficiencies. Generally there is no benefit to be gained from excess or 'mega-doses' of vitamins or minerals. Guidance on safe upper levels for vitamins and minerals is given by the Food Standards Agency (FSA, 2003).

The evidence for nutritional support in the surgical patient

Preoperative nutritional support

If a severely malnourished patient requires surgical intervention, attempts should be made to provide a period of nutritional support, although improving nutritional status may be difficult due to the underlying disease process, such as cancer or inflammatory bowel disease (Weimann et al, 2017).

Traditionally, patients used to be fasted for at least 12 hours preoperatively. These delays have been shown to be unnecessary and most patients should now be allowed clear fluids until 2 hours before anaesthesia (Brady et al, 2003).

Postoperative nutritional support

The European Society of Parenteral & Enteral Nutrition (ESPEN) recommend that oral nutritional supplements or enteral tube feeding should be provided if it is anticipated that the patient will be unable to eat for more than 5 days or for those who cannot maintain oral intakes above 50% for more than 7 days (Weimman et al, 2017).

Timing of postoperative nutritional support

Historically, surgeons instigated strict protocols for the reintroduction of oral fluids/diet postoperatively, particularly after gastrointestinal surgery, normally starting with

small amounts of water (30−60 mL/h), before proceeding on to free fluids and a 'light diet' once bowel function has returned. Although there is no universal definition of a 'light diet', this often consists of foods which have a moderate fat and low fibre content, such as soup, eggs, fish, potatoes, yoghurt and ice cream. Although this practice is common, the benefits have never been confirmed by research. More recently, studies have compared early reintroduction of fluids/diet with routine care in surgical patients and in most cases oral nutrition can be reintroduced without delay (Lewis et al, 2001).

In some instances, such as following major upper gastrointestinal surgery (e.g. oesophagectomy or total gastrectomy), delays in resuming oral intake do occur and other forms of nutritional support should be considered. The use of enteral feeding tubes placed into the small bowel (nasojejunal or jejunostomy tubes inserted in the operating theatre) allows early postoperative feeding but variable practices exist regarding their routine use (Weijs et al, 2015).

Methods of nutritional support

It is not always easy for patients to meet their nutritional requirements. Once vulnerable patients have been identified, implementing a nutrition care plan and improving nutrient intake is essential to improve outcomes. The objectives of nutritional support in the surgical patient are to improve or maintain nutritional status, enhance wound healing, reduce postoperative complications and reduce the period of convalescence. Nutritional support can be provided by:

- oral intake: food and drink, oral liquid supplements
- enteral tube feeding: nasogastric, gastrostomy or jejunostomy
- parenteral feeding: via a central or peripheral vein.

Improving oral dietary intake

Treatment should always be tailored to the needs of the individual, but in general, if a person is able to swallow and digest food then the first step would to encourage this with a 'food first' approach. Recognizing the problem is an important first step. Once individuals and those involved in their care are aware of the problem, often simple measures to increase food intake may be enough to significantly improve nutritional intake. For success these have to be consistently delivered by the whole ward team, and good communication with all those who provide food to the patient will be required. There are many measures that can be taken at ward level to help improve a patient's food intake, including:

- *Food selection*. If a patient is helped to make a choice from the hospital menu, then it is more likely to be something they will eat, and be in line with their food preferences, ethnic and cultural needs. Specific dietary needs of the patient must be considered and there must be robust systems to ensure these are provided for (this would include, for example, patients with coeliac disease, food allergies, renal impairment, and diabetes). Patients with poor appetites should be encouraged to choose the high-calorie, high-protein options. Foods such as soup and ice cream on a hospital menu often provide only small amounts of protein and calories, and patients taking just these choices are unlikely to be meeting their nutritional requirements.
- *The ordering process*. Think about how the meal-ordering process will work for those patients you offer care to. Nutritionally vulnerable patients can often find this challenging, and those who are confused, have dementia or difficulty communicating their needs may require additional support or systems put in place. A meal planner sheet can be a useful resource that the patient's relatives and carers can help populate, and can then be used to ensure suitable choices are ordered.
- *Missed meals*. If a meal is missed (because the patient is away from the ward) then a replacement should be available. (If a hot meal is not available then a sandwich or snack box alternative should be provided.)
- *Provide encouragement*. Taking time to explain to patients that eating well will aid their recovery and demonstrating its importance by providing lots of encouragement can help.
- *Small frequent meals with snacks in between*. If a patient has a poor appetite they are probably not going to eat all the food available at a meal. It is far better to encourage a 'little and often' approach. High-energy and high-protein snacks should be available between meals to enhance dietary intake over the day. Some patients find that they are able to eat more at certain times of day and the most successful plan will take this into consideration.
- *Assistance with feeding*. Assistance with eating is important in improving food intake. A red tray system has been used as a way of identifying a patient who needs assistance and ensuring communication to all members of staff on the ward that help is needed (Age Concern, 2006; Bradley & Rees, 2003). The level of help required by patients can vary; some may just need the packaging opened, or adaptive cutlery, while others will require someone to feed them. Reports still highlight that patients are not always getting the support they need at mealtimes (Vizard & Burchard, 2015).

- *Consider the positioning of the food and the patient*. Studies have shown that placing food outside a patient's reach is not uncommon, and that trays of food are later removed untouched (Age Concern, 2006). Eating in bed can be difficult, and it is important that food intake is not limited by an inability to access the meal.
- *Speak to relatives*. Relatives are often happy to do what they can to help, providing extra encouragement and suitable foods from home. They can often provide useful information about which nutritional strategies will help.
- *Treat underlying conditions*. Ill-fitting dentures or inadequate oral status may be causing difficulties, and dental advice may help overcome these problems. Nausea, vomiting, constipation and depression all have an effect on food intake. Treatment with antiemetics, laxatives, antidepressants or appetite stimulants may be helpful.
- *Environment*. Food presentation, and the immediate environment with its smells, sounds and sights, can all have a big impact on the amount of food eaten. The idea of 'protected meal times' has been introduced to reduce non-urgent clinical activity at meal times to enable patients to eat their meal without interruption and to allow nurses time to supervise meals and offer assistance. Areas where this system has been instigated report a positive effect on patient care (National Patient Safety Agency [NPSA], 2008).
- *Nourishing drinks*. Drinks that are a better source of nourishment than just tea, coffee or water should be encouraged. This may include: full-cream milk; milky drinks such as drinking chocolate or malted milk drinks; soup, especially condensed or 'cream of' varieties; or milk-based supplement drinks (e.g. Complan, Aymes Retail, Meritene strength and vitality). These can be offered between meals, or when meals cannot be managed.
- *Document food intake*. It can be difficult to get a clear picture of the amount of food being consumed, as different members of staff will be involved in meal delivery and collection over the course of a day. Documentation of food intake should be made at the end of each meal, before it is removed, clearly describing what has been eaten, and the amount. The Nursing and Midwifery Council (NMC) (2018) make it clear in the Code that nurses must ensure that the care they offer people is recorded clearly, accurately and relevant to practice. These charts should then be reviewed to see if the food eaten is providing adequate nutrition for the patient. In cases of inadequacy a referral to a dietitian should be made. An appreciation of the amount and type of food a patient should be having is important. The 'Eatwell Guide' demonstrates

the types of food that should be eaten to provide a balanced intake (Public Health England, 2016). Completion of a food record chart is often considered a role for everyone to assist with; it is important to ensure it is not overlooked.

Improving food intake takes patience and good multidisciplinary teamwork. For success, it is important that nutrition and hydration are considered essential care, and as vital as medication and other types of treatment (Royal College of Nursing, 2011). It should not be underestimated how much difference lots of small simple changes can make to a patient's intake over the course of a day. It is important that when progress remains a concern, despite these measures, referral is made to a specialist.

There are four key themes associated with the Code (NMC, 2018). The nurse must prioritize people, practise effectively, preserve safety and promote professionalism and trust. The four themes are all relevant in ensuring that the patient's nutritional needs are met.

Nutritional supplements

If the shortfall in nutrients cannot be met by food alone, oral nutritional supplements can be used, some of which are prescribable. The benefits of oral nutritional supplements in both hospital and community settings have been shown, improving energy and protein intakes, body composition, function and clinical outcome (Stratton et al, 2003). There are many steps that can be taken to help with patient concordance, and ensure that the potential benefit from the supplement is realized.

Many of the supplement drinks taste much better when chilled, so giving them to patients from the fridge when they are ready to drink them is best. Patients may need assistance with opening cartons, and they should be given out at an appropriate time – between meals is usually best. It also helps to present the supplement positively, explaining about its contents and how it will help recovery. Many patients find that they prefer to sip these slowly over a period of time (check manufacturer's guidance on how long they can be left at ward temperature for). Most supplements will be available in a range of flavours, and it is important to find those which suit the patient. In addition to supplement drinks, powders, puddings and small-volume shots are available.

Oral nutritional supplements have a role in the treatment of surgical patients, but should be used once food intake has been properly assessed and nutritional goals set. A dietitian's input will ensure the most appropriate products are used.

Enteral tube feeding

The provision of enteral nutrition via the placement of feeding tubes into the stomach (nasogastric or gastrostomy) or the small intestine (nasojejunal or jejunostomy) may be necessary in patients who have a functional gastrointestinal tract and are:

- unable to eat, e.g. due to oral surgery, upper gastrointestinal surgery or dysphagia
- able to eat but not in sufficient amounts to achieve an adequate nutritional intake, e.g. severely malnourished patients; those with raised requirements due to malabsorption; or those who have undergone gastrointestinal surgery and have a limited capacity to eat.

The choice of feeding tube is dependent on numerous factors, including the patient's anatomy, expected length of treatment, comfort, and the expertise of the clinician placing the tube. Management requirements of each type of enteral feeding tube also differ, for example how the tube is replaced if it becomes displaced will depend on whether it was initially placed at the bedside or via endoscopy, radiological or surgical placement and how it is retained (internal balloon or sutured).

Nasogastric feeding

A nasogastric tube (NGT) is often used when tube feeding is required for a period of less than 3–4 weeks. A NGT used for administration of nutrition, fluid and/or medication should be EnFIT compliant (not IV compatible) (International Standard (ISO) 80369-3). For most patients a fine-bore tube is used. During placement, tubes may coil in the pharynx or pass into the respiratory system; therefore, gastric placement must be confirmed prior to use by either testing the pH of the aspirate or performing a chest X-ray (NHS Improvement, 2016). The safe range for pH is 0–5.5 (NPSA, 2005). Although an abdominal X-ray used to be considered the gold standard, it only confirms the position of the tube at the time of the procedure. Auscultation is not reliable and must never be used as the sole method of confirming tube position (Methany et al, 1990).

Gastrostomy feeding

When longer-term feeding is anticipated, a gastrostomy tube may be placed directly into the stomach, during surgery or under radiological or endoscopic control. The latter tube is known as a percutaneous endoscopic gastrostomy (PEG). The tube is held in the stomach by an internal flange or balloon, and an external retention device prevents internal migration of the tube.

Contraindications to PEG placement include previous gastric surgery, obstruction to the oesophagus (such as cancer) and clotting disorders. Goals of therapy, the expected length of treatment and the longer-term impact of using the feeding tube should be considered prior to placement. It is recommended that patients are referred to a multidisciplinary team for assessment to avoid complications/inappropriate placements (National Confidential Enquiry into Patient Outcome And Death, 2004).

Postpyloric feeding

Enteral feeding beyond the stomach may be used to allow feeding after upper gastrointestinal surgery (oesophagectomy), or in situations where there is a delay in gastric emptying.

Tubes may be introduced through the nose and advanced through the pylorus for nasoduodenal or nasojejunal feeding. Double-lumen tubes are available which allow duodenal/jejunal feeding in conjunction with gastric aspiration.

Longer-term tubes inserted directly into the jejunum and brought out through the anterior abdominal wall are useful for patients who have undergone surgery to the stomach or have pyloric obstruction.

Administration of enteral feeding

There are several methods available to administer enteral feed and the most appropriate method should be assessed on an individual basis. Enteral feed can be given either via an electronic feeding pump or using an enteral syringe.

- *Enteral feeding pump.* This method is commonly used for patients starting enteral tube feeding, for patients in intensive care, or for patients with poor tolerance. It avoids the administration of a large volume of feed into the gastrointestinal tract at one time. Common infusion rates are 25–100 mL/hr. Patients are normally fed for 18–24 hours a day but feeding can be given for shorter infusion periods. Overnight feeding may be used to supplement a patient's oral intake.
- *Bolus feeding.* This involves the administration of 200–400 mL of feed via a syringe. Feed or fluid is either poured into the syringe, which is attached to the giving set and the clamp released to allow it to flow through, or the feed is drawn up into the syringe and then slowly pushed into the feeding tube over 15–30 minutes, depending on the volume and patient tolerance. This technique is not common in the hospital setting but it does mimic normal eating patterns more and allows greater flexibility of movement for the patient. This technique is rarely used in patients being fed directly into their small bowel, as the stomach reservoir has been bypassed.

Additional fluids can be given as water flushes during the day and help prevent tube blockages. If medicines are to be administered via the enteral feeding tube, liquid preparations should be used and there should be liaison with the pharmacy regarding the route and mode of action (i.e. it may not be suitable to give some drugs via the jejunal route).

Enteral feed is a sterile, specifically designed nutritional liquid that is licensed to be administered via an enteral feeding tube. A variety of different enteral feeding formulations are available with different nutritional profiles (such as high energy, fibre-containing). Some are designed to be better tolerated for some patients, such as peptide-based feeds for patients with reduced pancreatic function/malabsorption. All patients' enteral feeding regimen should be designed following an individual assessment, although standard protocols may be used in certain situations such as during the first few days of enteral feeding or in critical care.

Parenteral nutrition

Parenteral feeding is the provision of nutrients directly into the bloodstream, bypassing ingestion, digestion and absorption. It is indicated where there is a failure of intestinal function to a degree where nutrients cannot be delivered or adequately absorbed via oral or enteral nutrition (NICE, 2006). Surgical patients who may require parenteral feeding include those who:

- have an intestinal fistula or perforation necessitating bowel rest
- have pre- or postoperative bowel obstruction
- have undergone extensive surgical resection resulting in a short bowel
- have a paralytic ileus
- are intolerant to enteral feeding, e.g. uncontrolled vomiting or diarrhoea.

Although it is an effective method of nutritional support, it should only be used under the guidance of an expert nutritional support or intestinal failure team, as it is associated with life-threatening septic, metabolic and thrombotic complications. Parenteral nutrition may be administered via a central or peripheral vein. The choice is dictated by venous access, the predicted length of treatment and the patient's nutritional requirements. Ideally, a single-lumen dedicated catheter of known history should be used, accessed by nursing staff trained in aseptic techniques, (Loveday et al, 2014). Strict protocols for managing patients on parenteral nutrition should be adhered to at all times.

Parenteral nutrition bags should be made in an aseptic unit in the pharmacy, with ideally no further additions made at ward level. While a range of 'all in one' off-the-shelf bags are available, these do not contain micronutrients and are not recommended unless further additions are made (NICE, 2006). The high strength (hypertonicity) of some parenteral nutrition fluids necessitates their administration via the central venous route, where rapid dilution occurs due to the high blood flow. Other, less hypertonic mixtures are available for short-term peripheral administration but these may not meet the patient's full nutritional and electrolyte requirements.

Most causes of intestinal failure are short term and self-limiting but some patients may require parenteral nutrition for prolonged periods and these are often very ill, with multiple clinical problems. Emotional support for the patient and family is vital, as poor morale can be a major problem. Patients requiring long-term parenteral nutrition at home may wish to contact a patient support group such as Patients on Intravenous and Nasogastric Nutrition Treatment (www.PINNT.com).

Ethics

Ethical considerations underpin every aspect of nutritional care. Nutritional screening is an ethical action because failure to identify and treat malnourished patients has been shown to increase the risk of complications. When planning care, the wishes of the patient are paramount and health professionals must carefully explain, in an unbiased and clear way, the rationale for any proposed nutritional therapy. A patient who is competent to make an informed decision regarding their care may refuse any intervention, and sensitivity is needed to determine the reason why. In current English law, feeding through a tube is viewed as medical therapy. As with any other medical intervention, the benefit must be balanced against the risk or burden it imposes. Complex situations, such as artificial feeding when patients are approaching the end of life or when they lack capacity, are often helped by establishing a goal for nutritional management, assisted by an ethical framework (Royal College of Physicians, 2010; British Medical Association, 2018).

Monitoring nutritional support

Monitoring is important to ensure administration of nutritional support is effective and safe, and to detect and treat any complications. Individual monitoring plans will take into consideration the underlying diagnosis of the patient, aims of treatment and the route/type of feeding and encompass an assessment of nutritional status (weight, anthropometric measures), nutritional intake, hydration status, laboratory measures (serum biochemistry), and if applicable any concerns with gastrointestinal tolerance and the enteral/parenteral feeding device (NICE, 2006). The compliance, acceptability, and effectiveness against goals need to be measured; this will help decide if the current strategy is still required or other forms need to be considered.

SUMMARY OF KEY POINTS

- Good nutritional status is essential to reduce complications, promote wound healing and reduce length of hospital stay.
- Malnutrition is common, under-recognized and undertreated in surgical patients.
- All surgical patients should undergo nutritional screening prior to and after surgery.
- Any patient identified as malnourished, or at risk of becoming malnourished, must have an individualized care plan to address their needs which should be regularly reviewed.
- The provision of nutritional support may be (a) oral: diet and nutritional supplements; (b) enteral tube feeding; or (c) parenteral feeding.
- Malnourished patients should have access to a dietitian and specialist hospital nutrition team.

REFLECTIVE LEARNING POINTS

Having read this chapter, think about what you now know and what you still need to find out about. These questions may help:

- What strategy would you employ in order to encourage a person who has recently undergone gastrointestinal surgery to eat and drink?
- How is a person's nutritional status assessed in the care area where you are working?
- Undertake a literature review regarding the safe and effective evidence-based method of ensuring that a nasogastric tube has been correctly placed or when parenteral nutrition is indicated in surgical patients.

References

Age Concern. (2006). *Hungry to be heard. The scandal of malnourished older people in hospital*. London: Age Concern. Available at: < https://www.ageuk.org. uk/documents/en-gb/hungry_to_be_ heard_inf.pdf?dtrk = true > .

Barak, N., Wall-Alonso, E., & Sitrin, M. D. (2002). Evaluation of stress factors and body weight adjustments currently used to estimate energy expenditure in hospitalised patients. *JPEN Journal of Parenteral and Enteral Nutrition, 26*(4), 231–238.

Bradley, L., & Rees, C. (2003). Reducing nutritional risk in hospital: the red tray. *Nursing Standard*, 17(26), 33–37.

Brady, M., Kinn, S., & Stuart, P. (2003). Preoperative fasting for adults to prevent perioperative complications. *The Cochrane Database of Systematic Reviews* (4), CD004423.

Brandstrup, B., Tonnesen, H., Beier-Holgersen, R., et al. (2003). Effects of intravenous fluid restriction on postoperative complications: comparison of two perioperative fluid regimens: a randomised assessor-blinded multicenter trial. *Annals of Surgery*, 238(5), 641–648.

British Association Parenteral and Enteral Nutrition (BAPEN). (2018). *Introduction to malnutrition: Who is at risk?* Available at: < https://www.bapen.org.uk/malnutrition-undernutrition/introduction-to-malnutrition?start = 1 >

British Medical Association. (2018). Clinically-assisted nutrition and hydration guidance. Available at: < https://www.bma.org.uk/advice/employment/ethics/mental-capacity/clinically-assisted-nutrition-and-hydration/clinically-assisted-nutrition-and-hydration-canh-guidance >

Cuthbertson, D. P., & Tompsett, S. L. (1935). Note on the effect of injury on the level of plasma proteins. *British Journal of Experimental Pathology*, 16, 417–475.

Department of Health. (2014). *The Hospital Food Standards Panel's report on standards for food and drink in NHS hospitals.* London: Department of Health.

Elia, M. (2003). *The MUST Report. Nutritional screening for adults: A multidisciplinary responsibility. A report by the Malnutrition Advisory Group of the British Association for Parenteral and Enteral Nutrition.* Available at: < https://www.bapen.org.uk/screening-and-must/must/must-report >

Elia, M. (2015). *The cost of malnutrition in England and potential cost savings from nutritional interventions, on behalf of BAPEN.* Redditch: BAPEN.

Finch, S., Doyle, W., Lowe, C., et al. (1998). *National diet and nutrition survey: Older people aged 65 years and over. Volume 1: Report of the diet and nutrition survey.* London: HMSO.

Fleck, A., Colley, C. M., & Myer, M. A. (1985). Liver export proteins and trauma. *British Medical Bulletin*, 41(3), 265–273.

Food Standards Agency (FSA). (2003). *Safe upper levels for vitamin and minerals. Expert Group on Vitamin and Minerals.* London: FSA.

Friedli, N., Stanga, Z., Sobotka, L., et al. (2017). Revisiting the refeeding syndrome: Results of a systematic review. *Nutrition*, 35, 151–160.

Hall, C., Norris, L., Dixon, L., et al. (2018). A randomized, phase II, unblinded trial of an Exercise and Nutrition-based Rehabilitation programme (ENeRgy) versus standard care in patients with cancer: Feasibility trial protocol. *Pilot Feasibility Studies*, 27(4), 192.

Ho, J. W., Wu, A. H., Lee, M. W., Lau, S. Y., Lam, P. S., Lau, W. S., et al. (2015). Malnutrition risk predicts surgical outcome in patients undergoing gastrointestinal operations: Results of a prospective study. *Clinical Nutrition*, 34 (4), 679–684.

Ishibashi, N., Plank, L., Sando, K., et al. (1998). Optimal protein requirements during the first 2 weeks after the onset of critical illness. *Critical Care Medicine*, 26(9), 1529–1535.

Lee, J. L., Oh, E. S., Lee, R. W., et al. (2015). Serum albumin and pre-albumin in calorically restricted, non-diseased individuals: A systemic review. *The American Journal of Medicine*, 128 (9), 1023.e1–22.

Lewis, S. J., Egger, M., Sylvester, P. A., et al. (2001). Enteral feeding versus "nil by mouth" after gastrointestinal surgery: systematic review and meta-analysis of controlled trials. *BMJ*, 323, 773.

Llop, J. M., Cobo, S., Padulles, A., et al. (2012). Nutritional support and risk factors of appearance of enterocutaneous fistulas. *Nutrition in Hospital*, 27 (1), 213–218.

Lobo, D. N., Bostock, K. A., Neal, K. R., et al. (2002). Effect of salt and water balance on recovery of gastrointestinal function after elective colonic resection: a randomised controlled trial. *Lancet*, 359(9320), 1812–1818.

Loveday, H. P., Wilson, J. A., Pratt, R. J., et al. (2014). epic3: National Evidence-Based Guidelines for preventing healthcare-associated infections in NHS Hospitals in England. *Journal of Hospital Infection*, 86, S1–S70.

Methany, M., McSweeney, M., Wehrle, M. A., et al. (1990). Effectiveness of the auscultatory method in predicting feeding tube location. *Nursing Research*, 39 (5), 262–267.

National Confidential Enquiry into Patient Outcome and Death. (2004). *Scoping our practice: The 2004 report.* Available at: < www.ncepod.org.uk/2004report/index.htm >

National Health Service Improvement. (2016). *Nasogastric tube misplacement continuing risk of death and severe harm.* Available at: < https://improvement.nhs.uk/news-alerts/nasogastric-tube-misplacement-continuing-risk-of-death-severe-harm/ >

National Institute for Health and Care Excellence (NICE). (2006). *Nutrition support for adults: Oral nutritional support, enteral tube feeding and parenteral nutrition.* London: NICE.

National Institute for Health and Care Excellence (NICE). (2012). *Nutrition support in adults. Quality standard [QS24].* London: NICE.

National Patient Safety Agency. (2005). *Patient Safety Alert 05: Advice to the NHS on Reducing Harm Caused by the Misplacement of Nasogastric Feeding Tubes.* Available at: < http://www.npsa.nhs.uk/patientsafety/alerts-and-directives/alerts/nasogastric-feeding-tubes/ >

National Patient Safety Agency (NPSA). (2008). *Protected meal times: Findings and recommendations report.* Available at: < www.npsa.nhs.uk/nrls/improvingpatientsaftey/cleaning-and-nutrition/nutrition/protectedmealtimes/ >

Nursing and Midwifery Council. (2018). *The Code. Professional standards of practice and behaviour for nurses, midwives and nursing associates.* Available at: < https://www.nmc.org.uk/standards/code/ >

Panis, Y., Maggiori, L., Caranhac, G., et al. (2011). Mortality after colorectal cancer surgery: a French survey of more than 84,000 patients. *Annals of Surgery*, 254(5), 738–743.

Pichard, C., & Jeejeebhoy, K. N. (1994). Nutritional management of clinical undernutrition. In J. S. Garrow, & W. P. T. James (Eds.), *Human nutrition and dietetics* (9th ed.). Edinburgh: Churchill Livingstone.

Public Health England. (2016). *The eatwell guide.* Available at: < https://www.gov.uk/government/publications/the-eatwell-guide >

Royal College of Nursing. (2011). *Nutrition now: Enhancing nutritional care.* London: RCN.

Royal College of Physicians. (2010). *Oral feeding difficulties and dilemmas: a guide to practical care, particularly towards the end of life.* London: Royal College Physicians.

Russell, C. A., & Elia, M. (2014). *Nutrition screening survey in hospitals in the UK, 2007–11. A report by BAPEN.* Redditch: BAPEN.

Sanders, J., Smith, T., & Stroud, M. (2019). Malnutrition & undernutrition. *Medicine Journal, 47*(3), 152–158.

Stratton, R., Green, C., & Elia, M. (2003). *Disease-related malnutrition: an evidence based approach to treatment.* Wallingford: CABI Publishing.

Studley, H. O. (1936). Percentage of weight loss, a basic indicator of surgical risk in patients with chronic peptic ulcer. *Journal of the American Medical Association, 106,* 458–460.

Varadhan, K. K., Neal, K. R., Dejong, C. H. C., et al. (2010). The enhanced recovery after surgery (ERAS) pathway for patients undergoing major elective open colorectal surgery: a meta-analysis of randomized controlled trials. *Clinical Nutrition, 29*(4), 434–440.

Verma, S., Patil, S. M., & Bhardwaj, A. (2018). Study of risk factors in post-laparotomy wound dehiscence. *International Surgical Journal, 5*(7), 2513–2517.

Vizard, P., Burchard, T. (2015). *Older peoples experiences of dignity and nutrition during hospital stays: secondary data analysis using the adult inpatient survey.* Case report 91. London: Centre for the Analysis of Social Exclusion (CASE): London School of Economics and Political Science (LSE).

Weijs, T. J., Berkelmans, G. H., Nieuwenhuijzen, G. A., et al. (2015). Routes for early enteral nutrition after esophagectomy. A systematic review. *Clinical Nutrition, 34*(1), 1–6.

Weimann, A., Braga, M., Franco, C., et al. (2017). ESPEN guideline: Clinical Nutrition in Surgery. *Clinical Nutrition, 36,* 623–650.

List of useful resources

- British Association of Parenteral & Enteral Nutrition including:
  - MUST tool kit – https://www.bapen.org.uk/pdfs/must/must-full.pdf
  - BAPEN good nutrition practice decision trees – https://www.bapen.org.uk/resources-and-education/education-and-guidance/bapen-principles-of-good-nutritional-practice

- European Society of Parenteral and Enteral Nutrition – https://www.espen.org/
- 10 key characteristics to good nutrition and hydration care – https://www.england.nhs.uk/commissioning/nut-hyd/10-key-characteristics/
- State of the nation: older people and malnutrition in the UK 2017 – https://www.malnutritiontaskforce.org.uk/sites/default/files/2019-09/State%20of%20the%20Nation.pdf; or Malnutrition task force website as useful resource – http://www.malnutritiontaskforce.org.uk/
- The Hospital Food Standards Panel's report on standards for food and drink in NHS hospitals – https://assets.publishing.service.gov.uk/government/uploads/system/uploads/attachment_data/file/523049/Hospital_Food_Panel_May_2016.pdf

Chapter | 7 |

Altered body image and the surgical patient

Adèle Atkinson

KEY OBJECTIVES OF THE CHAPTER

At the end of the chapter the reader should be able to:

- discuss the meaning of body image and altered body image
- discuss perceptions of body image
- discuss the effects of surgery on body image
- identify the effects of altered body image on body reality, body presentation and body ideal
- discuss social support and coping strategies
- highlight the role of the surgical nurse in supporting the patient with an altered body image.

Areas to think about before reading the chapter

- What do you understand by the term body image?
- Provide an overview of the grief response.
- What is the difference between coping and defence mechanisms?

Introduction

Physical appearance as an aspect of our identity is closely allied with the notion of who we are as people. Body image carries significant meaning, and is consistent with self-concept, self-esteem and identity. The very nature of surgery is a traumatic invasion of the body and the self, and will invariably cause temporary or permanent changes. Some of these changes may not be anticipated or only emerge after the patient has been discharged. The issue of altered body image, and the degree to which it might affect a patient's quality of life and self-concept, has become an increasingly important factor to consider when caring for patients undergoing surgery. This chapter will predominantly discuss issues related to patients undergoing planned/elective surgery, but will highlight other matters related to patients undergoing emergency surgical procedures, where appropriate.

What is meant by body image?

Body image is a widely used but poorly defined term. The concept of body image is generally taken to include the psychological and social aspects of behaviour. At the simplest level, body image has been described as how we think and feel about our bodies (Schilder, 1935 cited in Newell, 1999). It is also believed to be multifaceted, reflecting the perception and attitude of one's physical functioning and appearance (Cash et al, 2005).

Other authors have emphasized the dynamic and ever-changing nature of body image and the external changes that can alter perceptions of body image (Bailey et al, 2016; Ferrer-Garcia & Gutierrez-Maldonado, 2012)

Physical appearance and behaviour are influenced by society, and the predominant sociocultural values of youth, physical attractiveness, health and wholeness are constantly reinforced through the media and by social contact. Even in the 21st century there is still evidence that regardless of other variables such as sex, age, intelligence and socioeconomic status, the physically attractive are favoured over others across a wide range of situations (Converse et al, 2016).

Further evidence has shown that perceptions and feelings about body size, function and appearance are also part of body image and have an impact on levels of self-esteem (Bailey et al, 2016). This means that body image is a psychological experience focusing on conscious and unconscious attitudes and feelings. There is no single static image of the body, as body image is always in the process of revision, being shaped according to the current situation of the individual.

Price (1990a) identified three major aspects of body image which, when in balance, constitute a healthy body image and a sense of well-being (Fig. 7.1). These three components are described as:

- *body reality*, i.e. the physical body as it is, which is influenced by life changes such as growth, pregnancy, scars, smoking and so on
- *body ideal*, i.e. the individual's desired body image, which is influenced by the media (including social media), societies norms and so forth
- *body presentation*, i.e. the body as it is presented to the world, which is influenced by fashion, peer pressure, etc.

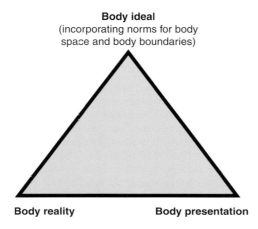

Body ideal
(incorporating norms for body space and body boundaries)

Body reality   **Body presentation**

Figure 7.1 A body image model.

Most people experience dissatisfaction in all three areas at one time or another due to the natural consequences of their genetic make-up, or the processes of physical maturation, ageing or other environmental events which cause changes in body image and subsequently in self-concept.

The influence of body image on personal self-image is an easier concept to comprehend, as it suggests that self-image is built upon valuing the opinions and respect of others and that body image is used in society to negotiate and develop a sense of self-worth. Views on what constitutes the 'self' are the subject of endless debate, but perhaps it is fair to say that self-image is our own assessment of our social worth and is important for our self-confidence, motivation and sense of achievement.

Perceptions of altered body image

Body image perceptions adapt to the naturally changing events in life such as puberty, pregnancy and ageing. However, unpredictable or unavoidable changes to body image, such as those that can occur due to the trauma of surgery, sometimes precipitate long-term consequences. These may alter perceptions of body presentation and consequently self-image.

Body image is a very personal matter and depends upon the experiences and the adaptability of the individual. Mind and body are closely linked, so that what happens to the body can have an effect on emotional health and vice versa. It can also determine a person's behaviour, as a result of the effect on self-concept. If people are not feeling well, they may not take as much care with their personal appearance, e.g. not washing hair, not wearing make-up or not shaving. This has the effect that when people look at themselves in the mirror their physical appearance reinforces how they feel. Since body image disturbance is the state in which an individual experiences a disruption in the way in which the body is perceived, it could be assumed that the consequences of surgery might have an effect on that individual's quality of life. At the same time, the individual may have to come to terms with the fact that the surgery is not a question of choice and that the treatment can be as bad as the disease, e.g. formation of a stoma following removal of a bowel tumour.

Certain operations can arouse specific fears in addition to the fear of pain and even the threat to life — e.g. mastectomy, formation of an ileostomy, colostomy or urostomy, amputation and certain types of plastic surgery — where fears of mutilation can be highly stressful. These fears can be related to the consequences of the change in daily life, and thus the perceived alteration of a concept of self.

Both the concept and the psychological effects of altered body image have been well studied, particularly in relation to the more obvious states of illness or injury, such as from the perspectives of oncology, burns, stomas, mastectomy and skin diseases (Lehmann et al, 2015; Ablett & Thompson, 2016; Fang et al, 2013; Williams, 2013; Pellard, 2006).

Changes that occur because of a surgical procedure, such as the insertion of a wound drain, nasogastric tube or intravenous infusion, may cause a disruption in body image; thus, a holistic approach to care should always consider the issue of altered body image as an integral part of a person's well-being. The nurse is in a unique position to engage the patient in conversation while caring for them, seeking in these dialogues to re-examine the meaning, if any, of altered body image and its impact on the patient. Perceptions of damaged or altered body image, and thus self-image, may significantly affect the patient's rehabilitation. This presupposes that health professionals are fully aware of the many meanings that changes in body image could have for the patient, the burdens that are carried by the individual and the factors that affect those burdens.

A person's experiences shape their perceptions and behaviours. Nurses need to help patients to cope with their reactions to the effects of surgery, and, since nurses are involved in determining patient needs, it is important that they have an insight not only into the obvious but also into the less obvious aspects of psychological perceptions. For example, in some situations a small scar may cause a patient more anxiety than a larger scar. Altered body image is therefore defined by the patient and not by health professionals.

Assessment of the perceived effects of altered body image is also complex because of the subjective nature of the phenomenon of body image. The nurse may have had some experience in reviewing their own body image, as well as the nature of body image in general, as they will have cared for others who have suffered physical trauma or who are dying. These experiences usually give a greater insight and empathy with the patient.

Reactions to altered body image

Being a patient in hospital can be identified as a threat to body image, because of the potential changes in body presentation and the body ideal (Bolton et al, 2010). How a person responds when faced with changes in body image depends on many factors. These are mainly bound up with their personality and the way in which that person perceives and values their own body, and their ability to adapt to stress. It also depends on the nature of the change to their body image, how it was brought about, and whether the change is visible, prominent, or hidden

as in the case of a woman having a hysterectomy. This may involve making adjustments for the future or it could be life-threatening. The significance of this change in body image may impact on the person's work, social or sex life and be perceived to have a negative effect on their future lifestyle. However, there are some patients who do not perceive a change in body image as a threatening disability or a problem, and this should be recognized by the nurse. It may be that the patient believes that surgery may help to give a more positive body image, e.g. in the case of bariatric surgery. It should therefore not be an assumption that the surgical patient will interpret a change in body image in a negative fashion.

Cultural issues are also associated with body image, and need to be taken into consideration when caring for patients from different cultures. Kocan and Gursoy (2016) identified that the female breast is important in society, and women undergoing mastectomy may no longer feel attractive and change the clothing that they would normally wear. They also found that some women avoided social situations. This highlights that a change in body image can affect how patients may perceive they are viewed by family members and the community they live or work in. Britain is a multicultural society and therefore different cultural needs must be taken into consideration; for example, there may be anxieties within the Afro-Caribbean population regarding the potential of keloid scarring. However, all patients should be treated as individuals and cultural stereotypes should be avoided.

Surgery on specific parts of the body also impacts on body image. Wounds resulting from surgery on the breast, uterus or genitalia can have significant meaning for women, as they are connected to their reproductive functions, while surgery on the male genitalia links to reproduction and sexual prowess. Women may see the surgery as a loss of their femininity and a loss of body ideal, while men undergoing prostatic surgery or an orchidectomy may fear impotence and loss of their manhood, also affecting their body ideal.

Breast surgery, either a lumpectomy or mastectomy, changes the shape of the breast and so affects body reality, and may impact on the woman's role in society (Kocan & Gursoy, 2016). In Western society, much emphasis is put on the shape and size of the perfect breast, so a change in shape or size following breast surgery can cause psychological trauma in some women.

If patients have a stoma formed — either temporary or permanent — it appears to contribute to a deterioration in body image (Bullen et al, 2012). It may alter their position in their social/cultural community and may lead to a life of isolation; separation from their family in relation to cooking, eating and caring; and preclusion from their place of worship. In some instances, they may be seen as permanently unclean and untouchable.

The face is also extremely important. This is because the face equates with attractiveness, so surgery to the face may alter the patient's perception of their attractiveness. This may lead to concerns that others view them with disgust (Shanmugarajah et al, 2012). If surgery to the face interferes with eating or talking, then this may further reinforce feelings of unattractiveness and helplessness.

Amputation of a limb not only alters body image (Holzer et al, 2014), but also extends it, as a prosthesis has to be worn, and crutches, a walking stick or wheelchair may be used to get around.

Hidden body image changes should not be forgotten, as these may also impact on the patient. This may include gynaecological surgery, or loss of fertility following hysterectomy. Also, areas of skin normally covered by clothing are more likely to be exposed in the summer months and when undertaking certain sporting activities such as swimming. A patient with a scar on the top of the arm may not want to expose it and prefer to wear short-sleeved tops rather than sleeveless tops, or a scar on the top of the leg may mean that a man will not wear shorts.

However, if there is conflict, and anxiety as a result of an altered body image, the nurse is well placed to recognize reactions, which are often manifested in the form of a grief response (Kubler-Ross, 1969; Parkes, 1972). Some surgical procedures may make a person look or feel 'different', presenting a major challenge. Patients may grieve for the loss of their 'old' body image and this is particularly exacerbated for the patient with a stoma, amputation or any mutilating surgery. However, this is not just limited to individuals with a visibly altered body image, as many patients may grieve for less obvious losses, such as changes in relationships, lifestyle and loss of personal freedom. A woman may have a sense of loss following a hysterectomy, as she may feel that she has lost her femininity. Likewise, a man may have a sense of loss following an orchidectomy, as he may feel that his masculinity has been affected by the surgery.

Loss of body image causes a grief reaction which will release in the afflicted person feelings of insecurity, particularly if the person perceives the change as a crisis. Tension and depression are typical reactions, and their recognition is the key to understanding the person's stress, sometimes perceived by the health team as being out of proportion to the magnitude of the actual surgical event. Yet grief, loss and mourning are all terms which have been associated with changes in body image, regardless of the cause, and can continue long after the patient has been discharged.

Bereavement may also be encountered by patients with an altered body image, and Dewing (1989) identified four stages of bereavement:

1. *Impact* — the initial shock and anger which can precipitate depression and pessimism regarding recovery. This reaction is exacerbated by those patients who have experienced sudden traumatic changes in body image and have had little or no time to receive information about, or prepare themselves for, the implications of the surgery, e.g. patients undergoing emergency surgery.
2. *Retreat* — a phase of mourning for the affected part and a desire to return to the previous self. There is often denial, avoidance and emotional withdrawal.
3. *Acknowledgement* — confrontation of the problem, reliving events, searching for a cause and seeking information to aid coping mechanisms.
4. *Reconstruction* — recognition of implications, accepting the use of aids and planning for the future.

Coping mechanisms are often employed unconsciously and are a normal human reaction to control fear and anxiety. A crisis associated with body image might be revealed by certain types of behavioural defence mechanisms, which have been observed by Wright (1993) (Box 7.1). Adjustment can be enhanced by the nurse with the appropriate skills to care for patients with an altered body image.

Regardless of the cause of altered body image, patients who have had a sudden traumatic change, e.g. following emergency surgery, may experience greater difficulty in

---

Box 7.1 Types of behavioural defence mechanisms

- *Passivity.* A change of mood or affect which can lead to sadness or withdrawal. The patient does not wish to be involved with their own care and may feel they are unacceptable. Motivation is poor and there is a loss of purpose and initiative.
- *Denial.* The patient refuses to look at or touch the altered part and may even deny its absence, trying to carry on as before. This dissociation from changes in body image demonstrates a distortion of reality which is a clear sign of psychological disequilibrium. The therapeutic relationship may be threatened by this resistance.
- *Reassurance.* The patient persistently seeks attention to check that they are still acceptable, sometimes making self-denigrating remarks to initiate a compliment. This can be a powerful affirmation that a person's attraction does not depend on a wholesome body reality.
- *Isolation.* This may be self-imposed because the patient feels unacceptable and fears risking rejection.
- *Hostility.* This may be due to a strong protest about what has been perpetrated on that person. It can also be a manifestation of anger against the medical profession and is often associated with grief and loss.

Source: Wright (1993).

coming to terms with the perception of loss, and will need more time to accept the event and their feelings regarding it. If a person can discuss – and, more importantly, be allowed to discuss – the fears and anxieties of forthcoming surgical procedures, it can promote healthier coping mechanisms and better reintegration of body image. Preoperative assessment clinics provide a place where this can be facilitated. Price (1990b) identified that support networks are also important in helping patients to adapt to a change in body image.

The preoperative phase

The prospect of imminent surgery and its hidden consequences naturally causes fear for the patient. The preoperative phase is a time when the nurse can discuss the patient's fears and anxieties and the events that are likely to occur during their hospital stay, and patients are able to express any concerns regarding a change in their body image. An important piece of research which has had an impact on nursing practice focused on giving information about the physical experiences that may be expected following surgery, with the result that postoperative pain was generally found to be reduced (Hayward, 1975). Garretson (2004) found that giving patients information preoperatively about their future care and treatment reduced stress in patients postoperatively. As this will reduce the amount of circulating adrenaline (epinephrine), pain should therefore be reduced. Some patients may have 'Googled' their surgery and time should be spent discussing any differences between the information they have found and what will actually happen. If a patient is coming into a day surgery unit, they will still be nervous and although there is shorter time before surgery, time must still be spent discussing their concerns. If a patient is admitted for emergency surgery, there is even less time for this to occur.

Four main stressors can be identified which can be seen during various stages in the preoperative period:
- loss of control over the events
- fear of the unknown
- loss of dignity
- lack of privacy.

Loss of control over the events

The patient's reaction to life in a hospital surgical ward and their adjustment to patient status can be stressful and the ward routine can undermine confidence. The loss of independence and a familiar environment poses a threat to the patient's body ideal. This is often not appreciated by ward staff, to whom the ward is a familiar and non-threatening environment. To fit into the ward environment, patients will often take the line of least resistance and become passive recipients of care.

The surgical procedure may be quite minor, such as the removal of a small cyst, or it may be a more substantial operation such as bowel surgery. Whatever the circumstances of the surgery, the surgical nurse needs to demonstrate that nursing care includes sensitivity to patient perceptions of possible changes in body image, no matter how small, and that facilitating patient control over events as much as possible can do much to sustain body ideal and self-esteem, e.g. giving patients information so that they are aware of the potential appearance of the scar in both immediately after healing and in the longer term (Case Study 7.1).

Effective preoperative assessment of patients undertaken in a holistic manner can gather valuable information on perceptions of their present body image, and can also elicit from the patient's own experiences something of the nature of their coping mechanisms in times of stress.

The patient and their family may also meet with specialist nurses who can give them more detailed information about the surgical procedure; discuss their expectations following the surgery; and give details of relevant support groups, if appropriate.

Giving the patient information on the forthcoming procedure helps them to feel involved and thus able to maintain a sense of control (Wilson-Barnett, 1978). Using photographs to illustrate how the patient may look after the surgery can help to reassure them. The admission procedure should ensure consultation with patients to encourage a sense of control over events and help patients make informed choices about the nursing care or therapy they will be receiving. This also helps to maintain their individuality within the hospital experience.

Case Study 7.1

Colin is a 24-year-old lorry driver who lives with his girlfriend and their two dogs. He has been diagnosed with a pilonidal sinus. A course of antibiotics has failed to improve the situation and Colin has been admitted for surgical excision of the pilonidal sinus.

Note: Pilonidal sinus is usually caused by ingrown hair around the natal cleft and causes an abscess. Post-surgery the wound can take up to three months to heal.

Questions for reflection

What anxieties may Colin have and how may the nurse, working with Colin, reduce these?

Think about how the wound may look? Will the wound be painful?

There will be times when the patient is unable to be in control, such as when they are anaesthetized or recovering from the anaesthetic, in which case the nurse is of necessity caring for the patient. It is important for patients to anticipate this and to feel confident that their needs will be dealt with respectfully. The surgical nurse should therefore be aware that this lack of control makes the patient feel vulnerable in this preoperative phase.

Fear of the unknown

Nurses need to recognize that patients may adopt defensive behaviours on admission due to their anxieties about forthcoming surgery which may affect their body image. Nurses appear to underestimate the impact of surgery on body image. This may be due to the familiarity of routine operations and their after-effects. Nurses may know the temporary nature of the ensuing scars, from previous experience, but the patient does not know this and has very real fears about their own body and the potential expected changes affecting it.

Patients typically have many concerns, and real anxieties, about what the operated part will look like and how other people might react to it, e.g. the partial or total loss of a breast, or formation of a stoma. These fears might be unfounded, but it is important to make time to discuss any concerns and listen to the patient's feelings. The nurse should be honest about the anticipated altered body image and allow the patient to talk through the reality of the forthcoming changes of body form and function, e.g. use of photographs to show before and after images. Patients also worry about how other people will react, fearing rejection, and it may be appropriate to discuss potential coping strategies with them at this point.

The transfer of the patient to the operating theatre can be the time of greatest stress for the patient, during which the surgical nurse needs to be conscious of the support that may be needed by the patient. Many patients are more concerned about the anaesthetic than they are about the surgery, as anaesthesia evokes fears due to loss of consciousness, which in some instances is equated with death.

Loss of dignity

One of the fears of surgical patients is the loss of bodily awareness while anaesthetized and of not being in control of their body. This fear can be exacerbated by previous bad experiences. It is important that the patient's dignity should always be respected by all healthcare professionals during the surgical experience.

Some of the more practical issues affecting body image arise from the need for physical preparation of the patient prior to surgery, which may affect body reality (Price, 1990b). This may involve procedures such as marking the skin at the planned operation site, and the removal of false teeth, contact lenses, make-up, nail polish and jewellery. These things can be an important aspect of a person's body presentation and self-worth.

The necessary removal of dentures can embarrass the patient and make them feel particularly vulnerable, as this is often only done in private and significantly alters body presentation. Another area that may make the patient feel vulnerable is the removal of their contact lenses/hearing aids. If contact lenses/hearing aids are removed too soon, the patient may feel anxious that they cannot see/hear what is going on around them. The removal of dentures and contact lenses should therefore be undertaken just before the patient leaves the ward/day surgery unit. Hearing aids should be removed in the anaesthetic room, so that the patient is aware of what is happening and can respond to any questions.

Lack of privacy

Marking the patient's skin to identify the operation site(s) is an important patient safety measure. Health professionals should have an understanding of how it might affect the patient's privacy and body image in relation to body reality and inform the patient as to why it is undertaken. The nurse should always adhere to local policy and procedure regarding prostheses and adjuncts to communication.

The patient in theatre

One of the identified patient fears, as stated previously, is the loss of bodily control under anaesthesia, coupled with the loss of dignity and privacy. Although it is vital for the surgeon to have optimal exposure to operate, it is the responsibility of the theatre nurse to act as the patient's advocate and ensure that the dignity of the patient is preserved as far as it is possible.

Increasing numbers of operations are performed under an epidural or local anaesthetic. It is therefore essential that the patient's dignity is maintained during their surgical procedure, and that patients have been fully informed in the preoperative phase as to the events that will occur during surgery. This is also pertinent for day surgery patients who may walk into the theatre.

Postoperative phase

Many of the factors discussed below will influence the patient's body reality, as surgery directly alters this. Body presentation may also be altered, to hide any drains, wound dressings or scars, for example. This may have a direct influence on patient's body ideal, as they may find it harder to achieve their body ideal by the way they present themselves to friends and the rest of society.

Following surgery, the assessment of the patient is primarily geared to the patient's physiological condition by the observation and monitoring of vital signs and level of consciousness, together with the relevant specific care, as described in other chapters concerned with specialist surgery.

Patient comfort and related perceptions in body image may not become apparent or be an issue until the patient has become alert enough to be aware of them. This may relate to gaining consciousness and becoming aware of an intravenous infusion *in situ*, or the long-term realization of the appearance of the scar, and this will alter the patient's body reality.

Following surgery, the patient may find their body image has extended or been breached, due to the necessity for tubes such as nasogastric tubes, urinary catheters, wound drains and intravenous infusions, so affecting their body presentation. As soon as possible, the nurse should reinforce the reasons why they are necessary, as well as whether they are of a temporary or permanent nature. The temporary nature of drains, for example, may result in minor threats to body image (Price, 1990a). This is probably because there is no need for long-term adjustment. Even so, it is important to realize that the patient may still grieve until the drains have been removed. If the changes are more permanent, then the aim is to help the patient to come to terms with their 'new' body image.

Nasogastric tubes are particularly distressing to the patient, as they occupy a facial position, make the face asymmetrical, and cannot be hidden. The angle of the tube should be as comfortable as possible, not pulling or distorting the nostril, and attention should be paid to nasal toilet, since it is not possible for the patient to blow their nose. This may alter the patient's body reality, as the patient becomes more dependent on the nurse, albeit for a short period of time. A minimal amount of tape to hold the tube in position should be used to keep the tube secure, and prevent pulling of the skin, which could cause distortion of the face. The nurse should also always check that the patient's view is not compromised by a loop of the tubing in front of the eyes.

For many patients the presence of a urinary catheter can be distressing, since it is invasive and can be seen by others. It is essential that the urinary catheter is appropriately secured, to reduce urethral trauma and possible pain or discomfort. The drainage bag attached to the catheter should be supported in a wire holder attached to the side of the bed. Once the patient is mobile, the presence of a urinary drainage bag to be carried around in a wire cradle can affect body presentation, and something more discreet, such as a leg bag, should be used.

Wound drains can also be a problem, particularly if attached to a drainage device, although their presence is often short term. If the patient is mobile and still has a wound drain *in situ*, the same discreet principle for carrying it around can be used as for the urinary catheter, thus helping to preserve the patient's body presentation.

Intravenous infusions should be positioned with some thought to the patient's comfort and abilities: for example, the non-dominant arm is the best choice unless there is some medical reason to do otherwise. This leaves the patient with the ability to use the dominant arm and preserves some independence, an important factor in maintaining some personal control.

Removing the operation gown and allowing the patient to wear an adaptation of their own clothing as soon as possible represents a limited return of control for the patient. Own clothing is preferable to their own nightdress/pyjamas as this not only enhances dignity but has been found to cut the length of time people spend in hospital (Stephenson, 2018). This also represents a limited return of control for the patient. A return to normality is also achieved when the patient can wear their own dentures/glasses/hearing aid, and so on, again.

Most surgical procedures will leave a wound. This may be an incisional wound or it may be a larger wound which will heal by secondary intention. If wounds are not hidden, then patients may go to great lengths to ensure that they are covered so that others do not see them (Neil, 2000). If patients do not want to draw attention to their wound, then the colour of the wound dressing is important, as few dressings actually blend into the skin. Some dressing products are bulky and may prevent patients from wearing the clothes or shoes that they wish to (Atkinson, 2002).

All wounds, including those from minimal invasive surgery, will heal leaving a scar. Brown et al (2010) found that the majority of patients who were concerned about scars had small or non-visible scars. This echoes an earlier study by Young and Hutchison (2009) which also found that scarring after surgery was just as much a concern for men as for women. Both studies found that people dressed differently to hide their scar. The importance of listening to the patient's worries cannot be overstated in the nursing care of a surgical patient. Using pictures of previous patients may help them appreciate the amount of scarring that they will have.

It must also be remembered that it may take years to adjust to a new body image if the body part that is affected has particular significance for the patient.

Pain following an operation is often one of the patient's greatest anxieties, and the fear of it should be discussed as part of the preoperative assessment, although this may not be possible for patients undergoing emergency surgery. Pain can be a challenge to body image because it is a body experience — sometimes unpredictable and always unpleasant. Price (1990b) believes that pain affects body image — the person can no longer trust their body, as they do not know when the pain will return. The surgical nurse must reassure the patient that, while pain is sometimes inevitable following the surgical procedure, it can be controlled, and no patient should be in pain or discomfort postoperatively. Assessment of, and nursing interventions for, the patient with postoperative pain are dealt with in more detail in Chapter 8.

Pain produces anxiety and reduces pain tolerance; therefore, increased pain is experienced by the anxious patient (Wall & Melzack, 1984). It is imperative to ensure that patients continue to be kept informed and can discuss their fears or anxieties. Early and prompt relief of postoperative pain usually results in decreased anxiety, less sensitivity to pain, earlier postoperative activity and a reduction in the total need for analgesics.

Social support and coping strategies

The desire to maintain body integrity is a profound need, which is usually internalized until it is threatened. People look for social approval of their appearance, especially when faced with illness, trauma or surgery. Alterations to the way body image is perceived can sometimes be so threatening that a crisis is precipitated. Many people have difficulty in coping with physical changes resulting from surgery, despite psychological support in the form of information-giving and listening to patients' anxieties. Helping patients to adjust psychologically through rehabilitation and to achieve a satisfactory body image will contribute to a more positive self-concept and feelings of self-worth.

People vary considerably in the way they cope psychologically with stress: sometimes confronting a problem directly and rationally (active coping strategies), and sometimes not facing up to the reality of the situation (avoidance coping strategies). The emotional and physical strain that accompanies stress is uncomfortable, upsetting the psychological equilibrium, and the response is to try to reduce that stress.

Social support can help to modify the impact of stress on the individual, and is referred to as the perceived comfort, caring, esteem or help a person receives from other people or groups (Sarafino & Smith, 2017). This can be through family or friends, work colleagues, or local support groups. Social support can be classified into five main types (Sarafino & Smith 2017):

- *Emotional support*: expression of empathy, caring and concern towards the individual, e.g. companionship; giving a shoulder to cry on.
- *Esteem support*: expression of positive regard for the individual; positive comparison of the individual with others. This encourages the individual's feelings of self-worth.
- *Tangible support*: direct assistance from someone in relation to finances or help in the home.
- *Information support*: giving advice/suggestions or feedback as to how the individual is doing.
- *Network support*: provides a feeling of membership in a group of individuals who share similar interests/activities.

Patients who can discuss their anxieties with someone who has experienced similar treatment are able to develop a more positive outlook. Partners, immediate family and close friends should also be included in counselling, to promote understanding of the loss and the patient's need for time to work through to acceptance. Both the patient and their partner and/or family frequently look to nurses for the opportunity to talk about their concerns; thus, the ability to build a good interpersonal relationship with both the patient and their immediate family can promote the adaptation and mature coping of all parties. The type of support the patient needs or receives will depend on the situation, although not all patients get the social support they need, e.g. elderly patients living alone; patients who are not sociable with others; or those patients who do not ask for help. However, social support can reduce the stress directly, e.g. changing how a person looks at a situation (a patient accepting a scar as body reality) or by giving a patient information which allows them to calm down and be less anxious.

What an individual actually does to manage the perceived stress is known as 'coping'. Coping is seen to be the process by which people try to manage a perceived discrepancy between the demands of the stressor and the resources available (Aust et al, 2016). Webb et al (2015) highlight individuality of coping, suggesting that a person's history and individual personality will determine what is perceived to be a stressor and what possible coping mechanisms are employed by the individual. Managing the stressful situation does not necessarily lead to a solution, but the coping efforts can help to alter the patient's perception of a discrepancy; to tolerate or accept the harm or threat; and to avoid or escape the situation. Coping is not a single event but is a dynamic series of continuous appraisals and reappraisals of the shifting person–environment relationships (Lazarus & Folkman, 1984). Thus, the re-evaluation of what is happening can influence subsequent coping efforts of adjustment and adaptation to perceived changes in body integrity.

The Lazarus model divides coping into two types:
- Problem-focused coping – in which a patient actively attempts to tackle the problem and tries to view the problem as manageable, e.g. purchasing and using a silicone gel sheet to reduce hypertrophic scar tissue following surgery.
- Emotional-focused coping – whereby the patient attempts to deal with the feelings associated with the problem. This can be through behavioural approaches such as drinking alcohol or talking to friends; or by using cognitive approaches such as rationalization; or

by denying unpleasant facts, e.g. denying that a breast lump is malignant and that it is only a cyst.

Problem-focused coping strategies appear to be more beneficial and more positive than emotional-focused coping strategies, with the internet being increasingly used as a key resource (Aust et al, 2016). Mindfulness may also help patients to pursue more problem-focused coping strategies (Atkinson, 2015). Mobile technology has brought a variety of health-related apps with it. Patients now have access to apps which may help them to cope with effects of surgery. Although these appear to be linked to specific concerns, for example, postoperative pain (Lalloo et al, 2017), it must be remembered that the evidence base for the effectiveness of these apps is unclear and therefore it may be helpful to discuss these with patients if they are wanting to use them.

The coping ability of the individual depends on two psychological factors, namely the degree of perceived threat and the person's ego strength, i.e. how someone uses their mental defence mechanisms. Think about the situation described in Case Study 7.2.

Anxiety and uncertainty of outcome can also lead to the use of defence mechanisms (Drageset & Lindstrøm, 2003) (see Box 7.1). Aust et al (2016) found that people who use more emotional-focused coping strategies tend to take longer to come to terms with the problem, in this case an alteration in body image. The nurse's caring role in helping patients and families cope with perceived changes in body image is important, and yet it is something that some nurses find difficult to address, preferring to deal with more concrete and familiar patient needs. Patients need to be able to express their feelings in an atmosphere of trust and confidence, and the nurse can help the facilitation of such expression, which in itself is therapeutic. The Nursing and Midwifery Council (NMC) requires all nurses, midwives and nursing associates to adhere to the professional and ethical standards that are encompassed in *The Code* (NMC, 2018). *The Code* is organized around four themes. These are:

- Prioritize people
- Practise effectively
- Preserve safety
- Promote professionalism and trust.

Assessing a patient's body image is complex, as there are many facets to it. On first meeting, the patient may not tell all, as information is usually disclosed over a period of time. Nurses can observe patients for their reactions and how they dress, and listen to the words that they use, e.g. patients may not maintain eye contact, or they may wear dark clothes to divert attention. Assessment will also take account of any potential threats to body image, e.g. anxiety due to surgery. It is also helpful for the nurse to reflect over what has caused problems in other patients and bear these in mind.

It is important that the nurse responds to the patient with 'positive-regard', to help build up a trusting relationship. When a patient starts to trust the nurse, it is possible to start to explore their body image with them. Price (1995) noticed that patients talked about how they felt about their bodies in terms of how they would perform in the future, rather than focusing on the now. Neil and Barrell (1998) found that one person in their study brought in photographs to show how she had looked before and after having a wound, to show how she felt her whole body had changed, even though the photographs were not of the area where the wound was.

It may be impractical, in a busy surgical ward, to use a lengthy assessment tool for assessing body image. Price (1990a) suggests that the need for extensive and formal assessment tools is much reduced where the nurse develops a patient profile through observation, reflection and effective communication, and can then formulate a tailored care plan which outlines the patient's concerns and perceptions.

Awareness of people's various coping strategies, and the different social resources that a patient can draw upon, will help the nurse to anticipate and understand the patient's reactions. The ability to communicate and actively listen will lead to trust. The knowledge and skills required by surgical nurses to comprehend why people react as they do, and the ability to help a patient overcome the problems of altered body image, are all concerned with good interpersonal skills, trust, empathy and touch.

Case Study 7.2

Mrs Brown is a 52-year-old woman who had a below-knee amputation when she was 20, after a horse-riding accident. She has been admitted for shaving of a neuroma on her amputation stump. Whilst you, the nurse, are talking to her about this, she mentions that she has never looked at her stump as she cannot bear to do so. On talking to her you discover that she blames the accident for preventing her from taking up nursing as a career.

Questions for reflection

How can the nurse, working with Mrs Brown, encourage her to start to look at her stump?

Think about how you would help her explore her feelings about the accident.

Conclusion

It is essential for surgical nurses to be aware of the invasive effects of surgery, however minor they may seem, and to have a clear understanding of the personal meaning of body image. This includes knowledge of the effects of the stress response, and the psychosocial adjustments needed for a patient to be able to cope in a positive manner when faced with perceived altered body image. Using strategies that will build up a trust with the patient, such as active-listening skills and 'positive-regard', will hopefully assist patients in coming to terms with their altered body image.

(cont'd)

- Pain following surgery can also be a challenge to a patient's body image.
- An individual patient's reaction to a perceived altered body image can be linked with reactions to grief.
- The surgical nurse has an important role in incorporating sensitive awareness and support strategies into the care of the surgical patient.

SUMMARY OF KEY POINTS

- Appearance is an important aspect of identity.
- Body image is related to self-esteem and self-worth.
- Perceptions of disruption, damage or changes in body image due to surgery differ between individuals, as do responses to an altered body image following surgery; therefore, care relating to body image must be individualized.
- Assessment of the surgical patient's concerns, anxieties and fears related to body image should be considered during the assessment process.
- Surgical nurses should be aware of potential pre-, peri- and postoperative situations that can cause an alteration in the patient's body image.

(Continued)

REFLECTIVE LEARNING POINTS

Having read this chapter, think about what you now know and what you still need to find out about. These questions may help:

- What key areas would you need to address preoperatively with the patient to help them cope with any differences in their body image postoperatively?
- How would you help patients come to terms with a new/different body image during the whole surgical process (preoperatively, perioperatively and postoperatively)?
- What is the role of social media in influencing people's body image?

References

Ablett, K., & Thompson, A. (2016). Parental, child and adolescent experiences of chronic skin conditions: A meta-ethnography and review of the qualitative literature. *Body Image, 19,* 175–185.

Atkinson, A. (2002). Body image considerations in patients with wounds. *Journal of Community Nursing, 16*(10), 32–38.

Atkinson, M. (2015). Mindfulness interventions for improving body image: a worthwhile pursuit? *Journal of Aesthetic Nursing, 4*(10), 498–500.

Aust, H., Rusch, D., Schuster, M., Sturm, T., Brehm, F., & Nestoriuc, N. (2016). Coping strategies in anxious surgical patients. *BMC Health Services Research, 16.* Available at: < https://www.ncbi.nlm.nih.gov/pmc/articles/PMC4941033/ >.

Bailey, K., Cline, L., & Gammage, K. (2016). Exploring the complexities of body image experiences in middle age and older adult women within exercise context: The simultaneous existence of negative and positive body images. *Body Image, 17,* 88–99.

Bolton, M., Lobben, I., & Stern, T. (2010). The impact of body image on patient care. *Primary Care Companion to the Journal of Clinical Psychiatry, 12*(2). Available at < https://www.ncbi.nlm.nih.gov/pmc/articles/PMC2911009/ >.

Brown, B., Moss, T., McGrouther, D., & Bayat, A. (2010). Skin scar preconceptions must be challenged: importance of self-perception in skin scarring. *Journal of Plastic, Reconstructive & Aesthetic Surgery, 63,* 1022–1029.

Bullen, T., Sharpe, L., Lawsin, C., Patel, D., Clarke, S., & Bokey, L. (2012). Body image as a predictor of psychopathology in surgical patients with colorectal disease. *Journal of Psychosomatic Research, 73,* 459–463.

Cash, T., Santos, M., & Eilliams, E. (2005). Coping with body-image threats and challenges: validation of the Body Image Coping Strategies Inventory. *Journal of Psychomatic Research, 58,* 191–199.

Converse, P., Thackray, M., Piccone, K., Sudduth, M., Tocci, M., & Miloslavic, S. (2016). Integrating self-control with

physical attractiveness and cognitive ability to examine pathways to career success. *Journal of Occupational & Organizational Psychology, 89*(1), 73–91.

Dewing, J. (1989). Altered body image. *Surgical Nurse, 2*(4), 17–20.

Drageset, S., & Lindstrøm, T. C. (2003). The mental health of women with suspected breast cancer: the relationship between social support, anxiety, coping and defence in maintaining health. *Journal of Psychiatric & Mental Health Nursing, 10*(4), 401–409.

Fang, S., Shu, B., & Chang, Y. (2013). The effect of breast reconstruction surgery on body image among women: a meta-analysis. *Breast Cancer Research and Treatment, 137*(1), 13–21.

Ferrer-Garcia, M., & Gutierrez-Maldonado, J. (2012). The use of virtual reality in the study, assessment, and treatment of body image in eating disorders and nonclinical samples: a review of the literature. *Body Image, 9,* 1–11.

Garretson, S. (2004). Benefits of pre-operative information programmes. *Nursing Standard, 18*(47), 33–37.

Hayward, J. (1975). *Information: A Prescription Against Pain*. London: Royal College of Nursing.

Holzer, L., Sevelda, F., Fraberger, G., Bluder, O., Kickinger, W., & Holzer, G. (2014). Body image and self-esteem in lower-limb amputees. *PLoS ONE, 9*(3). Available at: <https://www.ncbi.nlm.nih.gov/pmc/articles/PMC3963966/pdf/pone.0092943.pdf>.

Kocan, S., & Gursoy, A. (2016). Body image of women with breast cancer after mastectomy: a qualitative research. *Journal of Breast Health, 12*, 145—150.

Kubler-Ross, E. (1969). *On Death and Dying*. London: Tavistock.

Lalloo, C., Shah, U., Birnie, K., Davies-Chalmers, C., Rivera, J., Stinson, J., et al. (2017). Commercially available smartphone Apps to support post-operative pain self-management: a scoping review. *JMIR mHealth uHealth, 5*(10), e162. Available at: <https://www.ncbi.nlm.nih.gov/pmc/articles/PMC5673880/>.

Lazarus, R. S., & Folkman, S. (1984). Coping and adaptation. In W. D. Gentry (Ed.), *Handbook on Behavioural Medicine*. New York: Guilford.

Lehmann, V., Hagadoorn, M., & Tuinman, M. (2015). Body image in cancer survivors: a systematic review of case control studies. *Journal of Cancer Survivorship, 9*(2), 339—348.

Neil, J. A. (2000). The stigma scale: measuring body image and the skin. *Dermatology Nursing, 12*(1), 32—36.

Neil, J. A., & Barrell, L. M. (1998). Transition theory and its relevance to patients with chronic wounds. *Rehabilitation Nursing, 23*(6), 295—299.

Newell, R. (1999). Altered body image: a fear evidence model of psycho-social difficulties following disfigurement. *Journal of Advanced Nursing, 30*(5), 1230—1238.

Nursing and Midwifery Council. (2018). *The Code. Professional Standards of Practice and Behaviour for Nurses, Midwives and Nursing Associates*. Available at: https://www.nmc.org.uk/globalassets/sitedocuments/nmc-publications/nmc-code.pdf

Parkes, C. (1972). *Bereavement: Studies of Grief in Adult Life*. London: Tavistock.

Pellard, S. (2006). Body image and acute burn injuries: a literature review. *Journal of Wound Care, 15*, 129—132.

Price, B. (1990a). A model for body image care. *Journal of Advanced Nursing, 15*(5), 585—593.

Price, B. (1990b). *Body Image — Nursing Concepts and Care*. London: Prentice Hall.

Price, B. (1995). Assessing altered body image. *Journal of Psychiatric & Mental Health Nursing, 2*(3), 169—175.

Sarafino, E., & Smith, T. (2017). Health Psychology — Biopsychosocial

Interactions ((9th ed.). New York: John Wiley.

Schilder, P. (1935). *The Image and Appearance of the Human Body*. London: Kegan Paul.

Shanmugarajah, K., Gaind, S., Clarke, C., & Butler, P. (2012). The role of disgust emotions in the observer response to facial disfigurement. *Body Image, 9*, 455—461.

Stephenson, J. (2018). Campaign to end PJ Paralysis. *Nursing Times*. Available at: https://www.nursingtimes.net/news/hospital/campaign-to-end-pj-paralysis-saved-710000-hospital-days/7025689.article.

Wall, P. D., & Melzack, R. (1984). *Textbook of Pain*. New York: Churchill Livingstone.

Webb, J., Wood-Barcalow, N., & Tylka, T. (2015). Assessing positive body image: contemporary approaches and future directions. *Body Image, 14*, 130—145.

Williams, J. (2013). Stoma care: intimacy and body image issues. *Practice Nursing, 23*(2), 91—93.

Wilson-Barnett, J. (1978). Patients' emotional responses to barium X-rays. *Journal of Advanced Nursing, 3*(1), 37—46.

Wright, B. (1993). *Caring in Crisis* (2nd ed.). Edinburgh: Churchill Livingstone.

Young, V., & Hutchison, J. (2009). Insights into patients and clinician concerns about scar appearance. *Plastic and Reconstructive Surgery, 124*, 256—265.

Further reading

Burrows, N. (2013). *Body image — a rapid evidence assessment of the literature*. Government Equalities Office. Available at: https://assets.publishing.service.gov.uk/government/uploads/system/uploads/attachment_data/file/202946/120715_RAE_on_body_image_final.pdf.

Deeny, P., & Kirk-Smith, M. (2000). Colloqial descriptions of body image

in older surgical patients. *Intensive and critical care nursing, 16*, 304—309.

Gursoy, A., Candas, B., Guner, S., & Yilmaz, S. (2016). Preoperative stress: an operating room nurse intervention assessment. *Journal of perianesthesia nursing, 31*(6), 495—503.

Price, B. (2011). How to map a patient's social support network. *Nursing Older People, 23*, 28—35.

Price, B. (2016). Enabling patients to manage altered body image. *Nursing Standard, 31*, 60—69.

Strubel, J., & Petrie, T. (2017). Love me Tinder: Body image and psychosocial functioning among men and women. *Body Image, 21*, 34—38.

Tiggermann, M. (2015). Considerations of positive body image across various social identities and special populations. *Body Image, 14*, 168—176.

Chapter | **8** |

Concepts of pain and the surgical patient

Sarah McKenna

KEY OBJECTIVES OF THE CHAPTER

At the end of the chapter the reader should be able to discuss the following:

- the classification of pain
- general principles in the management of acute pain
- factors that can affect the experience of acute pain
- pain assessment
- the physiological response to pain and the dangers of poorly managed acute pain
- methods of administering postoperative analgesia
- pharmacology in acute postoperative pain management
- the Acute Pain Service team.

Areas to think about before reading the chapter

- Pain is not just a symptom; it is also a condition. What do you understand by this?
- What pain assessment tools are available to the nurse?
- How might having pain make a person feel isolated?

Introduction

Pain is a complex, multidimensional experience and it is unique to the person experiencing it. Pain is often seen as a warning sign that something is wrong and is a common reason for people to consult their healthcare provider.

Although it would be an unrealistic expectation for patients to believe that they will be pain free after a surgical intervention, postoperative pain should not be seen as an inevitable part of recovery and it can be assumed that patients should not suffer unnecessarily. Nurses have an ethical duty to provide pain relief, and this is reinforced in Article 3 of the *Human Rights Act* (1998), which states: 'No one shall be subjected to torture or to inhuman or degrading treatment or punishment.'

In addition, poorly managed postoperative pain can activate several physiological responses which can be harmful and may delay recovery from surgery and ultimately the patient's discharge. It is difficult to state that good pain relief alone will reduce length of stay, as this is only one part of the patient's journey, but it is reasonable to expect that a patient who experiences a manageable level of pain is less likely to experience postoperative complications and hence is likely to recover more quickly.

Classification of pain

The British Pain Society (2019) states that pain is transmitted via signals that use the spinal cord and specialized nerve fibres to travel to the brain. These signals jump along the nerve fibres through a release of a chemical and these are called neurotransmitters. Furthermore, they classify pain into three different categories:

- Acute pain – short-term pain, e.g. a sprained ankle
- Chronic pain – long-term pain, such as back troubles or arthritis
- Recurrent or intermittent pain – pain that comes and goes, e.g. as in a tooth ache.

Acute pain is pain of recent onset and limited duration. It usually has an identifiable cause and an identifiable beginning and end. Acute postoperative pain is nociceptive pain. Nociception is the term used to describe the processing of noxious or damaging stimuli, and nociceptive information is transmitted by specific pain fibres called nociceptors. Tissue injury starts the process of inflammation as local swelling compresses sensory nerve endings. This is exacerbated by chemical mediators of the inflammatory process, such as bradykinin, histamine and prostaglandins, which potentiate the sensitivity of the nerve endings to painful stimuli. Although it can be appreciated that pain is not a pleasant experience, it has been suggested that it indirectly promotes healing by encouraging protection of the damaged area (Waugh & Grant, 2018).

However, this process heightens the likelihood of the nociceptors to have increased sensitivity to pain. This nociceptive pain can feel different depending on whether it is coming from the skin, muscles and soft tissues (classified as somatic pain). Pain coming from the internal organs is classified as visceral pain.

Acute pain is also associated with the stimulation of the sympathetic nervous system, which can lead to the activation of several potentially harmful physiological responses.

Chronic pain may be defined as that pain which has persisted, either continuously or intermittently, for 3 months or more and does not respond to traditional medical or surgical treatment. Chronic pain usually presents for months to years beyond the expected duration of time it should take for an injury to heal or disease to be treated. Chronic pain can totally disrupt normal life by taking over the life of the person experiencing it and of those close to them. Chronic pain can be complex and multidimensional in nature, which can lead to the person seeking many different treatment modalities. It is important to note that inadequately controlled acute pain can lead to chronic pain. Correll (2017) states that chronic postoperative pain is poorly recognized as a potential outcome from surgery within the healthcare sector and that it affects millions of patients each year, with pain lasting for months to years. Correll also identified that the highest incidences of chronic postoperative pain are associated with amputations, thoracotomies, cardiac surgery and breast surgery, and that other risk factors include preoperative pain, psychological factors and the intensity of acute postoperative pain.

Neuropathic pain can be described as pain initiated or caused by a primary lesion or dysfunction in the nervous system. Patients will often describe neuropathic pain as burning, shooting or stabbing in nature and the pain may also be associated with abnormal sensations such as numbness and hyperalgesia. Neuropathic pain can occur following a viral infection such as shingles, following surgery such as amputation, or it may be linked to a medical condition such as diabetes (diabetic neuropathy). An important part of postoperative pain management is the recognition of neuropathic pain. Staff should be alerted to signs of an increase in pain and if the pain is requiring increasing amounts of opioids with little or no effect, this may be a sign of neuropathic pain. The British National Formulary (Joint Formulary Committee, 2019) notes that there is some evidence this pain responds to opioid analgesics such as tramadol hydrochloride, morphine and oxycodone hydrochloride. However, treatment with morphine and oxycodone should only be administered under specialist supervision and tramadol should only be used when other treatments have been unsuccessful.

Many other types of pain have been identified in recent years, as defined by Action on Pain (2019), a charity that supports and offers advice to people in pain (Table 8.1).

It is important to note that any kind of pain can be complicated by psychological factors. It should be acknowledged that pain caused or made worse by such psychological factors is real to the person experiencing it. Such pain may require both medicated treatment as well as psychological treatment.

General principles in the management of acute pain

The patient-driven outcome in relation to pain relief should be for the patient to report that they are comfortable, or that their pain is at a level which is acceptable to them, with minimal side-effects such as nausea and vomiting or oversedation. Pain must be assessed and recorded regularly, and the assessment of that should be acted upon in a timely manner. Pain assessment must involve the patient, where possible, and should be a dynamic pain assessment, measured on moving or coughing, or during procedures which might cause pain.

Recording of pain scores can be inconsistent. The Royal College of Physicians introduced the National Early Warning Scoring (NEWS) system in 2012, which was used across most of the healthcare sector, and pain was included in this scoring system in an attempt to enhance consistency. In December 2017, NEWS 2 was introduced; it has increased compliance and patient safety in relation to pain management in the acute hospital setting (Royal College of Physicians, 2017).

Table 8.1 Types of pain

Allodynia	Pain caused by stimuli which are not deemed to be painful, or pain that is in a different site than the stimulated area.
Anaesthesia dolorosa	A complication of neurosurgery that is irreversible. It occurs when a nerve (usually the trigeminal nerve) is damaged by surgery or physical trauma and as a result the sensation in part of the body is reduced or eliminated entirely, however pain still presents.
Breakthrough pain	Aggravation or worsening of pre-existing chronic pain that is being treated. Adjustments of treatments may need to be applied to relieve the pain as it often comes on quickly and can last minutes to hours.
Complex regional pain syndrome 1 (reflex sympathetic dystrophy)	A chronic condition that is believed to be the result of dysfunction in the central or peripheral nervous systems. Dramatic changes in the colour and temperature of the skin occur over the affected area. The pain does not correspond to the distribution of a single nerve and is worse on movement.
Complex regional pain syndrome 2 (causalgia)	This is a burning type of pain associated with a partially damaged peripheral nerve. The skin of the affected person is usually cold, moist and swollen and later becomes atrophic.
Hyperalgesia	This is a condition of altered perception whereby stimuli that would normally cause trivial discomfort are perceived to cause significant pain. Hyperalgesia is often a component of neuropathic pain syndrome.
Hyperpathia	This is also a condition of altered perception arising from repetitive and prolonged stimulation of neurons.
Idiopathic pain	This is a diagnosis of pain which is suffered by a patient for longer than 6 months for which there is no physical cause and no specific psychological disorder.
Malignant pain	This pain is associated with diseases such as cancer caused by the tumour affecting the surrounding tissues (more common in bone tumours). It can be a result of the tumour itself or the treatments of the tumour such as radiotherapy or chemotherapy.
Paraesthesia	A sensation of tingling, pricking or numbness of a person's skin with no apparent long-term physical effect. Chronic paraesthesia indicates a problem with the function of nerve cells or neurons.
Phantom limb pain	Severe pain and tingling sensation which continues to be experienced from the perceived existence of the limb that has been amputated. It is more common in cases where amputation was delayed after the initial injury.
Psychogenic pain	This pain is entirely or mostly related to a psychological disorder where a person has persistent pain with evidence of psychological disturbances but no evidence of a disorder that could cause pain.

As part of pain assessment, it is essential that the effects of analgesics must also be evaluated and reviewed regularly. Historically the strongest available analgesic should be used, and opioid analgesics are the mainstay in the management of moderate to severe pain. However, the Royal College of Anaesthetists (RCOA, 2019) state that it should be noted that opioids may be less effective for acute pain than medicines with other mechanisms of action. However, despite promoting intravenous opioid delivery for acute pain they advocate that the most appropriate route for administering opioids must be used at the time pain is assessed as severe, although local policies will guide this. Epidural analgesia and patient-controlled analgesia may be used in all surgical areas, whereas the administration of intravenous opioids by intermittent bolus may be limited to a postoperative recovery area or a critical care area, as opposed to a ward environment.

Multimodal analgesia involves the use of different types of drugs that each contribute to analgesia in different ways. Paracetamol regularly administered either intravenously or orally will provide effective analgesia; administered concurrently with an opioid, paracetamol improves the quality of pain relief (Furyk et al, 2018).

What can affect the experience of acute pain?

Pain is a complex interaction of both mind and body, and the outcome of postoperative pain management is subject to many contributing factors. For example, staff and patient attitudes may prevent a patient from receiving adequate analgesics. A study revealed that patients' experiences of pain influenced their attitudes and strategies for postoperative pain management. The results from this study acknowledge that pain experiences and coping strategies are highly diverse and individual. Therefore, staff must approach pain management in a patient-centred manner, ensuring it is personalized and objective in order to optimize pain relief (Angelini et al, 2018). Education of all staff involved in the care of patients postoperatively is essential, to ensure that unhelpful attitudes are challenged.

It is important to undertake a full assessment of the patient's pain history. This should include questions about any previous surgery, previous and current analgesic use, and any fears or misunderstandings about analgesics, such as addiction or side-effects.

Patients who have an existing opioid requirement or a substance abuse disorder will have a higher opioid requirement if they have surgery. This is because tolerance leads to a decrease in opioid potency when repeatedly administered (Volkow & McLellan, 2016). Other factors, such as the age of the patient, will affect analgesia requirements. The elderly patient may have other ongoing pain problems due to conditions such as arthritis. They may take a variety of different types of medicines in addition to analgesics (polypharmacy) and they may be stoic about pain, perhaps feeling that it is simply to be expected as part of an ageing life.

A patient's personality can strongly influence the way in which pain is expressed. A patient who appears quiet and comfortable may not necessarily be and the patient who is rolling around verbally expressing their pain could be experiencing something different to pain. People with extroverted personality types are more likely to complain and to express their pain than introverted personality types. If this is so, then it could be argued that extroverts will probably receive more analgesics. Chester et al (2019) found that patients with more confidence experienced less pain than those who lacked confidence, and believed their pain could improve.

A nurse's own cultural experience and background can influence how they assess pain and it is important for all professionals to recognize how a cultural bias on their part can affect this, and reflection on and in practice is encouraged. In addition, a person's culture can also strongly influence perception of pain and how pain is expressed, which will affect the outcome of treatment. Givler and Maani-Fogelman (2019) acknowledge how cultural difference can influence pain and palliative care decisions. They also recommend that cultural beliefs should guide professionals in how, when and sometimes even if the patient's pain should be treated. The Nursing and Midwifery Council (2018) makes clear that the nurse must accurately identify, observe and assess signs of normal or worsening physical and mental health in the person receiving care, and this also includes the assessment of a person's pain.

Unfortunately, some cultures do not openly accept the use of opioids, which are commonly used in pain management. Although this situation could prove challenging in relation to surgical interventions and pain management, it should be respected by healthcare professionals and alternative methods of pain management should be sought (Yim & Parsa, 2018).

Previous pain experience may also be reflected in the response of an individual to pain. Many of these responses are learnt during childhood and carried through into adult life, with associated personal beliefs and coping mechanisms. Therefore, comparable stimuli in different people do not necessarily produce the same pain, either in duration or intensity. Therefore, there is a misconception that a particular surgical procedure or injury will produce a predictable level of pain on different patients. Recently, Yang et al (2019) determined that there are nine predictors of poor postoperative pain control and suggested that these predictors should be considered when developing discipline-specific clinical care pathways to improve pain outcomes and guide future surgical pain research. The nine predictors are:

1. Younger age
2. Female sex
3. Smoking
4. History of depression
5. History of anxiety symptoms
6. Sleeping difficulties
7. Higher body mass index (BMI)
8. Presence of preoperative pain
9. Use of preoperative analgesia.

It is important to consider what the pain means to the patient and how this aligns with the meaning of the surgery. For example, a patient undergoing a joint replacement will know that this is likely to improve their quality of life, whereas a patient who has had surgery related to cancer may have many anxieties due to the potential impact of their condition.

Pain assessment

Pain assessment is the core of effective pain management and it is important that the patient is involved wherever possible. Multidisciplinary care that is well integrated with supporting specialties should be offered to patients but with a focus on self-management strategies, therefore making the patient an expert in their own pain management (Royal College of Anaesthetists, 2015).

It is important to ascertain what words patients use to describe their pain so that communication between the patient and nurse is effective. The nurse and other healthcare professionals may use the term 'pain', which the patient may consider to mean only severe or excruciating pain rather than soreness or aching, which can also prevent them from performing their daily activities.

Pain assessment in the acute or postoperative setting tends to focus on pain intensity. Although this may appear to be an overly simplistic measure, it offers a tool to help provide treatment as quickly as possible. One of the most common measures in the acute care pain setting is the categorical scale (Bedinger & Plunkett, 2016). This uses phrases such as 'no pain', 'mild pain', 'moderate pain' and 'severe pain' to describe the magnitude of pain. Numbers can be added alongside this verbal description to help the patient to use the tool and for the nurse to begin to understand the patient's degree of pain.

Pain assessment using the categorical scale (Fig. 8.1) may be difficult for some patients, such as the elderly or cognitively impaired. Pain assessment in the elderly is not only complex from a cognitive-impaired stance but other coexisting pain issues can also be present alongside postoperative pain. Cognitively impaired patients may face challenges in making known that they are in pain and this can make pain assessment difficult. Therefore, it is appropriate and Schofield (2018) recommended that other pain assessment tools are used, such as a facial expression or behavioural assessment tool. The Abbey Pain Scale is a behavioural assessment tool that uses six indicators to help measure pain in patients with dementia, and the Association of Anaesthetists in Great Britain and Ireland (AAGBI) have recently made recommendations that all patients undergoing surgery with dementia who cannot vocalize their pain must have their pain assessed using the Abbey Pain Scale (AAGBI, 2019).

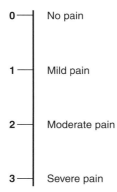

Figure 8.1 Categorical pain scale.

Despite variation among patients in their ability to use some tools, it is often necessary to standardize pain assessment tools, to avoid uncertainty when staff move between areas in one hospital. Patients undergoing elective surgery should be introduced to a pain assessment tool preoperatively and written information given to them about how to use the tool and what to do if their pain is not controlled. The preoperative assessment clinic may be an ideal environment for the dissemination of this preoperative information, although it must be recognized that patients are given a great deal of information at that time and this will need revisiting on admission.

The physiological response to pain and the dangers of poorly managed pain

Severe acute pain can be physiologically harmful due to the stimulation of the sympathetic nervous system. The role of the sympathetic nervous system is to protect the body in times of stress, and stimulation causes several physiological responses known as the 'surgical stress response'. These include the release of hormones such as cortisol and growth hormone; increased levels of blood glucose; and fluid and electrolyte imbalances. Increased metabolism will lead to an increased catabolism, requiring higher levels of oxygen.

Poorly managed acute pain may be particularly harmful to the elderly or those with pre-existing cardiac morbidity, because of the resulting increased workload on the heart. More oxygen will be required if the heart is forced to work harder and this could be compounded further if the patient is unable to breath properly due to pain, resulting in lower oxygen availability. Because of their age, elderly patients may have lower circulating blood volume, reduced muscle mass and reduced renal function, thereby leading to a reduction in medication clearance (Wu, 2018). Wu (2018) also states that since elderly patients are at higher risk of drug accumulation because of decreased renal function, there is a narrow window between dosages of opioids that are safe and those that could lead to respiratory depression or overdose. In addition, frequent polypharmacy in the elderly patient may make them more susceptible to adverse drug reactions.

Methods of administering postoperative analgesia

The administration of strong opioids is the first-line treatment for pain following surgery. The route of analgesic administration will be dependent on the type of surgery and on the environment in which the patient is being cared for. For example, patients with continuous epidural analgesia may need to be nursed in a high-dependency setting, while patients undergoing day case surgery will require shorter-acting opioids to enable them to go home as planned.

Oral administration

Oral administration of analgesics is the most acceptable route for patients, and it should be the first choice if possible. However, this route is seldom appropriate in the immediate postoperative phase, as gut motility is often reduced or the type of surgery may make this route impossible. If the oral route is used inappropriately, then there can be delayed absorption at an unpredictable time and if the patient is nauseated or is vomiting, there will be very little absorption of the drug.

Rectal administration

Analgesics such as paracetamol and non-steroidal anti-inflammatory drugs (NSAIDs) can be administered rectally, although this method may not be acceptable to patients and it is therefore essential that verbal consent is obtained and recorded prior to administering drugs rectally. Absorption may be unpredictable and some NSAID suppositories can directly irritate the rectal tissues. The wide availability of intravenous forms of paracetamol and NSAIDs should reduce the need to use the rectal route in the postoperative setting.

The intravenous route

The intravenous route is a rapid way of administering analgesics, including opioids, paracetamol and some NSAIDs. The administration of opioids by this route is often limited to clinical areas where there are high staff-to-patient ratios, such as the post-anaesthetic care unit (PACU). The intravenous route is fast acting and easy to titrate to pain levels, but it requires the nurse to stay with the patient during administration and for some time afterwards. Best practice is that naloxone should be immediately available during administration, and that the nurse administering the opioid would remain responsible for the safekeeping of any unused portion of the drug until no more was required; any remainder could be discarded and documented according to local policy and procedure.

The intramuscular route

The intramuscular route can be used for the intermittent 'as required' dosing of opioids, this method is rarely used, due to the wider use of more effective methods of analgesia. The intramuscular route commonly fails for several reasons. Most patients do not like injections, because they are painful. The nurse has control of the analgesia instead of the patient, and many patients worry about bothering the nurses if they are in pain, especially if the nurses look busy. Additionally, the prescribing and administration of intramuscular opioids may be inadequate and the pharmacokinetics are unpredictable.

Patient-controlled analgesia (PCA)

PCA is a common method of administering postoperative analgesia and many patients have benefited from using it. PCA empowers the patient to self-administer analgesics quickly within set parameters. Patients may also prefer PCA to other methods of analgesia as they are in control and do not have to alert the nurse caring for them in order to receive pain relief quickly. The aim of PCA is to keep plasma levels of opioid at a consistent, effective level without causing peaks and troughs of analgesia.

PCA is frequently used for both adults and children postoperatively. The most obvious criteria for its use are that the patient is physically able to use the chosen device and that they have the ability to understand the concept. Some patients may not feel that PCA is appropriate for them, as they may not wish to take control of this part of their care or they may associate the use of an opioid with drug addiction.

To help ensure best practice in the use of PCA, every step must be taken to reduce risk, such as the standardization of equipment and the use of prescribing guidelines or protocols. Any changes made within these guidelines or protocols to allow for individual patient need must be made absolutely clear by the prescriber, and observation parameters may need to be altered as well. Administration lines used must be designed for PCA use, incorporating a one-way valve port for the safe attachment of intravenous infusions plus an anti-siphon valve to prevent gravity-induced siphoning, which could occur if the PCA pump is placed too high. All staff using PCA equipment must be trained in its use, and this training must be provided as an ongoing programme.

It is important that all staff caring for patients using PCA can confidently manage the equipment. This must include being able to check the pump settings against the prescription chart, and monitor and confirm the amount of drug administered and the number of bolus demands, including unsuccessful demands. This information should be recorded with each set of observations, and each time a different nurse takes over the care of the patient. Staff must also be able to troubleshoot potential problems with the equipment and replace PCA syringes or infusion bags as needed, to ensure that the patient does not have a break in analgesia, constantly evaluating the effectiveness of the pain relief.

Description of terms used in patient-controlled analgesia

It is important to understand the terminology used for PCA. The *bolus dose* is the amount of analgesic drug that the patient will self-administer on a successful demand with PCA. The bolus should be enough to provide good analgesia with minimal side-effects. Morphine is frequently used for PCA and a 1-mg dose every 5 minutes, if required, appears to be a fairly standard dose for most adult patients. This would appear to go against the argument that we should be providing analgesia which is tailored to the individual, but consistency in prescribing is necessary to help reduce risk.

The *lockout time* is the time during which the PCA pump will not deliver any dose of analgesic. The patient must be reassured that the PCA will not give a dose of analgesic during this time, no matter how many times the demand button is pressed. Lockout times of between 5 and 10 minutes are commonly used.

When setting up a PCA, initial analgesia in the form of an intravenous *loading dose* may be needed, as the small amount of drug given with each patient bolus may not be adequate for a patient who is in severe pain. The loading dose will help to establish an effective level of analgesia which the patient can then maintain with PCA. The loading dose is given by a doctor or a nurse who has received the appropriate training. The amount of analgesic given as a loading dose will depend on the individual analgesic requirement for each patient. The loading dose can be given as a separate injection but ideally it should be given by utilizing the 'clinician override' facility on an electronic PCA pump (Anaesthesia UK, 2017).

Patient education

Patients must have been provided with a clear understanding of how to use the PCA equipment prior to using it. This may be difficult if the patient is undergoing emergency surgery or if they are given information too far in advance and their understanding of how to use the PCA is not rechecked. Ocay et al (2018) note that although PCA use has many advantages, concerns towards safety of the devices are still present and they recommend careful patient selection and assessment, and comprehensive education for patients, families and healthcare providers.

Common problems with patient-controlled analgesia

If the patient is not receiving adequate analgesia, the nurse should check that the patient is using the PCA equipment correctly. The pump history must be checked, as the patient may not be using the pump enough due to a lack of understanding. If the patient is not using the PCA appropriately, then further advice and support can be given to help the patient to get the greatest benefit.

The nurse should also ensure that the patient has simple analgesics such as paracetamol prescribed alongside the PCA and ensure that these are given. If no regular, simple analgesics are prescribed, then it is the responsibility of the nurse to request that the analgesic prescription is reviewed. If the patient has used the PCA to the maximum and has received other analgesics but the level of pain remains unacceptable to them, then their drug regimen must be reviewed. An intravenous 'rescue' dose may be required to reinstate analgesia or the bolus dose may need to be increased for that patient. Maintenance of their usual opioid requirement in addition to postoperative analgesics can be provided with a background infusion plus PCA or by prescribing a higher PCA dose. This approach may also be appropriate for other patients who take regular opioid-based analgesics, including those with cancer or chronic non-malignant pain problems.

It is not appropriate to give an opioid intramuscularly as an addition to PCA, as the effect of this may be unpredictable and could lead to over sedation and respiratory depression. Whilst morphine is the most common drug used for PCA, other drugs are also used, including diamorphine, fentanyl and oxycodone.

All opioids administered by any route have the potential to cause oversedation and respiratory depression. Whenever PCA is prescribed and used, those staff caring for the patient must be able to recognize problems early on and follow clear guidelines for subsequent management and care of the patient. Patients using PCA must only be nursed throughout the 24-hour period in clinical areas where the staff have received the appropriate training. This must be understood by and strictly adhered to by all staff, including the prescriber. It is still considered good practice to prescribe oxygen therapy for all patients who are receiving PCA, but if the respiratory rate drops to less than 8 breaths per minute, the oxygen should be increased to 15 L immediately and a doctor must be called to review the patient (Royal Cornwall Hospital NHS Trust, 2018).

It could be argued that if the patient is using the PCA unaided, then the natural control would be that they would stop using it if oversedation occurred. However, oversedation is a possibility, particularly if another person is pressing the demand button on behalf of the patient or if it is mistaken for the call bell. The basic principle of PCA requires only the patient to press the button and if they became too drowsy to press the demand button, then they would not do so. However, if another person, such as a family member or a healthcare professional, presses the button, this would override the natural control loop and the patient could easily become overdosed. Visitors are to be actively discouraged from pressing the PCA demand for a patient and must be informed of the potential dangers of doing so. If the patient is unable to understand how to use the PCA or is unable to press the demand for themselves without prompting, then the PCA must be discontinued and an alternative method of analgesia prescribed (Soffin & Liu, 2018).

If a patient becomes sedated at such a level that they are difficult to rouse or they are unrousable, then the PCA handset must be removed and the patient closely observed until they become less sedated. Close observation means direct observation by a nurse who is competent and is also able to constantly monitor sedation, respiratory rate and oxygen saturations. A reduced level of consciousness due to sedation occurring in a situation such as this is likely to be accompanied by a reduction in respiratory function, such as is evidenced by reduced oxygen saturations and respiratory rate. If the nurse is concerned about the patient's respiratory function and level of sedation, then the nurse must communicate this to medical staff immediately and ensure that naloxone is available and ready for rapid use, if required, to reverse the action of the opioid. Local policies will dictate at which point naloxone should be used and whether nursing staff are able to administer it.

The patient may show other signs of opioid overdose, such as constricted pupils (myosis) and cyanosis. Other potential side-effects of opioids, such as pruritus, nausea and vomiting, hypotension and constipation, are discussed in the pharmacology section of this chapter.

Regional analgesia

Spinal injections

Drugs injected below the dura, directly into the cerebrospinal fluid (CSF), are called 'spinal' or 'intraspinal/intrathecal' injections. Injection of a local anaesthetic is called 'spinal anaesthesia', whereas injection of an opioid is called 'spinal analgesia'. Some patients will have their surgery carried out under spinal anaesthesia (instead of or in addition to a general anaesthetic) and the effect of the drugs may last for several hours. Some patients may have a combined spinal epidural (CSE); this is a spinal injection followed by an epidural using the same catheter.

Spinal anaesthesia provides a dense motor block which can last for several hours. Staff may be concerned about sitting patients up or allowing them to mobilize following this procedure. Patients can sit up as their general condition allows, but they should not mobilize until they have full motor power in their legs and, even then, initial mobilization must be under the supervision of two members of the clinical staff. Motor power is tested by asking patients to bend their knees and to perform a straight leg raise, which will demonstrate quadriceps strength. Patients may also experience urinary retention due to blocking of the sacral autonomic fibres. Opioids administered spinally without a local anaesthetic will not cause a motor block.

Potential complications following a spinal injection/spinal anaesthesia

A potential complication following a spinal injection is the development of a postdural puncture headache, commonly known as a spinal headache. The headache is due to leakage of cerebrospinal fluid through the hole punctured in the dura by the spinal needle – cerebrospinal fluid leaks out through the dura, leading to a drop in the pressure of the cerebrospinal fluid. The headache can be severe and is classically worse on sitting up, as this causes a further drop in the pressure of the cerebrospinal fluid. The patient may also feel nauseated, be photophobic and have pain when flexing the neck. Patients are encouraged to rest lying down and to gradually sit up as they feel able, and must be reassured that the condition is not life-threatening. Administration of simple analgesics such as paracetamol may help, and the patient should also be encouraged to drink plenty of fluids to help increase the levels of cerebrospinal fluid. If the patient is unable to drink, then an intravenous infusion will be necessary to maintain hydration. If the headache does not resolve, then administration of a 'blood patch' may be required. During this procedure, a small blood sample is taken from the patient and injected into the epidural space to seal the hole in the dura. Drinks containing caffeine may also help to relieve a spinal headache, as the headache is caused by the dilation of blood vessels and caffeine constricts them, which should help relieve symptoms.

Epidural analgesia

Epidural analgesia involves the injection of drugs into the epidural space. *Epi* means above; therefore, this means that the injection is administered into the space above the dura. Many patients receive epidural analgesia following major surgery and most centres use a mixture of opioids and local anaesthetics in a continuous infusion to deliver balanced analgesia. Opioid analgesics administered epidurally will be partly absorbed through the epidural veins and fat, but the majority will diffuse across the dura into the cerebrospinal fluid. They ascend rostrally in an upward spiral to the brain but also act upon opioid receptors in the dorsal horn of the spinal cord, mimicking the action of endogenous opioids. A continuous epidural infusion containing both an opioid and a local anaesthetic has the potential to provide excellent analgesia, while providing sympathetic blockade.

Patients receiving a continuous epidural infusion containing an opioid should not receive opioids by any other route for the duration that they have the epidural, as this may lead to an accidental opioid overdose. The exception to this may be for patients who have an existing opioid requirement, for whom the maintenance of their usual opioid requirement will be necessary in addition to the epidural analgesia.

An epidural will not be appropriate for all patients. The risks and possible side-effects should be explained to the patient by an anaesthetist, who will also assess whether it is safe to undertake the procedure. The absolute contraindication to an epidural is if the patient does not consent to the procedure. The patient should be given all the information before admission if their procedure is elective and must give verbal consent prior to the procedure, which is to be documented accordingly as per the latest AAGBI guidelines on consent and anaesthesia (AAGBI, 2017).

Caution should be exercised in the following situations (although these are not necessarily absolute contraindications):

- The presence of a clotting disorder, or if the patient is being anticoagulated, may increase the risk of bleeding into the epidural space.
- Any abnormal spinal anatomy can narrow the vertebral canal or the epidural space, and may make it difficult to site the epidural catheter.
- The presence of aortic valve stenosis may reduce the ability of the body to compensate in situations of hypotension. Equally, any untreated hypovolaemia can compound the hypotension caused by epidural local anaesthetic agents.
- Patients with any head injury may not be suitable for epidural placement in case of damage to the dura.
- The presence of any local or generalized infection may put the patient at risk of meningitis or an epidural abscess.

Caring for the patient with an epidural

A major role of an Acute Pain Service, where this is available, is the management of a ward-based epidural service. Key tasks for the acute pain nurse are to minimize risk by educating staff in the management of epidurals, standardizing equipment, auditing problems and ensuring that appropriate observation of the patient is carried out in accordance with local policy. All nurses caring for patients with epidurals must be aware of the potential effects of local anaesthetics and opioids and how to manage potential problems, including the management of the epidural equipment.

Local policy will dictate the type and frequency of observations carried out for patients with continuous epidural analgesia. It would be realistic to suggest that blood pressure, heart rate, respiratory rate and oxygen saturations, pain levels, sedation, and any nausea and vomiting are measured and recorded at least 2-hourly during the first 24 hours and 4-hourly for the remainder of the time that the epidural infusion is in progress. In addition, monitoring of sensory and motor block must be carried out at least 4-hourly, plus observation of the epidural site whenever a different nurse takes over the care of the patient or if the patient reports an increase in pain.

An epidural should enable patients to achieve relief from dynamic pain; they should be able to move and be able to take a deep breath and cough with minimal, if any, pain. If a patient has pain that prevents these activities, staff should follow their local guidelines to manage the situation before calling for assistance from anaesthetic staff or from the Acute Pain Service. Patients will rarely report a sudden increase in pain unless the epidural catheter has fallen out, become disconnected or the infusion has been interrupted for any other reason. An increase in pain is likely to be accompanied by increased blood pressure, heart rate and a sensory block that is below the level of the surgery. If the patient reports pain, then the nurse must check the sensory level, the epidural site and general observations, and also whether other analgesics such as regular paracetamol have been administered. It may be helpful to change the patient's position to encourage the flow of the epidural towards gravity and to increase the rate of the epidural infusion. However, if these actions fail to improve the level of pain within 30 minutes, then advice should be sought, as the patient may require a 'top up' administered by the Acute Pain Service or an anaesthetist, depending on local guidelines.

A 'top up' involves the administration of a further dose of analgesics via the epidural to reinstate analgesia. If a strong solution of local anaesthetic is used, then the patient must be advised that there may be increased numbness around the wound site following the 'top up'. If the patient has a lumbar epidural, then it is possible that they will experience a motor block for approximately two hours post 'top up' and that their feet will feel warm due to the vasodilatory effect (NHS, 2017). A 'top up' may cause hypotension due to the vasodilatory action of local anaesthetics and this may occur very quickly due to the speed of administration of the bolus. It is therefore essential to monitor and record the patient's blood pressure in addition to their heart rate, sedation and pain level at 3- to 5-minute intervals. The sensory level and motor function should also be monitored. It is reasonable to suggest that if a 'top up' fails to help the patient's pain levels within a timescale of about an hour, then an alternative method of analgesia will be required, as any more time spent trying to rectify the pain may result in the patient losing confidence in the epidural. The administration of 'top ups' is time-consuming and patients may not have timely access to such an intervention at all times, such as during the night and at weekends. Methods such as patient-controlled epidural analgesia can reduce the requirement for 'top ups'.

Hypotension is a possible side-effect of all epidurals containing a local anaesthetic and can occur at any time. Hypotension can lead to cerebral hypoxia and to poor perfusion to other organs such as the kidneys, heart and the gut. Although local anaesthetic agents have the ability to cause hypotension due to their vasodilatory action, this is less likely with more sophisticated epidural solutions using lower concentrations of local anaesthetic and adjuvants. If a patient becomes hypotensive in relation to their normal systolic blood pressure, accompanied by a reduced urinary output, then a review of their fluid balance and administration of a colloid solution may be all that is required, particularly if they feel well otherwise. However, if the patient becomes symptomatic, feels faint, nauseated or becomes unresponsive, then they must be reviewed urgently as they may require more expert intervention. If hypotension is not responsive to an increase in fluid administration, then it may be necessary to give a vasoconstrictor such as ephedrine. Ephedrine stimulates alpha- and beta-adrenergic receptors, causing vasoconstriction, and it must be available for intravenous use in all areas where patients with epidurals are nursed, and all staff must be familiar with its preparation and administration.

If a patient with an epidural feels nauseated or is actually vomiting, this could be due to the opioid in the epidural, particularly if it is accompanied by a feeling of light-headedness or dizziness. However, nausea and vomiting may also be due to hypotension, and the patient's blood pressure should always be checked if vomiting occurs. Urinary retention can occur as a side-effect of opioids as they reduce detrusor contractions or interfere with relaxation of the urethra and can increase tone in the bladder (NICE, 2019).

Nursing staff caring for patients receiving epidural analgesia must also be able to recognize signs of local anaesthetic toxicity. This could occur due to overdose or due to accidental intravenous administration. Signs and symptom of this are shown in Box 8.1 (Sekimoto et al, 2017) and if a patient reports any of the early symptoms, then the epidural must be stopped and medical help sought immediately.

The presence of a headache in the patient who has an epidural may be due to several causes and should be investigated. The anaesthetic record will detail any problems encountered during the siting of the epidural, such as a dural puncture, or whether a combined spinal epidural injection was used. Both of these would pierce the dura, possibly leading to a spinal headache. The anaesthetic record should be part of the handover from theatre to recovery and from recovery to the ward or day surgery unit, to ensure that all staff members are aware of the patient's intraoperative treatment.

Epidural analgesia can be further improved by techniques such as patient-controlled epidural analgesia. Patient-controlled epidural analgesia allows the patient to self-administer an epidural bolus using a handset attached to the epidural infusion pump in addition to a continuous infusion. This may lead to less intervention by nursing staff as the patient can self-administer a bolus as soon as they start to feel pain, rather than waiting for clinical intervention. Epidurals can also be improved by adding other drugs, such as clonidine or adrenaline (epinephrine), to enhance the action of the opioid and/or the local anaesthetic, meaning that lower concentrations of analgesics can be used, thus reducing the likelihood of side-effects from those drugs.

Testing the level of sensory block

A specific observation recorded for patients with continuous epidural analgesia is the sensory level, although local policy will dictate how much emphasis is given to this particular observation. The anaesthetist will site an epidural to provide the appropriate level of sensory block and it is expected that the sensory block will spread approximately two to three dermatomes above and below the level of insertion. For example, an epidural sited between the eighth and ninth thoracic vertebrae would be expected to block the area supplied between the sixth and twelfth thoracic vertebrae.

Box 8.1 Symptoms of local anaesthetic toxicity

Early neurological symptoms

- Circumoral and/or tongue numbness
- Metallic taste
- Lightheadedness
- Dizziness
- Visual and auditory disturbances (difficulties focusing and tinnitus)
- Disorientation
- Drowsiness

Severe respiratory and cardiovascular symptoms

- Hypotension
- Arrhythmia
- Bradycardia
- Cardiac arrest
- Respiratory arrest

The sensory level can be tested using ice or a neurological testing pin to ascertain a change in sensation on the skin. The rationale for carrying out this test is that patients would have reduced sensation to cold or pinprick at the dermatome levels covered by the spread of the epidural solution and so would not feel pain at that same level. It would seem logical, therefore, that the height of the sensory block should be at least to the top of the surgical wound and regular checks of the sensory level will help to monitor this, ensuring that the rate of the epidural infusion can be adjusted as needed. This test will vary in different care environments and it may not be consistent due to staff education, patient understanding and also the type of epidural solution used, as those containing lower concentrations of local anaesthetic may make this a difficult test.

Conversely, a different reason for checking the sensory level could be proposed – namely, to ensure that the sensory level has not risen above the dermatomal level supplied by the fourth thoracic nerve (T4). This could occur if the epidural had been topped up or if the epidural catheter had migrated. An epidural sensory level of above T4 could block the cardioaccelerator nerves, causing respiratory difficulty, bradycardia and hypotension. The epidural infusion should be stopped and the patient reviewed urgently, to prevent this leading to respiratory and/or cardiac arrest.

Possible complications of epidural analgesia

Epidural analgesics should provide analgesia by blocking sensory nerves with minimal effect on motor nerves. The presence of a persistent bilateral motor block must be investigated without delay, as it could be an indication of a complication such as an epidural haematoma or migration of the epidural catheter. If the catheter has migrated, the motor block will be accompanied by a sudden drop in systolic blood pressure. It may be necessary to temporarily stop the epidural infusion to ensure that normal motor function is present and the epidural infusion can then be restarted at a lower rate to prevent this recurring.

Some degree of motor block may be inevitable if a patient has a lumbar epidural, and this is often unilateral. A motor block can impede recovery by delaying mobilization and may lead to the development of sacral or decubital pressure ulcers due to reduced sensation. Regular checking of pressure areas must be an integral part of care for the patient with a lumbar epidural. The motor block must be tested by asking patients to move their feet, flex their knees and perform a straight leg raise. If an epidural haematoma is suspected, then this demands immediate investigation. An epidural haematoma may cause severe back pain at the epidural insertion site and this would be accompanied by a change in sensation and movement in the legs. If left untreated, an epidural haematoma can lead to permanent paralysis. A haematoma is most likely to form following the siting or removal of the epidural catheter; therefore, the administration of any anticoagulants must be timed to ensure that the epidural procedure can be carried out and local policies relating to epidurals and the use of anticoagulants, including the administration of subcutaneous heparin, should be in place to help reduce this risk.

Pharmacology in acute pain management

Opioids

Opioids are potent analgesics used for moderate to severe pain. They exert their action by binding to opioid receptors in the central nervous system, mimicking the actions of endogenous opioids. The receptors can be classified into three main types: mu (μ), kappa (κ) and delta (δ). Most opioids bind with varying degrees of affinity to μ-receptors – hence, this receptor type is associated with pain, respiratory depression and euphoria; δ-receptors are associated with pain at higher levels; and κ-receptors are linked with dysphoric effects. The degree of affinity to a receptor determines whether an opioid is classed as an agonist (has the maximum effect), partial agonist (has less effect), antagonist (has a blocking effect) or agonist/antagonist (has an effect at one receptor but blocks another).

The efficacy of an opioid will vary between patients and is also dependent on the route used and the frequency with which it is administered. Wherever possible, opioid dosages should be tailored to the individual patient. Opioids have a direct action on opioid receptors in the central nervous system and therefore have the potential to cause several side-effects, including respiratory depression, sedation, nausea, vomiting, and constipation (NICE, 2016). Respiratory depression can occur due to depression of the respiratory centre in the medulla, potentially leading to a reduction in tidal volume and respiratory rate and a reduced response to hypoxia. As already discussed, measurement of respiratory rate can be a late indicator of respiratory function and the sedation level of the patient should be considered first.

Opioids given by any route can cause nausea and vomiting, as they stimulate the chemotrigger receptor zone in the medulla oblongata. The nausea related to postoperative opioid administration needs to be acknowledged as a postoperative issue, as nausea and vomiting postoperatively are not only an unpleasant experience, they can also lead to complications such as bleeding, wound dehiscence, aspiration pneumonitis, and fluid and electrolyte imbalance (Lim et al, 2016).

113

The action of all opioids is reversed by the opioid antagonist naloxone. The half-life of naloxone is approximately one hour, which is shorter than most opioids (Scarth & Smith, 2016). Therefore, the patient's level of sedation must be closely monitored during this time, as further doses of naloxone may be required if the patient becomes sedated again. Naloxone is also a treatment for pruritus (itching). This can occur due to histamine release caused by opioids. Pruritus can be relieved with an antihistamine drug such as chlorphenamine, but if the itching is very distressing for the patient, the administration of low-dose naloxone may be considered to help reverse this effect. Administration of naloxone in this way must be carefully titrated to avoid reversing the analgesic effect of the opioid.

Morphine remains the most frequently used opioid in postoperative pain management and the effects of other parenteral analgesics are measured against it. Morphine is a pure μ-receptor agonist and it can be given parenterally or orally.

Fentanyl is also commonly used in the postoperative setting. It is a synthetic, lipid-soluble opioid with a high affinity for the μ-receptor and it is 50–100 times more potent than morphine. Fentanyl cannot be administered orally, as it is subjected to high first-pass metabolism, but it can be administered epidurally, intraspinally or intravenously.

Once a patient is able to take oral analgesics, this should be encouraged. However, it should not be assumed that the patient will no longer need a potent analgesic. Morphine can be administered orally as a tablet or as an elixir. The potential side-effects are the same as with other routes of administration.

Oxycodone is an alternative oral opioid preparation that can be given orally or parenterally in the postoperative setting. Oxycodone is a semi-synthetic opioid, structurally related to morphine, and is a full opioid agonist with an affinity for μ- and κ-receptors. When given orally, it is less subject to first-pass metabolism than other oral opioids and is twice as potent as oral morphine (Scarth & Smith, 2016).

Tramadol is a centrally acting analgesic with a multimode of action used to treat moderate to severe pain and it acts on serotonergic and noradrenergic nociception. Tramadol as standalone pain relief does not usually provide adequate analgesia, and in non-cancer pain there is little evidence for using tramadol for longer than three months (World Health Organization, 2014).

Both oxycodone and tramadol substances are involved in pain modulation in the central nervous system. Tramadol is an effective analgesic for moderate to severe pain, can be administered orally or parenterally, and is useful in the management of neuropathic pain. It has advantages over morphine in the postoperative setting, as it has less affinity for the μ-receptor and therefore is likely to cause less respiratory depression, and less slowing of the gut. Tramadol is not a controlled drug even though it has μ-receptor activity; hence, it is more convenient for staff to administer. Tramadol should not be prescribed for patients with epilepsy as it can reduce the seizure threshold, and it should be prescribed with caution for patients who are taking selective serotonin reuptake inhibitor medicines (SSRIs) as there would be an increased risk of sedation and possible serotonin syndrome due to increased serotonin levels.

Non-steroidal anti-inflammatory drugs (NSAIDs)

NSAIDs are familiar to most patients and are a useful addition to the range of medicines used in acute pain management. NSAIDs alone are unlikely to be adequate for postoperative analgesia but the quality of opioid analgesia can be enhanced by their use. NSAIDs have analgesic, antipyretic and anti-inflammatory actions and they work by inhibiting the action of enzymes called cyclo-oxygenase (COX). This action inhibits the synthesis of prostaglandins. There are two isoforms of COX: COX-1 and COX-2. COX-1 is a normal constituent with a protective role and is always active, synthesizing prostaglandins for regulation and maintenance of homeostasis. Inhibition of COX-1 will lead to a reduction in this protective function of particular prostaglandins. COX-2 is only active during tissue damage or inflammation, when large numbers of prostaglandins are produced as part of the inflammatory process.

The analgesic action of NSAIDs is directly related to the anti-inflammatory action and is mainly peripheral at the site of injury, although there is some central action. Prostaglandins are only a part of the inflammatory process; therefore, the inhibition of prostaglandin synthesis will only reduce the inflammatory response, because other mediators such as bradykinin and histamine are unaffected. The antipyretic effect is achieved by blocking prostaglandins in the hypothalamus, which regulates normal body temperature. The role of prostaglandins and the actions of NSAIDs in blocking prostaglandins are illustrated more fully in Table 8.2. The full prostaglandin-blocking effect may not occur for several days; therefore, the incidence of side-effects may be reduced if NSAIDs are prescribed for a limited number of days. Side-effects will be more likely with longer-term use and higher doses.

Most NSAIDs will block both COX-1 and COX-2 to some degree, but newer NSAID agents are available that concentrate on blocking COX-2. These are called COX-2-selective anti-inflammatory drugs. Low-dose ibuprofen is considered to be an appropriate first-choice NSAID in terms of low gastrointestinal and cardiovascular risk and is a frequently prescribed simple NSAID for postoperative

Table 8.2 Side-effects of non-steroidal anti-inflammatory drugs (NSAIDs)

Area in which prostaglandins are present	Protective function of prostaglandins	NSAID effect	Additional information and cautions in NSAID use
Gastrointestinal tract	Decrease acid production; inhibit pepsinogen release; stimulate mucus and bicarbonate secretion and mucosal blood flow.	Will inhibit the protective gastric functions of the prostaglandins, which may lead to gastric erosions, gastritis, bleeding. The drugs themselves are also acid-based — if they embed themselves into the gastric mucosa, then they can directly irritate the gastrointestinal tract.	Patients may require gastric protection agents. The NSAID called Arthrotec contains a prostaglandin analogue called misoprostol to reduce gastric irritation. The lowest possible dose of NSAID should be prescribed for the shortest possible time. NSAIDs must not be administered to patients with a history of dyspepsia or gastric ulcers. Patients must be advised to take these medicines with or after food and to stop taking the drug if they have dyspepsia, abdominal pains, vomiting blood, blood in stools. NSAIDs administered by any route have the ability to cause side-effects.
Renal system	Renal blood flow is dependent on prostaglandin E_2. Prostaglandins also help to regulate sodium and water balance and glomerular filtration rate.	May decrease renal blood flow, glomerular filtration rate and urine output. Sodium and water imbalance may lead to water retention and hypertension.	NSAIDs should not be administered to patients who are hypovolaemic, have deranged serum urea and electrolyte levels, are dehydrated or have cardiac failure. Caution should be exercised in patients who are taking angiotensin-converting enzyme (ACE) inhibitor or diuretic medications. Caution in patients over the age of 65 years.
Blood	Role in the regulation and aggregation of platelets. Production of thromboxanes when tissue damage occurs.	May lead to prolonged bleeding times and inhibition of platelet formation (reversible). Reduction in platelet adhesiveness. Inhibition of thromboxane production.	Should not be prescribed for patients with coagulation problems or patients taking warfarin. Advise patient to report any unexplained bruising or bleeding.
Respiratory system	Protective mechanism not clear	Inhibition can lead to mild or severe responses. Adults with a history of asthma more likely to react, also patients with nasal polyps.	If patients have previously taken aspirin or any 'over the counter' NSAIDs without a reaction then likely to be able to tolerate other NSAIDs. Advise patients to stop taking the NSAID if they develop shortness of breath, wheezing, pruritus, facial swelling and/or rashes on the body.

pain in patients who can take oral medication. All NSAIDs have the ability to cause side-effects but the likelihood of these occurring can be reduced by taking a careful history from the patient, by prescribing the lowest effective dose for as short a time as possible, and by giving clear and concise patient information.

There is some debate regarding the use of NSAIDs for patients undergoing orthopaedic surgery or patients who have bone fractures, due to the possibility that NSAIDs may have a negative effect on bone healing in adults in particular. NSAIDs have been found to have less of an effect on bone healing in paediatrics (Wheatley et al, 2019).

Paracetamol

Paracetamol is a simple analgesic which is used for the management of mild to moderate pain. It is a drug that is likely to be familiar to most patients and the majority will report taking it at some time in their lives. Paracetamol is frequently administered regularly as part of multimodal analgesia in acute pain management, as it can be administered orally, rectally, and intravenously as the prodrug propacetamol, therefore making it easy to administer to a diverse range of patient groups and situations.

Oral paracetamol can be combined with a weak opioid to form a compound oral analgesic preparation. Examples of a compound drug are co-codamol, which is paracetamol with codeine, and co-dydramol, which contains paracetamol and dihydrocodeine. Codeine is metabolized to morphine by liver enzymes. However, it is important for practitioners to recognize that some people have a variation of the enzyme that can cause a small amount of morphine to be metabolized or none at all and consequently, it will not provide enough pain relief.

Paracetamol is very dangerous and as little as 5 g of paracetamol taken over a 24-hour period can cause liver problems. Statistics show that, in 2016, deaths from overdosing with paracetamol increased by 11% compared to 2015; the report states deaths could have increased due to accidental poisoning and because paracetamol is easily accessible (Office for National Statistics, 2017). Paracetamol is not contraindicated in patients with liver disease or those who have a heavy alcohol intake, but these patients may require reduced doses.

Local anaesthetic agents

Local anaesthetic agents are used routinely in epidural solutions but some patients may have local anaesthetic nerve blocks performed as part of the anaesthetic to provide balanced postoperative analgesia. Examples of local anaesthetic blocks are femoral nerve blocks for lower limb surgery and brachial plexus blocks for upper limb surgery. Local anaesthetics work by reversibly blocking sodium

channels within nerve cells. The flow of ions across the nerve membrane is then reduced, inhibiting the conduction of impulses and consequent sensory input into the central nervous system. Adrenaline (epinephrine) can be added to a local anaesthetic if vasoconstriction is required. Constriction of blood vessels will prolong the action of the block by reducing absorption into the general circulation, and will also reduce the risk of system toxicity.

Potential risks of local anaesthetic use include toxicity, which is most likely if inadvertent intravenous injection occurs. Bupivacaine is a common local anaesthetic agent, used in epidurals and for local anaesthetic blocks. Bupivacaine binds readily to sodium channels in the nerve cells but it is slow to dissociate. If a patient was given a toxic dose of bupivacaine, the slow dissociation could lead to fatal arrhythmias. Other local anaesthetic agents may be less cardiotoxic but they may have reduced potency.

Adjuvants

Other medicines are often used in addition to analgesics in the management of acute pain. Medicines that enhance the action of analgesics while not actually having an analgesic effect are known as adjuvants. Tricyclic antidepressant medicines such as amitriptyline are frequently used, although their use in pain management is 'off label', which means that they are prescribed outside the manufacturers' licensed use and this must be explained to patients before treatment commences. Anticonvulsant medicines such as carbamazepine, gabapentin and pregabalin can be used for acute neuropathic pain and N-methyl-D-aspartate (NMDA) receptor antagonist drugs such as ketamine are also being seen in clinical practice for acute pain that is opioid-resistant.

The Acute Pain Service team

An Acute Pain Service team should be available in the hospital setting and sets a standard to ensure that patients receive 'safe, effective, optimal pain relief without increasing side-effects'. It achieves this is by educating staff and patients on pain management and equipment. The emphasis should be on the education and support of clinical staff, particularly nurses in the various areas, to ensure that practice is enhanced at local level, rather than staff becoming deskilled by the Acute Pain Service team. Education can be delivered in the clinical setting, including during ward rounds, as well as in formal study days; whatever format is used, education must always include the relevant practical skills, including management of the equipment. This is supported by the use of a skills competency framework. Critical incidents involving pain management must be managed in a supportive way, using reflection to ensure that the incident is used as a learning experience. Acute Pain Services are embedded within the health service and are involved in the education of other health professionals, including trainee anaesthetists, medical students, pharmacy students and physiotherapists.

The practitioner in the clinical area is likely to spend the most time with patients postoperatively compared to other team members. It could be proposed that it is the practitioner who is best placed to enable the patient to get optimal pain relief: hence the importance of the supporting role of the Acute Pain Service team.

Many acute pain teams are advanced practitioner-led on a day-to-day basis. Leadership of an Acute Pain Service requires expert clinical skills and knowledge in the specialty, and roles are constantly developing to support the growing number of patients and the methods used for postoperative pain management. Acute Pain Service teams also help in the care of non-postoperative acute pain patients, such as those with acute back pain, and practitioners on the Acute Pain Service team may be undertaking advanced roles such as nurse prescribing, physical assessment and siting nerve block catheters. Using and developing these skills can bring great job satisfaction, but it is important that the core purpose of undertaking them is to improve patient access to treatment.

The Acute Pain Service team has a responsibility not only to challenge the 'old' ways of doing things but also to find the solutions to do them more effectively while maintaining safety at all times. Only then should the ongoing development of the service, such as the introduction of new drugs and of new techniques, such as patient-controlled epidural analgesia, be considered. All postoperative analgesic practices should be supported by written guidelines, including guidelines for prescribing analgesics.

Finally, the Acute Pain Service team does not work in isolation. The team may work closely with other teams involved in pain, such as the chronic pain team and the palliative care team. The team is also part of the wider hospital team, and good communication by team members is essential to ensure safety and consistency in practice. Until recently, the Acute Pain Service team was almost unique in its set up, but this has changed with the introduction of critical care outreach teams.

SUMMARY OF KEY POINTS

- Pain is a subjective and complex experience: an interaction of both mind and body. Past experiences, culture and background will affect the pain response.
- Pain must be assessed, involving the patient where possible, and this must be a dynamic pain assessment.
- The physiological response to acute pain can be harmful.
- Poorly managed acute pain can lead to the development of chronic pain.
- The use of epidural analgesia containing a local anaesthetic agent may help to reduce the stress response to surgery.
- Multimodal analgesia forms the basis of good postoperative analgesia. Potent opioid analgesics should be used with the addition of regularly prescribed simple analgesics, which will provide an opioid-sparing effect.

REFLECTIVE LEARNING POINTS

Having read this chapter, think about what you now know and what you still need to find out about. These questions may help:
- What are the key differences between acute and chronic pain?
- How might you define pain?
- How can pain have different qualities in some patients?

References

Action on Pain. (2019). *Different types of pain.* Available at: < http://www.action-on-pain.co.uk/you-and-chronic-pain/different-types-of-pain/ >

Anaesthesia UK. (2017). *Patient-controlled analgesia (PCA).* Available at: < https://www.frca.co.uk/article.aspx?articleid = 101344 >

Angelini, E., Wijk, H., Brisby, H., & Baranto, A. (2018). Patients' experience of pain have an impact on their pain management attitudes and strategies.

Pain Management Nursing, 19(5), 464–473.

Association of Anaesthetists of Great Britain and Ireland (AAGBI). (2017). *AABGI: Consent for Anaesthesia 2017.* London: AAGBI.

Association of Anaesthetists of Great Britain and Ireland (AAGBI). (2019). *Dementia and anaesthetics supplementary information.* Available at: < https://www.aagbi.org/sites/default/files/Dementia%20anae14530-sup-0001-Supinfo1-3.pdf >

Bedinger, T., & Plunkett, N. (2016). Measurement in pain medicine. *BJA Education, 16*(9), 310–315.

Chester, R., Khondoker, M., Shepstone, L., Lewis, J., & Jerosch-Herold, C. (2019). Self-efficacy and risk of persistent shoulder pain: results of a Classification and Regression Tree (CART) analysis. *British Journal of Sports Medicine, 53*(13), 825–834.

Correll, D. (2017). *Chronic postoperative pain: recent findings in understanding and management.* Available at:

< https://www.ncbi.nlm.nih.gov/pmc/articles/PMC5499782/pdf/f1000research-6-11975.pdf >

Furyk, J., Levas, D., Close, B., Laspina, K., Fitzpatrick, M., Robinson, K., et al. (2018). Intravenous versus oral paracetamol for acute pain in adults in the emergency department setting: a prospective, double-blind, double-dummy, randomized controlled trial. *Emergency Medicine Journal, 35*(3), 163−168.

Givler, A. & Maani-Fogelman, P. (2019). *The importance of cultural competence in pain and palliative care.* Available at: < https://www.ncbi.nlm.nih.gov/books/NBK493154/ >

Human Rights Act. (1998). *Article 3: Prohibition of torture.* London: HMSO.

Joint Formulary Committee. (2019). *British National Formulary.* London: BMJ Group and Pharmaceutical Press.

Lim, H., Doo, A., Son, J., Kim, K., Lee, K., Kim, D., et al. (2016). Effects of intraoperative signal bolus fentanyl administration and remifentanil infusion on postoperative nausea and vomiting. *Korean Journal of Anaesthesiology, 69*(1), 51−56.

National Institute for Health & Care Excellence (NICE). (2016). *Managing common side effects of opioids for pain relief in palliative care.* Available at: https://pathways.nice.org.uk/pathways/opioids-for-pain-relief-in-palliative-care/managing-common-side-effects-of-opioids-for-pain-relief-in-palliative-care#content = view-node%3Anodes-managing-nausea

National Institute for Health & Care Excellence (NICE). (2019). *Urinary retention.* Available at: < https://bnfc.nice.org.uk/treatment-summary/urinary-retention.html >

NHS. (2017). *Overview: Epidural.* Available at: < https://www.nhs.uk/conditions/epidural/ >

Nursing and Midwifery Council. (2018). *The Code. Professional standards of practice and behaviour for nurses, midwives and nursing associates.* < https://www.nmc.org.uk/globalassets/sitedocuments/nmc-publications/nmc-code.pdf >

Ocay, D., Otis, A., Teles, A., & Ferland, C. (2018). Safety of patient-controlled analgesia after surgery in children and adolescence: concerns and potential solutions. *Frontiers in Paediatrics, 6,* 336.

Office of National Statistics. (2017). *Deaths related to drug poisoning in England and Wales: 2016 registrations.* Available at: < https://www.ons.gov.uk/peoplepopulationandcommunity/birthsdeathsandmarriages/deaths/bulletins/deathsrelatedtodrugpoisoninginenglandandwales/2016registrations >

Royal College of Anaesthetists. (2015). *Core standards for pain management services in the UK.* London: Royal College of Anaesthetists.

Royal College of Anaesthetists. (2019). *Opioids and acute pain management.* Available at: < https://fpm.ac.uk/opioids-aware-clinical-use-opioids/opioids-and-acute-pain-management >

Royal College of Physicians. (2017). *National Early Warning Score (NEWS) 2: Standardising the assessment of acute-illness severity in the NHS.* London: RCP.

Royal Cornwall Hospitals NHS Trust. (2018). *Patient-Controlled Analgesia (PCA) Adult Clinical Guidance.* Truro: Royal Cornwall Hospitals NHS Trust.

Scarth, E., & Smith, S. (2016). *Drugs in anaesthesia and intensive care* (5th ed.). Oxford: Oxford University Press.

Schofield, P. (2018). The assessment of pain in older people: UK National Guidelines. *Age and Ageing, 47,* i1−i22.

Sekimoto, K., Tobe, M., & Santo, S. (2017). Local anesthetic toxicity: acute and chronic management. *Acute Medicine and Surgery, 4*(2), 152−160.

Soffin, E., & Liu, S. (2018). *Chapter 12: Patient-controlled analgesia. Essentials of Pain Medicine* (2nd ed.). London: Elsevier.

The British Pain Society. (2019) *What is Pain?* Available at: < https://www.britishpainsociety.org/about/what-is-pain/ >

Volkow, N., & McLellan, A. (2016). Opioid abuse in chronic pain — misconceptions and mitigation strategies. *The New England Journal of Medicine, 374,* 1253−1263.

Waugh, A., & Grant, A. (2018). *Ross and Wilson's Anatomy and physiology in health and Illness* (13th ed.). London: Elsevier.

Wheatley, B., Nappo, K., Christensen, D., Holman, A., Brooks, D., & Potter, B. (2019). Effect of NSAIDs on bone healing rates. *Journal of the American Academy of Orthopedic Surgeons, 27*(7), 330−336.

World Health Organization. (2014). *Tramadol: Update review report.* Available at: < https://www.who.int/medicines/areas/quality_safety/6_1_Update.pdf >

Wu, A. (2018). Special considerations for opioid use in elderly patients with chronic pain. *US Pharmacist, 43*(3), 26−30.

Yang, M., Hartley, R., Leung, A., Ronksley, P., Jette, N., Casha, S., et al. (2019). Preoperative predictors of poor acute postoperative pain control: a systematic review and meta-analysis. *BMJ Open, 9* (4), e025091.

Yim, N. & Parsa, F. (2018). From the origins of the opioid use (and misuse) to the challenge of opioid-free pain management in surgery. Available at: < https://www.intechopen.com/online-first/from-the-origins-of-the-opioid-use-and-misuse-to-the-challenge-of-opioid-free-pain-management-in-sur >

Chapter 9

Discharge planning following surgery

Julie McLaren

KEY OBJECTIVES OF THE CHAPTER

At the end of the chapter the reader will be able to:

- define and describe the process of discharge planning and relate it to a variety of healthcare environments
- understand the differences in discharge planning for a diverse range of patients
- recognize the importance of communication, multidisciplinary team working and patient/carer involvement in successful discharging.

Areas to think about before reading the chapter

- Who might be involved in discharge planning and what might their roles and responsibilities be?
- What is the role of the nurse during discharge planning?
- When should discharge planning begin and fitness/suitability of discharge be assessed?
- What barriers and/or challenges might be faced during the discharge planning process?

Introduction

This chapter will describe the background, purpose and various considerations related to the patient discharge planning process with the aim of providing knowledge to aid in discharge 'best practice' following all types of surgery.

According to the National Health Service (NHS) Improvement Report (2018), discharging a patient should be a process rather than a one-off occurrence and every patient should have a discharge plan, which should be commenced from the moment of admission. The aim of successful discharge planning is to provide a smooth transition from hospital to home following any form of surgery including bridging any gaps that exist amongst complex cases. Well-planned discharges can also help to provide positive patient outcomes, promote care in the community, and help reduce the cost of care.

After any surgery, the postoperative recovery stage may be hard for the patient. During this time patients can find themselves particularly vulnerable. Every patient admitted to hospital regardless of healthcare setting, or whether they are an emergency or elective admission, should have a discharge plan put in place and this plan should always have the patient at its centre. However, when the discharge planning process does not consider the patient's individual needs, there is a risk of increased length of hospital stay or even readmission following discharge. With this is mind, it is essential that healthcare staff plan for a successful, efficient and well-timed patient discharge.

Over the years, the key principles of how to discharge patients may not have changed. However, the course and management of discharges from hospital have been transformed with particular emphasis on a shortened available length of time to undertake discharge planning. This is because the average inpatient stay has become shorter with patients being sent home at an earlier stage of their recovery, therefore the time permitted for planning discharges appropriately has been significantly reduced. Nevertheless, there has been continued debate about the existence of a good discharge process – what is an efficient means of discharge planning, and what is the right way to undertake this task so the best health, social and economic outcomes are reached for every patient.

With an increasing ageing patient population within hospitals as a result of developments in healthcare services and surgery, consideration needs to be given to patients' increasing vulnerability and often the presence of multi-morbidities. As such, this patient group can often bring with them complexities, and they may also be vulnerable within the discharge planning process. This chapter will consider their needs in detail. The chapter also discusses what discharge planning is and the various elements required to make this a successful process, as well as suggesting some complexities and challenges to consider.

Previous research (Shepperd et al, 2013; Mabire et al, 2018; Kothari & Guzik, 2019) has suggested that patients discharged from hospital often fail to receive the care they need. This can in turn result in readmission which is often costly for the patient, the family and the care provider. This chapter will also discuss ways in which failures in the discharge process can happen and how they can be prevented. Emphasis has been placed on areas identified as directly attributable to poor discharge planning, such as:

- Poor communication between patients and professionals
- Communication breakdown between the multidisciplinary team
- Lack of appropriate patient assessment
- Overreliance on informal care and lack of, or slow provision of, community care
- Inattention to the special needs of the most vulnerable.

What is discharge planning?

According to Weiss et al (2015), discharge planning is: 'The development of an individualized discharge plan prior to leaving the hospital, with the aim of improving patient outcomes and reducing costs of care through timely discharge and coordination of providers and services following hospital discharge to reduce readmission risk and promote community-based health management.' (p. 4)

A Cochrane review undertaken by Shepperd et al (2013) describes discharge planning as being a common element amongst healthcare systems throughout the world. The aim of this discharge planning is to reduce the patient's length of stay as an inpatient, help combat unnecessary readmissions, and enhance the use and management of post-discharge patient services. This can be achieved through the use of individualized patient discharge plans.

For patient discharge to be successful, planning should be undertaken in a timely manner. Consideration of the most appropriate point in the hospital stay to discharge each individual patient should be assessed regularly and communication between hospital and post-discharge services must be well-coordinated.

Assessment

Discharge planning, to ensure a smooth transition from hospital to home, requires the assessment of many areas such as physical, psychological and social, and at a variety of different times from the starting point of admission to the end point of discharge. Some of these assessments, such as motor function, cognition, home circumstances, family/caregiver support and psychosocial and cultural influences, can often be undertaken at the point of admission. Whereas other risk assessments, such as knowledge and information shortfalls, will often be completed nearer to the point of discharge. Assessment and evaluation of relevant aspects of the patient's care and circumstances should also be undertaken by a member of the multidisciplinary team (MDT) at an appropriate time during admission, including psychological status, intravenous medications (i.e. antibiotics/chemotherapy), home environment, and surrounding support from family, friends and/or carers. Part of this assessment process should also include continuous consideration of the patient's readiness for discharge including their needs, desires and abilities, and if they are appropriately prepared and equipped to be discharged effectively and safely. The correct timing and management of assessment can have a direct impact on successful patient discharge. As a rule, assessment should be continuously undertaken throughout the hospital stay to ensure an informed decision is made regarding readiness for discharge and the need for additional care post-discharge. However, like all areas of healthcare, if assessment is not undertaken and/or communicated efficiently, then this can impact on discharge planning due to misunderstandings concerning individual circumstances and personal requirements (including social environment, transport needs and community service requests).

Patients undergoing elective surgery

When coming into hospital for elective surgery, patients often attend a pre-admission appointment, which can be days or even weeks before the planned date of surgery. During this appointment, an ideal opportunity exists to begin the discussion and organization of discharge with the patient and their families/carers (if appropriate), making every contact count. This discussion should include a conversation about expectations of discharge and possible delays to the process from both the patient and the healthcare perspective. This will allow plans and support, if or where needed, to be put in place as early as possible. This will also ensure that any unnecessary delays do not happen at the point of discharge.

Patients undergoing emergency surgery

In a situation or setting in which emergency admissions exist it is challenging and often not possible to start discharge planning immediately. However, this should still be carried out as quickly as possible after admission and, where appropriate and feasible, undertaken within 24 hours of the patient's admission for surgery.

Policy and guidelines: discharge planning

Regardless of elective or emergency admission, a set of discharge guidelines should be followed to ensure a smooth process. These guidelines should consider the following as a baseline:

- Indicate an approximate date and time for discharge as early as possible
- Identify if the patient will be a straightforward or complex discharge
- Determine what the patient's needs are (if any) post-discharge and how they can be supported
- Confirm what requirements are expected to be met by that patient to be safely discharged.

There may be occasion, particularly in settings such as day surgery, in which there are a high number of straightforward and uncomplicated discharges. In this case, the nurse undertaking the discharge should follow a fairly standardized process that is usual for their particular area of practice but generally based upon the following guidelines according to the NHS Improvement (2018):

1. Start planning before or on admission:
   - This should be continuously updated and assessed.
2. Identify whether the patient has simple or complex needs and their likely care pathway:
   - A simple discharge is one that can be executed at ward level with the MDT

- Funding issues, changes of residence, increased health or social needs and vulnerable patients can make discharge complex.
3. Develop a clinical management plan within 24 hours of admission. This management plan should aim to combine the thoughts of the MDT and the patient on aspects of discharge care.
4. Coordinate the discharge or transfer process using administrative staff or specially trained nurses.
5. Set an expected date of discharge within 48 hours of admission – this should be estimated as early as possible to guide the discharge planning process. The date can then be reassessed and changed according to ongoing patient assessment.
6. Review the clinical management plan daily.
7. Involve the patient and their family/carers if appropriate – this is to ensure that expectations and complexities can be managed.
8. Plan discharges and transfers to take place over 7 days.
9. Complete the discharge checklist (often available amongst patient electronic or paper notes) 48 hours prior to the expected discharge date.
10. Make decisions regarding transfer and discharge every day.

Communication and collaboration

To provide successful discharge planning it is essential that input has been gained from all appropriate professionals involved (for example, nurses, doctors, physiotherapists, dieticians). Part of this encompasses the successful coming together of all areas of care and support to provide a smooth transition from hospital to home or a secondary care facility. Efficacious discharge coordination includes effective communication between the MDT, good post-discharge care arrangements, and successful sharing of patient information between care providers. The extent of MDT involvement will vary depending on when the admission takes place throughout the working day, i.e. admissions after 1700h will often not be reviewed by medical or allied health professional (i.e. physiotherapists, dieticians) staff until the ward round the following day.

Inadequate communications and coordination between nursing staff, the MDT, and other professionals and services involved in the care of the patient being discharged can lead to the risk of an adverse event such as delayed discharge, readmission and inadequate postoperative care.

National Institute for Health and Care Excellence (NICE) guidelines (2013) explain that deficiencies in the communication between care services both during the inpatient stay and post-discharge can lead to important patient information being miscommunicated and in turn delays in discharge or poor management once back in the community.

Roles and responsibilities

Discharge planning is something that should be undertaken by a registered nurse, social worker or other healthcare professional. The decision that a patient is medically fit for discharge is usually made by the doctor responsible for the care of the patient. However, it is often the case that the nurse, although not generally responsible for making the decision to discharge, is the most appropriate person to undertake the planning and execution of the actual discharge (Nordmark et al, 2016). This is often a nominated nursing duty accepted by the MDT, primarily because nurses tend to be at the forefront of patient care on a daily basis and they are best placed to prepare patients and their families/carers for discharge. The nurse observes the everyday needs and the individual situation of each patient as well as any changes in their condition that occur.

Although nurses and social workers have been seen as the key roles in discharge planning, successful discharge planning must also hold at its core valuable collaboration between the various members of the MDT and anyone else involved in the discharge of a particular patient, e.g. pharmacists, transport services and appropriate therapists. Within this collaboration, the communication and sharing of essential information should always happen effectively.

It is also essential for the nominated person responsible for the discharge planning process, usually the nurse or discharge coordinator, to ensure that any follow-up care or appointments are organized efficiently and within the appropriate timescales. This nominated person should also be responsible for the identification of any other services needed for successful discharge. These services may include health and social care practitioners and family members and ensure that their contact details are available within the discharge plan.

There must also be effective communications with other services that may be provided within the community setting, and in particular, appropriate information sharing with the patient's general practitioner (GP). Any healthcare professionals, i.e. any member of the MDT, responsible for the care of the patient should ensure they complete and update the discharge summary which provides details of the admission and any plans decided on for successful discharge. This summary should be made available to community services involved in the care of the patient, in particular the patient's GP. A copy of this should also be provided to the patient on the day of discharge.

Patient/family/carer involvement

All patients (and, if appropriate, carers and family) should have the opportunity to participate in decision-making related to their care needs prior to, during and after surgery, including discharge planning decision-making. Patients themselves are often best placed to know and discuss their potential postoperative needs and should be given the opportunity to ask questions or mention concerns. The earlier that this discussion can happen, the better equipped and more organized the MDT are for planning the discharge.

Families and carers play a vital role during discharge planning and often particularly at times when decisions surrounding discharge are required when the patient is still ill. This is an important element of a successful discharge and is linked to improved patient satisfaction and postoperative outcome. All members of the MDT involved in patient care and discharge planning should recognize that carers and family members provide an enriched knowledge base regarding the patient and may be able to offer detailed information regarding the patient's individual circumstances and requirements. When patients and family members/carers are not involved in this process, this can often lead to lack of knowledge and increased risks in relation to self-management after discharge.

Patient-centred discharge planning

Patient-centred care is vital throughout healthcare and should be integrated into the process of discharge planning. NICE guidelines (2015) state that every patient should be seen as an individual and an equal who can make choices about their own care, and they should be treated with dignity and respect throughout their transition. NICE guidelines (2016) also suggest that transition from hospital to home/care facility is patient-centred and is directed by recovery. During discharge planning, healthcare professionals should pay attention to the holistic needs of each individual patient, and patient participation should be encouraged. However, this can often be let down by the healthcare practitioner's own limitations, attitudes and behaviours in practice. Nonetheless, the question of what matters to the patient should always be asked; gathering all relevant information relating to the patient is essential and should include their personal motivations and goals, their social and financial situation, and their specific care needs, including any requirement for additional support services to allow for discharge. A discharge plan that is patient-centred and tailored to the individual can often lead to a reduction in the risk of readmission post-surgery (Shepperd et al, 2013), suggesting that individualized discharge planning and tailored support can drastically reduce unnecessary hospital readmissions.

Patients with complex needs

There may be some occasions when consideration needs to be given to patients with complex needs who undergo surgery, for example vulnerable or elderly patients. These patients will often need enhanced support and input from additional areas, such as social work, physiotherapy and occupational therapy. There may also be a requirement for extra care needs to be met by services available out in the community, such as the provision of specialist equipment (e.g. hospital-style bed), daily support from carers to help complete activities of living, or regular district nurse visits (e.g. to administer medication). It is this inclusion of supplementary services that can make discharge a complicated and involved process. NICE guidelines (2018) explain that the delivery of an efficient and well-timed discharge built upon a robust plan is vital to the successful transition of patients with complex needs from hospital to home or to a care facility. A poorly planned and executed discharge could result in poor patient outcomes, including increased length of stay in hospital. It could also have dangerous implications, directly impacting on patient safety.

Like any other discharge planning process, the successful and safe discharge of a patient with complex needs relies heavily on the coming together of all healthcare professionals involved in the care of the patient both within the hospital setting and also in the community setting. To mirror other aspects of healthcare the discharge planning of patients with complex needs must consider the holistic patient-centred situation including personal circumstances, preferences, functional ability, past medical history and available support on discharge. The Nursing and Midwifery Council (2018) stipulates that nurses must listen to patients and respond to their preferences and concerns. The nurse must work in partnership with people ensuring that care is delivered effectively and must recognize and respect the contribution that people can make to their own health and well-being.

When a patient requires any kind of additional support for discharge there must be certain steps followed to ensure this is done safely and correctly:

1. If the patient resided in social care (e.g. care home or supported living), then details of this should be noted during admission and regular updates and plans for discharge provided to them.

2. During the patient's stay and after surgery, an assessment of the patient's support needs should be undertaken.

3. A discharge summary or other appropriate form of communication should be sent to areas of support prior to discharge, advising of expected discharge time and date, and the patient's expected ability and support requirements.

An important thing to remember when discharging patients with complex needs is that no important decisions, for example, changes to current care arrangements and the choice to move into long-term care, are made by patients during times of vulnerability. In the case of any patient who is homeless on admission, it is helpful to liaise with the local government authority (or equivalent) to ensure that the person has the right support at the point of discharge. The Queen's Nursing Institute (2015) provides guidance for the care of homeless people using a health assessment tool.

Caring for the older person

As a result of advances in surgical technologies and the provision of improved health and social care, there is an increasingly ageing population in the UK. As people live longer, patients are often admitted with multi-morbidities, chronic diseases, cognitive decline and complex needs. According to the Department of Health (2016), older patients make up the highest percentage (62%) of beds within hospital settings. This patient group can often be vulnerable and at risk of a slower recovery, and evidence shows an increase in unnecessary hospital stays amongst elderly patients aged 65 years and over (Department of Health, 2016). Pellet (2016), in a Queen's Nursing Institute report, has suggested that patients aged 75 years and over are at greater risk of readmission, particularly if they are not provided with adequate support upon discharge, compared with other age groups. Age UK (2016) have explained that delayed discharges and unnecessary stays in hospital often negate the original reason for admission and frequently elderly patients are discharged home in a less independent state than when they were admitted. The Department of Health (2016) agreed with this, explaining that for older patients a lengthier hospital stay can often worsen their original predicted health outcome and increase their care needs long term. The Department of Health (2016) also comment that increasing inpatient stays for elderly patients can impact on the financial pressures of the NHS and local government. Therefore, it is essential, that elderly patients have a clear and well-planned discharge put in place at the point of admission. Otherwise the consequences faced may be dangerous and costly including a higher rate of readmission.

Challenges in caring for the older surgical patient

One of the biggest challenges faced postoperatively by elderly patients is a decline in food and/or fluid intake. For some patients, this may be further exacerbated by malnutrition on admission. This nutritional deficit means that patients pose a risk of unnecessarily long hospital stays, susceptibility to readmission and significantly poorer quality of life. It is for this reason that extra emphasis should be placed on the nutritional intake of elderly patients during their stay in hospital with dietician input (where necessary), from the point of admission and throughout discharge planning.

Further issues must also be considered by the nurse with regards to independence and surgical intervention. Independence is the ability to undertake the activities of living with little or no interference. However, surgical intervention has the potential to take away a person's independence (temporarily or long term) and this can result in a dependence on others for health and social care needs, which can impact negatively on a person's health and wellbeing. The RCN (2018) have made the implications of delayed discharge amongst elderly patients clear and explain explicitly that it is the responsibility of the whole nursing team to understand these negative implications.

Elderly patients who remain in hospital unnecessarily, for example due to delayed discharge after surgery, may be exposed to the risk of some form of muscle wastage, which in turn can make the person more susceptible to falls, and makes activities such as climbing stairs and getting out of bed difficult. This complex area of care, if not acknowledged during admission and discharge planning, can lead to recurrent admissions postoperatively, and in some extreme cases death following discharge (Berian et al, 2016). An example of good practice to encourage independence is to help patients get out of bed and get dressed each day. However, it may still be that elderly patients require some short- or even long-term care support in the community to live as independently as possible, such as providing care services to their home or staying in supportive living accommodation or a care home facility.

Guidelines for the discharge of patients with additional care needs

Some guidelines for the successful discharge of patients requiring additional care support can include:

- Early informal notification to the care facility of the patient's level of functionality and expected date of discharge.
- The inclusion of care home managers in the discharge planning process (if applicable).

- Provide or obtain a single named contact from each area or service involved in the patient's care.
- Ensure comprehensive communications with all services and appropriate documentation is provided to care providers.
- Take home medications should be organized, ordered and made available the day before discharge.
- Make timely transport arrangements for safe transition of the patient from hospital to home/care facility.
- Clear communication with patients and family and/or carers giving accurate information, expectations and timescales.

Teaching and education

An important aspect to ensuring that the patient and their family and/or carers are ready for discharge is the offer of effective patient education. The provision of a supportive educational discharge structure can ensure that patients feel empowered in the discharge process and gain confidence in the ability to self-manage their post-discharge care. During education, patients can be given important information regarding what to expect during their postoperative recovery including possible complications and their warning signs. The first 30 days of recovery is when postoperative patients are at their most vulnerable to postoperative complications such as haemorrhage and infection, which can often not present until after discharge (Kang et al, 2018). If patients do not receive an adequate level of education during their admission in preparation for discharge, then the risks of complication and readmission is heightened.

In essence, the provision of effective postoperative education could potentially prevent up to half of hospital readmissions following surgery. If postoperative education is not provided at the right level or the right amount, it is possible that patients can become vulnerable to postoperative complications, such as wound infection, pulmonary embolism and deep vein thrombosis, which in turn increases negative outcomes, including readmission.

How and when to teach postoperative patients

How and when this teaching is communicated to patients, and the content of the discussion, can have a direct link to the patient's ability to recover successfully at home. Factors to be considered when thinking about the level of education and teaching are gender, age and type of surgery, which could affect the person's ability to learn. The success of discharge education and teaching can also be linked to patients' varying levels of health literacy (Weiss et al, 2015). People who are health literate, for example, often communicate more effectively with the healthcare team and are able to express their needs and their decisions to aid in their post-surgery recovery period compared to those with limited health literacy (McMurray et al, 2007). For those less health literate, communication and discussing their needs can prove to be a challenge and can cause barriers when discussing or teaching around discharge planning. Consideration must also be given to the learning needs and capabilities of the individual patient. Education must be delivered at a level and in a language that the person will understand whilst ensuring that it provides all the key and important information. This may mean that standard information needs to be tailored to the individual patient; for example, some patients may prefer verbal instruction, some may relate better to visual aids, and some may need to be provided with the information more than once to allow the information to be assimilated.

Kang et al (2018) have suggested that the most effective way to include patient education and teaching is to incorporate it throughout the whole of the patient's stay, which provides the person with the ability to make informed decisions about their care and discharge. However, it must not be something that occurs solely on the day of discharge, as other factors on that day may result in a learning environment that is not conducive to retaining information offered. When undertaking moments of patient education, the nurse should consider the patient holistically, and explain and demonstrate to the person in a person-centred manner taking into account the individual's personal circumstances rather than providing a 'one size fits all' explanation. This can help the patient to gain an effective understanding of the key issues whilst the nurse is gaining an understanding of potential barriers or challenges that the patient may have.

What to teach postoperative patients

In terms of the content of discharge education, it is essential for patients and family/carers to understand how to care for themselves or their relative, and to understand what the normal healing process is and how to monitor for symptoms of postoperative complications. Patients should also be provided with advice on appropriate support and community services available to them as well as contact details and practical advice should they be worried at all about their recovery.

Discharge medication

Historically, the input of a pharmacist in the discharge process has been limited, often only occurring at the very last minute. However, pharmacy input into the discharge planning process is essential. Medications required to take home on discharge should be organized and made available in a timely manner, with preference to this being on the day prior to discharge in order to combat long waits and delays on the day of discharge. According to NICE guidelines (2013), most UK healthcare trusts encourage early dispensing of discharge medications during inpatient hospital stays. Most UK healthcare trusts also rely heavily on the use and availability of patients' own drugs, which they are requested to bring into hospital prior to admission. The responsibilities of the nurse in the organization of discharge medication remain vital, with nurses being in the best position to identify any drugs requiring to be ordered for discharge.

The effective organization and ordering of discharge medication by both the nursing and pharmacy staff provides overall benefit to the patient experience and can ensure a timely patient discharge.

Barriers and challenges to discharge planning

A constant pressure to empty inpatient beds provides an unfortunate opportunity to discharge patients too soon in their recovery. In addition to this, the increasing pressure on healthcare economies and minimally invasive procedures can mean that patients can be subjected to faster discharges often as soon as they have regained their baseline mobility. These pressures should not mean that there are unplanned or uncoordinated discharges happening within healthcare. However, bed management often causes discharges that are poorly organized (NHS Executive, 2000). Faster discharges can bring with them less time to discuss, teach and plan suitable and safe discharges. When discharges are rushed, there are often time constraints on arranging community support, such as district nurse visits. There may also be less time to offer a patient-centred approach to discharging. This is often a concern of the nursing team along with sufficient time to gather all relevant information, which would ensure efficient patient-centred discharge planning.

NICE (2015) details barriers to successful discharge planning including poor communication, poor provision of specialist equipment, lack of care (particularly home care packages), and delay in the provision of discharge medication and transport from hospital. NICE (2015) also reported on lack of time to ensure that the appropriate people are identified to ensure the plan is patient-centred.

Conclusion

In contemporary healthcare practice the motivation to improve discharge planning has never been greater. This is because advances in technology now mean that potentially life-enhancing surgery is possible particularly due to the overall ageing population. Simultaneously, pressure on acute hospital beds and emphasis on standards of care delivery within community settings has encouraged rapid patient discharge. Paradoxically, just as the need for thorough and efficient discharge planning is heightened, the available time in which to achieve this is significantly reduced.

In looking to the future, goals such as improved discharge planning with reductions in readmission could be enhanced by better interprofessional communication and more consideration of patient-centred discharge planning.

This chapter has discussed the various themes, principles and goals of discharge planning, which must be addressed when nurses and other healthcare professionals are considering 'best practice' methods of discharge planning, particularly for the older patient following surgery.

SUMMARY OF KEY POINTS

- Discharge planning is a complex process which must involve all members of the multidisciplinary team.
  (Continued)

(cont'd)

- Poor discharge planning can lead to readmission to hospital, at considerable cost — both emotionally and financially — to patients, relatives of the patients, and the healthcare economy.
- Discharge planning is important for all patients leaving hospital, but certain groups of patients, e.g. the elderly, those living alone, those who are homeless and those whose carers are elderly, are particularly vulnerable.
- Discharge planning must start early, possibly even before admission to hospital, and must address physical, psychological, emotional and social health needs.

REFLECTIVE LEARNING POINTS

Having read this chapter, think about what you now know and what you still need to find out about. These questions may help:

- Outline the key factors that must be given consideration when providing patient-centred discharge.
- In the area where you are working, what is the local policy and procedure regarding a referral to the community healthcare team?
- How will you provide information to other members of the health and social care team with regard to a patient's discharge without breaching confidentiality?

References

Age UK. (2016). *Behind the headlines: Are older people and their families really to blame when their hospital discharges are delayed?* Available at: < https://www.ageuk.org.uk/Documents/EN-GB/Press%20releases/Behind_the_Headlines.pdf?dtrk = true >

Berian, J. R., Mohanty, S., Ko, C. Y., Rosenthal, R. A., & Robinson, T. N. (2016). Association of loss of independence with readmission and death after discharge in older patients after surgical procedures. *JAMA Surgery, 151*(9), e161689—e161689.

Department of Health. (2016). *Discharging older patients from hospital.* London: National Audit Office.

Kang, E., Gillespie, B. M., Tobiano, G., & Chaboyer, W. (2018). Discharge education delivered to general surgical patients in their management of recovery post discharge — a systematic mixed studies review. *International Journal of Nursing Studies, 87,* 1—13.

Kothari, P., & Guzik, J. (2019). *Health care provider perpectives on discharge planning: from hospital to skilled nursing facility.* Quality Institute, United Hospital Fund.

Mabire, C., Dwyer, A., Garnier, A., & Pellet, J. (2018). Meta-analysis of the effectiveness of nursing discharge planning interventions for older inpatients discharged home. *Journal of Advanced Nursing, 74*(4), 788—799.

McMurray, A., Johnson, P., Wallis, M., Patterson, E., & Griffiths, S. (2007). General surgical patients' perspectives of the adequacy and appropriateness of discharge planning to facilitate health decision-making at home. *Journal of Clinical Nursing, 16*(9), 1602—1609.

National Health Service (NHS) Executive. (2000). *Inpatient admissions and bed management in NHS acute hospitals.* London: The Stationery Office.

National Health Service (NHS) Improvement. (2018). *Quality, service improvement and redesign tools: Discharge planning.* Available at: < https://improvement.nhs.uk/resources/discharge-planning/ >

National Institute for Health and Care Excellence (NICE). (2013). *Pharmacy management and nurse-led medicines ordering: To improve efficiency and aid patient discharge.* Available at: < https://arms.evidence.nhs.uk/resources/qipp/588825/attachment >

National Institute for Health and Care Excellence (NICE). (2015). *Transition between inpatient hospital settings and community or care home settings for adults with social care needs.* Available from <https://www.nice.org.uk/guidance/ng27>

National Institute for Health and Care Excellence (NICE). (2016). *Transition between inpatient mental health settings and community or care home settings.* Available at: <https://www.nice.org.uk/guidance/ng53>

National Institute for Health and Care Excellence (NICE). (2018). *Chapter 35 Discharge planning — emergency and acute medical care in over 16s: service delivery and organization.* Available at: <https://www.nice.org.uk/guidance/ng94/evidence/35.discharge-planning-pdf-172397464674>

Nordmark, S., Zingmark, K., & Lindberg, I. (2016). Process evaluation of discharge planning implementation in healthcare using normalization process theory. *BMC Medical Informatics and Decision Making, 16*(1), 48.

Nursing and Midwifery Council. (2018). *The Code. Professional standards of practice and behavior for nurses, midwives and nursing associates.* Available at: <https://www.nmc.org.uk/globalassets/sitedocuments/nmc-publications/nmc-code.pdf>

Pellet, C. (2016). *Discharge planning: best practice in transitions of care.* Available at: <https://www.qni.org.uk/resources/discharge-planning-best-practice-transitions-care/>

Royal College of Nursing (RCN). (2018). *Delayed discharge.* Available at: <https://www.rcn.org.uk/magazines/health%20and%20care/2018/delayed-discharge>

Shepperd, S., Lannin, N. A., Clemson, L. M., McCluskey, A., Cameron, I. D., & Barras, S. L. (2013). Discharge planning from hospital to home. *Cochrane Database of Systematic Reviews* (1), CD000313.

The Queen's Nursing Institute. (2015). *Assessing the healthcare needs of people who are homeless.* Available at: <https://www.qni.org.uk/wp-content/uploads/2016/10/HAT_final_web.pdf>

Weiss, M. E., Bobay, K. L., Bahr, S. J., Costa, L., Hughes, R. G., & Holland, D. E. (2015). A model for hospital discharge preparation: from case management to care transition. *Journal of Nursing Administration, 45*(12), 606—614.

Further reading

Cameron, B. (2018). The impact of pharmacy discharge planning on continuity of care. *The Canadian Journal of Hospital Pharmacy, 47*(3), 101—109.

Department of Health and Social Care. (2018). *The Delayed Discharges (Continuing Care) Directions 2013.* Available at: <https://www.gov.uk/government/publications/delayed-discharges-continuing-care-directions>

Goncalves-Bradley, D. C., Lannin, N. A., Clemson, L. M., Cameron, I. D., & Shepperd, S. (2016). Discharge planning from hospital. *Cochrane Database of Systematic Reviews* (1), CD000313.

Hesselink, G., Schoonhoven, L., Barach, P., Spijker, A., Gademan, P., Kalkman, C., et al. (2012). Improving patient handovers from hospital to primary care. *Ann Intern Med, 157*(6), 417—428.

Jones, D., Musselman, R., Pearsall, E., McKenzie, M., Huang, H., & McLeod, R. S. (2017). Ready to go home? Patients' experiences of the discharge process in an enhanced recovery after surgery (ERAS) program for colorectal surgery. *Journal of Gastrointestinal Surgery, 21*(11), 1865—1878.

Lees, L. (2013). The key principles of effective discharge planning. *Nursing Times, 109*(3), 18.

Lithner, M., Klefsgard, R., Johansson, J., & Andersson, E. (2015). The significance of information after discharge for colorectal cancer surgery—a qualitative study. *BMC Nursing, 14*(1), 36.

Murphy, T., Butler, M., & Kidd, J. (2018). Losing something of value: An exploration of risk in discharge planning with older people. *New Zealand Journal of Occupational Therapy, 65*(2), 13.

Thoma, J. E., & Waite, M. A. (2018). Experiences of nurse case managers within a central discharge planning role of collaboration between physicians, patients and other healthcare professionals: A sociocultural qualitative study. *Journal of Clinical Nursing, 27*(5-6), 1198—1208.

Ulin, K., Olsson, L. E., Wolf, A., & Ekman, I. (2016). Person-centred care—An approach that improves the discharge process. *European Journal of Cardiovascular Nursing, 15*(3), e19—e26.

Young, A. M., Mudge, A. M., Banks, M. D., Rogers, L., Demedio, K., & Isenring, E. (2018). Improving nutritional discharge planning and follow up in older medical inpatients: Hospital to Home Outreach for Malnourished Elders. *Nutrition & Dietetics, 75*(3), 283—290.

Section | 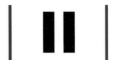 |

Nursing care for specific surgical procedures

Chapter 10

Patients requiring neurosurgery

Chris Brunker

KEY OBJECTIVES OF THE CHAPTER

At the end of the chapter the reader should be able to:

- Give a brief overview of the anatomy of the skull and brain.
- Discuss the phenomenon of intracranial pressure and the danger of raised intracranial pressure.
- Discuss the indications for neurosurgery, different operative approaches and neurosurgical operations.
- Describe the common symptoms and presentations of neurological disease and the investigations patients may undergo.

- Describe preoperative assessment, specialist neurological observations and the special significance of basic observations in neurological disease.
- Describe the holistic care of patients undergoing intracranial surgery, showing an increased awareness of neurological deficits and the longer-term consequences of neurological disease.

Areas to think about before reading the chapter

- How can brain disease affect activities of living, such as eating and drinking and maintaining personal hygiene?
- What can cause raised pressure within the skull (intracranial pressure)?
- How can brain disease affect work and family life?

Introduction

Imagine walking along a busy pavement on a cold sunny day. Now consider what your brain must do to accomplish this basic task. You move head, trunk, arms and legs in a smooth sequence, constantly adjusting to the uneven surface of the pavement beneath you and the slope of the street. You integrate vision and hearing as you decide the positions and predict the paths of people and vehicles. You make decision after decision: move a little to the left to avoid someone, speed up to squeeze through that gap and overtake the person dawdling in front of you. Are the lights at the next crossing going to change in time or should you walk further along the street? You register the adverts on the sides of the buses and the conversations of strangers. Your pupils constrict and dilate as you move between shade and light, you pull your coat a little tighter around you against the cold and you smell the traffic fumes and taste the remains of your breakfast. Every now and then you swallow the saliva in your mouth and your breathing, heart rate and blood pressure change as you speed up or slow down. And you are not thinking about any of this: you're just walking along.

We usually overlook the fabulous complexity of what our brains do (what we do, for we are our brains) all of the time. It is sometimes only when disease changes our brains and how we perceive, experience and act in the world that we can see just how much we have taken for granted. The brain makes everything possible, from chewing a mouthful of food to writing an opera. The brain is the memory, the personality, the hopes and fears of each human and every brain is unique.

Overview of the anatomy and function of the brain

The human brain is a mass of around 10 billion nerve cells (neurons), each of which has around 10,000 possible connections (synapses) to other neurons, creating a system of unimaginable complexity. Yet this astounding organ is small: about 1350 g. It is soft and easily damaged, it needs a constant supply of oxygen and glucose and only functions well within narrow ranges of temperature, acid–base balance, and fluid and electrolyte levels.

The skull

The brain is completely encased in the skull. Fused pairs of bones form a vault over the upper surface and continue under the brain to complete the base. The spinal cord emerges from an opening in the skull base (the foramen magnum).

The meninges

There are three meningeal layers. The dura mater is fairly thick (like fine leather) and adheres to the inside surface of the skull, with two folds projecting inwards: the falx cerebri separates the left and right cerebral hemispheres while the tentorium cerebri separates the upper brain (cerebrum) from the brain stem and cerebellum. Below the dura is the subdural space. The arachnoid mater is much finer than the dura, like a spider's web, and follows the contours of the brain surface. Under the arachnoid is the subarachnoid space. The pia mater is a very fine membrane adhering to the brain surface.

Cerebrospinal fluid and the cerebral ventricles

The subarachnoid space is filled with a light straw-coloured cerebrospinal fluid (CSF). In the middle of the brain's structures are four CSF-filled ventricles: two (left and right lateral) in the cerebral hemispheres, a third deeper and midline and the fourth midline at the level of the brainstem. CSF circulates around the system via narrow aqueducts. CSF helps maintain a narrow range of pressure, temperature and chemical balance and the ventricles maintain the brain's shape.

The cerebrovascular system

Two pairs of arteries supply the brain. The vertebral arteries run up the anterior surface of the spine, enter the skull and join to form the basilar artery which feeds the brainstem and cerebellum. Two internal carotid arteries enter the skull further forward. Pairs of communicating arteries link these feeding vessels to form the circle of Willis and the cerebral arteries branch off to supply the cerebrum. The brain controls the flow and pressure of arterial blood inside the skull, buffering the cerebral circulation from surges or drops in systemic blood pressure (BP). This auto-regulation can become impaired in acute brain disease, leading to under- or overperfusion.

Venous blood drains into sinuses in the dura and then into the jugular veins and down to the subclavian veins and back to the heart. There are no valves in the system: effective drainage depends on patency of the vessels, gravity and the difference between the intracranial and intrathoracic pressures.

The brain stem

The brain stem handles the most basic and essential functions. There are three parts. The midbrain relays motor signals from the upper brain to the spinal cord and processes visual and auditory information. The pons is involved in sensory analysis, movement and posture and is the origin of the reticular activating network, a pathway linking to the cerebral cortex which generates alertness. The medulla oblongata is the site of the cardiovascular centres, which control heart rate and blood pressure, and the respiratory centre, which controls breathing.

The cranial nerves

The cranial nerves form direct neural pathways connecting the brain to other parts of the body and to the outside world. There are twelve pairs of nerves, ten of which join the brain stem; the other two enter the anterior skull and join the cerebrum directly.

The cerebellum

The cerebellum is a distinct region behind the brain stem whose major function is the coordination of movement. It integrates eye movement with bodily movement and allows visual tracking of moving objects.

The limbic system and the hypothalamus

The limbic system comprises structures (thalamus, hypothalamus, amygdala and hippocampus) deep in the brain which help coordinate movement, maintain bodily homeostasis and are the seat of our most basic drives and emotions: hunger, thirst, attraction and aggression. The limbic system is also involved in the formation and retrieval of memory.

The pituitary gland

Projecting down from the hypothalamus is the pituitary gland, a small bulb attached by a stalk. The hypothalamus and pituitary are critical to the autonomic and hormonal systems of the body. The pituitary sits in a small bony cavity on the skull floor, close to the crossing of the optic nerves; the first sign of a pituitary tumour may be a problem with vision.

The cerebral cortex

The cerebrum, or cerebral cortex, is divided into four pairs of lobes: frontal, temporal, parietal and occipital. The left side of the brain manages the right side of the body and vice versa. Much of the complex work of the brain depends on the integrated working of multiple regions, but specific areas do show significant specialization. The occipital lobes deal with vision, the parietal lobes with sensory information and perception, the temporal lobes with hearing and balance and the frontal lobes with movement as well as higher-level functions such as attention, decision-making and judgement and personality. Vocabulary and grammar are usually controlled by the left side of the brain and other aspects of language (stress and intonation) by the right.

Grey and white matter

The cell bodies of the cortical neurons are concentrated in a thick outer layer: the grey matter, with its characteristic wrinkles and folds. Connecting axonal fibres, which carry the neuronal impulses, are bundled together in the deeper, paler core known as white matter. On a CT scan the grey matter, being denser, appears paler than the white matter.

Box 10.1 Causes of raised intracranial pressure

- Haematomas
- Abscesses
- Cerebral oedema
- Tumours
- Arteriovenous malformations
- Hydrocephalus

Intracranial pressure

The skull is a rigid box completely filled by its normal contents: brain, blood vessels and CSF. In fact, the skull is slightly overfilled, with a slight internal pressure: the intracranial pressure (ICP), which in normal circumstances is between 0 and 15 mmHg. If one of the skull's contents expands and occupies more space (Box 10.1), one of the others must take up less space or the ICP will rise. Raised ICP is significant because it compresses the capillaries and reduces the flow of oxygenated blood, causing secondary ischaemia, which leads to swelling and further rises in ICP. If this cycle is not stopped the pressure will build up to such an extent that the brain will decompress itself through the tentorium cerebri. The pressure 'cone' this creates crushes the brain stem, killing the patient.

Indications for neurosurgery

Tumours

Tumours inside the skull occupy space, raising the ICP and disrupting adjacent structures. A brain tumour will be fatal if its growth cannot be controlled.

Neurons do not divide and multiply in adult brains and so do not form tumours. But primary tumours may grow from glial cells (support cells interspersed with the neurons) or from the meningeal layers. Gliomas are graded depending on how invasive they are (Santosh, 2014; Kleihues et al, 2017): a low-grade glioma is benign and relatively easy to separate from healthy tissue. High-grade gliomas are invasive and malignant, they cannot be removed completely and prognosis is poor. Meningiomas are benign, relatively slow-growing and clearly distinct from brain tissue. This makes them relatively easy to remove although, depending on their location, complete removal is not always possible (Jalali et al, 2017). Tumours may also develop from support cells associated with the cranial nerves, particularly the acoustic nerve. Secondary tumours (metastases) are sites of spread from cancers elsewhere in the body. Prognosis depends on the

133

course of the primary disease and the extent of the cerebral spread.

Spontaneous haematomas

Spontaneous intracranial haemorrhage can be the result of a cerebrovascular abnormality (see below), a tumour or hypertensive bleeding. Haematomas damage the surrounding tissue and raise the ICP. Surgery to evacuate a haematoma may save life but will not correct the damage done to the brain by the bleed.

Hydrocephalus

Hydrocephalus is an excess of CSF within the skull, caused by overproduction, underabsorption or a block in circulation. Hydrocephalus can be acute (blood in the CSF from a haemorrhage slows re-absorption and blocks the aqueducts, for example), chronic (infection may scar the aqueducts, reducing flow), or congenital (some people are born without patent aqueducts). Hydrocephalus creates a rise in ICP which may be fatal if not treated by diverting the excess CSF.

Infection

Bacterial infection can cause an abscess or empyema to form. This sort of infection may result from a breach in the skull (such as a penetrating wound or infected surgical site) or from infections invading the skull from nearby structures: the ears, nasal sinuses or mouth. Systemic infections such as tuberculosis and HIV can also produce cerebral abscesses. Infections of the meninges (meningitis) or the brain tissue (encephalitis) rarely require surgery.

Trauma

Trauma to the head can fracture the skull, cause bleeding between skull and brain and damage the brain tissue (Table 10.1). Damaged tissue swells, raising the ICP and creating the conditions for secondary ischaemia and further damage which, if not halted, may kill the patient. Surgery may be necessary to repair the skull, evacuate a haematoma, resect swollen damaged brain tissue or decompress dangerously high ICP.

Cerebrovascular abnormalities

Cerebral arteries may develop aneurysms (thin-walled weaknesses at the junctions of vessels) or form bundles of abnormal vessels called arteriovenous malformations (AVMs). In many cases these are only detected when they rupture, causing subarachnoid or intracerebral haemorrhage, conditions with high mortality and morbidity. Surgery and interventional radiology aim to prevent further rupture by blocking, bypassing or removing the abnormality. Subarachnoid haemorrhage carries the additional risk of cerebral vasospasm: prolonged constriction of cerebral arteries risking additional cerebral ischaemia and infarction leading to disability or death (Mestecky, 2011).

Parkinson's disease

Parkinson's disease is a disorder of movement caused by poor functioning of the cells of the basal ganglia, deep in the cerebral hemispheres. The condition is typically managed with drugs, but a surgical approach is possible (Owen, 2014). Electrodes are positioned deep in the brain and connected to a battery-powered pulse generator. This deep brain stimulation technique has also been used to treat neuropathic pain (Sayat et al, 2019), anorexia (Whiting et al, 2018) and obsessive–compulsive disorder (Kohl et al, 2014).

Epilepsy

Patients with very frequent seizures may be offered neurosurgery to ablate the site in the brain where the seizures begin if investigations can pinpoint the area responsible (Anderson et al, 2017).

Table 10.1 Sites of intracranial haemorrhage

Extradural	Between the skull and the dura	Arterial bleeding, usually associated with trauma to the skull. Rapid expansion under high pressure.
Subdural	Between the dura and the arachnoid	Venous bleeding, occasionally spontaneous but usually the result of trauma. Slower expansion.
Subarachnoid	Between the arachnoid and the pia	Arterial bleeding. May be traumatic or from a ruptured aneurysm.
Intraventricular	In the cerebral ventricles	Usually an extension of a subarachnoid bleed.
Intracerebral/ intraparenchymal	In the brain tissue	May be traumatic (contusion), aneurysmal, hypertensive, or from a tumour or arteriovenous malformation.

Symptoms and presentations

Onset of disease in the brain can be sudden or slow and insidious. Traumatic injury and spontaneous haemorrhage happen in seconds while tumours may grow over years. Such is the complexity of the brain's function that changes in how someone experiences and acts in the world may be subtle or dramatic, even bizarre.

Headache

Spontaneous intracranial haemorrhage typically begins with sudden severe headache, often described as like being hit with a bat. Headache is also a feature of intracranial infection and raised ICP caused by, for example, hydrocephalus or a tumour. It is worth remembering that all of these neurological conditions are rare: most headaches are unpleasant but not serious.

Posture, movement and balance

Sudden weakness or loss of sensation on one side of the body is hard to ignore: clearly something is seriously wrong. However, changes can be more subtle: leaning to one side when sitting, for example, or unaccustomed clumsiness.

Sensation

We tend to think of altered sensation in terms of numbness or pins and needles in the limbs. But other senses can be affected: loss or distortion of smell or taste, vision and hearing may all indicate intracranial pathology.

Seizures

Seizures have many possible causes, not all of them originating in the brain: careful investigation is essential. Seizures may be the first sign of serious brain disease such as infection, tumour or AVM. Generalized seizures affect the whole brain and typically cause unconsciousness and tonic–clonic movements of the whole body. A new onset of this sort of seizure is an obvious sign that something is seriously wrong. Some seizures are partial, affecting only one part of the brain, and these produce a variety of often subtle symptoms including disordered movement or sensation, strange visions, sounds, tastes or smells, or unusual behaviour. Epilepsy is a common chronic consequence of brain disease.

Hormonal change

Pituitary tumours can cause either overexcretion or underexcretion of hormones. The effects may seem to have little to do with the brain, such as unexpected bone growth or lactation (in either sex), fatigue, weight gain, hirsutism, erectile dysfunction or polyuria.

Language

Aphasia is the term given to a range of disorders in the use of language and is broadly separated into receptive (reduced understanding of language) and expressive (reduced ability to generate language), reflecting the fact that these two aspects of communication are controlled by different areas of the brain. Deficits may be obvious, or subtle and difficult to detect without careful assessment by a speech and language therapist (Ager & Little, 2018). Note that the term *aphasia* is preferred to *dysphasia*, even when the deficit is only partial. This avoids confusion with *dysphagia*: difficulty with swallowing.

Cognition

New difficulties in thinking skills such as problem-solving, planning, switching attention when appropriate, reasoning, or dealing with complex information may indicate intracranial disease.

Mood, personality and behaviour

Intracranial disease can produce changes in mood, personality and behaviour, but so can many other things: changes in life circumstances or relationships, mental illness, substance misuse and so on. Changes may not be obvious except to those closest to the patient and can be difficult to describe. Statements that someone 'isn't normally like this' should be taken seriously.

Insight

You are your brain and you assume that your experience of the world is the way the world is. Brain disease, however, can alter the way you encounter the world and it is difficult to accept that you are no longer your own best guide to what is going on. Many people with newly acquired brain injury lack insight into their predicament and struggle to accept that anything is wrong.

Investigation and diagnosis

History

Accounts given by patients and those who know them well are typically the starting point. It is important to remember that people rarely describe signs and symptoms

135

in professional language: nurses must listen and ask questions carefully and with imagination.

Examination

Neurosurgical emergencies such as intracranial haemorrhage or traumatic brain injury do not allow clinicians time to carry out a detailed examination: depressed conscious levels, abnormal pupil reactions and gross motor weakness are sufficient signs that a CT scan is needed urgently. When disease progression is more gradual, a careful physical examination is essential. This is not limited to the nervous system: signs and symptoms from all the body's systems may be relevant to diagnosis, treatment and recovery.

CT scanning

Computerized axial tomography (CT scanning) is the basic neurological investigation and a brain CT can be done in a matter of minutes. CT uses X-rays to render images in slices showing relative densities of tissue. Dense bone shows as white on CT, CSF as black and brain tissue as shades of grey. CT is excellent for showing the compression of raised ICP and abnormalities of different densities to normal tissue, such as the dense white appearance of fresh blood. Contrast medium may be given to highlight abnormalities such as tumours, or to capture serial images of blood flowing through the arterial and venous systems (CT angiography and CT venography).

MRI scanning

Magnetic resonance imaging (MRI) uses radio waves in a powerful magnetic field to generate images. MRI gives a more detailed picture than CT and is the key investigation for brain tumours and for damage at the grey–white matter junctions.

PET scanning

In positron emission tomography (PET) the patient is given a radioactive tracer substance. This gathers in different areas of tissue in proportion to their level of metabolic activity and the scanner detects the different radiation signals in fine detail, generating a 3D image which can detect abnormalities too small to show up on MRI or CT.

EEG

For an electro-encephalogram (EEG), electrodes attached to the scalp map electrical waves generated by cortical neurons as they signal to each other. EEG shows details of seizures as they happen, demonstrating where the seizure begins and how it spreads. EEG also distinguishes between seizures and other non-epileptic disorders.

Lumbar puncture

Using aseptic technique a cannula is placed into the spinal canal below the end of the spinal cord and CSF is drawn off for analysis. Lumbar puncture (LP) is used to investigate possible infection, immune disorders, haemorrhage or cancer.

Cerebral angiography

A long catheter is inserted, usually via the femoral artery. Using X-ray guidance, the catheter is steered up to the carotid or vertebral arteries (a 4-vessel exam will image each vessel in turn) and radio-opaque contrast is injected while a rapid series of X-ray images is captured. The flow of the contrast shows abnormalities such as aneurysms or AVMs as well as restricted flow through sclerotic or spastic vessels or the blood supply to a tumour.

Neurosurgery

Neurosurgery is inherently risky. The skull cavity is small and crowded with vital structures. The target of surgery may be tiny and poorly differentiated from surrounding structures, and many neurosurgical operations are carried out under a microscope. Bleeding must be minutely controlled: even small haematomas have a serious effect in the closed space of the skull. Errors are potentially devastating: death and severe disability are real possibilities in even the most routine procedure. The surgeon must also consider whether operating is the right thing to do: an operation may save life but leave the patient so severely disabled that meaningful recovery is impossible. Surgeons must also consider that they may have very different ideas from patients and families as to what kind of survival is worthwhile. Discussion of risks and benefits with patients (when possible) and families is essential but in the end the surgeon carries a grave responsibility.

Operative approaches

Burr holes

A small circular hole (about the size of a penny) is drilled into the skull vault. This gives limited access, sufficient for placing a ventricular drain or taking a tissue biopsy. Burr holes are also used to evacuate chronic subdural haematomas.

Craniotomy

An area of the skull is exposed by lifting the scalp (one edge remains attached). Burr holes drilled into the skull are joined with a pneumatic saw and the flap lifted. The surgeon then cuts through the dura to expose the brain surface (Fig. 10.1). At the end of the procedure the dura is sealed, the bone re-sited and fixed and the scalp replaced. Craniotomy is the standard approach to lesions in the frontal, temporal and parietal lobes.

Craniectomy

A craniectomy proceeds in the same way as a craniotomy, but the skull flap is not replaced at the end of the operation: the dura and scalp are closed over the gap. This lets any swelling expand, minimizing raised ICP. The flap may be 'marsupialized' (placed in the peritoneal cavity where it will receive a blood supply), or disposed of and replaced later with a titanium or acrylic plate (cranioplasty).

Post-fossa craniectomy

The post-fossa cavity is small and densely packed with the brain stem, cerebellum, cranial nerves and blood vessels. Surgeons typically approach this area from the rear, under the bulge of the occiput, chipping away bone around the foramen magnum to make a small window.

Trans-sphenoidal surgery

Lesions under the anterior brain are difficult to reach via a craniotomy. One answer is to gain access from beneath. In trans-sphenoidal surgery access is gained via the nostril,

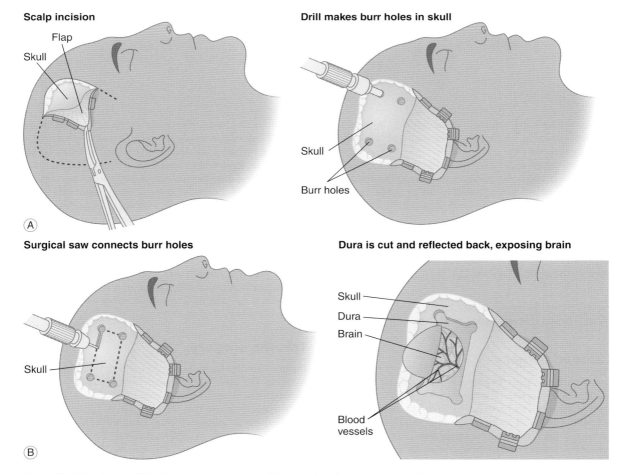

Figure 10.1 Craniotomy. (Reprinted with permission of Medtronic Sofamor Danek, Inc.)

137

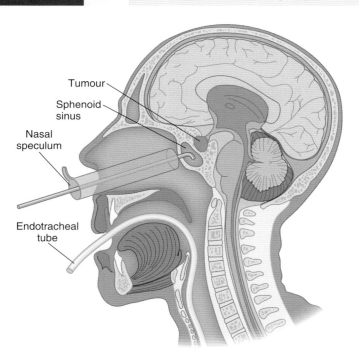

Figure 10.2 Trans-sphenoidal surgery. (Reproduced from Andrew H. Kaye, *Essential Neurosurgery*. Wiley-Blackwell, with permission.)

cutting through the sphenoid bone which forms part of the skull base (Fig. 10.2). This is the standard approach to pituitary tumours.

It is important to bear in mind that the choice of surgical approach affects the patient's postoperative experience. Patients are placed supine, on one side or prone in operations which last hours. The skull is held still with clamps pinned into the skull. Some posterior-fossa operations are done with the patient in a sitting position with the head angled forward. Swelling from a frontal craniotomy may close up one eye and retraction of the muscles may make opening the mouth painful.

Neurosurgical operations

Tumour surgery

Tumour surgery aims to remove the entire tumour or as much of it as possible. Careful planning with CT and MRI scans is essential and techniques to guide the surgeon are available. Gliolan is a drug with an affinity for high-grade gliomas. It fluoresces under a special light, making mapping the tumour easier. A stereotactic frame can be used with CT mapping to pinpoint the site and depth of a lesion relative to reference points marked on the scalp (Lindsay et al, 2010; Mohan & Ramamurthy, 2014). When a patient has a tumour in or around the motor or speech centres of the frontal lobes, one possibility is to perform an awake craniotomy. The patient is sedated to begin with, but then woken up. The surgeon uses a probe to stimulate questionable areas while asking the patient to perform movements or speech tasks. If the probe is stimulating brain rather than tumour, the patient will have a transient impairment. This allows the surgeon to map the border between tumour and brain with great accuracy, minimizing damage to healthy tissue (Brown et al, 2013). It is not always possible to remove an entire tumour without causing serious damage and in many cases the surgeon must settle for partial resection, relieving symptoms and delaying progression. For all the advances in imaging and technique, much depends on the experience and skill of the surgeon.

Trauma surgery

Trauma neurosurgery is aimed at relieving raised ICP, reducing the cycle of secondary damage, ischaemia and pressure which may kill the patient. Extradural and subdural haematomas can be evacuated by craniotomy. Where there is serious cerebral swelling a decompressive craniectomy may be necessary. It should be noted that not all traumatic brain injuries are suitable for surgery: some traumatic damage is diffuse and microscopic in scale (Rajkumar et al, 2014) and some injuries are too severe for survival to be possible.

Labels on figure: Tumour, Sphenoid sinus, Nasal speculum, Endotracheal tube

Haematoma surgery

Spontaneous haematomas can be evacuated by craniotomy. However, depending on the site of the haematoma, the extent of any swelling and the age of the patient, surgery may not always improve outcome (Jha & Gupta, 2014).

Aneurysm surgery

Aneurysms are typically sited at junctions of arteries around the circle of Willis, deep under the brain. Aneurysms are small, thin-walled sacs bulging out of the artery wall, prone to rupture if disturbed. The surgeon approaches and exposes the aneurysm and its feeding vessels with great care. The aim is to slide a small clip across the aneurysm neck, sealing it off. Should the aneurysm burst before the clip is placed, the situation is critical: the rapid loss of blood fills the operating field and obscures the surgeon's view. The surgeon must clamp the arteries to stop the bleeding and then clip the aneurysm very quickly before unclamping the arteries and restoring flow. Too long a delay will cause a stroke (Buckley & Hickey, 2014).

Arteriovenous malformations

The vascular complexity of AVMs, with arterial and venous supplies poorly distinguished, makes surgery difficult. If the feeding vessels can be clearly distinguished, the AVM can be excised like a tumour. Many cases require a combined approach involving selective embolization of vessels, surgery and radiation therapy (Ramamurthi & Kapu, 2014).

Surgery for hydrocephalus

Acute hydrocephalus is relieved by placing an external ventricular catheter into one of the lateral ventricles via a burr-hole. The catheter is connected to a drainage apparatus: CSF pressure is controlled by varying the height of the drain relative to the head (Humphrey, 2018). Chronic hydrocephalus is treated by placing a ventriculo-peritoneal shunt. A catheter is placed in the ventricle and tunnelled subcutaneously down to the peritoneal cavity. Drainage is controlled by a pressure valve (Vacca, 2018). An alternative is endoscopic ventriculostomy, a procedure in which an endoscope is introduced through a burr hole to cut a fistula in the floor of the third ventricle (Jiang et al, 2018).

Interventional radiology

More and more intracranial procedures are carried out by interventional radiology. Most cerebral aneurysms are now treated by coil embolization, using an angiogram catheter to place tiny platinum coils into the aneurysm from within the artery, blocking the flow of blood into the aneurysm (Mestecky, 2011). Stents can be placed (Murchison et al, 2018), thrombi removed (De Sousa, 2016) and arterial flow diverted around aneurysms (Wakhloo & Gounis, 2014). Drugs can be given intra-arterially to dilate spastic vessels or dissolve thrombi. Embolization techniques are also used as an adjunct to surgery for tumours and AVMs.

Preoperative assessment

It is important to have as clear a picture as possible of a patient's background and presentation before surgery. Assessment in neurological disease is not a quick or simple process. It is important to observe carefully and listen attentively to patients and their families. Many neurosurgical operations are emergencies with only a few hours between first symptoms and surgery. In such cases, preoperative assessment is based on the principles of resuscitation: ABCDE. It is after surgery that the background information becomes relevant.

Pain

Patients with intracranial bleeding typically suffer a sudden severe onset of headache, which may reduce but is likely to continue, aggravated by bright light (photophobia), noise or movement. Neck pain and stiffness are common. Patients with slower-growing lesions such as tumours may experience headaches over long periods, especially in the early mornings.

Breathing

Essential background information includes respiratory history (disease, smoking) and daily function (exercise tolerance). It is essential to assess respiration by watching the patient breathe at rest, counting for a minute. Disease affecting the brain stem can produce erratic breathing patterns: changes can only be detected promptly if the baseline pattern is clearly established. Saturation monitoring is important but secondary.

Maintaining a safe environment

Neurological disease can generate a range of safety concerns.

Seizures pose an obvious safety risk. It is important to establish what kind of seizures the patient has had, how long they last, how long it takes to recover and what medication the patient is taking.

Safety can also be compromised by subtler changes, including visual impairment, poor balance or loss of coordination, confusion, impulsiveness and deficits in memory or attention. Patients may lack insight into their problems and collateral history from family and friends is important.

Communication

Patients or relatives may report difficulties with language. These may be subtle and some patients mask difficulties very effectively. Sometimes the assessing nurse is the first person to detect a problem and assessment by a speech and language therapist (SLT) may be needed.

Eating and drinking

Disease in and around the brain stem and cranial nerves, or affecting the sensory and motor cortex, can compromise safe swallowing. Dribbling, a 'wet voice', difficulty swallowing, and choking or coughing when eating or drinking, as well as difficulty articulating speech clearly (dysarthria) are all significant signs indicating the need for SLT assessment (Atkinson, 2019)

Disease in and around the brain stem and the temporal lobes can also impair balance and vestibular—ocular function with resulting nausea.

Patients should be weighed on admission and any recent weight change noted. Urine should be tested for glycosuria. Patients and families should be asked about any changes in eating and drinking habits. Sensory and perception problems, limb weakness or poor coordination can make the mechanics of eating difficult: watching a patient eat can be revealing.

Elimination

It is important to obtain a history of bladder and bowel habits, noting any recent changes. Incontinence can be the result of a loss of control but also of language or cognitive deficits: patients may simply not be able to ask for the toilet.

Washing and dressing

Limb weakness, poor coordination and balance and cognitive problems (memory and attention) can compromise basic self-care, as can changes in personality and mood. Recent changes in washing or dressing habits are significant.

Mobilization

Motor deficits are a common sign of neurological disease. It is useful, whenever possible, to watch a patient walking: is there anything abnormal about the gait, do they lean to one side, are they unsteady and do they seem to be aware of obstacles on both sides?

Working and playing

Neurological disease is likely to affect someone's work and leisure activities. Listening to patients and families talking about how life has changed is important in itself and may elicit new information about the disease.

Expressing sexuality

Neurological disease can create both physical problems and changes in behaviour, including libido, which can in turn cause emotional stress.

Sleeping

Sleep patterns can be disrupted by neurological disease and by some treatments, particularly steroid therapy for brain tumours.

Death and dying

Disease of the brain is inherently dangerous and neurosurgery carries a significant risk of death and serious disability. Anxiety and fear can have a profound effect on all aspects of life.

Observations

Conscious level: the Glasgow Coma Scale

The Glasgow Coma Scale (GCS) assesses consciousness: the brain's ability to engage with the world (Table 10.2) (Teasdale & Jennett, 1974; Jennett & Teasdale, 1977). It is not a numerical scale (the numbers are just a shorthand code) but a description of a patient's interaction with the world in three key aspects. Eye opening denotes arousal, the brain's receptivity to stimulus. Verbal response assesses the brain's ability to engage with the world through language. Motor response tests the brain's ability to organize movement. When using the GCS it is important to report the results in full, specifying any deficits: the summary score is too ambiguous to be clinically useful — there are 17 different ways to reach a GCS 'score' of 8 (Teasdale et al 1983).

Pupil responses

The pupils of the eye should be circular and equal in size. Pupil diameter should be appropriate to the ambient light

Table 10.2 The Glasgow Coma Scale

	Level	Description	Abbreviation
Eyes open	Spontaneously	Eyes are open before the assessment starts.	E4
	To speech	Eyes open on speaking or shouting to the patient.	E3
	To pain	Eyes open on physical contact: shaking or trapezius pinch.	E2
	None	Eyes do not open even to strong pain.	E1
Verbal response	Orientated	Recalls own name, day, date and current location.	V5
	Sentences	Uses coherent word combinations.	V4
	Words	Single or unconnected words, random or meaningless.	V3
	Sounds	Noises, but no discernible words.	V2
	None	Patient makes no sound, even in response to pain.	V1
Motor response (record best arm)	Obeys commands	Follows simple motor commands.	M6
	Localizes	Patient moves a hand to the source of a noxious stimulus.	M5
	Normal flexion	The elbow bends and there is no rotation of the arm or unnatural posturing at the wrist. The movement is not clearly aimed at locating the pain source.	M4
	Abnormal flexion	The elbow bends, but the arm rotates inwards and there may be posturing at the wrist; a clearly abnormal movement.	M3
	Extension	The elbow straightens. There is often internal rotation of the arms and posturing at the wrist and the whole body may stiffen.	M2
	None	There is no movement, even on pain stimulus.	M1

conditions and pupils should constrict briskly to bright light. In the context of low or deteriorating consciousness, fixed and dilated pupils are a sign of critically high intracranial pressure.

Limb strength

Left–right differences in limb strength can indicate a lesion on one side of the brain. A left-sided tumour, haematoma or stroke will cause a right-sided weakness. A clear baseline is important: changes in relative strength are a common early sign of postoperative complications, typically preceding changes in conscious level.

Vital signs

Airway, breathing and circulation all affect the central nervous system and all are in turn affected by it. Methodical observation of breathing, pulse, temperature and blood pressure is essential. If intracranial pressure becomes critically high, vital signs become highly disordered with extreme hypertension, bradycardia and Cheyne–Stokes breathing: Cushing's triad (Cushing, 1902, 1903). The

relationship between ICP, neurological signs and vital signs is shown in Figure 10.3.

Fluid and electrolyte balance

Careful recording of fluid balance is essential for all surgical patients. Some neurological disorders pose specific problems (Cook, 2011). Subarachnoid haemorrhage can lead to cerebral salt wasting, with high urine output and falling serum sodium. Pituitary disorders can cause diabetes insipidus, with very high urine output and rising serum sodium. Syndrome of inappropriate ADH secretion (SIADH) is a complication of intracranial infection, resulting in low urine output and falling serum sodium. In all such cases the urine specific gravity should be tested and urine sent for urea and electrolyte analysis.

Preoperative preparation

The extent of preoperative preparation depends on the urgency of the surgery. In many cases, patients and

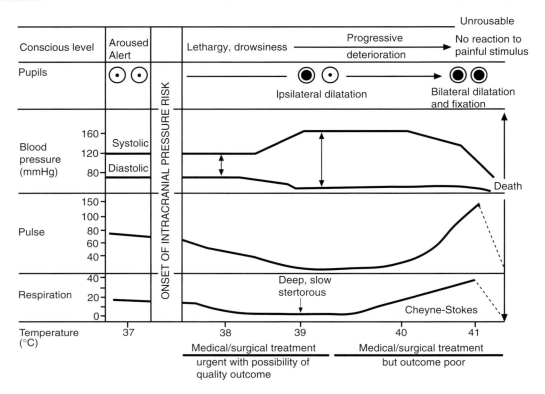

| Conscious level | Aroused Alert | | Lethargy, drowsiness | Progressive deterioration | Unrousable No reaction to painful stimulus |
| Pupils | ⊙ ⊙ | | ● ⊙ Ipsilateral dilatation | | ● ● Bilateral dilatation and fixation |

Figure 10.3 Rising intracranial pressure (ICP).

families are told that a dangerous operation must be performed at once to save life: they have little time to process the information and absorb the shock. Even when surgery is planned in advance, the time between diagnosis and operation is typically days to weeks at most.

Information, capacity and consent

Whenever possible, the neurosurgeon must give patients all the information they need to decide whether to undergo the proposed operation. This includes estimates of risk of death and disability, information about how the surgery is done and what the patient is likely to experience. The alternatives to operating, and the consequences of not operating, must be spelled out. All of this must be clearly documented. If there are concerns about a patient's ability to give or refuse meaningful consent to treatment, a capacity assessment should be undertaken. If a patient lacks capacity, the surgeon will make a decision based on the patient's best interests: whenever possible this should be based on information from the patient and those close to them (Department of Health, 2005).

Anaesthetic assessment

The anaesthetist assesses the patient's anatomy and physiology, specifically respiratory, cardiovascular and metabolic health. This involves taking a history, reviewing observations and blood tests. Other tests, including chest X-ray and ECG, may be required.

Special preparations

Some neurosurgical operations require specific preparation. CT and MRI scans are used to place markers on the patient's head for stereotactic surgery (Mohan & Ramamurthy, 2014). Speech therapy assessment is needed if the patient is undergoing awake craniotomy for a tumour near the brain's speech centres.

Steroid therapy is commonly prescribed for patients with brain tumours in the period between diagnosis and surgery (Townsley, 2011). Steroids reduce the reactive swelling in brain tissue around the tumour. This often relieves symptoms but steroids can have significant side effects, including irritability, insomnia, increased appetite, hyperglycaemia and fluid retention.

Incision lines are often above the hairline and the surgeon may need to clip or shave hair to prepare the site, although practice varies. Hair removal is usually done in the operating theatre.

The nurses role

Preparation for an operation follows a protocol designed to ensure patients arrive in the operating theatre fully ready for surgery. Every element of the protocol from patient identification to nil-by-mouth procedures is important but nurses should also be alert to the emotional needs of patients and families. Anxiety and fear are rational responses to the situation. Nurses should be attentive to signs that patients and families do not fully understand what is going on. They will have been given a lot of complex information at a time of great stress and may not have absorbed it fully, or may have questions which only occur to them when they have time to think. The Nursing and Midwifery Council (2018) stipulates that nurses must 'act in partnership with those receiving care, helping them to access relevant health and social care, information and support when they need it.'

Postoperative care

The principles of immediate post-anaesthetic care are covered elsewhere in this book, but neurosurgery poses specific risks. Haematomas below the skull flap do not have to be very big before they compress adjacent brain and cause rises in ICP. Exposure and manipulation of the brain raises the risk of seizures, and surgery may have damaged the brain or cranial nerves.

Airway

Airway patency can be compromised by poor consciousness. This in turn may be the result of incomplete reversal of anaesthesia or of rising ICP. Surgery to or around the brain stem and cranial nerves involves a high risk of airway failure.

Breathing

Altered respiratory rate and depth can be caused by incompletely reversed anaesthesia or high ICP. Again, surgery to or around the brain stem carries a high risk of respiratory failure.

Circulation

Neurosurgery can involve high blood loss, although this is unusual. Damage to the brain stem can lead to cardiac instability. The neurosurgeon may set a narrow target range for postoperative blood pressure: hypertension risks bleeding in the operation site but hypotension may compromise cerebral perfusion.

Neurological

Neurosurgeons want to see patients awake as quickly as possible after surgery to check for any new neurological deficits. As well as overall function tested by the standard observations, nurses should look for potential deficits specific to the surgery: contralateral weakness or sensory loss, facial droop, visual deficits, speech and language problems, difficulty swallowing and so on. Seizures are a risk even in patients with no history of epilepsy (Oscroft & Ram, 2017). Any deterioration from the patient's preoperative baseline must be promptly reported to the neurosurgeon.

Frequency of observations

Risk of complications is highest in the immediate postoperative period and observations will be as frequent as every 15 minutes. If there are no problems with airway, breathing and circulation and if the patient recovers to their preoperative conscious level, observation frequency may be steadily reduced. Each change in frequency is a clinical decision for an individual patient.

Patient care location

Patients undergoing more minor procedures may be able to go back to a ward after a period in the recovery suite. But even minor neurosurgical operations carry risks and patients should be nursed where they will be seen regularly for at least the first 24 hours. Patients who have had longer or more dangerous operations are usually cared for in a high-dependency setting for at least the first night after surgery. In either case, nurses caring for such patients must have a good knowledge of neuroscience nursing: early signs of serious deterioration may be missed by staff lacking experience of this patient group.

Recovering from neurosurgery

Many neurosurgical operations are carried out on patients who are already very seriously ill. In such cases surgery is aimed at preventing death and reducing disability, but cannot reverse the damage done to the brain by the original insult. These patients are likely to be in a serious or critical condition for days to weeks after surgery; complications are common and survival cannot be assumed.

For patients who are less acutely ill at the time of surgery, recovery from the operation can be surprisingly rapid, although there will often be considerable challenges ahead.

Observations

Neurological and vital signs observations will continue during the patient's stay but frequency should be kept under review. Neurological observations require nurses to disturb patients. Over-frequent observation over too long a time results in patients with sleep deprivation, which can lead to fatigue, reduced tolerance for rehabilitation and even delirium. Observations which require inflicting painful stimulus are only justified if they elicit information which is likely to affect the patient's management.

Existing, persisting and new deficits

Surgery may improve a patient's preoperative symptoms, by removing a tumour, for instance. But preoperative deficits can persist and new problems may emerge. Certain operations carry specific risks: operating on tumours on the acoustic nerve, for example, may worsen existing hearing loss and damage the adjacent facial nerve with resulting facial palsy. Neuroscience nurses should be aware of the expected risks but also be alert to the possibility of the unexpected.

Mobilizing

Many post-neurosurgery patients will be able to mobilize fairly soon after surgery, often the next day. The neurosurgeon should be consulted before the patient gets up and care should be taken, even if the patient was fully mobile preoperatively. If patients had problems with mobility, balance or vision before surgery or seem to have such problems after surgery, they should be reviewed by a physiotherapist.

Drains and sutures

Wound drains should be removed on the surgeon's instructions, typically at 24 hours postoperatively. Patients often go home before clips or sutures are due to come out, in which case the patient must be informed of arrangements for removal. Wounds above the hairline are difficult to dress: existing or re-growing hair makes it difficult get an adhesive dressing to stick and head bandages are hot, cumbersome and rarely stay in place for long. Wounds should be reviewed and cleaned regularly: infection of a cranial wound is a potentially very serious complication. Nurses must follow local policies and procedures for wound care.

Early rehabilitation and the multidisciplinary team

Early rehabilitation

Rehabilitation should begin as soon as possible after admission. In the initial stages, the emphasis will be on conservative management, preventing complications such as loss of joint range. But more positive rehabilitation can begin very early in most cases (Ntoumenopoulos, 2015).

Neuroplasticity

The brain functions by passing signals between neurons in synaptic networks and pathways. The brain is able to learn throughout life: new demands create new synaptic connections, and if these are reinforced by repetition the connections become stronger and faster making our performance of tasks quicker, smoother and more efficient. This is how anything new is learned, from knitting to a new route from work to home. This adaptive property is called neuroplasticity and underlies modern concepts of rehabilitation (Young & Tolentino, 2011). The adult brain does not grow new neurons: damaged cells are not replaced and disrupted synaptic pathways lead to functional deficits. Nonetheless, if the brain is given the right stimulation it can learn new ways to do old things. There are limits to this and deficits may endure, but in the large majority of patients valuable progress is possible. In this light, rehabilitation and recovery must be understood as open-ended and lifelong: we are all learning from birth to death.

Physiotherapist

Posture, balance and mobility can all be problematic for some people recovering from neurological disease. Specialist physiotherapy helps patients regain as much independence as possible (Duysens et al, 2015). There is a wide range of potential needs, from advising on exercise routines to recovering something as basic as the ability to sit up unsupported. Physiotherapists also play a key role in respiratory management and rehabilitation, particularly for patients who have needed ventilatory support in the acute phase (Hellweg, 2012).

Occupational therapist

Occupational therapy helps patients regain the ability to function in their lives and to adjust successfully to new challenges posed by the effects of their illness (Wheeler et al, 2017). The occupational therapist's work reveals the overlooked complexity of daily life. Can someone complete household tasks such as making a cup of tea or are they too easily distracted to finish the job? Is someone safe to cross a busy road? Can they cope with all the choices in a shop and buy the ingredients for a meal, and can they find their way back to the ward? Do patients have the insight to understand their new limitations and what strategies they can use to manage them? What is the home environment like and are changes needed to make it safe?

Speech and language therapist

Speech and language therapists have two vital roles. The assessment and rehabilitation of swallowing problems (dysphagia) in neuroscience patients requires specialist knowledge. Close cooperation between SLTs, physiotherapists and nurses is essential to keep patients safe, prevent complications and promote independence (Waterhouse, 2016). Language and speech deficits can be disabling in themselves and impede all aspects of rehabilitation. Skilled intervention is needed to help patients recover function or manage life with persisting deficits (Ager & Little, 2018).

Dietician

Neurological disease can affect nutrition in various ways, while poor nutrition impedes recovery and rehabilitation. Acute brain injury leads to a hypercatabolic state resulting in high energy and protein requirement (Hickey & Jacobs, 2014, p. 184). Dysphagia is an obvious barrier to safe independent eating and drinking (Somerville et al, 2016), but other deficits also pose problems. A distractible patient may fail to finish meals, someone with weakness in the hands or poor coordination may not be able to manage a knife and fork, a patient with severe one-sided neglect may eat only one half of a plate of food, unaware that the other half of the plate is even there. Nutritional strategies must be specific to both needs and abilities, changing where necessary as patients recover function.

Neuropsychologist

Neuropsychologists look at cognitive deficits in depth along with problems with managing mood and emotion, including the patient's role in a family and the family's role in rehabilitation (Ptak & Schnider, 2015).

Multidisciplinary working and the nurses role

Successful rehabilitation requires close cooperation between disciplines and the nurse's role is central, an example of the cooperative working required of nurses by the NMC (2018). Strategies learned in therapy need reinforcement between sessions and nurses are best placed to manage this, integrating them into the patient's day (Aries & Hunter, 2014). Of all the disciplines, nurses spend the most time with patients and families; they are the eyes and ears of the team and it is essential that nurses are not only aware of rehabilitation goals and strategies and the rationale behind them but that they contribute fully to discussions and plans.

The future

Further treatment

For many patients, neurosurgery is part of a treatment course which may require radiotherapy or chemotherapy, further surgery or interventional radiology. Periodic surveillance imaging may be needed to detect recurring disease.

Rehabilitation

The major work of rehabilitation is done when patients no longer need close medical care. In some cases rehabilitation is community-based, others benefit from inpatient rehabilitation. Rehabilitation programmes should be tailored to individual needs, including a patient's tolerance for therapy: someone who is exhausted after 15 minutes will need a slower approach than someone who copes well with hour-long sessions.

Returning home

Most patients will be able to go home. Some need adaptations such as rails or accessible bathrooms, some need care in the home and some patients with cognitive deficits cannot be left alone if they are to be safe. Neurological disease often changes a whole family's life. A small minority of patients are unable to go home and need ongoing institutional care.

Returning to work

Returning to work or study is often a patient's major goal, but some find they can no longer function at their previous level and fatigue is a serious problem for many (Welch & Mead, 2015). Specialist vocational rehabilitation can help people adapt to new limitations and develop new skills (Vining Radomski et al, 2016).

Driving

Drivers who have had brain disease must report their condition to the relevant authority. A medical report will be required and licences are typically suspended at least temporarily. Insurance companies must also be notified.

A new me

It can seem that neurological disease is all about loss. Certainly many will lose abilities they once took for granted, as well as accustomed roles in employment, family and society. Many will undergo changes in personality, tastes and habits. Loss is undeniable and difficult to accommodate. But many people with acquired brain injury come to see 'a new me' with a new life, different but not always inferior and in some ways better than the old.

Conclusion: nursing the neurosurgical patient

Caring for neurosurgical patients requires knowledge and a range of skills. Many patients are suddenly and unexpectedly completely dependent on nursing staff for fundamental aspects of their care. Some are confused or cognitively impaired, a few exhibit challenging, even violent, behaviour. All neurosurgical patients and their families are facing a crisis, a time of uncertainty and unexpected change. Caring for neurosurgical patients requires energy, imagination and resilience. At the same time, neurosurgical patients offer remarkable insights into what it is to be human and it is a privilege to be able to care for people at the most vulnerable moments of their lives.

SUMMARY OF KEY POINTS

- Knowledge of the structures of the skull and brain is essential to understanding patients' signs and symptoms.
- Neurological disease and its treatments pose a serious risk of death and often change the lives of patients and those around them. Anxiety and fear are natural responses.
- Nurses play a key role in the continuing assessment of neurosurgical patients and their care planning.
- A neurosurgical operation is only one stage in a patient's progress.
- Caring for neurosurgical patients requires a team approach with nursing at its centre.

REFLECTIVE LEARNING POINTS

Having read this chapter, think about what you now know and what you still need to learn. These questions may help:

- Which two pairs of arteries supply the brain?
- What is meant by Cushing's triad?
- What is the most common cause of subarachnoid haemorrhage?
- What sort of problems might someone have after damage to the frontal lobes of the brain?
- What is neuroplasticity?

Care plans

Two sample care plans are given, covering preoperative and postoperative care. The plans use the Mead model of care (McClune & Franklin, 1987). The Mead model was derived from the Roper, Logan and Tierney model (Roper et al, 1985) and was developed for intensive care. It is particularly suited to highly acute patients in all settings. The patient in the care plans is fictitious.

PREOPERATIVE CARE PLAN

Care plan for emergency admission

Ms Renuka Chaudhary, aged 52, had a sudden onset of severe headache late at night followed by a collapse witnessed by her husband who promptly called an ambulance. When the paramedics arrived she was eye opening to speech, speaking in sentences but not orientated, and following commands. She vomited on the journey to hospital. In the emergency department (ED) her conscious level was unchanged and she had persisting severe headache with increasing photophobia (headache worsened by bright light) and nausea. A CT scan and CT angiogram showed a subarachnoid haemorrhage (SAH) from a right middle cerebral artery aneurysm. She was admitted to the neurosurgical ward in the early hours. An angiogram and coil embolization of the aneurysm under general anaesthetic was planned for later that day.

Problems or potential problems	Nursing goals	Nursing actions	Rationale
Airway			
• Although Ms Chaudhary vomited on the way to hospital, she was able to clear her own mouth. On admission to the ward she had a patent and safe airway. • Neurological deterioration would create a high risk of airway insufficiency or obstruction.			
Risk of loss of airway patency	Early detection and prompt intervention	• Nurse Ms Chaudhary in a bed close to the nurses' station • Check suction is working and immediately available • Check airway patency with respiratory observations (look, listen, feel) • Loss of patent airway is an EMERGENCY. Call the resuscitation team AT ONCE. Clear and support airway as needed: suction, manual manoeuvres, airway adjuncts • Once airway is re-established, assess breathing, circulation and disability.	Delayed response to deterioration may be fatal.
Breathing			
• On admission, Ms Chaudhary had a normal respiratory pattern with a rate of 14–18 breaths per minute and a peripheral oxygen saturation (SpO2) of 97% on air. A chest X-ray taken in the ED was clear and she has no history of respiratory disease or smoking. • Neurological deterioration would create a high risk of altered respiration.			

Risk of altered respiratory function	Early detection and prompt intervention	• Nurse Ms Chaudhary in a bed close to the nurses' station
		• Check oxygen is working and mask and tubing are immediately available.
		• Half-hourly respiratory observations and SpO2. Report if:
		  • Respiratory rate <12 or >20 breaths per minute
		  • Irregular respiratory pattern
		  • SpO2 <96% on air
		• In the event of altered respiratory function:
		  • Call the responsible medical team
		  • Assess airway (see above).
		  • Oxygen at 15 L/min via a non-rebreathe reservoir mask, titrating to maintain SpO2 97–100%
		  • Continuous saturation monitoring
		• If you cannot stabilize the respiratory function, the situation is an EMERGENCY: call the resuscitation team AT ONCE.
		  • Once breathing is stabilized, assess circulation and disability
			Delayed response to deterioration may be fatal.

Circulation			
• Ms Chaudhary has no history of cardiovascular disease. On admission her pulse was 82 beats per minute and regular and her BP was 140/85 mmHg. An ECG in ED was normal. Her temperature is 36.7°C.			

(Continued)

(cont'd)

- Hypertension creates a high risk of aneurysmal re-bleed. Hypotension may impair cerebral perfusion.
- Neurological deterioration may be accompanied by reactive hypertension, cardiac arrhythmia or cardiac arrest.

| Risk of re-bleed or cerebral hypoperfusion | Prevention | <ul><li>Nurse Ms Chaudhary in a bed close to the nurses' station</li><li>Half-hourly observation of pulse rate and rhythm and BP. Two-hourly temperature. Report if:<ul><li>Pulse rate <51 or >90 beats per minute</li><li>Irregular pulse</li><li>Systolic BP <130 or >160 mmHg</li><li>Temp <36.0 or >38.0°C</li></ul></li><li>In the event of altered cardiovascular function:<ul><li>Call the responsible medical team</li><li>Assess airway and breathing (above)</li><li>Continuous cardiac monitoring</li><li>BP every 5 minutes until stable</li><li>Assess disability</li></ul></li><li>If you cannot stabilize the cardiovascular function, the situation is an EMERGENCY: call the resuscitation team AT ONCE.</li></ul> | Delayed response to deterioration may be fatal. |

Disability

- On admission to the ward Ms Chaudhary was eye opening to speech (E3), orientated (V5) and following commands (M6). Her pupils were equal at 4 mm and reacting briskly to light. She had no limb weakness. She has no history of diabetes and her blood sugar was 5.9 mmol/L.
- Ms Chaudhary has suffered a ruptured cerebral aneurysm. There is a high risk of re-bleed in the first 72 hours. Re-bleeding carries a high risk of critical neurological deterioration and death.
- Ms Chaudhary is at risk of developing hydrocephalus caused by blood in the CSF space. Hydrocephalus causes rising ICP and requires urgent surgical intervention.
- Ms Chaudhary is at risk of seizures.
- There is a risk of hypoglycaemia (patient is nil-by-mouth) and hyperglycaemia (stress response). Altered blood glucose can impair consciousness.

| Risk of neurological deterioration | Early detection of deterioration | <ul><li>Nurse Ms Chaudhary in a bed close to the nurses' station</li><li>Close and frequent supervision. Half-hourly neurological observations. Report if:<ul><li>Deterioration in GCS</li><li>Unequal or unreactive pupils</li><li>Any one-sided limb weakness</li><li>Any seizure</li><li>Blood sugar <4 or >7 mmol/L.</li></ul></li><li>In the event of any neurological deterioration:<ul><li>Call the responsible medical team</li><li>Check airway, breathing and circulation</li><li>Check blood sugar.</li></ul></li></ul> | Delayed response to deterioration may be fatal. |

Pain

- On admission Ms Chaudhary had a persisting headache with a stiff neck and photophobia. In addition to the distress this causes, pain may exacerbate hypertension, risking re-bleeding of the aneurysm. Overuse of opiates risks depressing the conscious level.

(Continued)

(cont'd)

| Pain | Relief of pain | • Ask Ms Chaudhary if she is in pain whenever taking her observations.
• Regular analgesia as prescribed, with as-required analgesia following the WHO pain ladder:
  • Paracetamol
  • Mild opiate, e.g. dihydrocodeine, codeine phosphate, Oramorph.
• Shield Ms Chaudhary from bright light
• If pain is not relieved, report to the responsible medical team. | Patients should be as free from pain as safely possible. |

Nutrition & hydration

• Ms Chaudhary is to be kept nil-by-mouth prior to an anaesthetic.

| Risk of dehydration | Adequate hydration | • Intravenous fluids as prescribed. | Dehydration may compromise blood pressure. |

Elimination

• A careful fluid balance is needed to monitor the risk of dehydration.

| Risk of dehydration | Early detection | • Monitor urine output. Report if <1 mL/kg/hr or >3 mL/kg/hr. | Dehydration may compromise blood pressure. |

Hygiene

• Ms Chaudhary is confined to bed until her aneurysm is treated. She is at increased risk of pressure damage to the skin and deep vein thrombosis. Anti-coagulant therapy is contra-indicated until the aneurysm is treated.

Risk of pressure sores	Prevent pressure sores	• Encourage Ms Chaudhary to change position 2–3 hourly.	Pressure sores cause pain, risk serious complications and delay recovery.
Risk of deep vein thrombosis (DVT)	Prevent DVT	• Mechanical thrombo-prophylaxis devices as ordered.	DVTs risk pulmonary embolus
Unable to manage own hygiene needs without help	Maintain hygiene	• Assist Ms Chaudhary with all care as required.	Adequate hygiene reduces infection and promotes a sense of well-being.

Psychological/social

• Ms Chaudhary was accompanied on her admission by her husband. Both are anxious about her diagnosis and treatment and the uncertain nature of the outcome.

| Fear and anxiety | Reduce fear and anxiety | • Brief, clear explanations of all interventions and changes
  • Explain any equipment alarms so that Ms Chaudhary and her husband do not worry unduly
• Allow Ms Chaudhary to express herself as she chooses. | A brain haemorrhage is a serious illness with high risks of death and disability. The treatment carries |

(Continued)

(cont'd)

		• Reassure Ms Chaudhary and her husband but do not mislead them as to the seriousness of the situation. • If Ms Chaudhary or her husband asks about her condition, treatment and prognosis, ensure that the responsible doctor speaks to them. Ms Chaudhary must be party to all such conversations unless she chooses otherwise.	significant risks. It is reasonable to be frightened.
Loss of privacy and dignity	Maintain privacy and dignity	• Ensure bed curtains are fully closed during interventions. • As far as possible, do not discuss Ms Chaudhary in the hearing of other patients or visitors. • Maintain the security of all patient records.	Ms Chaudhary is entitled to privacy and dignity.
Preparation for interventional radiology			
Inadequate preparation for procedure under anaesthetic	Ensure full preparation completed	• Complete hospital preoperative check-list. • Ensure consent is properly documented.	Complete preparation avoids delays and reduces risks of error.

POSTOPERATIVE CARE PLAN

Ms Chaudhary underwent a right-sided craniotomy and clipping of a middle cerebral artery aneurysm and then spent 48 hours in the high-dependency unit before returning to the ward. She developed a left arm weakness after her craniotomy but this has resolved. Otherwise she has been stable neurologically and has not required
(Continued)

(cont'd)

respiratory or cardiovascular support. Her headaches persist and she has had bouts of nausea.

Additional information has been obtained: Ms Chaudhary is self-employed, working as a book illustrator. She and her husband have three children, aged 17, 15 and 12 years. She does not normally snore.

Problems or potential problems	Nursing goals	Nursing actions	Rationale
Airway			
• Ms Chaudhary's airway is intact. • Neurological deterioration would create a risk of airway insufficiency or obstruction.			

Risk of loss of airway patency due to neurological deterioration	Early detection and prompt intervention	• Check suction is working and immediately available
		 • Check airway patency with respiratory observations (look, listen, feel)
		 • Report if:
		   • Snoring when asleep or stridor when awake
		   • Dribbling, choking or coughing on food or drink.
			Compromised airway may lead to aspiration and chest infection.

(Continued)

(cont'd)

Breathing

- Ms Chaudhary has a baseline respiratory rate of 12–16 breaths per minute with a regular pattern and an SpO2 of 96–98% on air. She had no respiratory problems in HDU.
- Neurological deterioration would create a high risk of altered respiration.
- Ms Chaudhary is at risk of hospital-acquired chest infection.

Risk of altered respiratory function	Early detection and prompt intervention	• 4-hourly respiratory observations and SpO2.
		Report if:
		  • Resp rate <12 or >20 breaths per minute
		  • Irregular respiratory pattern
		  • SpO2 <96% on air
		• In the event of altered respiratory function:
		  • Call the responsible medical team
		  • Oxygen as prescribed
		  • Continuous saturation monitoring
		  • Increase observation frequency.
			Chest infections prolong hospital stay, delay neurological recovery and may become critical illnesses.

Circulation

- Ms Chaudhary's cardiovascular function was stable in HDU, with a baseline heart rate of 70–90 beats per minute and a systolic BP 130–150 mmHg. She has been apyrexial.
- Ms Chaudhary will be at risk of cerebral vasospasm for up to 3 weeks after the initial haemorrhage. Hypotension may exacerbate this.

Risk of cerebral hypoperfusion due to vasospasm if she becomes hypotensive	Early detection	• 4-hourly observation of pulse rate and rhythm, temperature and BP.
		  • Pulse rate <51 or >90 beats per minute
		  • Irregular pulse
		  • Systolic BP <130 or >160 mmHg
		  • Temp <36.0 or >38.0°C
		• In the event of altered cardiovascular function:
		  • Call the responsible medical team
		  • Increase observation frequency
			Poor cerebral perfusion may lead to avoidable neurological damage and death.

Disability

- In HDU Ms Chaudhary has been eye opening to speech (E3), orientated (V5) and following commands (M6). Her pupils were equal at 2–5 mm and reacting briskly to light. She developed a left arm weakness after her craniotomy, which has resolved.
- Ms Chaudhary is at risk of delayed cerebral ischaemia due to cerebral vasospasm. The risk period is up to 21 days after the original bleed. She has been prescribed nimodipine (a calcium-channel blocker) to reduce the risk.
- Ms Chaudhary is at risk of seizures.

Risk of neurological deterioration	Early detection of deterioration	• 4-hourly neurological observations. Report if:
		  • Deterioration in GCS
		  • Unequal or unreactive pupils
		  • Any one-sided limb weakness
		  • Any seizure
		• Nimodipine as prescribed.
		• In the event of any neurological deterioration:
		  • Call the responsible medical team
		  • Check airway, breathing and circulation
		  • Check blood sugar.
		• Daily urinalysis. Report if glycosuric.
			Delayed response to deterioration may lead to avoidable neurological damage and death.

(Continued)

(cont'd)

Pain

- Ms Chaudhary has persisting headaches.

Pain	Relief of pain	• Ask Ms Chaudhary if she is in pain when taking her observations or if her behaviour and demeanour suggest she may be in pain.
		• Regular analgesia as prescribed, with as-required analgesia following the WHO pain ladder:
		  • Paracetamol
		  • Mild opiate, e.g. dihydrocodeine, codeine phosphate, Oramorph.
		• If pain is not relieved, report to the responsible medical team.
			Patients should be as free from pain as safely possible. Pain hinders effective rehabilitation.

Nutrition & hydration

- Ms Chaudhary has been eating and drinking in HDU and has no problems with swallowing.
- Ms Chaudhary's appetite has been poor: she is nauseous at times and seems uninterested in eating and drinking. The dietician has prescribed nutritional supplements.

Risk of dehydration Risk of poor nutrition	Adequate hydration	• Dietician to review post-HDU discharge • Encourage Ms Chaudhary to drink • Record a fluid balance. • Anti-emetic medication as prescribed. • Offer Ms Chaudhary light meals and snacks. If she prefers food brought in from home or outside, encourage this. Record food intake.	Dehydration may compromise blood pressure. Poor nutrition delays recovery and increases infection risk. Independence in nutrition is a rehabilitation goal.

Elimination

- Cerebral salt wasting is a possible complication of subarachnoid haemorrhage, causing high urine output and overexcretion of sodium.
- Ms Chaudhary has not opened her bowels since admission. She is taking opiate drugs which exacerbate constipation and is prescribed aperients.

Risk of dehydration	Early detection	• Monitor urine output. Report if:
		  • output <1 mL/kg/hr or >3 mL/kg/hr.
		  • 24-hour balance is negative.
			Dehydration may compromise blood pressure.

Constipation	Return to normal bowel habit	• Encourage food and fluid intake • Aperient drugs as prescribed. • Record bowel function on the stool chart.	Constipation is uncomfortable and may hinder effective rehabilitation.

Hygiene

- Ms Chaudhary may mobilize but needs a physiotherapy assessment of her movement and balance. On HDU she did some self-care of her hygiene needs but only when prompted: she appeared to lack motivation.
- Ms Chaudhary has a right-sided craniotomy wound which was closed with clips. The wound drain has been removed.

Complications of reduced mobility	Return to independent mobility	• Physio assessment of movement and balance. • Encourage mobilization as prescribed by the physio.	Immobility risks avoidable complications. Return to independent mobility is a rehabilitation goal.

(Continued)

(cont'd)

Risk of DVT	Prevent DVT	• Mechanical thrombo-prophylaxis devices as ordered.	DVTs risk pulmonary embolus.
Reduced self-care	Maintain hygiene and promote independent self-care	• Occupational therapy (OT) assessment • Encourage self-care as per OT plan: negotiate as necessary to extend what she does each day. • Record Ms Chaudhary's level of activity in self-care	Adequate hygiene reduces infection and promotes a sense of well-being. Independent self-care is a rehabilitation goal.
Risk of infected craniotomy wound	Prevent infection	• Daily inspection and cleaning of the wound (aseptic non-touch technique). Report if any leakage, inflammation or discharge. • Clips to be removed on postoperative day 10.	Wound infection risks intracranial infection.

Psychological/social

- Ms Chaudhary seems passive at times, lacking motivation. Although orientated when assessed for the GCS, she seems reluctant to engage in conversation. She sleeps for much of the day and often seems listless when awake.
- Mr Chaudhary is caring for their children with help from other relatives and there are no concerns about their welfare. They have visited their mother.
- Mr Chaudhary is concerned about the impact his wife's illness will have on her role in the family and her ability to work, although he is aware it is too early to predict what may happen.

Possible cognitive deficit following subarachnoid haemorrhage	Assessment of cognition and rehabilitation of any deficits	• OT to assess cognition • Neuro-psychology assessment if required.	OT assessment screens for higher cognitive deficits not apparent on basic tests such as GCS. Neuro-psychology intervention may be needed.
Fatigue	Avoid over-tiring and improve activity level	• MDT discussion and plan for rehabilitation programme 　• Short sessions with rest between 　• Avoid over-scheduling activity • Monitor and record sleep pattern 　• Discuss sleep pattern with medical staff: is medication indicated? • Ms Chaudhary should go outside every day.	Fatigue will hamper progress in recovery and rehabilitation. Sleep patterns can be disrupted by brain injury Exposure to daylight promotes a normal sleep pattern.
Family and career disruption	Help the Chaudhary family to adjust	• Ask Ms and Mr Chaudhary if they would like to meet the social worker to discuss any immediate needs regarding: 　• Childcare arrangements 　• Benefit entitlements • Preliminary MDT family meeting to discuss current issues and future concerns.	Early discussion of potential problems allows families to clarify their concerns and plan to make any necessary changes. The situation is likely to change as Ms Chaudhary's recovery and rehabilitation progress.

References

Ager, K., & Little, L. (2018). Understanding aphasia and improving communication. *British Journal of Neuroscience Nursing, 14*(suppl 5), S13–17.

Anderson, I., Sivakumar, G., & Chumas, P. (2017). The role of the neurosurgeon in the treatment of epilepsy. *British Journal of Hospital Medicine, 78*(3), C41–44.

Aries, A., & Hunter, S. M. (2014). Optimising rehabilitation potential after stroke: a 24-hour interdisciplinary approach. *British Journal of Neuroscience Nursing, 10*(6), 268–273.

Atkinson, K. (2019). Neurological conditions and acute dysphagia. *British Journal of Nursing, 28*(8), 490–492.

Brown, T., Shah, A. H., Bregy, A., et al. (2013). Awake craniotomy for tumour resection: the rule rather than the exception? *Journal of Neurosurgical Anesthesiology, 25*(3), 240–247.

Buckley, D. A., & Hickey, J. V. (2014). Cerebral aneurysms. In J. V. Hickey (Ed.), *The clinical practice of neurological and neurosurgical nursing* (7th ed.). Philadelphia: Lippincott, Williams & Wilkins.

Cook, N. (2011). Assessment and management of fluid, electrolytes and nutrition in the neurological patient. In S. Woodward, & A.-M. Mestecky (Eds.), *Neuroscience nursing: An evidence-based guide*. Oxford: Blackwell.

Cushing, H. (1902). Some experimental and clinical observations concerning states of increased intracranial tension. *The American Journal of the Medical Sciences, 124*(3), 375–400.

Cushing, H. (1903). The blood pressure reaction of acute cerebral compression, illustrated by cases of intracranial haemorrhage. *The American Journal of the Medical Sciences, 125*, 1017–1045.

Department of Health. (2005). *The mental capacity act 2005*. Chapter 9. Available at: <http://webarchive.nationalarchives.gov.uk/20100407181935/http://opsi.gov.uk/acts/acts2005/pdf/ukpga_20050009_en.pdf>

De Sousa, I. (2016). Thrombectomy in acute ischaemic stroke and the implications for nursing practice. *British Journal of Neuroscience Nursing, 12*(S5). Available at: <https://doi.org/10.12968/bjnn.2016.12.Sup5.S28>.

Duysens, J., Verheyden, G., Massaad., et al. (2015). Rehabilitation of gait and balance after CNS damage. In V. Dietz, & N. S. Ward (Eds.), *Oxford textbook of neurorehabilitation*. Oxford: Oxford University Press.

Hellweg, S. (2012). Effectiveness of physiotherapy and occupational therapy after traumatic brain injury in the intensive care unit. *Critical Care Research and Practice, 2012*, 768456.

Hickey, J. V., & Jacobs, E. O. (2014). Nutritional support for neuroscience patients. In J. V. Hickey (Ed.), *The clinical practice of neurological and neurosurgical nursing* (7th ed.). Philadelphia: Lippincott, Williams & Wilkins.

Humphrey, E. (2018). Caring for neurosurgical patients with external ventricular drains. *Nursing Times, 114* (4), 52–56.

Jalali, R., Wen, P. Y., & Fujimaki, T. (2017). Meningiomas. In T. T. Batchelor, R. Nishikawa, N. Tarbell, & M. Weller (Eds.), *Oxford textbook of neuro-oncology*. Oxford: Oxford University Press.

Jennett, B., & Teasdale, G. (1977). Aspects of coma after severe head injury. *Lancet, 1*(8017), 878–881.

Jha, A. N., & Gupta, V. (2014). Spontaneous intracerebral haemorrhage. In P. N. Tandon, R. Ramamurthi, & P. K. Jain (Eds.), *Manual of neurosurgery*. New Delhi: Jaypee Brothers.

Jiang, L., Gao, G., & Zhou, Y. (2018). Endoscopic third ventriculostomy and ventriculoperitoneal shunt for patients with noncommunicating hydrocephalus: A PRISMA-compliant meta-analysis. *Medicine, 97*(40). Available at: <https://doi.org/10.1097/MD.0000000000012139>.

Kleihues, P., Rushing, E., & Ohgaki, H. (2017). The 2016 revision of the WHO classification of tumours of the central nervous system. In T. T. Batchelor, R. Nishikawa, N. Tarbell, & M. Weller (Eds.), *Oxford textbook of neuro-oncology*. Oxford: Oxford University Press.

Kohl, S., Schönherr, D. M., Luigjes, J., et al. (2014). Deep brain stimulation for treatment-refractory obsessive-compulsive disorder: a review. *BMC Psychiatry, 14*, 214.

Lindsay, K. W., Bone, I., Fuller, G., & Callander, R. (2010). *Neurology and neurosurgery illustrated* (5th ed.). Edinburgh: Churchill Livingstone.

McClune, B., & Franklin, K. (1987). The Mead model of nursing. *Intensive Care Nursing, 3*(3), 97–105.

Mestecky, A.-M. (2011). Management of patients with intracranial aneurysms and vascular malformations. In S. Woodward, & A.-M. Mestecky (Eds.), *Neuroscience nursing: an evidence-based guide*. Oxford: Blackwell.

Mohan, M., & Ramamurthy, R. (2014). Stereotaxy – brain tumours. In P. N. Tandon, R. Ramamurthi, & P. K. Jain (Eds.), *Manual of neurosurgery*. New Delhi: Jaypee Brothers.

Murchison, A. G., Young, V., Djurdjevic, T., et al. (2018). Stent placement in patients with acute subrachnoid haemorrhage: when is it justified? *Neuroradiology, 60*(7), 735–744.

Ntoumenopoulos, G. (2015). Rehabilitation during mechanical ventilation: Review of the recent literature. *Intensive and Critical Care Nursing, 31* (3), 125–132.

Nursing and Midwifery Council. (2018). *The code: Professional standards of practice and behaviour for nurses, midwives and nursing associates*. Available at: <https://www.nmc.org.uk/globalassets/sitedocuments/nmc-publications/nmc-code.pdf>

Oscroft, O., & Ram, F. S. F. (2017). Rate of seizure reduction after surgical resection of brain tumour: levetiracetam versus phenytoin. *British Journal of Neuroscience Nursing, 13*(2), 59–62.

Owen, S. L. F. (2014). Treating Parkinson's disease: deep brain stimulation. *Journal of Operating Department Practitioners, 2* (1). Available at: <https://doi.org/10.12968/jodp.2014.2.1.36>).

Ptak, R., & Schnider, A. (2015). Neuropsychological rehabilitation of higher cortical functions after brain damage. In V. Dietz, & N. S. Ward (Eds.), *Oxford textbook of neurorehabilitation*. Oxford: Oxford University Press.

Rajkumar., Vaid, V. K., & Mahapatra, A. K. (2014). Diffuse axonal injury. In P. N. Tandon, R. Ramamurthi, & P. K. Jain (Eds.), *Manual of neurosurgery*. New Delhi: Jaypee Brothers.

Ramamurthi, R., & Kapu, R. (2014). Surgical management of cerebral AVMs. In P. N. Tandon, R. Ramamurthi, & P. K. Jain (Eds.), *Manual of neurosurgery*. New Delhi: Jaypee Brothers.

Roper, N., Logan, W. W., & Tierney, A. J. (1985). *The elements of nursing*. Edinburgh: Churchill Livingstone.

Santosh, V. (2014). Classification of tumours of the nervous system. In P. N. Tandon, R. Ramamurthi, & P. K. Jain (Eds.), *Manual of neurosurgery*. New Delhi: Jaypee Brothers.

Sayat, A. R. G., Mestecky, A.-M., & Hassanzadeh, A. (2019). Assessment and management of central post-stroke pain: an overview. *British Journal of Neuroscience Nursing*, 15(suppl 2). Available at: <https://doi.org/10.12968/bjnn.2019.15.Sup2.S4>.

Somerville, P., Lang, A., Nightingale, S., & Birns, J. (2016). Dysphagia after stroke and feeding with acknowledged risk. *British Journal of Neuroscience Nursing*, 12(4), 162–170.

Teasdale, G., & Jennett, B. (1974). Assessment of coma and impaired consciousness. A practical scale. *Lancet*, 2 (7872), 81–84.

Teasdale, G., Jennett, B., Murray, L., et al. (1983). Glasgow coma scale: to sum or not to sum? *Lancet*, 2(8351), 678.

Townsley, E. (2011). Management of patients with intracranial tumours. In S. Woodward, & A.-M. Mestecky (Eds.), *Neuroscience Nursing: an Evidence-based Guide*. Oxford: Blackwell.

Vacca, V. M. (2018). Ventriculoperitoneal shunts: what nurses need to know. *Nursing*, 48(12), 20–27.

Vining Radomski, M. V., Anheluk, M., Bartzen, M. P., et al. (2016). Effectiveness of interventions to address cognitive impairments and improve occupational performance after traumatic brain injury: a systematic review. *American Journal of Occupational Therapy*, 70(3), 7003180050. Available at: https://ajot.aota.org/article.aspx?articleid=2512802.

Wakhloo, A. K., & Gounis, M. J. (2014). Revolution in aneurysm treatment: flow diversion to cure aneurysms: a paradigm shift. *Neurosurgery*, 61 (Suppl), 111–120.

Waterhouse, C. (2016). A basic understanding of dysphagia in neuroscience nursing. *British Journal of Neuroscience Nursing*, 12(Suppl 2), S10–14.

Welch, K., & Mead, G. (2015). The impact of fatigue on neurorehabilitation. In V. Dietz, & N. S. Ward (Eds.), *Oxford textbook of neurorehabilitation*. Oxford: Oxford University Press.

Wheeler, S., Acord-Vira, A., Arbesman., et al. (2017). Occupational therapy interventions for adults with traumatic brain injury. *American Journal of Occupational Therapy*, 71(3). Available at: https://doi.org/10.5014/ajot.2017.713005.

Whiting, A. C., Oh, M. Y., & Whiting, D. M. (2018). Deep brain stimulation for appetite disorders: a review. *Neurosurgical Focus*, 25(2), e9. Available at: https://doi.org/10.3171/2018.4.FOCUS18141.

Young, J. A., & Tolentino, M. (2011). Neuroplasticity and its applications for rehabilitation. *American Journal of Therapeutics*, 18(1), 70–80.

Further reading

Eagleman, D. (2015). *The brain: the story of you*. Edinburgh: Canongate.

Gorelick, P. B., Testai, F. D., Hankey, G. J., & Wardlaw, J. N. (Eds.), (2014). *Hankey's clinical neurology*. Boca Raton: CRC.

Marsh, H. (2014). *Do no harm: Stories of life, death and brain surgery*. London: Weidenfeld and Nicolson.

Sacks, O. (2015). *The man who mistook his wife for a hat*. London: Picador.

Chapter 11

Patients requiring ophthalmic surgery

Helen Gibbons

KEY OBJECTIVES OF THE CHAPTER

At the end of the chapter the reader will be able to:

• understand the basic structure and function of the eye
• understand the causal relationship between altered physiology and patients' visual problems
• demonstrate an awareness of the special needs of patients undergoing ophthalmic surgery
• recognize the importance of continuity of care between hospital and the community
• acknowledge the need for effective patient education.

Areas to think about before reading the chapter

• What is a Snellen's chart and how does the nurse use it?
• What is the role and function of the nurse in assessing a person's vision?
• Discuss the term mydriatic.

Introduction

Nursing patients with a real or potential visual handicap requires perception, patience and good communication skills, as well as the implementation of good nursing care. The majority of elective ophthalmic surgery is carried out on a day care basis and under local anaesthesia.

Individual ophthalmic units have their own protocols regarding patient selection for day care or overnight stay, and there should be a specialist facility for those who need longer periods of care. The Royal College of Ophthalmologists (2017) no longer recommends that all units have inpatient facilities that are separate from other surgical activity, but do recommend that infected cases are isolated from other surgical ophthalmic cases to reduce the risk of infection.

The medical and nursing care that patients receive will also vary from unit to unit, and the following discussion is intended as a guide to key principles of care.

Many patients requiring ophthalmic surgery are in the older age group and may have other medical conditions; these facts must be considered when planning their admission, care and discharge.

Surgery can take many forms, because within the eye there are many structures that affect vision and require surgical intervention to correct or halt a decrease in visual acuity. Knowledge of the structure and function of the eye and its component parts aids understanding of the abnormalities that can occur and the operations that are performed.

Both eyes consist of a globe, cushioned by orbital fat within a cone-shaped bony orbit, and protected anteriorly by the lids, lashes and tear flow.

The eye has three layers:

- sclera and cornea – outer layer
- iris, ciliary body and choroid – middle layer, also known as the uveal tract
- retina – inner layer.

Sclera

The sclera is an opaque, dense layer of tough fibrous tissue with a high collagen content which prevents light entering the eye inadvertently. The opaque nature of the sclera is due to the haphazard positioning of the collagen fibres. It is 0.6–1 mm thick except at the insertion of the recti muscles, where it is only 0.3 mm in depth. The blood supply comes from the posterior ciliary arteries in the elastic episclera that covers the sclera. The nerve supply is derived from the ciliary branch of the oculomotor nerve.

The weakest part of the sclera is the posterior area where it is pierced by the optic nerve fibres, resulting in a sieve-like structure known as the lamina cribrosa, and where the sclera becomes continuous with the dural layer of the meninges. Anteriorly, the sclera merges with the cornea at the limbus. The sclera is a protective layer; it is more elastic in children, becoming tougher with increasing age.

Cornea

The cornea constitutes the anterior one-sixth of the eye; it is 0.5 mm thick centrally and thicker at the periphery; it averages 12 mm × 11 mm in adults. It is a transparent layer with a convex anterior curve, allowing the passage of light rays to focus on the retina.

It is divided into five layers:

- *Epithelium* is composed of five to six layers of squamous stratified epithelium which is continuous with the epithelium of the conjunctiva, and is the only regenerative layer. Damage results in bacteria being able to penetrate corneal tissue.
- *Bowman's membrane* is the anterior elastic membrane, consisting of a thin layer of collagen which is tough, forming a protective layer that does not regenerate if damaged, resulting in scarring.
- *Stroma* accounts for 90% of corneal tissue and consists of modified collagen fibres and keratinocytes.

- *Descemet's membrane* is the posterior elastic membrane, acting as a barrier against invasion by micro-organisms, chemicals and changes in intraocular pressure.
- *Endothelium* is a single layer of cells that lines the posterior surface of the cornea and 'pumps' fluid from the cornea into the anterior chamber. Interference with this function results in corneal oedema and loss of transparency.

There has been evidence to suggest that there is a further layer to the cornea, called the Dua layer (Dua et al, 2013), situated between the stroma and Descemet's membrane. This layer is of particular relevance to corneal specialists and does not affect how the cornea is assessed in everyday practice.

The cornea is essentially avascular; nutrition and oxygen is obtained from the vascular arcades of the anterior ciliary arteries at the limbus, the aqueous via diffusion at the endothelium and from atmospheric oxygen. Corneal nerve supply is derived from the ophthalmic division of the trigeminal nerve.

The cornea has two functions:

- protection
- refraction: it is the most powerful refractive part of the eye, and essential to this function is corneal clarity, which is maintained by:
  - avascularity
  - uniformity of structure
  - efficient epithelial function.

Iris

The iris is a pigmented disc with a central opening, the pupil. It is situated in front of the lens and behind the cornea, so separating the anterior and posterior chambers, and is a forward extension of the ciliary body.

There are three layers:

- endothelium
- stroma, consisting of pigmented cells, blood vessels, nerves and muscles
- pigmented epithelium, continuous with the pigmented epithelium of the retina.

The colour of the iris results from the presence of melanin and is genetically predetermined. Initially, babies only have pigment in the epithelial layer, but, over the first few weeks of life, pigment is laid down in the stroma and the eyes acquire their adult colour.

There are two muscle groups in the iris: the radial dilators and the central sphincter constrictor, the latter being the more powerful. The nerve supply is derived from the short ciliary branch of the oculomotor nerve for the sphincter pupillae and from the long ciliary branch of the trigeminal nerve for the radial pupillae. The arterial capillaries of the long posterior ciliary arteries and the anterior ciliary arteries join to form a circular vascular network.

The iris acts as a regulator, controlling the amount of light that reaches the retina, and this is determined by the environment, emotion and the intensity of surrounding light.

Ciliary body

The ciliary body is triangular, lying between the choroid and the iris. It is continuous with the iris and has numerous folds on its inner surface, the ciliary processes, where secretion of aqueous takes place.

Most of the ciliary body consists of circular and longitudinal muscle fibres whose function is to alter the shape of the lens, i.e. accommodation, by exerting an equal force on the suspensory ligaments that run from the margin of the ciliary body to the periphery of the lens.

The ciliary body can be divided into three areas:
- The pars plicata contains the 70—80 radiating strips that constitute the ciliary processes and secrete aqueous into the posterior chamber.
- The pars plana is continuous with the pars plicata.
- The ciliary muscles are situated on the anterior surface of the ciliary body and are composed of circular and longitudinal fibres. They contract and relax to bring about accommodation, resulting in light rays being focused on the retina. Contraction of the ciliary muscles results in the relaxation of the suspensory ligaments, and the lens becomes more bulbous, so increasing refraction, as when viewing near objects.

The nerve supply is derived from the short ciliary branch of the oculomotor nerve. The blood supply is the long posterior ciliary artery and vein, the anterior ciliary artery and vein, and the vortex vein. The ciliary body produces and secretes aqueous, as well as altering the shape of the lens.

The choroid

The choroid is a pigmented, highly vascular layer lying between the sclera and the retina. It extends from its junction with the ciliary body, the ora serrata, posteriorly to the optic disc.

It is composed of four layers:
- suprachoroid — contains elastic tissue, pigment cells and collagen
- vascular layer — large and small blood vessels supported within a pigmented stromal tissue
- choriocapillaries — capillaries
- Bruch's membrane — a protective, supporting sheath.

The nerve supply is derived from the posterior ciliary branch of the oculomotor nerve. Blood supply is from the short posterior ciliary artery and is drained away by the choroidal and vortex veins.

The choroid provides nutrients for retinal cells adjacent to the choroid, especially the rods and cones. The pigment in the choroid prevents light rays scattering and causing internal reflection of light, so aiding focusing of light rays on the retina.

The retina

The retina is a complex structure consisting of 10 layers of cells, divided into two separate parts. One part is made up of nine layers, the transparent neural division; this lies on the single pigmented epithelial layer which is adjacent to the choroid (Shaw & Lee, 2017). These two parts are firmly attached to each other only at the optic disc and the ora serrata.

Three specific areas of the retina must be considered:
- The macula lies in the central area of the retina, 3 mm to the temporal side of the optic disc, and is 1.5 mm in diameter. It consists mainly of cones, and in its centre is the fovea, an area consisting entirely of cones. Macular function is to give very precise, coloured, central vision, and it lies on the visual axis.
- The rest of the retina consists of a mix of cones and rods, the latter being responsible for the perception of light and dark.
- The optic disc is found at the point where the retinal veins and nerve fibres leave the eye and the retinal artery enters. There are no light receptors in this area, so it is insensitive to light and is consequently known as the 'blind spot'.
- Once a nerve impulse is initiated, it is transmitted along the visual pathway, via the optic nerve to the occipital cortex. Impulses from the nasal fibres of each eye cross at the optic chiasma to the branch of the optic nerve on the other side of the brain.
- The ora serrata is the anterior edge of the retina, where the retinal pigmented layer merges with the ciliary epithelium and the neural layers end.

The blood supply of the retina is derived from two main sources: the anterior one-third is from the choriocapillaries of the choroid, and the posterior two-thirds is from the central retinal artery. The retina is one of the few areas in the body where the blood vessels can be viewed directly.

The retina reacts to the presence of light and initiates impulses that are then transmitted to the visual cortex of the brain for interpretation.

The transparent media of the eye

This consists of the cornea plus the aqueous and vitreous humours and the lens.

Aqueous fluid

Aqueous fluid consists mainly of water, with some proteins and chlorides, and is produced by the ciliary processes of the ciliary body. It is secreted into the posterior chamber and flows around the lens, through the pupil and circulates around the anterior chamber before draining via the trabecular meshwork into the canal of Schlemm and so into the venous return of the eye. Aqueous also drains out through the ciliary body into the episcleral vessels, i.e. the uveal scleral route. The openings to the trabecular meshwork are located in the drainage angle of the anterior chamber, formed by the junction of the cornea and the iris.

The aqueous is responsible for maintaining intraocular pressure at approximately 15–20 mmHg (Shaw & Lee, 2017). It nourishes the lens and posterior surface of the cornea and provides a clear medium for refraction.

Lens

The lens is a biconvex structure approximately 9 mm × 4 mm, lying between the posterior surface of the iris and the anterior surface of the vitreous. It is avascular, is not innervated, and is held in position by the suspensory ligaments or zonules.

It is composed of three parts: the elastic capsule, epithelial cells on the anterior surface, and the lens substance. The lens substance consists of a nucleus, layers of protein called crystallins arranged like an onion and 'Y' sutures that mark the junction of the protein fibres. Nutrition is provided by the aqueous, and the crystallins act as enzymes to convert sugar into energy. Depending on the position of the object being viewed, the lens 'accommodates', so allowing the light rays to focus on the retina.

Vitreous

Vitreous lies between the posterior capsule of the lens and the retina, in the posterior cavity, within the hyaloid membrane. The vitreous body consists of a semigelatinous substance that is produced during embryonic life and, if lost, cannot be replaced naturally. It is avascular, is not innervated, and receives nutrition from the blood vessels of the choroid, retina and ciliary body. It is attached to the ciliary body at the ora serrata and to the retina at the optic disc. The vitreous holds the retina in place, helps to maintain intraocular pressure and preserves the shape of the eye. It also assists in refraction.

Eyelids

The eyelids act as protection for the anterior portion of the eyes, and the epithelium of the lids is continuous with the conjunctiva lining the inner aspect of the lids. Their shape and strength is maintained by cartilaginous tissue forming the upper and lower tarsal plates; within these are found the meibomian glands, which secrete sebum, a substance necessary to control tear flow, lubricate the lid margins and prevent excessive evaporation of tears from the surface of the eye.

Eyelashes are situated along the lid margins and act as protective filters; they are kept supple by sebum secreted directly into the lash follicles by the glands of Zeis.

There are two main muscle groups in the eyelids: a sphincter called the orbicularis oculae, responsible for closing the eye, and the levator palpebrae, whose function is to raise the upper lid. Movement of the lids may be both voluntary and involuntary.

The nerve supply to the orbicularis muscle is from the facial nerve, and the oculomotor nerve supplies the levator palpebrae. The blood vessels to and from the lids are the lacrimal artery and vein, the superior and inferior medial palpebral artery and vein, and the supraorbital artery and vein.

The functions of the eyelids are to:
- protect the eyes from excessive light
- protect the eyes from foreign objects
- lubricate the anterior surface of the eye
- prevent the anterior surface of the eye from drying out, even during sleep.

The conjunctiva

The conjunctiva is a thin, transparent mucous membrane lining the lids; it reflects back over the anterior aspect of the eye and is continuous with the corneal epithelium. The point at which the bulbar and palpebral conjunctival layers meet is known as the fornix, and there is sufficient conjunctival tissue here to allow for movement of the globe.

The nerve supply is derived from the nasociliary branch of the trigeminal nerve. There is a rich blood supply from the anterior ciliary artery and vein, the superior and inferior medial palpebral artery and vein, and the conjunctival artery and vein.

The conjunctiva:
- produces the mucin layer of the tear film, so reducing the rate of tear evaporation
- facilitates movement by moistening the surface of the eye and lids
- protects the eye against damage and infection.

Lacrimal apparatus

The lacrimal apparatus consists of the lacrimal gland, ducts, superior and inferior puncta and canaliculi, common canaliculus, lacrimal sac and nasolacrimal duct.

Tears are produced in the lacrimal gland, which is situated in the upper outer quadrant of the orbit, and then drain via the tear ducts onto the anterior surface of the eye. Blinking causes the tears to be distributed across the cornea, towards the puncta at the inner aspect of the eye. They then drain into the canaliculi via the puncta and collect in the lacrimal sac before draining into the nose via the nasolacrimal duct. Tears consist of water, protein, glucose, sodium, potassium, chloride, urea and lysozymes. Mucin from the goblet cells of the conjunctiva and an oily layer from the meibomian glands facilitate movements, slow down evaporation and prevent overflow onto the cheeks.

The nerve supply to all parts of the lacrimal apparatus is from branches of the trigeminal nerve. The blood supply to the lacrimal gland is from the lacrimal artery and vein, whereas the rest of the system is supplied by the nasal artery and vein, and the superior and inferior medial palpebral artery and vein.

The lacrimal system produces tears which:

- aid refraction by providing an optically smooth corneal surface
- lubricate the anterior surface of the eye, so easing movement
- clean dust particles from the eye
- protect against infection by the action of lysozymes.

The orbit

The eye is protected by being situated in a pyramid-shaped bony cavity — the orbit. It consists of seven fused bones:

- ethmoid
- sphenoid
- frontal
- lacrimal
- zygomatic
- palatine
- maxilla.

Anteriorly, the orbit is open and its apex is positioned posteriorly. Each orbit is described as having a medial wall on the nasal side, a lateral wall, a roof and a floor, the floor and the lower part of the medial wall being the thinnest.

The orbit contains the eyeball, six extraocular muscles, ophthalmic artery and vein, the optic, oculomotor, trochlea, trigeminal and abducens cranial nerves, lacrimal gland, lacrimal sac, orbital fascia, fat and ligaments. There are three openings within the orbital wall, the largest of which is called the optic foramen, and it is here that the optic nerve and ophthalmic artery enter. The bony nature of the orbit acts as a very effective protection from most trauma, except anteriorly.

Extraocular muscles

There are six muscles concerned with the movement of each eye, and they work together to give the precise coordination of movement that is essential for good vision. They are mainly voluntary, and each one is involved in all ocular movement by a balance of contraction and relaxation.

All the muscles receive their blood supply from the muscular arteries, but innervation differs from muscle to muscle:

- oculomotor nerve — superior rectus, inferior rectus, medial rectus and inferior oblique muscles
- abducens nerve — lateral rectus muscle
- trochlea nerve — superior oblique muscle.

Assessment of the eye

Whenever anybody presents with an abnormality of vision, no matter how trivial it may seem, it can cause pain and a fundamental fear of losing sight (Walsh, 2005). This means that the nurse has to use all their psychological skills to reassure the individual and gain their cooperation in order to make an accurate assessment of their vision and the condition of their eye. All information gained should be clearly documented, as a written recording of all findings is a legal requirement (Khaw et al, 2004; Royal College of Nursing, 2018).

The first element of assessment should be the measurement of vision, unless this is not feasible because of the extent of injury, acute pain, or inability to participate, e.g. due to altered level of consciousness. This is done for medical, legal and diagnostic reasons, as visual acuity is a measure of macular function.

The most common way of testing visual acuity is with a Snellen's chart. This requires the patient to read letters of varying sizes on a chart 6 m away (this excludes all but a very small amount of accommodation). The letter size indicates at what distance a normal-sighted person should be able to see it:

- 6/60: normal-sighted person would see this 60 m away
- 6/6: normal-sighted person would see this 6 m away.

In younger people especially, vision may be better than this: e.g. 6/5, 6/4. However, if 6/60, being the largest letter on the chart, cannot be seen, then the person's ability to count the fingers on a hand held up a metre away (CF) or the appreciation of movement (HM) is recorded. If this is not achieved, then perception of a light source is determined and recorded as perception of light (PL) or no perception of light (NPL).

Each eye should be tested individually, the worst eye first, as there may be a degree of unconscious recall. A record should be made of whether glasses or contact lenses are being worn, as an apparent discrepancy in visual acuity may occur when it is recorded next time.

Improvement in visual acuity may be achieved by using a pinhole: the patient looks at the Snellen's chart through a small pinhole, which means that light only passes along the principal visual axis of the eye and so vision is less affected by any abnormality of refraction.

Assumptions must not be made about the patient's ability to read, especially if they appear to be able to see effectively, i.e. they have negotiated their way around obstacles with ease. They may be reluctant to admit they cannot read, but this can be overcome diplomatically by using a Snellen's chart based on the letter 'E' or with pictures rather than letters. Alternatively, use of a LogMAR chart (logarithm of the minimum angle of resolution) gives a more effective and precise record of visual acuity.

LogMAR chart

The LogMAR chart was designed originally by Ballie and Lovie and used in its early days in research for the Early Treatment Diabetic Retinopathy Study. The chart has the same number of letters on each line and the progression of letter sizes is linear, the spacing regular and the scoring method allows each letter to be scored.

The features of the Log MAR are that there are more letters for patients with low vision, each letter can be scored as each letter has a value of 0.02 log units. The test can be carried out at any distance but 4 m is standard. There are five letters per line, the spacing between letters and rows is consistent with the height and width of the letters. The letter size changes between each line by 0.1 unit; therefore, as there are five letters on each line, each letter has a score of 0.02.

Most age-related macular degeneration clinics use this method to test vision (Royal College of Ophthalmologists, 2017) as it is a more accurate way of testing a patient's vision, and many departments have now started to use this to test all their patients. Near vision is tested using ordinary printer's type. Colour vision can be assessed using the Ishihara colour plates.

Visual acuity should always be measured before instilling mydriatic drops, as many of them also have a cycloplegic effect and so paralyse the ciliary muscle and alter accommodation. This also applies when assessing a patient's visual field. If visual acuity is measured following instillation of mydriatics, this must be recorded in the notes.

A basic assessment of visual field can be done by asking the patient to say when they can see an object moving in from the side while focusing on a central object. More precise results can be obtained by using a perimetry machine, which plots peripheral vision by moving a target across a semicircle marked out in degrees. Computerized field analysers are also capable of interpreting results related to the intensity of light needed to stimulate retinal activity.

Mydriatics should not be used when raised intraocular pressure is suspected, as dilating the pupil decreases the amount of aqueous being drained and will increase intraocular pressure even more.

Intraocular pressure is measured most accurately by the use of an applanation tonometer attached to a slit lamp; as this requires the applanator head to be pushed against the cornea, local anaesthetic drops should always be instilled prior to use. Patients who cannot be positioned at a slit lamp can have their intraocular pressures measured using a handheld tonometer, such as a Tono-Pen. If this apparatus is not available, the presence of raised intraocular pressure may be identified by means of careful digital palpation, but this must be done with great care and never when a perforating injury is suspected.

Examination of the eye itself must be carried out systematically, with the cooperation of the patient. If the patient is photophobic, a darkened environment will facilitate matters. The process of examination may be along the following lines:

1. Head posture — abnormal positioning may indicate lid malalignment, squints or deficits of the visual field.
2. Facial appearance — any asymmetry, lacerations, skin disorders or bruising.
3. Lids — signs of inadequate closure, abnormal tear flow, ability to open the eye, alignment of the lid margins, position of the lashes, swelling, and any crusting or exudate along the lid margins.
4. The patient is seated with their head well supported, and analgesic drops, e.g. proxymetacaine 0.5%, oxybuprocaine 0.4% or tetracaine 0.5–1%, instilled if further examination would be difficult due to the level of ocular discomfort and there are no other contraindications such as a possible perforating injury.
5. While the anaesthetic is taking effect, careful explanation of the examination is given, and a detailed history of the condition/trauma is obtained.
6. Once the eyes can be seen, their position within the orbits is noted to ensure that there is no displacement and that both eyes are able to move together in parallel, horizontal and vertical planes. Any instance of double vision, i.e. diplopia, is recorded and reported.
7. Once the patient is comfortable and able to open their eyes, a bright light source (using a slit lamp or a pen torch) is used to examine the eyes themselves, commencing with the less affected one.

Care must be taken to continue the systematic examination by beginning with the outer aspect of the eye and then going on to the internal structures, to ensure an accurate assessment of the condition of the eye.

- *Conjunctiva* — observe for lacerations, degree and position of vascular injection, oedema (chemosis), foreign bodies, naevus, pinguecula and pterygium.
- *Cornea* — note any lacerations, foreign bodies, surface anomalies and the degree of corneal clarity. Identification of superficial damage may be assisted by the instillation of fluorescein sodium 2% drops, as the damaged area will then appear bright green when illuminated. Rose bengal 1% drops may also be used, as they stain all dead corneal tissue pink. If the patient complains of seeing haloes around lights, this may indicate the presence of corneal oedema.
- *Anterior chamber* — shining the beam of light in at an angle makes it is possible to estimate the depth of the anterior chamber. It is also important to note whether the chamber is clear or contains red or white cells and, if these are present, whether they are settled with a specific level or diffuse throughout the chamber.
- *Iris* — examine for any obvious bleeding points or any abnormal pigmentation, and ensure that it is moving freely and equally in all directions, is intact and in position.
- *Pupil* — examine both pupils to verify the existence of a consensual response and equality of size. Their shape, size and briskness of movement are also recorded. The pupil should be black in colour unless there is a reflection from the retina, in which case the pupil appears red. Sometimes the pupil may appear white, possibly indicating the presence of a cataract.
- *Lens* — Should be clear but on dilation varied degrees of opacification may be seen.
- *Retina* — the optic disc may be examined using a direct ophthalmoscope through a normal-sized pupil, but in order for the whole retina, especially the periphery, to be examined, the pupil needs to be dilated using mydriatic drops. The most efficient way of then examining the retina is with an indirect ophthalmoscope (Fig. 11.1).

Apart from the overall examination of the eye, more specific investigations may be carried out.

- Keratometry: measurement of the curvature of the cornea.
- Fluorescein angiography: injection of fluorescein dye, which allows the retinal vessels to be visualized.
- Gonioscopy: examination of the drainage angle.
- Biometry: measurement of the axial length of the eye.
- Ultrasound: measurement of blood flow and exclusion of retinal detachment/tear or tumour in the presence of opacity in the transparent media obscuring direct observation.
- Corneal topography: maps the corneal surface.

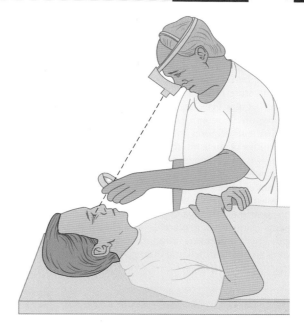

Figure 11.1 Indirect ophthalmoscopy.

- Pachymetry: measures the corneal thickness.
- Amsler grid test: monitors macular degeneration.
- Exophthalmometry: measures degree of proptosis.
- Refraction: determines strength of refractive elements of the eye.
- Schirmer's test: determines the amount of tears produced on a strip of filter paper over a 5 minute period.
- Ishihara colour plate: a series of coloured plates used to detect colour vision.

Preoperative assessment

It is now commonplace that patients are cared for as day cases. The decision about whether patients are suitable for day surgery or will need to stay in hospital is made at the preoperative assessment clinic, and in most units these are now nurse-led. Each day surgery unit has its own criteria for determining what care each patient will need, but some investigations and issues are common to all.

Most units require patients having day surgery to fulfil certain criteria (see Chapters 1 and 3). If the criteria are met, the patient's medical condition is monitored for suitability for local anaesthesia.

- The patient must be able to cooperate: for example, be capable of lying down and keeping still for a period of 20–40 minutes.

- Any medical condition, e.g. diabetes mellitus or hypertension, must be well controlled.

Specific ophthalmic investigations will depend on the type of surgery being undertaken. For cataract surgery with lens implant, keratometry will be undertaken to measure the curvature of the cornea, and biometry to measure the length of the eye's axis. These two measurements allow the required strength of the implant to be determined. If the patient requires surgery for glaucoma, a series of recordings of their intraocular pressure may be taken. This is known as phasing and usually takes place over a 12-hour period.

Careful observation of the eyes should be made, especially with patients having intraocular surgery, as any local infection must be treated prior to admission. These assessments normally take place 2–4 weeks prior to admission, and any community support required postoperatively needs to be identified and arranged at this stage.

Pre- and postoperative care of patients undergoing intraocular surgery

Care needs to be planned systematically for each patient having ocular surgery; whilst the surgery is routine in many cases, each patient has different needs. Each ophthalmic unit will have their own care pathways; however it is common practice to offer a pre-assessment visit which essentially allows all necessary investigations to be undertaken prior to the surgical procedure taking place. If no physical assessments (e.g. bloods, biometry or ECGs) are due to take place then some units will offer a telephone assessment rather than a face-to-face assessment, saving patients from making long journeys or often taking time away from their work commitments.

At the pre-assessment appointment the nurse will:

- Take a history from the patient
- Note general observations
- Carry out a visual acuity
- Perform a slit lamp examination to rule out any abnormalities. (If there are any lid infections the patient will have enough time to treat these prior to surgery.)
- Ascertain who will be instilling the eye drops post surgery, so that if the patient is instilling their own eye drops they can be taught and be encouraged to buy an over-the-counter lubricant to practise their technique at home. If the patient cannot manage their drops and has no one else to help, a district nurse will need to be involved, and the referral can be made at pre-assessment.

- Offer an opportunity for the patient to ask any questions about their condition or their pre-, peri- or postoperative care.
- Any other investigations, such as biometry measurements, will be carried out at this point and consent for surgery obtained.

The areas identified in the discussion on pre- and postoperative care are only meant as a guide (Tables 11.1 and 11.2), and focus on patients having their surgery under local anaesthesia, but they can be adapted to take into account the type of anaesthesia, medical condition, degree of visual handicap and social background, and should take into account that the patient may have difficulty reading, so time will be needed to discuss it with them.

Cleaning the eye

The eye should only be cleaned if there is exudate/secretions along the lid margins. The patient should be positioned comfortably, with their head well supported.

If both eyes require cleaning, they are cleaned one at a time, and if there is any sign of infection, separate packs should be used for each eye, with the potentially infected eye cleaned second.

Patients known to have an infected eye should not have their eyes cleaned until after all other dressings have been completed, and, where possible, cared for by a nurse who is not responsible for any pre- or postoperative ophthalmic patients, to reduce the risk of cross-infection.

Cleaning is carried out using lint/gauze soaked in normal saline 0.9% or cooled boiled water. Sterile packs containing lint/gauze squares, cotton buds, gallipot and a paper towel are usually available. The towel is used either to dry the nurse's hands after washing or to protect the patient's clothing. The eye is cleaned using a lint/gauze square folded into four, with the fluffy side of the lint square innermost, to prevent strands being left in the eye, causing irritation. The swab is held by the cut edges, the folded edges being used to actually clean along the lid margin. Gauze and cotton-wool balls should only be used wet to further reduce the likelihood of particles being left along the margins (Shaw & Lee, 2017).

Lid margins are cleaned from the inner canthus outwards, avoiding any potential infective agents being swept into the lacrimal drainage system via the puncta. Care should also be taken to avoid contact with the cornea, as this may cause the eyes to close involuntarily, due to pain, and may result in corneal abrasion. Each swab is used once and then discarded; four to six swabs are usually sufficient for this procedure.

If an eye pad is required, the eye must be closed and the pad applied firmly, as contact between the cornea and the pad will result in a corneal abrasion. This is especially important if local anaesthetic drops have been instilled.

Table 11.1 Preoperative care for patients undergoing intraocular surgery

Patient's problems	Intervention	Outcome
Communication		
New surroundings and unfamiliar routine	Introduce to staff and other patients. Orient patient and family to unit and explain expected course of events up to and including discharge	Well-oriented, relaxed patient; informed patient and family
Decreased vision and possible loss of independence	Explain that surgery may improve/maintain vision	Patient optimistic about outcome of surgery
Fear of anaesthesia and surgery	Explain exactly what is going to happen prior to, during and after surgery	Patient understands events
Maintaining a safe environment		
Potential risk of wrong operation	Check consent form has been signed and understood by patient	Correct operation performed
Potential risk of peri- and postoperative complications	Instil prescribed topical medication such as miotics, mydriatics or antibiotics. Give prescribed systemic premedication. Follow unit's preoperative protocol. Check for any allergies, e.g. latex, iodine	Surgery is performed without complications
Potential risk of deterioration in a pre-existing medical condition	After consultation with medical/anaesthetic staff, give necessary medication, e.g. insulin, hypotensive agents. Initiate supportive therapy, e.g. physiotherapy. Facilitate patient's involvement in own care	No deterioration in medical condition
Risk of corneal abrasion due to loss of sensation, secondary to application of local anaesthetic drops	Examine for signs of corneal trauma	Cornea is not abraded

Instillation of eye medication

Eye medications are prescribed in two main topical forms: drops or guttae (G.), or ointment or oculentum (Oc.).

Eye medication is instilled into the lower fornix, the 'gutter', which is formed by gently pulling down the lower lid. Drops are placed in the middle of the fornix, avoiding the puncta, as this can result in a dry mouth and unpleasant taste caused by the drops draining away via the lacrimal system. The eye dropper should not come into contact with the corneal surface, but should not be held too far away, as this increases the force with which the drop touches the eye, causing a sudden reflex squeezing which may increase intraocular pressure and so threaten the integrity of the incision, if present. This may also occur if the drops cause a stinging sensation, so the patient should be warned.

When instilling beta-blocking agents such as timolol, it is advisable to occlude the puncta with a fingertip for 2–3 minutes to reduce the risk of systemic uptake, and it is essential to understand which medications interact with each other (International Glaucoma Association, 2019).

Ointments are squeezed gently into the inner aspect of the fornix, being careful not to touch the eye with the nozzle of the tube. Only a small amount should be applied and the eye then closed gently; any excess should then be wiped away. Patients should be made aware that the ointment may create a film across the surface of the cornea and so blur vision.

Where a combination of drops is used, 5 minutes should be left between each to ensure effective uptake (International Glaucoma Association, 2019), and in the case of ointments, they should be placed next to each other in the fornix, not on top of each other, as one may be lost when the eye closes. Drops are instilled before ointment, otherwise absorption is reduced.

Contact between the dropper/nozzle and the cornea can result in a corneal abrasion, so any complaints of pain should be noted and the eye examined.

Table 11.2 Postoperative care following intraocular surgery under general anaesthetic

Patient's problem	Intervention	Outcome
Breathing		
Potential difficulty with breathing	Check that patient is able to maintain own airway Position patient comfortably and encourage effective breathing	Adequate respirations and no acquired chest infection
Maintaining a safe environment		
Difficulty with maintaining own safety	Assess orientation of patient; reorientate as required Educate staff and visitors about the importance of keeping things in the same place and avoiding leaving objects around that may cause injury or confusion Inform all appropriate departments and staff of patient's visual handicap Adjust lighting to suit individual needs; dark glasses may be worn as required	Orientated patient, able to look after self
Potential problem of ocular pain/discomfort	Observe for signs of pain/discomfort Offer prescribed analgesics, and monitor effect Report unrelieved or severe pain to the medical staff	Patient states that they are comfortable
Potential risk of delayed recovery due to ocular complications	Systematic examination of eye(s) Cleanse eye as required Advise patient not to rub or wipe eye with used handkerchief/tissue If necessary, apply 'shield' to eye to avoid inadvertent rubbing Instil, or educate patient/family to instil/administer, prescribed medication	Uneventful recovery
Risk of corneal abrasion due to loss of sensation secondary to application of local anaesthetic drops	Examine for signs of corneal trauma	Cornea is not abraded
Communication		
Difficulty due to poor vision reducing impact of non-verbal communication	Emphasize the importance of appropriate touch Use tone of voice to reinforce message Approach patient from the side with most vision, and speak as approaching or leaving	Establishes an effective rapport between nurse and patient Patient is not startled
Anxiety regarding success	Adequate information is given and questions answered	Patient is aware of outcome
Mobilization		
Difficulty with mobilization due to: anaesthesia; visual acuity	Mobilization is determined by operation and surgeon's preference, but should be as soon as possible Walking aids to be accessible and call-bell within patient's reach	Preoperative level of mobility restored Patient mobilizes safely

(Continued)

Table 11.2 Postoperative care following intraocular surgery under general anaesthetic—cont'd

Patient's problem	Intervention	Outcome
Eating and drinking		
Difficulty with eating and drinking due to: poor vision; effects of anaesthesia	Assist with selection of food and dietary intake Observe for signs of nausea Give antiemetic as required	Balanced diet eaten to facilitate healing Patient does not vomit, and subsequent raised intraocular pressure does not weaken the incision
Working and playing		
Potential problem of being unable to return to normal lifestyle	With the involvement and cooperation of patient and family/carer, an effective discharge plan (see p. 164) is devised and implemented	Patient is confident to return home

Corneal graft (keratoplasty)

A corneal graft is the replacement of scarred or degenerative corneal tissue by healthy tissue. This is a less complicated procedure than organ transplant, because of corneal avascularity, although this may have been compromised by new vessel growth from the corneal margins.

Corneal tissue can be obtained in three ways.

- *Autogenous* — when the patient's other eye is blind but has a healthy cornea, the eye can be used to provide donor material.
- *Live donor* — when another patient has undergone enucleation but the cornea is healthy, it can be used as donor material for someone requiring a graft.
- *Cadaver* — this is the most common and is the grafting of corneal tissue from donated eyes following death. Donated eyes should be removed within 24 hours of death and can be stored in short-term storage media for 3–7 days at 4°C, or for up to 30 days in an organ culture system at 34°C.

Removal and storage of donor material is subject to the Human Tissue Act (Department of Health, 2004).

Although most people are suitable donors, there are some exceptions:

- infections such as methicillin-resistant *Staphylococcus aureus*, HIV, hepatitis A, B and C, syphilis, and septicaemia
- unexplained neurological disease, because of the risk of infections such as Creutzfeldt–Jakob disease
- leukaemia, lymphoma and myeloma
- eye conditions such as uveitis, retinoblastoma, history of intraocular surgery, and malignancies of the ciliary body and iris
- jaundice
- death due to unknown cause, although donation may take place after a postmortem has been carried out.

Types of corneal graft

Partial-thickness or lamellar

Anterior lamellar keratoplasty. This is a partial-thickness graft that involves replacement of the abnormal corneal tissue down to the level of Descemet's layer (Fig. 11.2). It is used when the pathology is anterior to Descemet's membrane and has the advantage of preserving the healthy endothelium. The risk of rejection is decreased, as the endothelium is not involved (Kanski, 2015).

Posterior lamellar or endothelial keratoplasty. This is a partial-thickness graft that involves replacement of only the posterior layers of the cornea, namely Descemet's membrane and endothelium. It is used when the

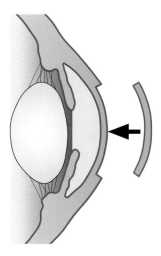

Figure 11.2 Lamellar keratoplasty.

pathology is confined to the corneal endothelium and where the anterior corneal structures are unaffected. The technique is relatively new and has the advantage of quicker visual recovery, increased corneal integrity and reduced risk of rejection. This approach is only available in a few specialist centres and, according to Mearza et al (2007), has a higher graft dislocation and failure rate.

Full-thickness or penetrating

This is the replacement of all five corneal layers (Fig. 11.3).

Reasons for corneal grafting

Reasons for corneal grafting are:
- keratoconus
- Fuchs' and other corneal dystrophies
- bullous keratopathy
- corneal scarring due to trauma or infection
- herpes simplex keratitis
- corneal melting syndromes/descemetoceles
- interstitial keratitis.

Specific preoperative care for penetrating/ lamellar grafts

Prior to preparing the patient for surgery, contact is made with one of the eye banks, to check availability of donor material and arrange for its delivery.

Surgery is usually carried out under a general anaesthetic, and, providing the patient has attended for preassessment, they are admitted on the day of surgery, having

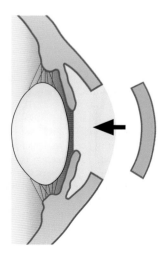

Figure 11.3 Penetrating keratoplasty.

fasted for 4 hours. Patients need considerable psychological support, as for some it may be the last chance of achieving useful vision. Topical medication consists of a miotic such as guttae pilocarpine 4% every 15 minutes for 1 hour. This constricts the pupil, and the iris acts as a protective barrier for the lens, so avoiding the risk of inadvertent cataract formation.

Specific postoperative care

The eye is examined, before instillation of any topical medication, for the following:
- position of graft and integrity of sutures
- depth of anterior chamber
- presence of red cells (hyphaema)
- presence of white cells (hypopyon)
- clarity of cornea.

If the condition of the eye is satisfactory, prescribed medication may be given, but if there is any cause for concern, medication should be withheld until medical opinion is sought.

Topical medication usually consists of:
- an antibiotic: e.g. guttae chloramphenicol 0.5% three to four times a day
- an anti-inflammatory: e.g. guttae dexamethasone 1% three to four times daily
- a mydriatic: e.g. guttae mydrilate (cyclopentolate) 1% twice a day may be given, as this dilates the pupil and rests the eye.

When opacification has been due to viral infection, systemic antiviral agents may be prescribed to reduce the risk of recurrence (Kanski, 2015).

Provided the suture line is not leaking aqueous, no dressing is required, but the eye may feel uncomfortable because of the presence of the sutures, although discomfort does decrease as the corneal epithelium regenerates over them. The level of discomfort can be reduced by wearing dark glasses or an eye shield.

Discharge home may take place on the actual day of operation, providing the condition of the eye and home circumstances are acceptable.

Potential complications of corneal graft

- Loose sutures lead to aqueous loss, diagnosed by Seidel's test, which demonstrates the passage of fluorescein from the exterior to the interior of the eye, and by the presence of a flat anterior chamber.
- Cataract formation.
- Intraocular/extraocular infection.
- Adhesions, known as synechiae, form between the iris and edge of the graft, and can result in blockage of the drainage angle, leading to post-keratoplasty glaucoma.

- Iris prolapse due to herniation through the incision.
- Rejection of graft may be 'early' or 'late' — 90% of grafts are successful and early rejection is unusual, but the highest risk is within the first 6 months (Kanski, 2015). The risk increases if the eye has been grafted before.
- Astigmatism is caused by the tension of the sutures and size of the graft altering the curvature of the cornea. Rigid contact lenses may be prescribed following removal of sutures.
- Growth of new blood vessels (neovascularization) around the graft can obscure vision if growth continues across the centre of the graft.

The cornea is avascular; therefore, healing takes considerably longer and the sutures may not be removed for up to 12 months. In the older patient, healing may take even longer. Removal of sutures is normally carried out under slit lamp illumination in the outpatient department, but if it is too uncomfortable for the patient, especially if a continuous suture has been used, then general anaesthesia may be considered.

Refractive surgery

The cornea and lens are the principal refracting structures of the eye. Until now, refractive errors have been corrected with lenses or spectacles, but, increasingly, people are opting for surgical correction, as the procedures have become safer and more readily available. The underlying principle involves altering the curvature of the cornea: flattening in myopia and making it steeper in hypermetropia.

The main approaches are:

- radial keratotomy — involves making radial incisions in the peripheral cornea and is used for low degrees of myopia (largely obsolete now)
- laser-assisted in situ keratomileusis (LASIK) — corrects refractive errors of hypermetropia, astigmatism and myopia
- photorefractive keratectomy (PRK) — corrects refractive errors but uses a slightly different technique that involves removing the corneal epithelium
- LASEK is a modified version of PRK that preserves the epithelial sheet
- implantable contact lenses — for people with severe levels of refractive abnormality.

Penetrating injuries

Patients giving a history of a sharp object entering the eye must be examined to exclude the possibility of a perforating injury, and lacerations to the globe need urgent admission to hospital and, usually, emergency surgery. Where possible, suspected perforating injuries should be treated in a specialist ophthalmic unit, as inexperienced care may result in a poorer visual outcome for the patient.

The commonest sites for such injuries are the sclera, cornea or corneoscleral junction, and the injuries range in severity from a slight puncture wound to a full-thickness laceration. Minor corneal perforations may heal themselves or resolve quickly following the application of a soft contact lens that acts as a 'bandage'. This has the advantage of maintaining the integrity of the eye without suturing, so reducing the risk of further scarring.

More severe injuries must be treated promptly, as they can potentially result in iris prolapse, damage to the lens, intraocular bleeding resulting in a hyphaema and the possibility of secondary glaucoma, and infection. Scleral perforation may lead to uveal damage, and uveal and vitreous prolapse. Gross perforating injury often leads to damage to and disorganization of most of the contents of the eye. The most common causes of penetrating injury are broken glass or pieces of metal travelling at speed, as in hammer, chisel and lathe injuries, and this type of injury is three times more common in males than in females (Kanski, 2015). Even though the Health and Safety at Work Act (HSE, 2019) requires goggles to be worn when working with certain tools and machines, many people ignore the law, because they find the glasses don't fit comfortably or mist up.

Some medical conditions may result in corneal perforation: for example, corneal ulceration and melting syndromes such as Mooren's ulcer.

Complications associated with perforating injuries mean it is important to take a detailed and accurate history and carry out a careful assessment. The latter may not be easy, as the eye is likely to be extremely painful; a local anaesthetic such as tetracaine 1% drops can be given once the possibility of glass being present in the eye has been excluded. In some cases, the pain may be so great that a systemic analgesic such as intramuscular morphine is necessary, and occasionally a full examination will be possible only under a general anaesthetic. In these cases, good documentation is vital as in cases of assault or injury at work there may be litigation concerns.

Sometimes, the perforation is visualized, but the nurse or doctor carrying out the examination should also look for an anterior chamber that is shallower than that in the unaffected eye, indicating aqueous leakage, hyphaema, an abnormally shaped pupil or absence of part of the iris. The eye may also feel soft, and great care must be taken not to exert pressure on the eye, as this may increase the degree of damage. DO NOT apply a pad that could put pressure on the eye; a cartella shield must be applied.

It is necessary to determine whether the object that caused the injury is still in or on the eye. The person carrying out the examination cannot rely on the presence of a foreign body sensation, as this may be due solely to the damage to the corneal or scleral surface. If the object cannot be visualized, then an X-ray is ordered to ascertain where the object is located, especially if there is reason to think it is in the eye itself. The X-rays should be taken at upward gaze, downward gaze and looking straight ahead, since, if there is an intraocular foreign body, it will move with the direction of gaze and so eliminate any radiological artefact. X-rays do not usually identify glass foreign bodies, unless the glass has a lead content. Once a definitive diagnosis has been made, then surgical intervention will probably be necessary to repair the perforation.

A metallic foreign body may be removed by using a magnet to draw the object back along its entry path; however, if the substance from the history obtained is thought to be inert, it may be left, as removal may cause more damage to adjacent structures.

At this early stage, the patient needs considerable psychological support, as it is extremely difficult to predict the ultimate visual outcome. Corneal avascularity means healing is prolonged, so the lens or sutures used to close the perforation may be left for up to 6 months. In cases where the perforation is relatively minor and does not affect other structures, mobilization and discharge will be quite rapid, providing there is no sign of aqueous leakage.

Specific postoperative care

Following surgery for more extensive wounds, treatment varies depending upon the extent of the injury and the parts of the eye involved. Psychological care is ongoing, because vision may be affected by actual trauma, bleeding into the vitreous or aqueous, or by the local medication being used. However, nursing and medical intervention may include the following aspects:

- The eye may be padded for 12–24 hours, depending on the surgeon's instructions. It is inadvisable to keep the eye padded for any longer than is necessary, as this provides a warm, moist environment that encourages bacterial growth. Dark glasses or a plastic shield may be worn for protection and to decrease photophobia. If the latter is a marked problem, then subdued lighting in the bed area may be required.
- Cleaning of the eye takes place as often as is necessary to maintain comfort, as an irritable eye may result in the patient rubbing it and causing further trauma.
- Eye examination identifies if there is blood present in the anterior chamber, how deep the chamber is and whether the pupil is the shape that it was at the end of surgery. If any iris was found to be missing or had to be removed during surgery, this should be recorded, and the appearance of the eye can be checked against the operation notes.
- Medication will be both local and systemic and, in the case of eyedrops, is likely to be given intensively for

the first 72 hours. If there is any concern that the patient may be at risk of endophthalmitis prophylaxis antibiotics will be given (Kanski, 2015). The types of drug that may be given are:
- antibiotics: e.g. cefuroxime or ceftazidime drops every hour; in severe cases, intravenous ceftazidime may be given for 5 days, otherwise oral ceftazidime, 750 mg twice daily for 5–7 days
- anti-inflammatories: e.g. dexamethasone drops decrease the swelling that results from the injury and the surgery and so reduce the risk of increasing intraocular pressure, decrease pain, and minimize the risk of sympathetic ophthalmitis
- mydriatic/cycloplegic: e.g. atropine drops dilate the pupil and paralyse the ciliary muscle, so inhibiting accommodation and fixing the lens at distant focus, thus resting the eye.
- If blood is seen in the anterior or vitreous chamber, the patient may be nursed sitting upright, or in a chair if more comfortable. This allows the blood to settle to the bottom of the chamber, a process that is much more rapid in the anterior chamber than in the vitreous, as is the actual absorption of the blood. Any signs of increased intraocular pressure, such as an increasingly hazy cornea, pain and redness around the corneal margin, must be reported, as blood cells can block the entrance to the trabecular meshwork and so decrease aqueous drainage. Sudden aggressive movement should be avoided as this may cause a recurrence of the bleeding.

Irritation to the eye caused by inflamed conjunctival and corneal surfaces, plus the presence of minute sutures, can result in epiphora and excessive tear production, and the patient may feel the need to be constantly wiping the eye(s). This is potentially problematical, as it may lead to corneal abrasion, introduce infective organisms or put undue pressure on the wound. Patients are educated to use disposable tissues once only, and to wipe below the lower lid, not on the eye itself. The problem can be eased by wearing dark glasses and the application of a small lint square/dental roll to the cheek immediately below the lower lid margin to act as a 'drip pad'.

Discharge arrangements

Discharge takes place when the wound is secure, i.e. not leaking causing a shallow anterior chamber, and low eye pressure bleeding has resolved and the level of pain can be controlled. The frequency of outpatient appointments will depend on the degree of injury and be determined by the consultant. The length of time for which these appointments carry on will depend upon the rate of recovery and the actual and potential risk of complications.

Complications of a penetrating injury

Incidence of complications appears to depend on the site and severity of the injury and includes the following:

- *Panophthalmitis*: intraocular infection involving the sclera (Shaw & Lee, 2017).
- *Cataract formation*: damage to the lens capsule leads to water being absorbed into the lens matter, which becomes opaque.
- *Corneal scarring*: clear corneal tissue scars as a result of either the injury itself or the sutures used to repair the injury. Scarring is inevitable if the injury penetrates the Bowman's membrane as it does not regenerate (Shaw & Lee, 2017).
- *Astigmatism*: curvature of the corneal surface can be altered by scarring or suture tension, so disrupting refraction.
- *Retinal detachment*: results from direct retinal trauma, traction from a vitreous haemorrhage, or a loss of pressure within the eye.
- *Secondary glaucoma*: rise in intraocular pressure due to occlusion of the drainage angle by red blood cells, white blood cells or scar tissue, or damage to the trabecular meshwork/canal of Schlemm.
- *Recurrent uveitis*: inflammation of the iris, ciliary body and choroid can be potentiated by the trauma itself, surgery or the presence of foreign bodies, or tissue material not normally in contact with the uveal tract.
- *Phthisis bulbi*: atrophy of the entire globe secondary to a non-functioning ciliary body, resulting in loss of aqueous production. The shrunken eye is sightless and painless.
- *Siderosis*: following injuries caused by iron fragments, deposits of iron are dissolved in the aqueous and vitreous and stain the surrounding tissues.
- *Sympathetic ophthalmitis*: a rare complication that may occur any time after the first two weeks following injury, even years later. It is a bilateral uveitis, probably resulting from an immune response to damage to the uveal tract, which exposes antigens unfamiliar to the body's defence mechanisms and leads to their destruction; the same process then takes place in the uninjured eye (James et al, 2016). If an eye is very badly injured, with no perception of light, and cosmesis is a problem, enucleation within nine days of the injury minimizes the risk of sympathetic ophthalmitis. If the condition does occur, then enucleation of the damaged, 'exciting' eye may be carried out.

Cataract

NICE (2017), in conjunction with the Royal College of Ophthalmologists, gives clear guidance on the management of patients with cataracts.

A cataract is an opacity of the lens which may interfere with vision. It results from denaturation of the lens protein, which may be caused by changes within the lens itself or by the lens capsule becoming no longer selectively semipermeable.

The lens epithelium continues to produce cell layers throughout life, so it increases in size. It is thought that, as the nutrients from the aqueous become less readily available to the lens nucleus, it hardens and accommodation becomes more difficult. This results in less efficient near vision, a condition known as 'presbyopia', which normally starts after the age of 40 years (Shaw & Lee, 2017).

In some people, lens changes continue, resulting in further deterioration of visual acuity, leading to loss of definition and colour appreciation, progressing to virtual blindness if not treated. During the development of the cataracts, vision may vary depending upon the light. Most difficulties arise in bright sunlight or at night, when headlights are being used. Cataracts are usually bilateral, one eye tending to be worse than the other, and are generally painless, unless the lens absorbs enough water from the aqueous to cause a marked increase in size, which can result in an increase in intraocular pressure, i.e. secondary glaucoma.

Causes of cataract

There are several causes of cataract formation:

- *Age-related*: these are the most frequent, are the result of the normal ageing process and are more common in people with diabetes mellitus.
- *Traumatic*: occur as a result of a 'blunt' injury, when a direct blow to the eye can cause a cataract by concussion; or after a penetrating injury, which results in perforation of the lens capsule, allowing aqueous to seep into the lens matter. Traumatic cataracts can develop very quickly, the opacity becoming apparent within 12–24 hours.
- *Metabolic*: can develop quickly in individuals with insulin-dependent diabetes mellitus (Kanski, 2015). They may also occur in people with hypoparathyroidism, as a result of a rise in calcium levels in the lens.
- *Inflammation*: local inflammation due to intraocular infection or chronic anterior uveitis causes changes in the lens function. Inflammation may also be secondary to skin disorders, e.g. rosacea.
- *Congenital*: can be secondary to maternal rubella, normally within the first trimester, or to the absorption of drugs across the placental barrier.
- *Genetic*: may be a manifestation of Down syndrome or can be one of the consequences of an enzyme deficiency that causes galactosaemia.

- *Drugs*: long-term medication using drugs such as steroids and thyroxine can lead to lens opacity.
- *Radiation*: ionizing radiation, especially if the patient is undergoing treatment for malignancies of the head and neck.

Types of surgery

To re-establish normal visual acuity, the opaque lens is removed and replaced with some means of optical correction. This ranges from insertion of an artificial lens in the eye, usually in the posterior chamber, to the fitting of corneal contact lenses, or to the wearing of glasses. These methods all correct aphakia, the condition of having no lens; the posterior chamber intraocular lens (Fig. 11.4) is the most efficient, as the focal distance is not altered, whereas aphakic glasses give only a central field of vision and a considerable degree of magnification.

The type of surgery is categorized by the way in which it is carried out.

Lens aspiration/lensectomy

This is used for removing congenital cataracts, as they have a soft nucleus that allows the lens matter to be sucked out through an incision in the anterior lens capsule. Any remaining lens matter is absorbed by the enzymes in the aqueous, and the posterior capsule is left in place. This operation must be carried out as early as possible, as failure to do so can result in amblyopia.

Phacoemulsification

Phacoemulsification is the most commonly used technique of extracapsular extraction and is the preferred method of cataract removal in the Western world (James et al, 2016). A 'stab' incision allows the phacoemulsifier to be passed into the lens, and high-frequency vibrations cause the hard nucleus to emulsify, allowing the lens contents to be 'sucked' out through an extraction tube which is part of the probe. The benefits of phacoemulsification, as opposed to a standard extracapsular extraction, are that healing is more rapid, less astigmatism occurs, and improved vision is achieved in a shorter length of time (Kanski, 2015). The wound is small − less than 5 mm − and usually doesn't need suturing. A foldable intraocular lens can usually be inserted, however if a non-folding lens is used, a larger incision will need to be made.

Extracapsular extraction

This is the technique of choice, since, by leaving the posterior capsule in place, there is less risk of vitreous loss and subsequent retinal damage. An incision is made in the anterior lens capsule, and the hardened nucleus is lifted out and as much as possible of the soft lens matter is removed by irrigation with saline (Fig. 11.5).

Intracapsular extraction

This used to be the most common method of cataract extraction but is now rarely used. The lens is removed in

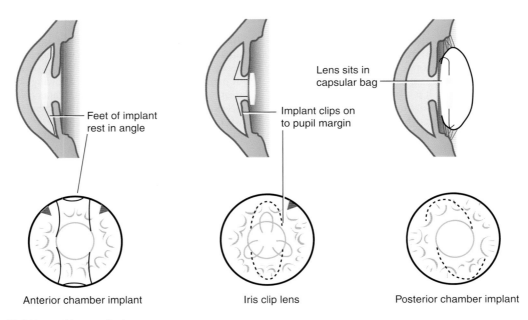

Feet of implant rest in angle

Lens sits in capsular bag

Implant clips on to pupil margin

Anterior chamber implant

Iris clip lens

Posterior chamber implant

Figure 11.4 Types of intraocular lens.

Specific preoperative care

Surgery should be offered at the point at which the individual's lifestyle is affected by their decrease in visual acuity — although, in reality, it is usually at this time that patients are added to the waiting list for surgery.

Patients are usually admitted as day cases but may stay in overnight if their medical background or social situation requires it. If they are having surgery under a general anaesthetic, then local protocols are followed and the pupil of the affected eye is well dilated, to facilitate access to the lens. This is done by using mydriatic drops such as mydrilate (cyclopentolate) 1%, phenylephrine 2.5–10% and homatropine 1–2%, in varying combinations, or by inserting a Mydriasert ophthalmic insert which means that the patient only has the insert applied once and achieves good mydriasis (depending upon the surgeon's wishes). In addition, if local anaesthesia is used, drops such as tetracaine 1% may be administered topically, either on the ward or in theatre. Sedation may sometimes be given, but is avoided where possible, as there is a risk of the patient falling asleep and then waking with a 'start' during the operation. The surgeon must be informed if the patient is taking or has taken Flomax (tamsulosin), doxazosin or alfuzosin, as this may result in floppy iris syndrome, which increases the risk of iris prolapse.

Specific postoperative care

On return from surgery, blood pressure and pulse are recorded, and are continued to be so at the nurse's discretion or as directed by local policy and procedure. Most patients can be mobile as soon as they return to the ward and feel safe to do so; it is usually the effect of sedation (if any administered) that necessitates their resting for a period of time. Patients may eat and drink as soon as they like, unless they are feeling nauseated or the anaesthetist gives instructions to the contrary.

The eye is usually covered with a cartella shield and the patient is educated not to rub it, as this may cause direct trauma to the incision, a rise in intraocular pressure or a corneal abrasion.

Timing and method of follow-up will vary from unit to unit, on the surgeon and on the time of surgery. It may be done prior to discharge, by telephone assessment, or at home the following day either by the patient or by a nurse, or in the outpatient department. If the assessment is face to face, the eye should be examined carefully and systematically (Table 11.3), and, providing the other eye is healthy, it is useful to use it for comparison. If the condition of the eye is satisfactory, no covering is necessary during the day, and patients complaining of photophobia are advised to wear dark glasses; they may be recommended to wear a shield at night, to avoid inadvertent rubbing.

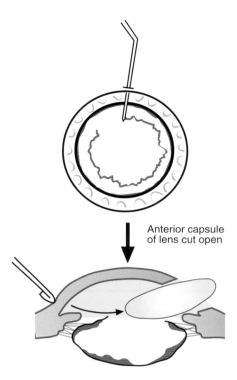

Anterior capsule of lens cut open

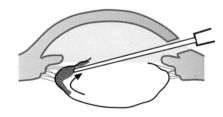

Nucleus of lens expressed from capsular bag

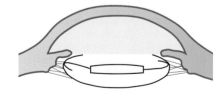

Lens remnants in capsule bag aspirated

Artificial lens implanted in capsular bag

Figure 11.5 Extracapsular extraction.

its entirety, and this is facilitated by the fact that, in an older person, the suspensory ligaments are weaker and can be easily broken to aid removal (Fig. 11.6).

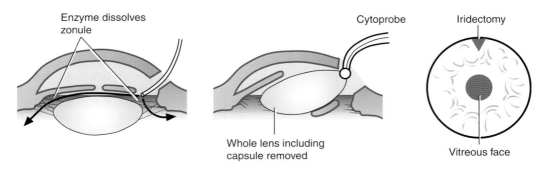

Figure 11.6 Intracapsular extraction.

Table 11.3 Postoperative examination of the eye following cataract extraction

Element of examination	Possible findings to be noted and recorded
Dressing	Any exudate, special note being taken of colour that might indicate bleeding or infection
Lids	Excessive swelling and redness, as this may indicate signs of an allergy or infection If the lid opening is small, this may make surgery more difficult, so a small cut may have been made at the outer junction of the lids. This is called a canthotomy, and its site should be checked Normally, sutures are not required, but, if present, are removed 5–7 days postoperatively
Conjunctiva	Any signs of a conjunctival haemorrhage or oedema
Incision	The integrity of the wound should be checked, and any gap, loose sutures, or prolapsed iris tissue should be reported immediately. Prolapsed iris is recognized by the presence of a tongue of pigmented tissue protruding through the incision and may be accompanied by an updrawn pupil adjacent to the incision. The incidence of this is less if a corneal incision is used
Cornea	The clarity of this normally transparent structure should be checked. If the cornea is hazy, this may indicate corneal oedema and could be secondary to raised intraocular pressure, damage to the corneal endothelium or intraocular infection. This should be reported immediately
Anterior chamber	Using a pen torch beam, the depth of the anterior chamber is estimated. This can be difficult to establish, when the nurse has had little experience in eye examination. It is important, as a shallow or absent anterior chamber may indicate the incision is not secure or the aqueous lost during surgery has not been replaced. The unoperated eye can be used as an indicator of the individual's normal chamber depth, provided there has been no previous surgery Visible accumulation of white blood cells, a hypopyon, indicates that a severe inflammation or infection is present. Occasionally, an accumulation of red blood cells, a hyphaema, indicates a blood vessel has ruptured. If a hyphaema is present, it is important to note whether the colour is bright red, a recent bleed, or dark, probably from the time of surgery. The hyphaema may also be diffuse, spread around the chamber, or may be settled, in which case the level should be recorded, as this will indicate whether it is resolving It is difficult to check the position of posterior chamber lenses without the aid of a slit lamp, whereas anterior chamber lenses can be seen on the surface of the iris
Iris	Sometimes there is a small triangular piece of iris missing at the periphery; this is known as a peripheral iridectomy, and is performed if there is a risk of the vitreous moving forward, resulting in pupil block and a sudden rise in intraocular pressure
Pupil	Its position, size and shape is noted, as an updrawn, peaked pupil may indicate an iris prolapse, or it may be caused by a capsule tag or adhesion of vitreous through the incision

Medication will depend upon the surgeon's wishes, type of operation and unit protocol, but usually consists of topical antibiotic and anti-inflammatory agents.

Changes to optical prescription are carried out once all postoperative inflammation has settled, usually at 4 weeks, and 6/12 vision or better is achieved in 80% of patients.

Complications of cataract surgery

- *Iris prolapse*: requires a return to the operating theatre to remove the prolapsed tissue and resuture the wound. This is carried out as soon as possible in order that the postoperative visual acuity is not affected.
- *Raised intraocular pressure*: usually due to postoperative inflammation, impairing the flow of aqueous through the trabecular meshwork, and normally resolves with intensive topical medication. The regimen will depend upon the degree of raised pressure, but could include Maxidex (dexamethasone) drops 2 hourly and acetazolamide 250 mg two to four times a day. Pressure may become raised as a result of 'pupil block', which occurs when aqueous is trapped in the posterior chamber owing to the forward protrusion of the vitreous or lens implant blocking the pupil.
- *Panophthalmitis*: an infection that rapidly involves all the eye and its surrounding structures. Signs and symptoms include rapid reduction in visual acuity, acute intraocular discomfort, lacrimation and severe intraocular inflammation. Incidence is rare, about 0.3% (James et al, 2016), but the consequences are severe.
- *Retinal detachment*: when vitreous is lost or prolapses forward, the pressure that holds the retina in position is reduced, resulting in detachment.
- *Cystoid macula oedema/Irvine−Gass syndrome*: 2−3 months after surgery, the patient presents with decreased visual acuity and possible photophobia and ocular irritation. It is more common in patients with diabetes, hypertension and those who have had complications such as vitreous loss and iris prolapse. Although the exact cause of this condition is not known, some units now prescribe non-steroidal anti-inflammatory drops both pre- and postoperatively, such as Acular (ketorolac tromethamine) or Ocufen (flurbiprofen sodium), as prostaglandins have been identified as a possible mediator (Kanski, 2015).
- *Posterior capsule opacification*: occurs when remnants of the lens epithelium cells fibrose behind the implanted intraocular lens. It occurs in up to 50% of eyes following cataract surgery. The lens is initially clear, but may become opaque, in which case a capsulotomy is performed, using a YAG laser (yttrium, aluminium, garnet) to allow light rays to pass to the retina (Coombes & Seward, 1999). The subsequent loss of vision can be rectified by capsulotomy.

Glaucoma

Glaucoma is the name given to a group of conditions characterized by damage to the optic nerve, loss of peripheral vision and, commonly, an increase in intraocular pressure. Normal intraocular pressure is usually identified as being between 15 and 20 mmHg (Shaw & Lee, 2017), but it has become increasingly clear that relying solely on intraocular pressure readings is not advisable. Ocular hypertension is a condition where the intraocular pressure is raised but the optic nerve is not damaged and the situation is monitored but not necessarily actively treated.

Cupping of the optic disc and loss of vision can sometimes be seen in people with a normal intraocular pressure. It may be due to changes in the local vasculature, resulting in a decreased blood supply to the vessels near to the optic nerve (Simmons et al, 2006).

Glaucoma is an age-related disease; in Western countries, primary open angle glaucoma occurs in approximately 1:100 people over 40 years of age (Chivers, 2003). There is a strong familial pattern with glaucoma: so much so, that in the UK free screening for glaucoma is available to the immediate families of those diagnosed with glaucoma. Child (2003) found that patients with different types of glaucoma have different causative genes. The International Glaucoma Association (2008) suggests that the most significant risk is to siblings, followed by parents and children. The Royal National Institute of Blind People (2015) identified that people of African origin are more at risk, the disease having an earlier onset and increased severity.

The surgery to be described is that associated with glaucoma resulting in a high intraocular pressure, of which there are several types, depending on the cause.

Glaucoma can be subdivided into:
- primary glaucoma:
  - primary open angle closure glaucoma
  - angle closure glaucoma
- secondary glaucoma
- congenital glaucoma.

Angle closure glaucoma (ACG)

This is an acute ophthalmic emergency and is due to obstruction of aqueous drainage by the closure of the angle formed by the iris and the cornea. It usually occurs in small, hypermetropic eyes with a shallow anterior chamber and narrow drainage angle and becomes more common as the lens ages, as it becomes harder, larger and is less mobile. Shaw and Lee (2017) also says that it becomes more common with age, as in people over 40 the incidence is 1:1000, with women four times more likely to be affected. The condition is usually bilateral, but one eye supersedes the other.

The attacks are episodic, and, in between, the intra-ocular pressure is normal. An attack usually happens when the pupil dilates and the iris root moves forward to block off the entrance to the trabecular meshwork. An attack may be precipitated by emotion, a decrease in light such as the onset of evening or in the dark, or the instillation of mydriatic drops.

There is a subacute stage when the angle is not completely blocked but the decrease in aqueous drainage causes a rise in intraocular pressure, resulting in corneal oedema. This causes the individual concerned to see haloes around lights and is often accompanied by mistiness of vision and frontal headaches.

If this stage is not recognized, then an acute attack is inevitable; the drainage angle becomes almost totally occluded, and the intraocular pressure rises massively to over 50 mmHg. This causes a sudden reduction in vision, severe pain in and around the eye, possible nausea and vomiting, photophobia and epiphora.

On examination the eye shows:

- a red, congested eye, worse around the limbus
- a hazy, green/grey cornea
- a shallow anterior chamber
- a moderately dilated immobile pupil, often irregular in shape.

The intraocular pressure must be reduced to within normal limits by intensive systemic and topical medical intervention in order to prevent irreparable loss of vision before any ocular procedure is performed. The intraocular pressure should initially be monitored hourly, and, once emergency treatment has finished, four-hourly.

If topical therapy is not successful, intravenous acetazolamide and/or mannitol may be considered, with oral glycerol as an additional treatment if the pressure is not reduced sufficiently (Marsden, 2017).

Open angle glaucoma (OAG)

This normally occurs in both eyes in both men and women over the age of 65 years, and there is a recognized association with raised systolic blood pressure and a familial link (Shaw & Lee, 2017). One eye usually develops the condition before the other, and the effect on vision is so gradual that the individual may have significant visual field loss, unnoticed by the patient, before diagnosis is made.

Changes in vision are sometimes wrongly attributed to the ageing process, rather than a specific pathology. There are often no obvious signs and symptoms, although, on questioning, the patient may give a history of frontal headaches.

Examination may reveal a consistently raised intraocular pressure of above 21 mmHg (except in normotensive glaucoma), a cupped optic disc and a reduced visual field

progressing to tunnel vision if not treated. Surgery is not indicated unless medical treatment fails to contain the rise in intraocular pressure, there is a continued reduction in the visual field, or patient concordance with medical treatment is poor.

A range of surgically derived drainage procedures have been carried out in the past, but currently the most common are trabeculectomy and trabeculoplasty.

Trabeculectomy

Trabeculectomy entails raising a conjunctival flap and then a partial-thickness scleral flap (Fig. 11.7). A section of underlying sclera and trabecular meshwork is then removed, so making a larger, permanent opening into the canal of Schlemm. This, plus an iridectomy, means that aqueous drainage should not be obstructed at any time. The scleral and conjunctival flaps are sutured back into position, but a small 'blister' of aqueous, a bleb, can be seen beneath the conjunctiva; this should result in a permanent maintenance of normal intraocular pressure.

Specific preoperative care. Patients may be treated as day cases or stay in overnight. If they are having surgery under a general anaesthetic, then local protocols are followed and the pupil of the affected eye may be constricted in order to make sure the drainage angle is as open as much as possible and the intraocular pressure is within normal limits. This is done by using miotic drops such as pilocarpine 4% plus the patient's current medication.

In addition, if local anaesthesia is used, drops such as tetracaine 1% may be administered topically, either on the ward or in theatre. Sedation may sometimes be given, but is avoided where possible, as there is a risk of the patient falling asleep and then waking with a 'start' during the operation.

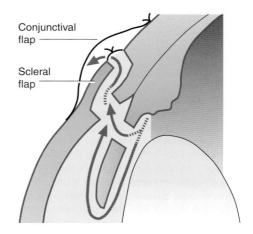

Conjunctival flap

Scleral flap

Figure 11.7 Trabeculectomy.

There is a risk that the development of scar tissue reduces the amount of aqueous drained, so sometimes steroids or antimetabolites such as 5-fluorouracil or mitomycin C may be given (Flammer, 2006); however, the latter group should be used with caution (Simmons et al, 2006).

Specific postoperative care. Care is similar to that following cataract surgery (see p. 164), except that patients are advised not to rub the eye, as this may cause direct trauma to the incision, resulting in a potentially damaging drop in intraocular pressure or a corneal abrasion.

Table 11.3 gives details of the postoperative examination, but the following specific findings should be considered:

- The integrity of the conjunctival flap is observed for the presence of a bleb, a small collection of aqueous under the conjunctiva. This may not always be visible to the naked eye.
- The peripheral iridectomy can be seen as a small triangular piece of iris missing at the periphery.
- The depth of the anterior chamber is checked to ensure that the flap is not over-draining.

If the eye is satisfactory, the procedures followed are similar to those following a cataract extraction, except that a topical mydriatic may be prescribed in order to avoid the formation of synechiae (adhesions) between the iris and cornea or lens. This must be suspected if, on subsequent examination, the pupil becomes irregular and immobile. Mydriatic therapy may cause blurring of vision because some mydriatics have a cycloplegic effect, paralysing the muscles of accommodation. This must be discussed with the patient to prevent unnecessary anxiety.

It is also essential that, if the second eye has not yet had surgery to correct glaucoma, the mydriatics prescribed for the operated eye are not inadvertently instilled into the wrong eye, so causing a rise in intraocular pressure. Current local and systemic therapy for the unoperated eye must continue.

Complications of surgery

- *Leaking wound*: if the situation is not rectified by application of a pressure dressing and mydriatic therapy, synechiae formation, corneal endothelial damage and cataract may occur.
- *Hypotony*: this occurs if there is excessive drainage via the bleb; this results in very low intraocular pressure and the eye may feel soft and can lead to choroidal detachment
- *Panophthalmitis*: infection enters through the bleb and quickly spreads throughout the ophthalmic tissues, causing acute pain and a dramatic loss of vision. It is very difficult to treat, even if diagnosed early.
- *Hyphaema*: bleeding from the ciliary and iris vessels can result in the collection of red blood cells in the anterior chamber, which obstruct the drainage angle and cause a secondary rise in intraocular pressure. Strenuous activity should be avoided until the follow-up appointment, as this may increase the risk of bleeding.
- *Cataract formation*: during surgery, inadvertent contact with the lens epithelium can lead to increased permeability and cataract formation.

Trabeculoplasty

This is a procedure that is carried out as an adjunct to medical treatment, which is the first line of treatment in older patients, and consists of laser therapy to the trabecular meshwork, usually as an outpatient procedure. This procedure increases the aqueous drainage of the trabecular meshwork. It is not usually carried out on patients under the age of 25 years, as its long-term effects are not known and it may only be a short-term solution. Flammer (2006) identified a 60% success rate, although its effect is thought to be short-lived, perhaps for only three years.

Although this is a non-invasive procedure, it causes considerable local inflammation, which may result in a rise in intraocular pressure, so oral acetazolamide 250–500 mg may be given prophylactically to reduce the amount of aqueous produced.

Secondary glaucoma

This is a rise in intraocular pressure resulting from mechanical blockage of the drainage angle. Presentation is similar to that of acute glaucoma, and initial treatment is usually medical, but surgery may be indicated in some cases.

The most common causes are listed below.

Lens matter

This can occur following extracapsular cataract extraction, in which case treatment consists of acetazolamide and topical intensive anti-inflammatory therapy until enzymes in the aqueous absorb the lens material.

Lens protein may also leak out of a hypermature lens, in which case lens extraction is necessary. Extraction is also carried out when the lens is dislocated, due to trauma or in Marfan's syndrome, as this may result in the lens dropping either into the posterior chamber and pushing the iris forward to obstruct the drainage angle, or into the anterior chamber, when there is direct obstruction of aqueous flow.

Haemorrhage

Red blood cells may be deposited in the drainage angle, following trauma or surgery. Surgery is not advocated, because of the risk of further bleeding, but an anterior chamber washout may be necessary if there is corneal involvement or synechiae formation that does not respond to medical intervention.

Uveitis

This inflammatory condition of the iris, ciliary body and choroid can cause secondary glaucoma by the presence of adhesions forming across the drainage angle and/or white cells in the aqueous (a hypopyon) collecting in the drainage angle. These are treated by intensive systemic and topical medications.

Adhesions may also develop between the posterior iris and the anterior lens surface, so obstructing the flow of aqueous into the anterior chamber and pushing the iris root forward to obscure the drainage angle. This is known as iris bombe (Fig. 11.8).

Infection

Infection can also result in the development of a hypopyon. Treatment is medical, with very intensive topical, subconjunctival and systemic antibiotic therapy.

Vitreous

Following cataract extraction, usually intracapsular or complicated extracapsular, the vitreous can move forwards and block the pupil, resulting in iris bombe.

Neovascularization

In conditions such as diabetic retinopathy and central retinal vein occlusion, in an attempt to establish a collateral blood supply, small blood vessels grow into the iris (rubeosis) and the drainage angle. The resultant rise in intraocular pressure is known as thrombotic glaucoma. Control is difficult to achieve, and, as a last resort, the production of aqueous may be reduced by destroying part of the ciliary body by either freezing (cyclocryotherapy) or with laser (cycloablation).

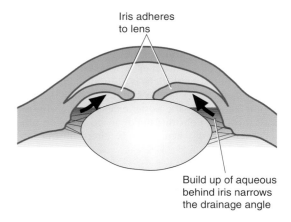

Iris adheres to lens

Build up of aqueous behind iris narrows the drainage angle

Figure 11.8 Iris bombe.

Tumours

Indirect pressure from a tumour outside the eye or actual tumour infiltration can obstruct aqueous drainage. Treatment will depend upon the extent of spread and size of the tumour, but excision may be necessary.

Congenital glaucoma

Congenital glaucoma is due to the absence or malformation of all or part of the trabecular meshwork, resulting in aqueous drainage being severely reduced or absent. The nature of a child's scleral tissue allows the eye to increase in size — hence, the name 'buphthalmos' or 'ox eye', as the corneal diameter may be greater than 12 mm.

Surgery should be carried out as soon as possible and usually consists of a goniotomy, where a direct channel between the anterior chamber and canal of Schlemm is opened up; this often needs repeating but has an eventual success rate of 85% (Kanski, 2015). Trabeculectomy and the insertion of aqueous shunts may also be undertaken.

Retinal surgery

Although small retinal breaks can be treated on an outpatient basis using laser therapy, more sophisticated, complicated surgery should be carried out in specialist units. Retinal breaks usually occur when the retinal tissue is ischaemic and breaks down. This can be due to tension on the peripheral retina, as in the case of myopia, or following trauma resulting in retinal bruising, known as commotio retinae. Breaks are usually found in the peripheral retina, immediately behind the ciliary body, as this is the least perfused area of the retina. They may also result from traction on the retina from the vitreous, especially if there has been intravitreal bleeding.

Breaks are treated depending upon their size and cause; if secondary to another condition, then that must be treated as well, but the break itself may be treated by laser therapy. This is usually an outpatient procedure, but the patient must be aware that they should not drive immediately following this treatment, as their pupils will have been dilated to allow good visualization of the retina, and the drops used can affect the ability to accommodate. Prior to the procedure, the patient should be warned that their eyes may feel slightly uncomfortable and may water; both symptoms should resolve within 24–36 hours.

Retinal detachments

Breaks may not be significant in themselves, but there is a high risk of detachment if left untreated. The term 'retinal detachment' is misleading, as it is the retinal neural division that separates from the retinal pavement epithelial layer, not the entire retina from the choroid below.

Stollery et al (2005) uses the terms 'float', 'pulled' and 'pushed' to differentiate the basic causes of retinal conditions requiring surgery.

- *Float*: following the formation of a retinal break, subretinal fluid or vitreous penetrates the space between the neural retina and the pigmented epithelial layer and lifts off the former.
- *Pulled*: fragile new blood vessels penetrate the normally avascular vitreous, as in diabetic retinopathy, or blood itself leaks into the vitreous, as in trauma. The fibrous strands, formed in the vitreous as the blood 'organizes' itself, contract, causing tension on the retina, resulting in the neural layer being pulled off the epithelial layer.
- *Pushed*: the detachment occurs because of exudate from an inflamed choroid or because of the presence of an intraocular tumour, such as a retinoblastoma or choroidal tumour.

The person may complain of one or all of the following:

- seeing non-existent flashing lights, i.e. photopsia, due to separation of the neural layers
- black spots or threads, as blood leaks out into the normally clear vitreous.
- loss of visual field, or shadows across their vision, due to the lifting off and, if in a superior position, the dropping down of the detached retinal tissue, across the line of vision; the person will see this as loss of the opposing visual field, due to the normal inversion of the image in the visual process.

On examination, there may be no obvious external signs of visual pathology, and visual acuity may not have changed, unless the detachment is extensive enough to have obscured or directly affected the macula.

The pupils are dilated with mydriatic drops such as tropicamide 0.5−1% and phenylephrine 2.5−10% to allow both retinae to be examined, as retinal changes are often bilateral. The most effective way of examining the retina is by using an indirect ophthalmoscope, as this makes it easier to see the periphery of the retina. The patient needs to have this procedure explained carefully, as some mydriatic drops may paralyse the muscles of accommodation and so reduce vision, and the bright light from the ophthalmoscope can be difficult to tolerate.

Types of surgery/treatment

Vitrectomy. This entails making an incision(s) into the vitreous chamber, usually through the pars plana. This allows vitreous to be removed if it has been infiltrated by blood that has not subsequently been absorbed naturally. It is also useful if the source of the detachment is too far back for treatment by plombage or encirclement, as a specially adapted laser can be used to seal any breaks in the posterior retina. Vitrectomy is often carried out in conjunction with other methods, such as the introduction of an intravitreal gas bubble, e.g. sulphur hexafluoride (SF), which is used to seal the break; the patient is positioned so that the bubble (tamponade) lies immediately next to the break and well away from the lens and cornea. This procedure carries a relatively high risk of retinal detachment and cataract formation.

Macular hole surgery. In the majority of cases, the development of macular holes is idiopathic, is more common in people in their sixth to eighth decades (Sundaram et al, 2016), and results in the loss of central vision. Surgery is now resulting in better visual outcomes, with 'anatomical closure in 80% and improvement in visual acuity in 60% of cases' (Sundaram et al, 2016).

Laser. Holes or tears are sealed by causing a localized inflammatory reaction that results in the layers adhering to one another, so preventing fluid seeping between them and pushing the layers apart. Where there is an actual detachment, laser therapy may be used to secure suspect areas around the periphery of the detached area.

Cryopexy. This is the application of extreme cold to the affected area, using a probe chilled by the use of carbon dioxide under pressure. It causes an inflammatory reaction and so seals the layers together, but, again, it is not effective when significant amounts of fluid are found between the detached layers, and so is often used to supplement other treatments.

Plombage/encirclement. Both methods physically isolate the source of the detachment, especially from the macula. Plombage is the application of a single piece of inert silastic material, which is sutured to the surface of the sclera over the site of the retinal break. The sutures are tightened, causing an indentation of the layers; this helps push the separated layers together by increasing the intraocular pressure and forming an intraocular barrier to prevent the detachment spreading.

Encirclement is used when there are several potential areas of weakness at the retinal periphery. Silastic straps, 2−3 mm, are used to encircle the eye and tightened fractionally to create an indentation all the way around, running underneath the extraocular muscles.

Subretinal fluid must be drained if it is felt that there is too much present for easy natural reabsorption, once its access to the potential space between the neural and pigmented layers has been closed.

Specific preoperative care

This will vary, depending upon the surgical procedure selected. The patient will have routine mydriatic drops, and further retinal examinations to allow the extent of the detachment to be accurately recorded, and a decision made about the type of surgery to be carried out. The patient may be encouraged to rest, lying in a certain position, depending upon the site of the detachment, as gravity may cause the area of detachment to increase.

It is important that the patient is told that certain procedures, such as encirclement, may cause considerable pain and discomfort and that analgesics can be prescribed.

Specific postoperative care

Vitrectomy and intravitreal tamponade. Patients may have to stay in the required position for approximately 7 days which can be difficult, especially in the case of macular involvement, as they may have to lie on their front, with the head facing down, as much as possible (dependent on the surgeon's preference and in most cases the patient is allowed a five to ten minute break every hour (Shaw & Lee, 2017). Consequently, considerable care and support is required when the patient is discharged home. This is especially true of those with other medical conditions, such as chronic obstructive airway disease. A support frame is available which is designed to hold the patient's head in the correct position and increase the patient's level of comfort.

Cryotherapy. The degree of reaction due to the application of extreme cold causes swelling and inflammation and may result in the eye being painful, so analgesics and an explanation of the cause of the pain must be given. Oral anti-inflammatory drugs such as ibuprofen 200–400 mg may also be given.

Encirclement. As the silastic strap encircles the whole eye, the subsequent swelling may cause an increase in intraocular pressure. The eye should be examined for any sign of corneal oedema, and complaints of increasing pain must be taken seriously. This is more likely to occur if cryotherapy has been used as an adjunct. Acetazolamide can be given to control the pressure until the swelling is reduced.

Depending upon the extent of the surgery, the eye may become oedematous, especially the conjunctiva, when the degree of swelling (chemosis) may mean that the lids cannot shut properly and exposure keratitis is a possibility. There is also considerable lacrimation and the eye may require frequent cleansing.

Short-term complications

Anterior segment necrosis: the blood supply to the anterior part of the eye may be obstructed if the encircling band is applied too tightly. This requires total revision of the surgery, with loosening of the encircling strap.

Long-term complications

Extrusion of the plombe: over a period of time, the plombe may work loose and find its way forward under the conjunctiva. This is removed and careful examination made to ensure that there is no focus of chronic infection.

Pre- and postoperative care of patients undergoing extraocular surgery

Squints

Squint (strabismus) occurs when the axis of one eye is not parallel with that of the other eye, and it can result in double vision. It is usually horizontal, the two images being side by side, but can be vertical. Squints can also be divergent (one eye deviates outwards) or convergent (one eye deviates inwards) and the manifestation depends on which muscles are involved, e.g. weakness of the lateral rectus will lead to a convergent squint. Children learn to control their eye movements in the first few years of life, and fusion of the images produced by each eye is brought about by a complicated, conditioned reflex.

The causes of squints fall into two main categories:
- *Concomitant* – the sensory components of eye movement are not functioning, e.g. refractive error. The commonest refractive error implicated is hypermetropia (long sight). Concomitant squints are more common in children and are predominantly horizontal and the angle of deviation is the same in all directions of gaze.
- *Paralytic (incomitant)* – the motor components of eye movement are not functioning, e.g. nerve or extraocular muscle damage, e.g. cerebrovascular accident, orbital trauma. Paralytic squints are more common in adults.

The diplopia that results is compensated for in one of two ways:
- The image of one eye is suppressed completely and, because of the subsequent lack of stimulus, the retina does not fully develop, resulting in amblyopia, the so-called 'lazy eye'.
- The images can be suppressed rapidly in turn, an alternating squint, meaning that full retinal development is achieved in both eyes.

In children, especially, treatment must be prompt, to prevent further deterioration in visual acuity, and in some cases simple correction of the refractive error is enough; however, if there is a risk of amblyopia, occlusion or 'patching' of the seeing eye may be necessary to improve the retinal function of the suppressed eye.

Every effort is made to correct the underlying cause of the squint before the child is of school age, as this increases the likelihood of a better visual outcome and because non-concordance can occur because of teasing at school. However, treatment is not always successful, and surgery may be necessary.

If the squint is paralytic in nature, the underlying cause should be identified and treated. The diplopia may be managed with prismatic glasses or occlusion, but corrective surgery may be required if there is insufficient improvement.

In adults who have concomitant squints which are either untreated or require further treatment, this may be carried out for purely cosmetic reasons.

Specific preoperative care

An orthoptic assessment is carried out to identify the muscles requiring surgery and the degree of correction needed. Surgery is usually carried out on a day care basis, under general anaesthesia. The most common corrective surgery involves resecting (shortening) a weak muscle, and so increasing its power, or recessing (weakening) an overactive muscle. Recession involves moving the insertion of the muscle further back on the eyeball, so reducing its power.

The balance achieved by these two processes swings the eye back onto a parallel axis, although sometimes the patient may be concerned postoperatively that they still have some double vision; however, this is usually due to postoperative oedema.

Specific postoperative care

The eye may require cleaning quite regularly, as conjunctival sutures can cause irritation and the eyes may be 'sticky'. Irritation may be exacerbated by dusty, dirty environments. The patient should be shown how to clean the eye using cooled, boiled water and moistened cotton wool. A sterile cleansing procedure is not required, as this is an extraocular operation and the risk of intraocular infection is minimal.

A combination of topical antibiotic and anti-inflammatory agents is given, according to the surgeon's preference. Mild analgesics may be required; this is especially so for patients who have had previous surgery to the same area. Padding of the eye is not necessary.

In more complex cases, where the goal is to improve cosmetic appearance or correct diplopia, use of adjustable suture techniques can improve the long-term results. The sutures are adjusted at the end of the list, once the patient is awake, or the following morning using a local anaesthetic (Kanski, 2015). This allows more precise adjustment of the extraocular muscles and a better visual outcome.

The patient may return to work or school as soon as the eye is comfortable, usually after a week.

They should be advised to take care, especially when hair washing, and to refrain from swimming for 3−4 weeks.

The continued use of occlusion patches (in children) and spectacles is determined for each individual, and appropriate information given prior to discharge.

Complications of squint surgery

- *Infection*: if the eye becomes increasingly red and painful and purulent discharge is noted, this probably indicates the presence of an infection. Swabs must be taken for microscopy, culture and sensitivity, and antibiotic therapy commenced.
- *Stitch granuloma*: there is a persistent red swelling immediately over the suture. This can cause concern but usually resolves spontaneously. If not, a combination of topical antibiotic/anti-inflammatory agents is prescribed.
- *Over-/undercorrection*: occasionally, muscles are recessed or resected inaccurately and further corrective surgery is required.
- *Slipped/lost muscle*: the muscle can slip back or be lost if it is not tightly and adequately sutured to the globe at the time of operation. This requires early surgery to retrieve the muscle.

Dacryocystorhinostomy

This is carried out to bypass a lacrimal drainage system blockage. Obstruction results from chronic inflammatory changes secondary to recurrent infections in the canaliculi or nasolacrimal duct. The surgery should never be carried out during an acute episode of dacryocystitis, as this increases the risk of orbital cellulitis.

The operation bypasses the obstruction in the nasolacrimal duct by an anastomosis of the lacrimal sac itself to adjacent nasal mucosa, a small area of bone having been removed to make the necessary opening (rhinostomy). If the obstruction is at the level of the common canaliculus, the patency of the drainage ducts is threatened by postoperative inflammation and adhesions. Therefore, silicone tubes are inserted via the punctum, through the rhinostomy and into the nose, and left in place for 3−4 months.

Surgery becomes necessary when:
- epiphora (watering) is so excessive that it interferes with lifestyle, due to continual wiping away of tears and excoriation of the skin below the affected eye
- there are recurrent episodes of dacryocystitis, which can be very painful
- congenital obstruction is not cured by syringing and probing of the canaliculi and nasolacrimal duct.

Prior to surgery it is important to determine where the obstruction is sited, and this can be done by syringing the ducts and monitoring the outcome. If there is a clear obstruction, an X-ray in the form of a dacryocystogram, when radio-opaque dye is injected into the lacrimal drainage system via the punctum, may be used to locate it. In situations where the blockage is due to a suspected functional obstruction such as lacrimal pump failure, a scintigram may be undertaken using a low-dose radionuclide test (Sundaram et al, 2016). Endoscopic procedures via the nasolacrimal duct have resulted in less trauma to the lacrimal sac and the surrounding bone. However, the administration of topical steroids is usually required post-operatively to reduce the degree of scarring and subsequent risk of blockage recurring.

Specific preoperative care

Surgery is usually performed under a general anaesthetic, so the patient is usually admitted on the day of surgery, having fasted for 4 hours prior to admission. However, when endoscopic dacryocystorhinostomy is undertaken, it may be carried out under local anaesthesia.

The preparation may vary according to surgeon's preference, and some patients have their noses packed with ribbon gauze soaked in a cocaine and adrenaline (epinephrine) solution to constrict blood vessels and reduce bleeding. This is usually done after induction of anaesthesia, but may be part of the ward preparation.

The patient should be warned that they may feel light-headed on mobilizing postoperatively, because of the possible use of hypotensive anaesthesia. It should also be made clear that marked bruising around the operation site is a possibility.

Specific postoperative care

As hypotensive agents may be used during anaesthesia to assist in reducing the blood flow to the surgical site, the patient may be kept in overnight for observation.

Haemorrhage is a possible complication, so regular and frequent observations of blood pressure, pulse and swallowing pattern are essential. This may not occur immediately but as the blood pressure returns to within the individual's normal limits. Patients do not routinely return to the ward with an intravenous infusion in progress, but if they do, then the cannula site should be observed for signs of extravasation, such as swelling and pain, and phlebitis, such as redness tracking along the course of the affected vein. The infusion is normally discontinued when the patient's blood pressure has returned to normal and when the anaesthetist is satisfied with the patient's condition.

A nasal bolster and/or pressure dressing may be applied in theatre, and this should be checked regularly for any signs of seepage. Any abnormal findings should be reported to the medical staff at once, as haemorrhage following a dacryocystorhinostomy is an ophthalmic emergency and may necessitate further surgery. In non-endoscopic surgery, the dressing should be taken down the following day and the incision cleaned if necessary, skin sutures being removed 5−7 days postoperatively.

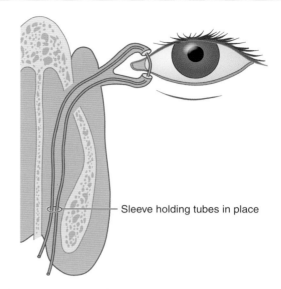

Figure 11.9 Position of silicone tubes following dacryocystorhinostomy.

Medication following surgery does vary, but antibiotic drops are usually prescribed alongside antibiotic ointment to apply to the suture line (Shaw & Lee, 2017). If silicone tubes have been inserted (Fig. 11.9), these are left *in situ* for 2−3 months, until all swelling has gone, and are removed in the outpatient department.

Patient education is important following dacryocystorhinostomy. Patients should be discouraged from sniffing, blowing their nose and sneezing for the first week, as these actions may result in perioperative surgical emphysema. If tubes are *in situ*, patients should also be taught to check that they are positioned properly, since, if they slip up the nose and out through the lacrimal passages, the tube may encroach on the cornea and cause an abrasion. The incision between the nose and the inner aspect of the eye may cause discomfort for patients wearing spectacles, and they may initially require help to carry out the activities of living because of reduced visual acuity.

Tumours of the eye and orbit

There is a wide range of benign and malignant tumours that can occur in and around the eye; see Table 11.4 for some of the most common types.

Types of surgery

- *Enucleation*: removal of the eye and, if a malignancy is diagnosed, part of the optic nerve.

Table 11.4 Tumours of the eye and orbit

Location/ type	Tumour	Description
Eyelids		
Benign	Xanthelasmata	Plate-like flat structures, often yellow tinged, that are thought to be indicative of hypercholesterolaemia. They are usually removed by simple excision, as an outpatient, but may recur
	Papillomata	Small growths; can be affected by the constant movement of the eyelid, becoming pedunculated. They are removed by excision, under a local anaesthetic, but may bleed and need cauterizing. These may also recur
Malignant	Basal cell carcinoma/ rodent ulcer	Mainly seen in the elderly, but increasingly in younger people exposed to sunshine. Patients need reassurance that, although the tumour invades surrounding tissues, it does not usually metastasize. It is the commonest malignancy of the eyelid, and there is usually a long history of the presence of a 'wart'. On examination, it has rolled edges and a crater in the centre covered by a scab and has grown slowly. These are treated by wide excision and/or radiotherapy. Pinch or Wolfe skin grafts may be needed following more extensive surgery
	Squamous cell carcinoma	Present as a wart-like growth that can cause eversion and induration of the lid margins. They are not as sensitive to radiotherapy as basal cell carcinoma, and wide excision of the tumour may need skin grafting in order to preserve the function of the eyelid
Orbit		
Benign	Meningioma	Arise from the meninges surrounding the optic nerve and may cause loss of vision due to involvement of the optic disc, or there may be direct pressure on the optic nerve from the meninges in the ethmoid region. The most common presenting sign is exophthalmos, with diplopia and downward or lateral deposition. Depending on the speed of tumour growth, surgical excision and radiotherapy are treatment options
Uveal tract		
Malignant	Melanoma	Can arise from a pigmented naevus and can be found anywhere in the iris, ciliary body or choroid, as they arise from the pigment cells of the uveal tissue. The patient must be referred to a specialist centre, where treatment options vary, ranging from chemotherapy and radiotherapy to evisceration
Retina and vitreous		
Malignant	Retinoblastoma	Tumour of the retinal layer which may be hereditary in origin, often affecting both eyes. It may also affect several members of the same family. If left untreated, it spreads to the orbital wall and surrounding structures

- *Evisceration*: removal of the contents of the eye, but the scleral shell is left behind. It is usually carried out following severe ocular trauma to reduce the risk of sympathetic ophthalmitis, or following intraocular infection to prevent infection tracking back to the meninges.
- *Exenteration*: this is radical surgery, involving removal of the entire contents of the orbit plus any bone suspected of having been infiltrated by the tumour.

Specific preoperative care

As all these operations will result in a degree of physical disfigurement, the psychological care of these patients is paramount. The amount of information given to each patient and their family will depend upon the individual, as some may find it very distressing to be given more information than they can absorb. It may be helpful for the patient to meet someone who has already had the type of surgery they are about to undergo.

183

Specific postoperative care

The amount of help and support the patient needs will vary, depending on the individual, the extent of the surgery and the reasons for it.

Initially, the socket may require frequent cleansing, using the same basic technique as following other ocular surgery, and antibiotic ointment/drops are instilled three to four times a day. A pressure dressing may be applied, in order to reduce bruising.

The size of the prosthesis will vary from a shell in enucleation/evisceration to a spectacle-mounted replacement of orbital bone and skin, plus an artificial eye, in exenteration.

The time it takes for patients to become proficient in caring for their prosthesis and socket will vary, and they must be allowed to take things at their own pace. This may mean that community services have to be involved and may need education themselves in caring for these patients. The family should be encouraged to participate in the care, as they may be the main line of support following discharge.

Patients may need the help of other professionals, such as prosthetic technicians and make-up therapists, to assist in fitting and applying the prosthesis and in restoring the patient's appearance and morale.

The final prosthesis will not be made until all swelling has reduced and the wound is completely healed.

Orbital fractures

The commonest orbital trauma is that of a 'blow-out' fracture. These occur when intraorbital pressure rises suddenly due to a blunt injury to the eye, resulting in either the medial or inferior wall of the orbit breaking and being pushed out into the relevant sinus. The latter is the most common, as it is the thinnest, and the patient may present with diplopia, restriction of elevation of the eye, decreased sensation over the maxilla and sinking of the globe further into the orbit (enophthalmos).

Where there is no evidence of displacement, treatment is usually conservative. However, if symptoms, especially diplopia and enophthalmos, persist, then surgical repair of the fracture, by insertion of a silicone implant, is carried out. This is often done in conjunction with the maxillofacial surgeons.

The eyelids

Blepharitis

Blepharitis is a common chronic condition of the eyelids and can occur at any age. It can be classified into anterior or posterior blepharitis by its appearance to the grey line.

The causes can be staphylococcal infections, seborrhoeic from eye lash debris of the scalp, eyebrows and lashes, or conditions such as acne rosacea and poor hygiene.

Patients will typically complain of irritating burning sensation in their eyes, which may be discharging if infected.

The lids may be red, there will be crustiness on the eyelashes, and prominent meibomian glands may be visible.

It is essential that patients are told how to manage this condition as if they do not comply it will just keep causing symptoms. Treatment is by warm compressions over closed eyelids (a specially designed heat mask is available which is easier and retains the heat better than a hot flannel), followed by eyelid cleaning with lid cleaning wipes. Some patients may be prescribed antibiotic ointment to their eyelids.

Entropion

The eyelid margins turn in, especially the lower lid, due to spasm of the orbicularis oculi muscle or scarring of the conjunctiva, so the lashes come into direct contact with the cornea, which is excruciatingly painful and leads to corneal abrasion and scarring (Marsden, 2007). Although temporary relief can be achieved by applying a strip of tape from the lower lid to the cheek, permanent improvement can only be achieved by surgery.

Treatment will depend on the cause of the entropion (Nerad, 2001). In the majority of cases, correction is achieved by excision of skin and/or muscle and/or the tarsal plate, effectively shortening the lower border of the eyelid and so pulling the upper aspect of the lid out. It is important not to overcorrect the entropion, as this can result in ectropion formation.

Ectropion

The eyelid margins turn out, usually due to loss of tone of the orbicularis oculi muscle or to scarring of the face near the eye. This causes a reduction in tear flow, as the puncta are no longer in apposition with the surface of the eye, and the tears flow down the cheek (epiphora), causing a red, uncomfortable eye due to exposure, and conjunctivitis caused by the ineffective tear flow and loss of lubrication of the ocular surface (Khaw et al, 2004). If there is only a minor degree of ectropion, a small amount of cautery to the area of the conjunctiva below the lower punctum is enough to scar the area sufficiently to pull the lid back into its proper alignment.

Greater degrees of ectropion are resolved by excising a wedge of the tarsal plate and conjunctiva, so shortening the upper margin of the tarsal plate of the lower lid, pulling it back into place.

Postoperative care

Both procedures are normally carried out under local anaesthesia. The eye is usually covered with an eye pad for 2–3 hours postoperatively, as there may be some bleeding. After the pad is removed, the patient applies antibiotic ointment two to three times a day for 4–5 days and returns to the outpatient department for the removal of sutures. The eye may need cleaning with cooled, boiled water, care being taken not to inadvertently remove the sutures.

Tarsorrhaphy

Tarsorrhaphy is performed when the patient is at risk of exposure keratitis and the use of lubricants and bandage contact lenses (large, soft lenses that have no other function than to protect the corneal surface and maintain the integrity of the eye) has been ineffective.

Ophthalmic conditions that may lead to tarsorrhaphy are exophthalmos, delayed healing of a corneal ulcer because of the constant blinking action of the upper eyelid disturbing the new corneal epithelium, and reduced ability to close the eye because of damage or malfunction of the facial nerve.

The patient is usually admitted for surgery, as this is usually the last resort of a planned course of treatment. They will need careful explanation of the procedure and may have some concern about their appearance following the procedure, as the size of the palpebral fissure will be decreased. This alteration in appearance is more marked if a central tarsorrhaphy is planned, as this means the lids are joined centrally; this is only done in extreme cases of exposure keratitis and may be a temporary measure. The patients often find that the relief of pain outweighs the cosmetic effect.

During the operation, the conjunctival epithelium of the upper and lower lid margins is excised, usually at the lateral aspect of the lid. This causes two rough edges, which will adhere together as they heal. The lids are sutured together, the sutures being passed through small rubber sleeves, so preventing them 'cheese wiring' out under the pressure of lid movement. As these sutures usually stay in for a minimum of 10 days, the patient is taught how to clean them, and how to apply antibiotic ointment. If the presence of the sutures and rubber sleeves is unacceptable to the patient, dark glasses can be worn. If tarsorrhaphy is done on a temporary basis, it is easily reversed.

Ptosis

Ptosis can affect one or both eyes, can be acquired or congenital, and means that the upper lid droops, sometimes resulting in loss of vision, or in the person developing an abnormal head posture, as they hold it back to allow them to peer out from under their lowered lids. It is usually due to a defective levator muscle, neural abnormality, or to abnormal weight upon the lid by oedema, tumour or scarring. Treatment will depend upon the cause.

Primary ptosis requires surgical intervention, but until this can be carried out, the ptosis may be corrected by the use of hook glasses or benched contact lenses that lift the lowered lid back to its normal position.

If the condition is secondary to a neurological disorder such as myasthenia gravis, then the primary cause has to be identified and treated where possible. If it is due to trauma, then surgery is delayed until all oedema and inflammation has subsided and reassessment of the situation can be done.

The operation of choice is usually resection of the levator muscle, either via the conjunctiva or the lid. The degree of resection depends upon the severity of the ptosis, but must be carefully estimated, as overcorrection can lead to exposure keratitis, although the use of adjustable sutures has reduced this risk.

Chalazion/meibomian cyst

Sebum blocks the duct leading from the meibomian gland, resulting in stagnation of sebaceous secretions, which are then frequently infected by *Staphylococcus aureus*. This presents as a hard rounded lump, often on the undersurface of the eyelid, causing irritation, and may be large enough to obstruct the vision and/or cause astigmatism by pressing on the cornea and altering the curvature.

Recurrent episodes may indicate diabetes mellitus, but if these are at the same site, malignancy such as sebaceous cell carcinoma must be excluded (Marsden, 2007). If the chalazion does not respond to antibiotic therapy, lancing and curetting of the infected gland is necessary, followed by antibiotic therapy.

Discharge planning

The move to day care surgery has increased dramatically over recent years, so effective discharge planning has become more important in order to ensure continuity of care and to reduce the risk of postoperative complications. Where possible, needs should be identified at the preassessment clinic or on admission, especially if community services are involved. The following factors need to be considered.

- *Medication*: nurses need to ensure that patients are capable of instilling their topical eye medication and understand the regime to be followed for both topical and systemic drugs. If patients are unable to give their own drops, then arrangements need to be made for this to be done by a carer or the community nursing service. Patients should also be told how to obtain further medication. A number of devices to assist the instillation of drops are available, but some of these are not suitable for use on recently operated eyes, as they may compromise the integrity of the wound.

- *Follow-up*: details of appointments for the outpatient clinic should be given to the patient prior to discharge.
- *Care of the eye*: patients or carers should be shown how to clean the eye and what they should use to do so. They should also be educated about recognizing possible complications and be given a contact number to ring if advice is required. Patients may return the next day for the first dressing, or they may be contacted by telephone to check there are no problems. Some ophthalmic units have nurses who visit the patient at home the following day, while others have short-term 'hotel' facilities and the patients return to the unit the next day or the nurses visit them in this facility.
- *Transport*: patients are advised to arrange for transport on discharge, and, if they are unable to do so, then hospital transport can be arranged. It is inadvisable for patients who have had eye surgery to drive themselves home afterwards, as even minor treatments can affect their ability to judge distances and may reduce their peripheral vision.
- *Community services*: help such as home help and meals on wheels may need to be reinstated or initiated. Patients should be given a contact number for social services, in case there are any problems or circumstances change.
- *Carers*: they should be involved in the discharge planning and informed of all arrangements made and information given.
- *Activities of living*: the restriction on activities will be determined by the type of surgery and the surgeon's personal preferences.

All information should be given verbally and supported with patient education booklets/sheets. These must be designed to take the patient's degree of visual impairment into account. It is important to assess the patient's and carer's understanding of the information given and to give further education if necessary.

Conclusion

This chapter has highlighted the specific needs and the care required by patients having both intra- and extra-ocular surgery.

Ophthalmic nursing involves caring for a wide range of patients with a variety of problems, and, to be effective, a holistic stance must be taken. The depth and complexity

of the role was first reflected in the competency framework developed by the Royal College of Nursing (2005), and now a multi-professional group competency (Royal College of Ophthalmologists, 2017).

Ophthalmic nursing care involves helping people who may have had their very independence threatened by the potential loss of vision, or, in a small number of cases, supporting those who have had to make some very fundamental changes to their lifestyle because of a visual handicap. This potential for change can mean that a situation/procedure that appears minor to the nurse can be very frightening for the patient. This need to see each patient as an individual is difficult with the rapid throughput of patients in most ophthalmic units today.

The effort that has to be put into supporting patients and carers is rewarded by seeing most people rediscovering their independence within the community.

SUMMARY OF KEY POINTS

- A knowledge of the basic structure and function of the eye is necessary for the nurse to appreciate the problems patients may have.
- An awareness of the special needs of patients undergoing ophthalmic surgery is important in the planning of efficient and effective care.
- Recognition of the importance of continuity of care between hospital and the community leads to an appropriately planned and implemented discharge.
- Effective patient education can result in a well-informed patient and a reduction in the incidence of readmission.

REFLECTIVE LEARNING POINTS

Having read this chapter, think about what you now know and what you still need to find out about. These questions may help:

- Why is it important to undertake patient examination in a systematic manner?
- What does the Amsler grid test monitor?
- What might be the causes of astigmatism?

Acknowledgements

Dawn Avery: Head Orthoptist, The Ipswich Hospital NHS Trust

Ali Mearza: Consultant Ophthalmologist, Charing Cross Hospital, Imperial College Healthcare NHS Foundation Trust

References

Child, A. (2003). Genetic basis for primary open angle glaucoma. *Glaucoma Forum – International Glaucoma Association, 4*, 22–23.

Chivers, J. (2003). Care of older people with visual impairment. *Nursing Older People, 15*(1), 22–26.

Coombes, A., & Seward, H. (1999). Posterior capsule opacification: IOL design and material. *British Journal of Ophthalmology, 83*(6), 640–641.

Department of Health. (2004). *Human tissue act 2004*. London: HMSO.

Dua, H. S., Faraj, L. A., Said, D. G., Gray, T., & Lowe, J. (2013). Human and corneal anatomy redefined: A novel pre descemets layer (Dua layer). *Ophthalmology, 120*, 1778–1785.

Flammer, J. (2006). *Glaucoma: a guide for patients, an introduction for care providers, a quick reference* (3rd ed.). Toronto: Hogrefe Nad Huber.

HSE. (2019). *Guidance on the personal protective equipment at work regulations*. London: HMSO.

International Glaucoma Association. (2008). *The risk to relatives from chronic (primary open angle) glaucoma*. Available at: <www.glaucoma-association.com/nqcontent.cfm?>

International Glaucoma Association. (2019). *Use your eye drops!* Available at: <https://www.glaucoma-association.com/about-glaucoma/treatments/eye-drops>

James, B., Chew, C., & Bron, A. (2016). *Lecture notes on ophthalmology* (12th edn). Oxford: Wiley Blackwell Publishing.

Kanski, J. (2015). *Clinical ophthalmology* (8th edn). London: Saunders.

Khaw, P., Shah, P., & Elkington, A. (2004). *ABC of eyes*. London: BMJ Publishing.

Marsden, J. (2007). *An evidence base for ophthalmic nursing practice*. Chichester: John Wiley.

Marsden, J. (2017). *Ophthalmic care*. Chichester: M & K Publishing.

Mearza, A. A., Qureshi, M. A., & Rostron, C. K. (2007). Experience and 12-month results of Descemet-stripping endothelial keratoplasty. *Cornea, 26*(3), 279–283.

Nerad, J. (2001). *Oculoplastic surgery: the requisites in ophthalmology*. London: Mosby.

National Institute for Health & Care Excellence (NICE). (2017). *Cataracts in adults: management*. (NG77). Available at: https://www.nice.org.uk/guidance/ng77

Royal College of Nursing. (2005). *Competencies: an integrated career and competency framework for ophthalmic nursing*. London: RCN. Available at: www.rcophth.ac.uk/professional-resources/new-common-clinical-competency-framework-to-standardise-competences-for-ophthalmic-non-medical-healthcare-professionals/.

Royal College of Nursing. (2018). *The Code: Professional standards of practice and behavior for nurses, midwives and nursing associates*. London: Nursing and Midwifery Council.

Royal College of Ophthalmologists. (2017). *Ophthalmic services guidance*. Available at: <www.rcophth.ac.uk/wp-content/uploads/2017/08/Emergency-eye-care-in-hospital-eye-units-and-secondary-care.pdf>

Royal National Institute of Blind People. (2015). *A glaucoma case finding pilot within the African Caribbean community*. Available at: www.rnib.org.uk

Shaw, M., & Lee, A. (2017). *Ophthalmic nursing* (5th ed.). Boca Raton: CRC Press.

Simmons, S. T., Cioffi, G. A. Gross, R. L., et al. (2006). *Glaucoma: Basic and clinical science course*. San Francisco: American Academy of Ophthalmology.

Stollery, R., Shaw, M. E., & Lee, A. (2005). *Ophthalmic nursing* (3rd edn). Oxford: Blackwell.

Sundaram, V., Barsam, A., Barker, L., & Khaw, P. T. (2016). *Training in ophthalmology the essential curriculum* (2nd ed). Oxford: Oxford University Press.

Walsh, M. (2005). *Nurse practitioners: clinical skills for health care professionals*. Edinburgh: Butterworth-Heinemann.

Further reading

Batterbury, M., & Bowling, B. (2018). *Ophthalmology: An illustrated colour text* (4th ed). London: Churchill Livingstone.

Brady, F. (1992). *A singular view: The art of seeing with one eye*. Toronto: Edgemore Enterprises.

Clark, A. (2003). Protocol-based care: 1. How integrated care pathways work. *Prof. Nurse, 18*(12), 694–697.

Fraser, S., Asaria, R., & Kon, C. (2000). *Eye know how*. London: BMJ Publishing.

Gordon, H. (2006). Preoperative assessment in ophthalmic regional anaesthesia. *Continuing Education in Anaesthesia, Critical Care and Pain, 6*(5), 203–206.

Marsden, J., & Shaw, M. (2003). Correct administration of topical eye treatment. *Nursing Standard, 17*(30), 42–44.

Richardson, M. (2007). The sense of sight: Part one – Structures and visual pathway. *Nursing Times, 103*(29), 26–27.

Richardson, M. (2007). The sense of sight: Part two – Seeing in colour, detail and depth. *Nursing Times, 103*(30), 24–25.

Richardson, M. (2007). The sense of sight: Part three – Testing vision. *Nursing Times, 103*(31), 26–27.

Strominger, M., & Richards, R. (2000). Adjustable sutures in pediatric ophthalmology. *Journal of Ophthalmic Nursing and Technology, 19*(3), 142–147.

Waldock, A., & Cook, S. D. (2000). Corneal transplantation: how successful are we? *British Journal of Ophthalmology, 84*(8), 813–815.

Walsh, M. (2005). *Nurse practitioners: Clinical skills for health care professionals*. Edinburgh: Butterworth-Heinemann.

Chapter | 12 |

Patients requiring surgery to the ear, nose and throat

Joseph Mahaffey

KEY OBJECTIVES OF THE CHAPTER

The aim of this chapter is to provide an overview of ear, nose and throat, head and neck surgery for healthcare professionals. At the end of the chapter the reader should be able to:

- describe the anatomy and physiology of the ear, nose and throat
- describe ear, nose and throat conditions that require surgery
- demonstrate knowledge of assessments specific to this specialty
- discuss pre- and postoperative care
- provide professional and caring patient education, including safe discharge planning
- be familiar with the terminology related to rhinology, otology and laryngology.

Areas to think about before reading the chapter

- Review the anatomy and physiology of the ear, nose and throat.

(Continued)

(cont'd)

- ENT surgery attracts a wide spectrum of ages and diseases. Make a list of common ENT surgical procedures and define them.
- What types of ENT surgery are best suited to be undertaken in a day surgery setting?

Introduction

The 19th century saw the establishment of ear, nose and throat (ENT) surgery as an independent specialty. Throughout the 20th century, major advances were made: the development of microscopic, endoscopic and laser techniques; day case surgery; and innovative approaches shown in reconstructive head and neck surgery. These have had a great impact on healthcare professionals working within an ENT unit. Surgery can be a less traumatic experience for the individual, recovery can be faster, and patient turnover is greater. In day surgical units, ENT surgery is now being performed on individuals who, having fulfilled certain criteria (as discussed in Chapter 3), are able to undergo general anaesthetic procedures and suffer only minimal disruption to their daily lives. The multidisciplinary ear, nose and throat, head and neck team can now offer a more optimistic future and improved quality of life for those patients suffering from extensive and malignant disease of the head and neck.

The diversity within ENT surgery provides practitioners working on an ENT ward with a wealth of opportunities and experience from which clinical skills and competencies can develop. It is hoped that the reader, upon following this chapter, will experience the rewards and challenges of otorhinolaryngology care.

This chapter is divided into four sections:

- The ear
- The nose and paranasal sinuses
- The throat
- Head and neck

The ear

Anatomy and physiology

The ear is divided into three parts:

- The external ear
- The middle ear
- The inner ear

The external ear

The pinna, composed of fibroelastic cartilage and skin, acts by localizing and amplifying sound and protecting the auditory canal from the environment and from trauma. This canal efficiently self-cleans by the continuous migration of epithelium from the inner to the outer aspect of its structure. Sound waves travel down the canal to the tympanic membrane, which transmits sound vibrations into the middle ear.

The middle ear

This is an air-containing cavity. It connects with the nasopharynx via the Eustachian tube, which ventilates and equalizes pressure within the cavity. The middle ear contains three ear ossicles: the malleus, incus and stapes. These transmit sound vibrations from the tympanic membrane to the cochlea of the inner ear. Posterior to the middle ear lie mastoid air cells. The mastoid process is closely related to the cerebellum, temporal lobe and the labyrinth of the inner ear. Portions of the facial nerve, which innervates facial movements, and the chorda tympani nerve, responsible for taste perception, are also located here (Luers & Hüttenbrink, 2016).

The inner ear

The inner ear consists of two sections: the cochlea (hearing canal) and the vestibular apparatus (balance canal), contained within the labyrinth (Van De Water, 2012).

Endolymph circulates in both canals to transmit sound and balance signals. The vestibulocochlear nerve has two branches and functions: the cochlear/auditory nerve for transmission of electrical impulses to the cerebral cortex, where sound is perceived; and the vestibular nerve, which transmits impulses from the inner ear and semicircular canals to the cerebellum, processing information regarding posture, movement and balance.

Conditions of the ear that require surgery

There are a variety of conditions and diseases that benefit from surgical intervention.

The following details the main examples, with types of surgery explained in Box 12.1.

- *Exostoses*: an overgrowth of bone in the external auditory canal. Repair is by canaloplasty.

Box 12.1 **Types of ear surgery**

- *Myringoplasty*: this is closure of a tympanic membrane perforation using a graft of temporalis fascia. The graft is tucked into place behind the membrane and is gently supported by pieces of Gelfoam, which are gradually absorbed over a few weeks. The graft is not completely stable until about 6 months later. There are two types of approach: end-aural and post-auricular. This procedure is also known as type I tympanoplasty.
- *Ossiculoplasty*: a connection is made between the stapes and malleus in order to improve ossicular conduction of sound. A myringoplasty may also be performed at the same time. This procedure is also known as type II tympanoplasty.
- *Mastoidectomy*: there are three types. A post-auricular approach is used.
  - Cortical: mastoid air cells are removed; hearing is unaffected.
  - Radical: more extensive than cortical; the eardrum, bony ear canal wall, middle ear mucosa and ossicles are removed; hearing is greatly affected.
  - Modified radical: preserves as much of the eardrum and ossicles as possible; hearing is less affected.
- *Stapedectomy*: a window in the footplate of the stapes is made, and the diseased stapes is removed. A prosthesis is inserted which is mobile, to allow for the vibration and conduction of sound.
- *Saccus decompression*: the endolymph that fills the membranous labyrinth of the inner ear is drained, in order to alleviate vestibular disturbance.
- *Labyrinthectomy*: the entire structure of the labyrinth in the inner ear is destroyed, resulting in total hearing loss on that side.

- *Perforated tympanic membrane*: due to trauma or otitis media (acute or chronic infection of the middle ear). Repair is by myringoplasty or tympanoplasty using a graft.
- *Ossicular discontinuity*: ossiculoplasty aims to repair the ossicular chain.
- *Otosclerosis*: an overgrowth of bone causing fixation of the stapes footplate and conductive deafness. This condition is familial, more common in women, and one which pregnancy appears to exacerbate. Repair is by stapedectomy.
- *Acoustic neuroma (schwannoma)*: a tumour of the vestibular element of the eighth cranial nerve. Its incidence is rare and progress can be slow; neurosurgeons and otologists often perform the surgery collaboratively.
- *Cholesteatoma*: a benign growth of squamous epithelial cells in the middle ear and mastoid air cells, which may lead to infection and suppuration, conductive and sensorineural hearing loss and facial nerve paralysis. Unless adequately treated, bony involvement (mastoiditis) occurs, which can lead to extra- and intracranial complications (Box 12.2). Surgery to remove cholesteatoma is mastoidectomy.
- *Ménière's disease*: aetiology is unknown. It affects the inner ear, causing vertigo, tinnitus and deafness. Endolymphatic sac decompression is occasionally performed, but a variety of medical treatments are first explored. No one treatment suits all Ménière's sufferers. Labyrinthectomy is performed if symptoms are severe and causing continued distress to the patient.
- *Profound sensorineural deafness*: may benefit from a cochlear implant.
- *Deafness*: a variety of deaf patients benefit from a bone-anchored hearing aid (BAHA) — a permanently implanted hearing aid.

Specific investigations

By a process of air conduction, sound waves pass through the ear canal to the ossicular chain. Bone conduction enables wave transmission to reach the inner ear, where sound energy is transformed into neural energy and interpreted by the brain. If a problem is identified within the external or middle ear, any hearing loss is termed conductive. If there is a cochlear, auditory nerve or central nervous system problem, hearing loss is sensorineural. Box 12.3 lists causes of specific hearing loss.

Clinical tests of hearing and ear disease

- *Simple audiometry*: i.e. use of tuning forks (Rinne and Weber tests) — these distinguish between conductive and sensorineural loss. It is inexpensive, simple and portable.
- *Auriscopy*: an examination of the inner aspect of the ear canal and tympanic membrane, to visualize and diagnose conditions such as wax (cerumen) accumulation, perforation, foreign body, otitis externa/media, exostosis, cholesteatoma and mastoiditis.
- *Pure tone audiometry*: a formal measurement of hearing, usually conducted by an audiologist. The patient wears earphones and signals when a sound is heard. Results are plotted on graphs, reflecting air conduction and bone conduction of sound.
- *Impedance audiometry*: gives information about middle ear pressure, Eustachian tube function and middle ear reflexes, and can provide measurement of any facial nerve dysfunction (Campbell, 2018).
- *Speech audiometry*: determines speech reception threshold and discrimination, and is effective in diagnosing sensorineural loss and evaluating for hearing aids.
- *Vestibulometry*: determines the functional state of the vestibular system; is useful in diagnosing dizziness.
- *Otoacoustic emissions*: assesses hearing in newborns to determine whether the cochlea is functioning. A probe with a speaker and a microphone is inserted into the ear canal. Tones are sent from the speaker through the middle ear, stimulating the hairs in the cochlea. The hairs respond by generating their own minute sounds,

---

Box 12.2 **Potential progression of severe middle ear infection**

Otologic complications

- Perforated tympanic membrane
- Mastoiditis
- Mastoid abscess
- Labyrinthitis

Head and neck complications

- Neck abscess
- Facial nerve palsy

Cerebral complications

- Extradural abscess
- Meningitis
- Subdural abscess
- Cerebral abscess

Box 12.3 **Causes of specific hearing loss**

Conductive hearing loss

- Impacted wax
- Foreign body in ear canal
- Damage to tympanic membrane
- Otosclerosis
- Cholesteatoma

Sensorineural hearing loss

- Arteriosclerosis
- Congenital
- Ototoxic drugs
- Acoustic neuroma
- Trauma from ear/head injury
- Overexposure to high-intensity noise
- Presbycusis

which are detected by the microphone. If there is a hearing loss, the hairs in the cochlea do not generate sound.

- *Brainstem auditory evoked responses*: measures the timing of electrical waves from the brainstem in response to clicks in the ear. Delays of one side relative to the other suggest a lesion in the eighth cranial nerve (such as acoustic neuroma), between the ear and brainstem, or the brainstem itself.
- *Radiology*: X-rays are useful to indicate stages of disease. Computed tomography (CT) and magnetic resonance imaging (MRI) scans are excellent diagnostic tools, particularly in determining middle ear and mastoid disease and acoustic neuroma.
- *Clinical test of balance*: the Romberg test is used to determine if a lesion is cerebellar or labyrinthine in origin. With feet together, the patient closes their eyes, standing erect. A labyrinthine lesion can cause the patient to sway to the side of the lesion, which is accentuated by closing the eyes. A cerebellar lesion may show symmetrical swaying unaffected by eye closure.
- *Clinical test of gait*: the patient walks in a straight line between two points and then quickly turns to return on the straight line. Patients with a labyrinthine lesion deviate to the side of the lesion. Marked imbalance on turning indicates a cerebellar lesion.
- *Clinical test of facial nerve*: the facial nerve is the main motor nerve to the facial muscles and the stapedius muscle in the middle ear and enables taste on the anterior two-thirds of the tongue. Facial nerve function in ear disease should always be assessed.

In relation to hearing loss, the presence of any otalgia (earache), otorrhoea (aural discharge) and tinnitus also aids diagnosis. Observing for nystagmus is also important; the eye moves slowly away from the affected side and then rapidly flicks back (horizontal nystagmus). This is common in inner ear disease.

Assessment of a patient requiring ear surgery

On admission, the practitioner gains a comprehensive assessment of the patient's physical and psychological status. The Nursing and Midwifery Council (2018) are clear in *The Code* that the nurses must ensure that a patient's physical, social and psychological needs are assessed and responded to; this is essential in ensuring that the care is safe and patient-centred. A model of nursing, such as that of Roper, Logan and Tierney, provides the framework for this (Holland, 2008). Specific to a patient requiring surgery to the ear and the subsequent postoperative care is the assessment of the following activities of living: communicating; working and socializing; expressing healthy body image; eating and drinking; and elimination.

Communicating

Hearing loss is a major disability that affects one's social, work and educational life. The healthcare professional needs to assess the patient's hearing loss by addressing the following issues:

Location and nature:
- Which side is affected?
- How severe is the loss?
- Is there distortion of sound or tinnitus?

Effects of the hearing loss:
- on socializing
- at work or study
- with routine activities, e.g. shopping, telephoning
- on body image and self-esteem.

Methods used to improve hearing/communicating:
- Is a hearing aid used?
- Is the aid working properly? When was it last cleaned? Is it comfortable to wear?
- Does the patient lip-read?

The practitioner should endeavour to provide the optimum environment for effective two-way communication (Box 12.4).

Encouraging the expression of any fears or concerns about surgery and aftercare is essential. Some types of surgery, e.g. stapedectomy and mastoidectomy, carry some degree of risk to that side of further, or even total, hearing loss.

Working and social

Establishing the patient's occupation and social situation helps the practitioner to assess care and plan safe

---

Box 12.4 Skills of communication for patients with impaired hearing

- Ensure a well-lit area to facilitate lip-reading and observation of facial expression.
- Ensure the patient's attention.
- Face the patient.
- Speak in a normal tone; shouting can cause distortion of sound.
- Speak clearly.
- Rephrase if misunderstood or misheard.
- Approach the better ear if not heard, but not too closely.
- Do not cover your face or lips or speak with anything in your mouth.
- Write down anything that is not well understood.
- Do not rush the conversation or show annoyance or frustration; patients with hearing loss are often sensitive to facial expression.
- Encourage the use of the patient's hearing aid and give time for the patient to adjust it.
- Involve the patient in doctors' rounds; ensure all members of the multidisciplinary team are aware of the hearing loss; avoid talking over the patient, and check for understanding.

---

discharge. Some occupations involve exposure to high levels of noise, e.g. builders or musicians, and this may have contributed to, or caused, the hearing loss. The surgeon may recommend changing occupation.

A certain amount of time (1–2 weeks) for full recovery is required in order to avoid complications. Arrangements will need to be made in advance for time off work and the caring of dependants, if maximum rest is to be achieved. Home and work life needs must be addressed preoperatively.

Body image

Body image and self-esteem can suffer if hearing loss interferes with the patient's life. Patients can feel sensitive, embarrassed, shy, and many lead isolated lives.

Scarring from surgery is minimal; incisions are either pre-auricular, via the tympanic membrane, or post-auricular (Fig. 12.1). The latter may involve shaving of hair, and this may cause the patient some concern.

Eating and drinking

Assessing the patient's normal diet and appetite is important. Due to labyrinth disturbance, postoperative complications may include dizziness, nausea and vomiting.

Elimination

The patient's normal bowel and bladder function is discussed. Postoperative dizziness and bedrest, in addition to the effects of anaesthesia, can all make this activity difficult, particularly for older patients. Embarrassment about using the urinal or bedpan may add to this.

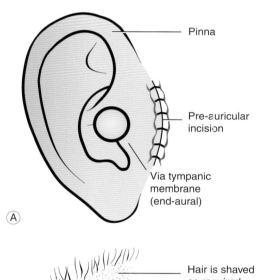

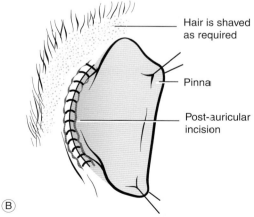

Figure 12.1 Types of incision in ear surgery. (A) Pre-auricular. (B) Post-auricular

Case study

The following case study aims to demonstrate both pre- and postoperative care for an individual undergoing a stapedectomy for otosclerosis.

Mrs Doris Marsh is a 42-year-old housewife and mother of two children (aged 9 and 14 years). Her husband, a businessman, works in France and returns home for weekends. Doris was electively admitted for a right-sided stapedectomy. Her symptoms include mild tinnitus and progressive right-sided hearing loss. Her two pregnancies may have exacerbated this loss.

Assessment

Box 12.5 identifies the assessment of Doris Marsh.

Specific preoperative preparation

The doctor admits and obtains informed consent from Doris. This includes a detailed discussion about any risks associated with surgery. The potential deterioration or total loss of hearing on her right side, due to failure of the prosthesis or surgical trauma, is of particular concern to Doris. The doctor seeks to allay such anxieties by providing realistic information and by confirming that Doris understands all aspects of the procedure.

Audiometry, unless performed within the previous 6 months, is repeated in order to obtain up-to-date information about Doris's current hearing function.

Postoperative care

Previous chapters have discussed general issues of postoperative care. For Doris, specific potential complications of surgery include displacement of the prosthesis, facial nerve palsy, dizziness, nausea and vomiting, and difficulties in communicating. Box 12.6 details the plan of care and evaluation of care given.

Discharge planning and patient education

The majority of patients who have undergone ear surgery are often discharged after 1–2 days; some procedures are undertaken as day cases.

Discharge planning and patient education begins in the pre-admission clinic, and issues are reinforced throughout the patient's hospital stay. Written advice sheets are an invaluable source of education and reassurance, as patients often experience difficulty in absorbing all the verbal information given by practitioners and doctors. Box 12.7 illustrates discharge advice given to patients following ear surgery.

Outpatient follow-up varies depending on the nature of the operation, and it can be between 1 and 6 weeks. Any aural packing is removed at the outpatient appointment, as well as a repeat aural examination and audiometry.

The nose

Anatomy and physiology

The nose is part of the respiratory system and is responsible for the sense of smell (olfaction). The nose also contributes major aesthetic features to the face (Behrbohm, 2015). The nasal passages link the face, the paranasal sinuses and the nasopharynx.

The external nose

The upper third of the external nose consists of two nasal bones, which are fused together. The lower two-thirds are cartilage, the tip of which is especially pliable and is protected by fibrofatty tissue.

The nasal cavity

This consists of twin passages, divided and supported by the osteocartilaginous septum. The anterior opening of each passage is the vestibule and is lined with skin and hair. The posterior opens into the nasopharynx and is termed the choana. Turbinates line the lateral wall of each side; there are usually three — superior, middle and inferior. They function to maximize the surface area of mucous membrane, enabling the warming and humidification of inhaled air. The space between the middle and inferior turbinates contains the ostiomeatal complex, which functions to drain the sinuses (Tysome & Kanegaonkar, 2017). Cilia contained in the epithelium beat constantly in order to transport mucus posteriorly to the nasopharynx (Freeman & Kahwaji, 2018).

Vascular supply

The rich arterial blood supply to the nose derives from the external and internal carotid systems serving the sphenopalatine artery and the anterior ethmoid artery. Venous drainage is via the sphenopalatine and ethmoid veins.

Nerve supply

The olfactory nerve innervates smell receptors in the nasal mucosa. Fibres of this nerve pass through the roof of the nasal cavity in the ethmoid sinus at the cribriform plate and form the olfactory bulb in the brain. Secretory glands of the nose are controlled by the autonomic nervous system. Sensory

Box 12.5 **Preoperative assessment of a patient undergoing a stapedectomy**

Maintaining a safe environment

- Observation of vital signs is performed: pulse, 72 beats per minute; blood pressure, 110/65 mmHg.
- Allergies: none known.
- Past medical history: caesarean section 9 years ago under general anaesthetic.
- Medication: Fybogel (fibre) sachet as required to maintain bowel regularity.
- Doris is anxious about surgery, in particular the potential but minimal risk to her existing right-sided hearing. She also expresses concern about speed of recovery, as her mother is caring for her children and her husband is away in France until the weekend (5 days away).

Breathing

- Respiratory rate: 14 respirations per minute.
- Doris smokes 10–15 cigarettes per day.
- Chest X-ray: no abnormalities.

Controlling body temperature

- Doris's temperature is 36.5°C.

Communicating

- Doris has normal vision.
- Normal hearing is present on the left side.
- Doris has pronounced right-sided hearing loss; mild tinnitus is present; she finds socializing difficult, particularly with large, noisy groups of people. It causes her some embarrassment; a hearing aid is not used.
- Doris expresses concern about surgery and home commitments.

Eating and drinking

- Doris is petite: height 1.55 m; weight 50 kg.
- Doris has a normal appetite and diet.

Elimination

- Doris is prone to constipation; bowels open every 2–3 days.
- She takes Fybogel to maintain this activity.
- Doris passes urine normally; urinalysis shows no abnormalities.

Personal hygiene and dressing

- Doris bathes every night and showers after exercise.

Mobility

- Doris is independent.
- Right-sided hearing loss makes her more cautious when driving, or out and about and in crowds.

Working and social

- Doris is a housewife and mother; her husband is only at home at weekends, so she leads a very busy home life.
- Doris swims twice per week and walks the dog every day.
- Doris expresses concern about the family's summer holiday in 4 months' time; they plan to fly to Spain.

Body image

- Doris is casual about her appearance and seems relaxed about the minimal expected surgical scarring.

Sleeping

- Doris sleeps well, about 7–8 hours per night.

Dying

- Doris feels a little apprehensive about the anaesthetic.

Box 12.6 Postoperative care of a patient following a stapedectomy

Doris Marsh returns to the ward following a right-sided stapedectomy. She is orientated but drowsy. Oxygen therapy is in progress at 4 L/min. An intravenous infusion is in progress. Doris is allowed to take oral fluids if not nauseous. A cotton-wool plug sits in the external ear canal and is covered by a light gauze dressing; it appears to be moderately bloodstained. The surgeon has instructed flat bedrest with one pillow until the following morning in order to maintain the integrity of the prosthesis.

Breathing

- *Problem*: Potential loss of clear airway and respiratory distress due to anaesthetic, drowsiness and flat bedrest.
- *Goal*: Doris maintains a clear airway and normal breathing.
- *Care*:
  - Ensure oxygen is given at the prescribed rate; provide oral care to prevent a dry mouth.
  - Encourage Doris to lie in the recovery position, with operated ear uppermost, until fully awake, to maintain optimum airway; one pillow is allowed for comfort.
  - Frequently observe respiration rate, depth and rhythm ($1/4$-hourly for first 2 hours, reducing to 1–2- to 4-hourly as condition stabilizes); also observe for cyanosis or respiratory difficulty and report at once to doctor.
  - Encourage deep breathing and coughing to clear secretions.
- *Evaluation*: Though drowsy for the first 2 hours, Doris showed no signs of respiratory distress. Oxygen therapy was stopped after the prescribed 4 hours. Though a smoker, her chest remained clear. Respiratory rate: 12–16 rpm.

Maintaining a safe environment

- *Problem*: Potential disturbance of middle ear prosthesis due to its initial vulnerability.
- *Goal*: To maintain integrity of prosthesis.
- *Care*:
  - Ensure Doris remains on flat bedrest as instructed; allow one pillow only.
  - Ensure Doris does not fall out of bed as she will feel dizzy and drowsy for the first few hours.
  - Place the call bell and necessities to hand, to minimize any inconvenience from the bedrest.
  - Assist Doris in meeting her daily needs, but reduce physical activity to the minimum; ensure Doris knows not to move suddenly or jerkily; offer the slipper bedpan for toileting; facilitate taking of diet and fluids by providing soft foods and drinking straws.
  - The following morning, ensure Doris mobilizes gently, at first with assistance in case of dizziness.
  - Advise Doris not to perform highly strenuous activity for the next 6 months.
- *Evaluation*: Doris found flat bedrest tiresome but maintained it well despite a few episodes of nausea. She successfully used the slipper bedpan and took fluids easily with a straw. The next morning, Doris cautiously but safely mobilized. The doctors advised her to continue restful activity for the next 2 weeks and that flying to Spain in 4 months' time was acceptable.
- *Problem*: Potential facial nerve palsy due to surgical trauma to the facial nerve.
- *Goal*: To promptly detect the onset of any facial nerve defect.
- *Care*:
  - Perform facial nerve checks when taking vital signs: observe Doris's face at rest for asymmetry; ask Doris to raise both eyebrows; ask Doris to smile; ask Doris to close both eyes tightly.
  - If any weakness or deficit is noted, inform the doctor immediately and continue monitoring.
  - Reassure Doris that any weakness is more than likely due to postoperative swelling causing nerve compression and that this tends to resolve completely.
- *Evaluation*: Regular checks were maintained and no weakness was noted. Therefore, facial nerve function remained intact.

Eating and drinking

- *Problem*: Doris feels unable to eat and drink normally because of postoperative dizziness, nausea and flat bedrest.
- *Goal*: To alleviate nausea, any vomiting and dizziness; for Doris to gain adequate hydration and return to a normal diet.
- *Care*:
  - Administer intravenous infusion as prescribed and check patency and integrity of cannula and site.
  - Maintain accurate fluid balance chart until intravenous infusion is complete and Doris is drinking normally.
  - Administer antiemetic therapy as prescribed/required and monitor effect; encourage Doris to inform staff if feeling nauseous or dizzy, and also frequently ask her how she feels.

(Continued)

Box 12.6 (cont'd)

- Oral fluids/diet are encouraged once nausea has subsided; first offer clear fluids, then light bland foods; then encourage relatives/friends to bring in favourite food and drink.
- *Evaluation*: Doris felt dizzy and nauseous upon returning to the ward. An antiemetic was given as prescribed, with good effect, though mild dizziness persisted. Doris then took oral fluids but declined diet until morning. The intravenous infusion was discontinued after breakfast was eaten. Doris was discharged home later that afternoon, once breakfast and lunch had been eaten and tolerated. She felt 'light-headed', but her family were there to take her home.

Communicating

- *Problem*: Doris states the hearing on her right side is worse than before surgery; she is anxious, particularly upon noting the bloodstained dressing.
- *Goal*: To alleviate Doris's anxiety.
- *Care*:
  - Reassure Doris that deterioration in hearing is normal; surgical oedema, aural packing and any middle ear drainage impairs existing hearing; effects of surgery are often not known for 2–6 weeks.
  - Some bleeding is expected; a moderate discharge of fresh blood onto the cotton wool can continue for the first 24 hours, and then this gradually declines.
  - Promote effective communication skills (see Box 12.4).
- *Evaluation*: Once the probable reason for Doris's worsened hearing was explained, she felt less anxious, and the postoperative visit by the surgeon was reassuring. Bleeding was moderate, and the cotton wool dressing was changed three times during the first 12 hours. By discharge, this had reduced to mild staining of slightly old blood. Doris was advised to change the dressing three times a day for the next 2 days and then daily until discharge had stopped. Doris communicated with staff and visitors by relying upon her left ear for hearing.

Box 12.7 Discharge advice for patients following ear surgery

- Change the cotton wool in the opening of your ear canal every day. Take care not to remove the ear pack. If the pack falls out, contact the hospital for advice.
- A small amount of reddish discharge from the ear is normal. If this becomes offensive, appears yellow/green, or fresh bleeding is noted, contact the hospital.
- Protect the ear, when bathing/showering, with cotton wool dabbed with Vaseline. Keep water out of the ear canal for at least 1 month, as this can cause infection. Use a dry shampoo for 1 week, and do not go swimming for 1 month or as advised.
- If there are any stitches, you will be advised upon their removal.
- Mild dizziness is common for a few days. If this worsens, contact the hospital. Do not drive if dizzy, and refrain from working and any strenuous activity for 1–2 weeks, or as advised. If applicable, do not fly for at least 1 month, but clarify this with your doctor before you leave. Do not blow your nose or play wind instruments for 1 month. Sneeze with your mouth open. These precautions protect the ear and surgery from trauma.
- Hearing is often reduced for the first few weeks because of packing, swelling or discharge. Follow-up hearing tests will be performed.
- Pain is usually mild. If pain increases, contact the hospital.
- If concerned about any matter regarding recovery and aftercare, do not hesitate to contact the hospital.

innervation of the nasal cavity is via the ophthalmic and maxillary divisions of the trigeminal nerve (Pires et al, 2009).

Functions of the nose

Functions of the nose are:
- Airway
- Filtration and protection – by nasal hairs, mucus transport and cilia; and antibacterial action within the mucus
- Humidification and warming – by blood and secretory glands
- Olfaction
- Resonance of sound.

The paranasal sinuses

The sinuses act as extensions of the nasal cavity. There are four pairs: frontal, sphenoid, ethmoid and maxillary.

Sinus functions include:

- mucus production
- air-filled cavities to reduce the weight of the skull
- protecting the eye and brain from trauma
- aiding sound resonance.

Conditions of the nose and sinuses that require surgery

There are a variety of conditions and diseases that benefit from surgical intervention. The following details the main examples, with types of surgery explained in Box 12.8.

- *Disorders of the nasal lining*: e.g. allergic rhinitis, sinusitis and nasal polyps.
- *Disorders of the autonomic nervous system*: namely, vasomotor rhinitis. An imbalance exists between parasympathetic and sympathetic nerve supplies to the nasal mucosa, resulting in increased vascularity of the turbinates and nasal obstruction.
- *Structural disorders*: e.g. deviated septum, septal haematoma, fractured nasal bones and irregular nasal bones.
- *Infection*: e.g. acute/chronic sinusitis. This is an inflammatory condition whereby the sinus ostia (natural sinus openings into the nasal cavity) become blocked. Mucus accumulates in the sinuses, is unable to drain and may become infected. If normal sinus clearance is not restored, this can lead to chronic mucosal thickening and subsequent nasal obstruction, headache, facial pain and purulent discharge.

Specific investigations

Physical examination and a thorough history need to be taken. Conservative treatment is the desired option, with

---

Box 12.8 Types of nasal and paranasal sinus surgery

Inferior turbinate surgery — for hypertrophy due to allergic/vasomotor rhinitis

- *Diathermy*: to scar/shrink mucosal lining of turbinate using bipolar, monopolar, laser or ablation methods.
- *Turbinoplasty*: to reduce size of turbinate from within using a microdebrider.
- *Turbinectomy*: partial or total removal — to increase airway patency.
- *Outfracture*: to reduce size and function — to alleviate obstruction and symptoms of rhinitis.

Septum surgery

- *Submucous resection of septum*: to straighten deviated septum, performed to increase nasal airflow.
- *Septoplasty*: maximum septal cartilage is preserved; performed to correct septal deviation. Cartilage tissue may be reinserted, straightened, as supporting graft.
- *Drainage of septal haematoma*: performed by either needle aspiration or formal incision.

Nasal bones

- *Rhinoplasty*: external and internal bony and cartilaginous deformity is corrected, for aesthetics and function.
- *Reduction of nasal fracture*: to restore patency of airway and aesthetics of nose.

Sinus surgery

- *Polypectomy*: nasal polyps can be removed using a microdebrider or surgical forceps.
- *Functional endoscopic sinus surgery (FESS)*: aims to restore normal functional drainage of the sinuses; includes gentle removal of diseased mucosal lining and widening of natural ostium of each sinus
  - Maxillary antrostomy.
  - Ethmoidectomy: posterior and anterior ethmoid sinuses gently debrided to improve mucus drainage.
  - Sphenoid sinus surgery: sphenoid ostia opened to minimize further obstruction.
  - Frontal sinus surgery: frontal recess opened to improve frontal sinus drainage.
- *External ethmoidectomy*: an external incision is made to facilitate disease clearance. Improved endoscopic techniques have lessened the need to perform this surgery routinely. A good approach for tumour clearance.
- *Antral washout*: saline is irrigated into the sinus via a cannula, and pus and mucus are expelled.
- *Caldwell–Luc procedure*: the maxillary antrum is cleared of disease via an antrostomy made inside the upper lip. Endoscopic sinus surgery has diminished the need for this type of antrostomy.

the prescribing of topical nasal and sinus preparations. The following investigations may be undertaken:

- *Allergy testing* – to locate and eliminate allergens.
- *Endoscopy* – to visualize the nasal anatomy.
- *Rhinomanometry* – objective measure of impaired nasal breathing.
- *X-rays* – reveal bony pathology.
- *CT scan* – gives a detailed image of bony and soft-tissue disease.
- *MRI scanning* – valuable in malignancy.

Assessment of a patient requiring nasal/sinus surgery

The majority of these procedures are performed as a day case or overnight admission. Referring to Roper, Logan and Tierney's model of nursing, the following activities of living need to be assessed on admission (Holland, 2008).

Maintaining a safe environment

Because of the rich blood supply of the nose, there is a risk of haemorrhage following nasal and sinus surgery. Preoperative observation of the patient's vital signs gives an accurate baseline for postoperative reference. A full medical and drug history may reveal conditions or medications that can exacerbate bleeding, e.g. blood clotting disorders or anticoagulant therapy.

Breathing

Conditions and diseases of the nose and sinuses often lead to nasal obstruction, snoring, obstructive sleep apnoea (cessation of breathing for intermittent periods while asleep) and mouth-breathing. Assessment of the patient's respiratory rate, depth and rhythm is therefore indicated. The surgical insertion of nasal packing forces the patient to mouth-breathe, and this may be distressing. Chest conditions which may lead to respiratory difficulty are also noted, e.g. asthma.

Eating and drinking

Nasal packing makes this activity awkward, as a partial vacuum is created; the patient may complain of a sucking sensation upon swallowing. Postnasal discharge, loss of sense of smell and the presence of blood in the mouth all hinder the desire to take diet and fluids.

Sleeping

Assessing the patient's normal sleep pattern is useful. As discussed, nasal and sinus conditions often cause nasal obstruction; this interferes with the activities of breathing and sleeping. The patient may be a snorer, suffer from interrupted sleep and dry mouth and may complain of fatigue. Postoperative nasal packing, swelling and discharge will also affect the patient's ability to sleep; this tends to improve as recovery progresses.

Body image

The presence of nasal dressings and/or nasal discharge can affect the patient's body image. Though present for only a short period, it can be distressing.

Case study

The following case study aims to demonstrate both pre- and postoperative care for an individual undergoing a septoplasty.

Mr Arnold Black is admitted to the ward at 10 a.m. as his surgery is planned for the afternoon. He is 52 years old, married and works as a chef. Arnold suffers with a deviated septum, causing nasal obstruction and snoring. He is also asthmatic, controlled by inhalers, and for this reason he was admitted for an overnight stay.

Assessment

Box 12.9 details the assessment of Arnold Black.

Specific preoperative preparation

Arnold has been 'nil by mouth' since an early breakfast at 6 a.m. Because of his asthma, Arnold has a chest X-ray to ensure fitness for anaesthetic and a peak flow to assess lung capacity. A premedication of three puffs of Arnold's asthma medication is prescribed and administered.

Postoperative care

Specific postoperative complications following septoplasty, and most types of nasal/sinus surgery, are:

- haemorrhage
- infection
- haematoma: e.g. septal or periorbital, i.e. around the eye
- difficulty in eating and drinking, due to nasal oedema and packing
- difficulty in breathing normally, due to nasal oedema and packing.

Box 12.10 outlines the postoperative care plan for Arnold.

Nasal packing and splinting
Nasal packing

As discussed previously, haemorrhage is the main postoperative complication following nasal and sinus surgery. For

Box 12.9 **Preoperative assessment of a patient undergoing a septoplasty**

Maintaining a safe environment

- Observation of vital signs is performed: pulse, 80 beats per minute; blood pressure, 150/80 mmHg.
- Allergies: none known.
- Past medical history: asthma since childhood; admitted with bronchitis and exacerbation of asthma 5 years ago; never had a general anaesthetic.
- Medication:
  - Salbutamol inhaler — two puffs three times per day and as required.
  - Becotide inhaler — two puffs twice a day.
- Arnold is anxious about the surgery, as he has never had a general anaesthetic; he is also concerned that his asthma will flare up.

Breathing

- Respiratory rate: 16 respirations per minute.
- Arnold gave up smoking 5 years ago when he required hospital admission and treatment for bronchitis and asthma.
- Arnold breathes through his mouth due to nasal obstruction.
- Chest X-ray: lungs clear; anaesthetist satisfied.
- Peak flow rate: 480 L/min.

Controlling body temperature

- Arnold's temperature is 36.8°C.

Communicating

- Arnold wears glasses for reading.
- Bilateral hearing is good.
- As discussed, Arnold expresses fears about the anaesthetic and the risk to his asthma.

Eating and drinking

- Arnold is of stocky build: height, 1.77 m; weight, 81 kg.
- He has a healthy appetite and, as he is a chef, enjoys cooking and dining with friends.
- Arnold is Jewish, so does not eat pork.

Elimination

- Arnold opens his bowels daily and passes urine normally.
- Urinalysis: nothing abnormal detected.

Personal cleansing and dressing

- Arnold is smartly dressed. Bathes daily.

Mobility

- Arnold is independent; avoids steep walks and climbing stairs because of his asthma.

Working and social

- Arnold works full time as a chef in a busy restaurant. He has arranged for 2 weeks' time off to recuperate.
- He enjoys swimming twice per week and visiting his family.

Body image

- Arnold is apprehensive about the presence of internal splinting and its appearance.
- He is aware that there will be no external scarring.

(Continued)

Box 12.9 (cont'd)

Sleeping

- Arnold breathes through his mouth, so awakes feeling very dry and uncomfortable.
- He snores and tends to have a restless night's sleep (about 6 hours), thus feeling unrefreshed.

Dying

- Arnold is a little anxious about the anaesthetic.

Box 12.10 Postoperative care of a patient following a septoplasty

Arnold Black returns to the ward following septoplasty. Nasal packing and internal splints are *in situ*. The packs are to be removed 6 hours after surgery if bleeding is not excessive. The splints are to remain in place for one week. Arnold is alert, orientated and receiving oxygen therapy at 2 L/min until the following morning. Moderate fresh blood is noted on the nasal bolster.

Breathing

- *Problem*: Potential loss of clear airway, and respiratory distress due to anaesthetic, nasal packing, splinting and asthma.
- *Goal*: Arnold is able to maintain a clear airway and mouth-breathe.
- *Care*:
  - Maintain upright position to facilitate respiration and nasal discharge.
  - Ensure oxygen therapy runs to prescribed regimen.
  - Observe respiratory rate, depth and rhythm, and for presence of wheeze/tightness so as to promptly detect any exacerbation of asthma and/or respiratory difficulty; adhere to appropriate frequency of observation.
  - Reassure Arnold that mouth-breathing ensures adequate airflow; provide mouthwash and care to help prevent dry mouth.
  - Administer asthma medications as prescribed and monitor effect.
  - Reassure Arnold that nose will feel blocked for 2–3 weeks due to surgical oedema.
- *Evaluation*: Arnold maintained oxygen therapy until morning. His respiratory observations remained within normal limits. Mouth-breathing was tolerated well, though a dry mouth was a little uncomfortable. A mild wheeze was heard upon returning to the ward, and two puffs from his salbutamol inhaler eased this. Arnold felt comfortable.

Maintaining a safe environment

- *Problem*: Potential haemorrhage following surgery to an area with a very rich blood supply.
- *Goal*: To minimize haemorrhage.
- *Care*:
  - Perform observations of vital signs as per recommended postoperative regimen; hypotension and tachycardia are signs of haemorrhage.
  - Observe nasal discharge; change nasal bolsters as required and chart frequency of dressing change; check back of throat for postnasal bleeding.
  - Apply ice packs to forehead, back of neck and bridge of nose if bleeding heavily – this will help vasoconstrict blood vessels.
  - Inform doctor if any of the above is apparent.
  - Remove packing as instructed but if bleeding heavily, do not remove packing until the doctor has reviewed Arnold first.
  - Ensure Arnold remains on bedrest until 1 hour after removal of pack, in order to minimize activity and risk of further bleeding; permit gentle mobility after that.
  - Reinforce no nose blowing or picking and advise Arnold to sneeze with his mouth open to reduce pressure within the nose.
- *Evaluation*: A steady moderate ooze of fresh blood continued for the first hour. An ice pack was applied, which appeared to reduce bleeding. After 4 hours, nasal discharge became minimal and haemoserous. Packing was removed as instructed, without complication. Observations were within normal limits. Arnold mobilized around the ward with no ill-effect.
- *Problem*: Potential infection of the nose due to surgery and insertion of splints.
- *Goal*: To prevent infection.

(Continued)

Box 12.10 (cont'd)

- *Care*:
  - Observe for signs of infection: purulent discharge, pyrexia and inflammation; report any signs.
  - Administer antibiotic therapy as prescribed and ensure Arnold knows to complete the course once discharged home.
  - Discourage contact with people with coughs/colds for 1 week once home.
- *Evaluation*: Arnold showed no signs of infection. Antibiotic therapy was administered and 'take-home' medication was arranged and explained.
- *Problem*: Potential septal haematoma due to collection of blood between the septum and mucous membrane.
- *Goal*: To detect onset promptly.
- *Care*:
  - Advise Arnold to inform staff if pain becomes worse and nasal blockage becomes severe after packing is removed.
  - Ensure splints remain *in situ* for 1 week as directed, to maintain septal position.
- *Evaluation*: There appeared to be no signs of haematoma. Pain was a mild discomfort (normal) that was relieved by paracetamol. Splints remained intact and were removed when Arnold attended follow-up at the outpatient clinic.

Eating and drinking

- *Problem*: Difficulty in swallowing due to the presence of nasal packs.
- *Goal*: To ensure adequate hydration/nutrition; for Arnold to return to swallowing normally.
- *Care*:
  - Maintain intravenous infusion as prescribed.
  - Encourage oral fluids/soft diet as able; provide supplement drinks if food is not taken.
  - Reassure that any difficulty in swallowing will pass once nasal packing has been removed.
  - Maintain an accurate fluid balance chart until intravenous infusion is completed and normal oral intake is achieved.
- *Evaluation*: Arnold complained of a sucking sensation at the back of his throat whenever he swallowed. His oral intake was poor at first (350 ml water in 5 hours) and he only managed soup at supper. The intravenous infusion was maintained until complete at 9 p.m. Once the nasal packing was removed at 8 p.m. his swallowing returned to normal. A late sandwich was eaten.

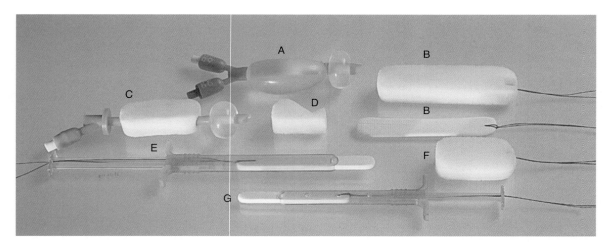

Figure 12.2 Examples of nasal packing. (A) Xomed Epistat nasal catheter. (B) Pope Flex-Pak nasal packing. (C) Xomed Epistat II nasal catheter. (D) Staxi-Stat pack without drawstring. (E) Large Fast-Pak nasal pack with applicator. (F) Weimert epistaxis packing. (G) Small Fast-Pak nasal pack with applicator. (From Roberts, J.R. & Hedges, J. (2009). *Clinical procedures in emergency medicine* (5th edn.). Elsevier Inc, with permission.)

some types of nasal surgery, packs are inserted at the end of the operation, to exert pressure against the mucosal wall, so reducing the risk of haemorrhage. It is now quite common for patients having nasal surgery to have no nasal packing postoperatively. Figure 12.2 illustrates types of nasal packing commonly used.

The surgeon determines when the packing is to be removed, and this may be 4, 12 or 24 hours later. Some

> ## Box 12.11 Discharge advice for patients following nasal/sinus surgery
>
> - The nose will feel more blocked due to swelling and can take 2—3 weeks to resolve. If prescribed, apply nasal drops to decongest the nose (Fig. 12.3 illustrates the correct method of instilling nasal drops).
> - Scabbing within the nose may occur as it heals; douching with warm water may soften the scabs; do not pick the nose, as this may precipitate bleeding.
> - Sneeze with your mouth open to reduce nasal pressure. Only wipe the nose, do not blow, until after the postoperative outpatient visit.
> - Nasal discharge can continue for a few days and is normally lightly bloodstained.
> - If fresh, steady bleeding occurs, pinch the fleshy part of the nose and lean forward; apply ice to the forehead and bridge of nose; avoid swallowing any blood as it can make you feel sick; if the bleeding does not stop after 15 minutes, ring the ward or casualty department for advice.
> - For the first few days, avoid very hot drinks, meals, baths and showers, as these can increase the risk of bleeding.
> - Avoid work and strenuous activity for at least 1 week or as advised.
> - Avoid smoking, crowded smoky places and people with colds or coughs, as infection can be picked up in the nose.
> - If nasal splints are *in situ*, do not touch; attend the outpatient appointment for removal.

fresh bleeding through the packs for the first 1—2 hours of recovery is normal. In order to monitor this, a nasal dressing (bolster) is applied, and this is changed as required. If the bleeding does not appear to be subsiding, the packing is left *in situ* and the doctor is notified.

Nasal packing may be removed by the practitioner. A basic dressing pack is prepared, as saline and gauze are used to gently clean the exterior of the nose once the packing has been removed. It is essential to outline the procedure to the patient in order to minimize anxiety. The patient needs to sit upright in the bed, as this facilitates pack removal and helps to avoid swallowing of any blood. The patient is then asked to breathe gently in and out in a steady rhythm; with each expiration, the pack is slowly eased out of the nose with the aid of forceps. If both sides are packed, one alternates from side to side, removing a little at a time. At first, some fresh bleeding is common, in the form of a trickle of blood. Gentle pressure on the nose and the application of ice packs to the forehead, bridge of nose and the back of the neck will enhance vasoconstriction. A nasal bolster is applied, and monitoring of nasal discharge continues. It is normal for nasal secretions to decrease to a minimal amount of haemoserous discharge over 2—3 days.

Nasal splinting

Internal silastic splints may be inserted into each nasal cavity following septoplasty. The splints maintain septal position and remain *in situ* for 1—2 weeks. They are sutured in place, and the patient is advised not to touch them. The surgeon removes the splints in the outpatient clinic.

If rhinoplasty is also performed, an external splint may be applied, to support the new position of the nasal bones following repair of nasal fractures and septorhinoplasty.

Splinting can be with layers of surgical tape, plaster of Paris, or a thermoplastic splint. The splint is removed by the doctor 1—2 weeks later, in the outpatient clinic.

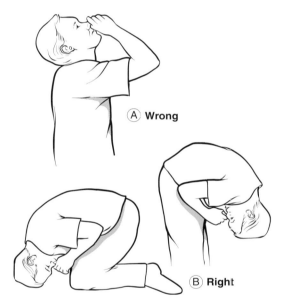

(A) Wrong

(B) Right

Figure 12.3 The correct method of instilling nasal medication. (A) If the wrong method is used, the nasal drops pass into the pharynx and avoid important internal nasal structures. (B) The correct method ensures the spread of nasal drops across important nasal membranes. *Drops:* staying with the head forward for a few minutes after instillation is advised. *Spray:* if medication is spray delivery, then upright position, no backward tilting, is recommended; the drug is delivered in a metered dose via a pump (Pires et al, 2009).

Discharge planning and patient education

Both written and verbal discharge advice are given to the patient (Box 12.11).

Outpatient follow-up varies from 1 to 6 weeks. Here, any nasal splinting is removed and examination of the nose and sinuses is performed. Assessing the benefits of the surgery is left until at least this time, as surgical swelling needs sufficient time to reduce.

The throat

Anatomy and physiology

Within the specialty of ENT surgery, the throat components are:
- Pharynx
  - Nasopharynx
  - Oropharynx
  - Hypopharynx
- Larynx
- Salivary glands.

Pharynx

The functions of the pharynx are:
- To deliver food, saliva and mucus to the oesophagus.
- To act as an airway from the nose and mouth to the larynx.
- To resonate sound produced in the larynx.

The nasopharynx lies above the soft palate at the rear of the nose, is lined with mucous membrane and contains the Eustachian tube orifice and the adenoids, which are sacs of lymphoid tissue. The oropharynx lies between the soft palate and the hyoid bone. The hyoid is a small U-shaped bone that lies below and supports the tongue; muscles and ligaments secure its position. The palatine tonsils are located within the oropharynx on either side of the base of the tongue. Like the adenoids, they are lymphoid tissue and their function is to protect against infection. The hypopharynx lies behind the larynx and connects with the oesophagus. Nerve supply to the pharynx is via branches of the glossopharyngeal (ninth cranial) nerve.

Larynx

The larynx is the organ of phonation, comprising rigid cartilage, ligament, muscle and membrane. The vocal cords consist of folds of mucous membrane, which adduct and abduct, producing controlled interference of airflow that results in audible vibrations, termed speech. The other important function of the larynx is to protect the tracheobronchial tree, and this is achieved by the following means:
- *The epiglottis:* a flap of cartilage and mucous membrane which occludes the larynx when swallowing.

- *The glottis:* the space between the vocal cords contained within the larynx, which can be closed in order to initiate a cough.

The vagus nerve supplies branches to the larynx, in the form of the superior and recurrent laryngeal nerve.

Salivary glands

There are three pairs of salivary glands.
- The *parotid glands* produce mainly serous saliva that secretes into the mouth via the parotid ducts near each second upper molar tooth.
- The *submandibular glands* produce seromucinous fluid that drains into the floor of the mouth via the submandibular ducts.
- The *sublingual glands* are principally mucous in nature and drain into the mouth via sublingual ducts.

Between 500 and 1000 mL of saliva is produced every 24 hours. The functions of saliva are listed in Box 12.12.

Blood supply

Arterial blood supply to the head and neck region derives from the arch of the aorta, to the internal and external carotid arteries. The internal carotid arteries deliver blood to the brain and the orbit of the eye; the external carotid arteries supply the more superficial tissues of the head and neck.

Venous blood from the face, neck and other superficial tissues drains into the external jugular veins.

Conditions of the throat that require surgery

The following are common examples of throat conditions that lead to surgery (Box 12.13).

Recurrent tonsillitis and peritonsillar abscess

Repeated bacterial infection, commonly streptococcal, can cause severe distress. Pain, pyrexia and difficulty in swallowing (dysphagia) are the problems experienced. The infection can localize over one of the tonsils, causing a peritonsillar abscess, known as a quinsy, which, if not

---

Box 12.12 Functions of saliva

- Facilitates chewing and swallowing
- Lubricates food
- Aids taste
- Protects the oral cavity from infection
- Aids speech

Box 12.13 Types of throat surgery

- *Tonsillectomy*: surgical removal of the palatine tonsils.
- *Uvulopalatopharyngoplasty* (UPPP): surgical resection of the uvula, soft palate, ± tonsils is performed to widen the upper airway.
- *Repair of pharyngeal pouch*: an endoscope is used to visualize the pharyngeal hernia (Zenker's diverticulum) and is repaired using staples; traditional technique of repair involves external neck incision and pharyngeal repair.
- *Pharyngoscopy*: endoscopic examination of the pharynx.
- *Oesophagoscopy*: endoscopic examination of the oesophagus.
- *Laryngoscopy*: endoscopic examination of the larynx.
- *Tracheostomy formation*: a small window of cartilage is removed between the second and third tracheal ring in order to create airway patency. The chosen tracheostomy tube is inserted and initially sutured in place.

---

adequately treated, can lead to the complication of a restricted, oedematous airway. For both conditions, a tonsillectomy is recommended.

Snoring and obstructive sleep apnoea

The temporary collapse of the upper airway on inspiration causes obstruction and snoring. The most common site of this problem is in the region of the soft palate.

Sleep apnoea is defined as 30 instances of stopping breathing, for at least 10 seconds each, over a period of 7 hours of sleep (Dhillon & East, 2013). Drinking alcohol, smoking and being overweight increase the risk of snoring and obstructive sleep apnoea, reducing pharyngeal muscle tone. Other factors include the following conditions: nasal polyps, deviated nasal septum, hypertrophied turbinates, enlarged adenoids and tonsils, floppy uvula and soft palate. Correcting these structural problems and addressing physiological obstruction should alleviate sleep apnoea and snoring.

The most common type of surgery for this condition is uvulopalatopharyngoplasty (UPPP), with or without tonsillectomy, a procedure designed to improve the upper airway (Fig. 12.4).

Pharyngeal pouch

This is a hernia of the pharyngeal mucosa in which food debris collects. The pouch can enlarge to cause oesophageal compression, regurgitation and dysphagia. Endoscopic surgery can repair the pouch using a purpose-built diverticuloscope and a stapling device. The patient can commence fluids and soft diet the next day and may be discharged home the following day.

Foreign body

Fish, lamb and chicken bones are the most common foreign bodies lodged in the pharynx or oesophagus of adult patients. This can cause pain and dysphagia and be distressing. Endoscopy to retrieve foreign bodies may include pharyngoscopy and oesophagoscopy.

Airway obstruction

Acute or potential airway obstruction is serious and can be caused by the following:

- Trauma to the trachea or larynx, causing oedema or structural injury.
- Oedema associated with head and neck surgery, and burns.
- Laryngeal incompetence (failure to function correctly).
- Loss of gag reflex and therefore risk of aspiration into the lungs.
- Inability to expectorate lung secretions.

A tracheostomy is performed to restore or maintain a clear airway for the above conditions. If a patient is receiving long-term artificial ventilation, a tracheostomy is often performed, as endotracheal intubation can cause laryngeal and tracheal injury (Myatt, 2015).

Types of tracheostomy tube

The most common makes are Portex, Shiley and Silver Negus, and they all come in a variety of sizes. Silver Negus tubes are now uncommon, as there are more durable and cost-effective alternatives. Tracheostomy tubes come in a variety of forms, and the patient's condition determines which type is used.

Plain or fenestrated. A hole or fenestration in the upper aspect of the tube enables passage of air from the trachea, through the larynx, into the pharynx: thus, when the end of the tube is occluded with either a finger or speaking valve, the patient can vocalize. Fenestrated tubes are therefore used in patients who have recovered from the acute period, have a functioning upper airway, have the functional ability to vocalize (laryngeal competence), and those who may be starting the process of weaning off the tracheostomy.

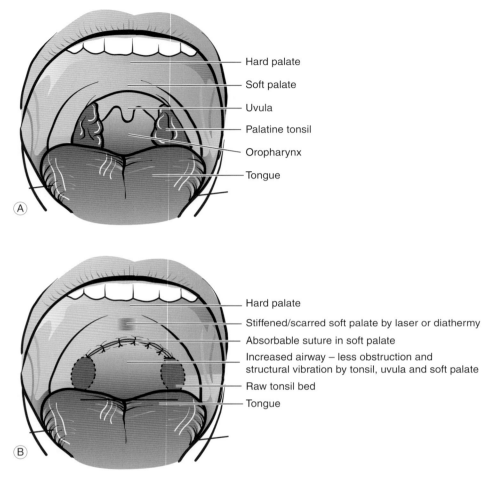

Hard palate
Soft palate
Uvula
Palatine tonsil
Oropharynx
Tongue

(A)

Hard palate
Stiffened/scarred soft palate by laser or diathermy
Absorbable suture in soft palate
Increased airway – less obstruction and structural vibration by tonsil, uvula and soft palate
Raw tonsil bed
Tongue

(B)

Figure 12.4 (A) The oropharynx in obstructive sleep apnoea. (B) UPPP with the large areas of painful raw tissue postoperatively, and the improved airway.

Plain tubes are inserted when the tracheostomy is initially performed. A plain tube has no hole; therefore, use of the upper airway or vocalization cannot be effectively achieved.

Cuffed or cuffless. The cuff sits at the base of the tube and is inflated with air via a valve, which is visible on the outside of the tube. Its purpose is to prevent aspiration of gastric/oral secretions by closing off the upper airway. It is inflated for long-term ventilation, ensuring maximum oxygenation of the lungs by preventing air leaks. The cuff must be deflated, or the tube changed to a cuffless type, if vocalization is desired, or if the process of weaning off the tracheostomy is to commence. Regular checks of cuff pressures when inflated are essential, as tracheal irritation and necrosis can occur with prolonged pressure; a specific manometer can measure this pressure.

With/without removable inner cannula. Tubes with inner cannulae are widely preferred, as they can be removed as often as necessary in order to clear secretions, they reduce the frequency of suctioning (which is traumatic to the patient), and they reduce the risk of tube occlusion and associated respiratory distress. Tubes without inner cannulae tend to accumulate viscous secretions that are difficult to clear, and so carry a greater risk of tube occlusion.

Tracheostomy care

This is more fully discussed in the case study for laryngectomy. Common aspects of care include the maintenance of a clear airway, with suctioning and humidification, and communicating.

Box 12.14 Specific issues of care for tracheostomy patients

- *A tracheostomy may be temporary.* Maintaining tube patency and security are essential in order to maintain airway. Sutures and/or tapes are used.
- *A tracheostomy bypasses the upper airway.* The body's natural humidification and warming systems of the mouth and nose are bypassed, so inhaled air is drier and cooler. Secretions become dry and viscous, and tracheal irritation can develop unless alternative methods of humidification and warming are applied, e.g. mechanical humidifiers, saline nebulizers and moist gauze veils.
- *A tracheostomy can impair the patient's cough reflex.* This causes an increase in tracheal irritation and sputum production. The ability to expectorate is reduced, so assistance is required in the form of physiotherapy and tracheal suctioning. Cleansing of inner cannula, if present, also clears secretions.
- *A tracheostomy impairs communication.* Patients can feel very anxious and isolated. Caring for them close to the nurses' station, having the call bell to hand, providing pen and paper and communication boards, and encouraging the use of mouthing and gesturing all alleviate difficulties in communicating. Patience and reassurance will establish the patient's confidence in their practitioner's ability to care for them. Once a speaking valve can be used or the patient can vocalize by occluding the end of the tube with a finger, the patient may feel more at ease.
- *A tracheostomy can make swallowing uncomfortable.* If allowed to take diet, soft foods are offered for ease of ingestion. For conditions where swallowing is greatly impaired, e.g. loss of gag reflex and aspiration, enteral feeding is provided.
- *A tracheostomy can cause infection.* Wound infection can occur at the incision site, requiring thorough attention to wound care. Using an aseptic technique, the area around the tube is cleansed with saline using gauze and cotton buds; a dressing is then placed under the flange of the tube, e.g. Lyofoam. This is performed as required, and at least once per shift.

Box 12.15 Step-by-step suctioning of a tracheostomy tube

- Ensure functioning suction equipment is set up at the bedside in order to use promptly as required.
- Recognize signs for suctioning: rhonchi (low-pitched gurgle), wheeze, dyspnoea, restlessness, restricted airflow felt on hand (Heidari & Shahbaz, 2017).
- Discuss all care with the patient in order to minimize anxiety.
- Remove inner cannula, if present, clear secretions and re-insert.
- If above signs persist, prepare equipment for suctioning.
- Attach suction catheter to tubing; its size has to be less than half the diameter of the tracheostomy tube, as too large a catheter removes too much oxygen and causes hypoxia.
- Turn suction on, pressure range being 80–120 mmHg; a high pressure can lead to hypoxia and trauma.
- Wear personal protective equipment – apron, goggles and gloves – to minimize risk of cross-infection.
- Remove catheter wrapping and insert catheter to only about one-third of its length, in order to minimize trachea trauma.
- Apply suction by occluding the catheter porthole. This should only be done during its withdrawal, and for no more than 15 seconds. Inappropriate technique increases the risk of hypoxia and trauma (Myatt, 2015).
- Discard the catheter and gloves into infectious waste and rinse the suction tubing with sterile water. These actions maintain high standards of infection control.
- Assess the patient's airway and, if further suctioning is required, repeat the process.

Boxes 12.14 and 12.15 outline key issues to be considered when caring for a patient with a tracheostomy.

Specific investigations for patients requiring surgery to the throat

The following investigations may be undertaken:
- Visual inspection with headlight and mirror, tongue depressor or laryngoscope.
- Sleep studies to diagnose sleep apnoea.
- Endoscopy to visualize structural abnormalities, e.g. pharyngeal pouch, laryngeal oedema.
- X-rays to demonstrate location and nature of foreign body.
- CT/MRI scan for traumatic injury to throat or soft-tissue lesions.
- Positron emission tomography (PET) scan to demonstrate cellular activity; also useful following radiotherapy.
- Barium swallow to reveal pharyngeal/oesophageal dysfunction, e.g. pooling in pharyngeal pouch.

The doctor takes a full history from the patient, and issues discussed include:

- Frequency of tonsillitis/quinsy and if hospitalized for treatment.
- Severity of sleep apnoea and snoring, and their effect on sleep quality and relationship with partner.
- Nature of dysphagia, types of food tolerated and presence of any weight loss.

Assessment of a patient requiring surgery to the throat

The following activities reflect the specific issues that need to be considered when assessing an individual admitted for throat surgery.

Breathing

Some types of throat surgery aim to improve the airway, e.g. UPPP and tracheostomy.

Thorough assessment of the patient's respiratory status, chest condition and blood oxygen saturation levels are documented to obtain an accurate baseline for postoperative reference.

Assessing the techniques used by the patient to make any difficult breathing easier is essential in order to provide individualized patient care. Methods used may include sitting upright, leaning across a table, throat-clearing, the use of nebulized drugs, oxygen therapy and relaxation techniques.

Maintaining a safe environment

For all patients, the practitioner needs to preoperatively assess vital signs and assess past medical history and current/recent medication for any bleeding tendencies.

The patient may experience discomfort or pain following throat surgery, particularly so after a tonsillectomy/UPPP. Preparing a patient preoperatively, with realistic expectations of postoperative pain, aims to improve recovery. Following tonsillectomy and UPPP, patients may experience moderate pain for up to 14 days.

Controlling body temperature

The swallowing of a foreign body, such as a sharply edged bone, carries a risk of pharyngeal/oesophageal perforation. The practitioner performs a thorough assessment of the patient's temperature, pulse and comfort level; pyrexia, tachycardia, and chest or upper back pain are signs of perforation (Lalwani, 2012). If the perforation remains undetected and oral diet is allowed, the patient can develop serious and possibly life-threatening complications, e.g. mediastinitis and empyema (pus in the pleural cavity).

Hence, a thorough assessment is of vital importance.

Eating and drinking

Assessing the patient's weight, body mass index, normal diet, fluid intake and general appetite are strongly indicated, as any condition of the throat affects an individual's ability to eat and drink. Repeated episodes of tonsillitis or quinsy may have led to weight loss, as can the dysphagia associated with a pharyngeal pouch and breathing difficulties. Obesity may be present in patients with obstructive sleep apnoea.

Communicating

Assessment of this activity is particularly pertinent for patients admitted with breathing difficulties and who may require a tracheostomy. The patient may be too exhausted to speak. Relevant issues that need to be explored include the following:

- Does the patient speak, understand and write English?
- Are there any hearing problems?
- Does the patient need spectacles, and for which activities?

Based on the above, alternative methods of communicating can be planned, e.g. the use of pen and paper, communication boards, mouthing words and gesturing.

Sleeping

Obstructive sleep apnoea, snoring and respiratory difficulties often result in poor sleeping patterns; some patients are admitted to hospital exhausted. A sleep assessment is necessary to obtain information about the quality, duration and style of sleeping, including methods used by the patient to improve sleep.

Postoperative care of patients who have had surgery to the throat

Specific postoperative complications following surgery to the throat involve the activities of breathing, maintaining a safe environment, controlling body temperature, and eating and drinking.

Potential loss of clear airway and difficulty in communicating

This applies especially to patients with airway obstruction or a tracheostomy. Specific aspects of care focus upon the alleviation of the respiratory distress, and the maintenance of adequate respiratory function. It is essential to monitor the patient's vital signs and blood oxygenation levels, as the patient's condition can deteriorate rapidly. Box 12.14 outlines key issues concerning tracheostomy care.

Haemorrhage, infection and pain, particularly following a tonsillectomy

Postoperative haemorrhage is a potential complication of all surgery. Following tonsillectomy, raw, vascular areas may bleed without warning. Regular observation of the patient's vital signs is indicated; hypotension and tachycardia are signs of haemorrhage. It is good practice to perform hourly pulse monitoring throughout the first postoperative night (not applicable if the patient is a day case), as a raised pulse while asleep is a reliable indicator of bleeding. Haematemesis and repeated swallowing may indicate bleeding from the tonsillar sites.

Infection can also cause bleeding. The patient should eat and drink as normally as possible (three meals per day with snacks, consisting of textured food, plus 2 L of fluids per day); the rationale being that this keeps the throat free of debris and infection, so minimizing the risk of bleeding.

Pharyngeal/oesophageal perforation following certain endoscopic procedures, including the retrieval of foreign bodies

As discussed earlier in the assessment process, close observation of vital signs is indicated. The surgeon dictates when the patient can commence oral fluids and diet; often only sterile water is allowed at first, and, providing the patient continues to demonstrate no signs of perforation, a soft diet is gradually introduced, usually by the next day.

Difficulty in eating and drinking

A patient with a tracheostomy may experience dysphagia due to oesophageal compression, so a soft diet is recommended. Following pharyngeal pouch repair or removal of foreign body, a soft diet is also advised in order to allow the affected area to heal comfortably. By contrast, the recommendation is to eat a normal, textured diet following tonsillectomy, for reasons discussed above.

Discharge planning and patient education

General advice is given to the patient regarding diet and pain control, and any take-home medication is explained. Patients having undergone a tonsillectomy receive written advice (Box 12.16) as a means of reinforcing important issues. Follow-up in the outpatient clinic ranges between 2 and 6 weeks.

Patients with a long-term tracheostomy are discharged with well-prepared community nursing support. Suctioning and nebulizing equipment may be delivered to the home, and the patient and family must have demonstrated competence in providing total tracheostomy care before discharge. Often, a trial at home, in the form of weekend or day leave, has been performed in order to assess the patient's and family's ability to cope.

Regular visits to the outpatient clinic are recommended, to facilitate tube change and assessment of the patient's progress (tube change is recommended on a monthly basis to prevent infection and tube occlusion). The patient and family are advised to contact the ward with any concerns or problems.

Head and neck

Conditions of the head and neck that require surgery

This branch of ENT surgery covers a wide range of conditions, often malignant, which require surgery and/or radiotherapy treatments. The activities of breathing, communicating, eating and drinking, and expressing healthy body image can be profoundly affected by both disease and treatment. Body image can be altered dramatically as a result of the disfiguring nature of the surgery. Care is specialized, with the aim of rehabilitating the patient to an altered way of life through education, and empathic support of the individual and family.

Head and neck neoplasms seem to occur more commonly in individuals who have been exposed to the following:

- smoking or snuff-taking
- alcohol
- hardwood dust
- heavy metals, e.g. chromium
- radiation
- viruses
  (Dhillon & East, 2013).

The following gives a brief overview of head and neck disease and surgery offered.

Salivary gland neoplasm

The majority of salivary gland tumours are in the parotid glands and are benign; incidence of malignancy is greater in the submandibular glands (American Cancer Society, 2019).

Parotidectomy is removal of the parotid gland. The risk of damage to the facial nerve is explained to the patient; often, facial weakness is temporary, due to surgical swelling.

Submandibular gland excision carries the risk of injuring the submandibular branches of the facial nerve; this can be permanent.

Box 12.16 **Discharge advice following a tonsillectomy**

- Rest for 2 weeks and take time off work.
- Eat a normal diet, as chewing and swallowing textured food relieves pain and cleanses the tonsillar beds, and this helps to prevent infection.
- Drink plenty of fluids (2−3 L per day).
- Be strict with hygiene and use a mouthwash and gargle after meals.
- This is a painful procedure. Discomfort may increase between the 4th and 8th day, when a membrane loosens off the tonsil beds, which is normal. Take regular analgesics, especially prior to meals.
- You may suffer earache. This is normal, as the nerve supply to the tonsil area and ears is connected.
- Avoid smoking and being in crowded places; keep away from people with colds and coughs. This will help to prevent local irritation and infection.
- White spots at the back of the throat are normal and are part of the healing process.
- The above advice is important; it is vital to eat and drink normally, in order to make a good recovery. If you experience any of the following symptoms, contact the ward or hospital emergency department, as these are signs of infection and may require readmission to hospital:
  - Severe and worsening pain.
  - Bleeding.
  - A raised temperature.

Neoplasm of the ear

Chronic ear infection may induce malignant disease in the pinna, ear canal and middle ear. Sun overexposure may lead to external ear malignancy.

Surgery ranges from a wedge-shaped excision of the pinna to radical resection of the total ear and surrounding tissues.

Neoplasms of the nose and sinuses

These are rare and may require ophthalmic, plastic, maxillofacial or neurosurgical collaboration. The close proximity to the eyes, face, jaw and brain requires delicate and precise resection, salvage and reconstruction. The ENT surgeon plays a key role in the management of these patients.

Nasopharyngeal neoplasm

Treatment for tumours arising in this region may involve surgical resection; clearance of disease is difficult, and radiotherapy may be a preferred treatment option.

Hypopharyngeal neoplasm

Benign tumours are rare. Typically, in malignant disease, patients are smokers and frequent users of alcohol. The disease can develop without severe symptoms; a mild sensation of 'something in the throat' is often the earliest complaint (Dhillon & East, 2013). Upon diagnosis, the tumour has grown sufficiently to require surgery and/or radiotherapy. The larynx, pharynx and possibly part of the oesophagus are removed; the oesophagus may be reconstructed with jejunum (Medina & Vasan, 2018). Between 30% and 40% of those treated survive 5 years (American Cancer Society, 2017).

Oropharyngeal neoplasia

The posterior third of the tongue, the floor of mouth, epiglottis, soft palate, uvula, tonsils and pharyngeal wall can be affected by malignancy, commonly squamous cell carcinoma. Metastatic spread to lymph nodes occurs because of the rich lymphatic supply in these areas. Surgical resection may involve removal of the affected oropharynx, part of the mandible if disease involves the bone, and reconstructive repair using muscle and skin flaps. Postoperative radiotherapy aims to eliminate residual malignant disease.

Laryngeal neoplasm

Benign tumours are rare, and squamous cell carcinoma is the most common malignant disease. Symptoms often include altered voice (dysphonia), dysphagia and, in advanced cases, breathing difficulties. Treatment may include endoscopic partial laryngectomy using a laser, or 'open' surgical removal of the larynx (laryngectomy) and neck dissection if neck nodes are affected. Postoperative radiotherapy may also be arranged. Fig. 12.5 demonstrates the altered anatomy following a laryngectomy.

Neck lumps

Commonly, lateral neck lumps are metastatic malignant disease, i.e. the distant spread of a malignant carcinoma, with its primary site often within the structures of the pharynx and larynx. In order to ascertain full diagnosis, a thorough clinical investigation is required.

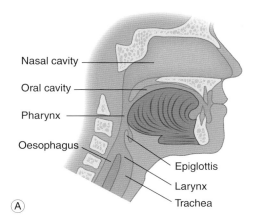

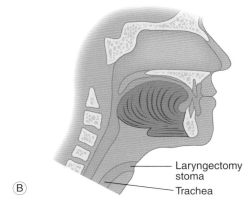

Figure 12.5 Altered anatomy following laryngectomy. (A) Before surgery. (B) After surgery.

Specific investigations for patients requiring head and neck surgery

Investigations include the following.
- Fine-needle aspiration of neck lump for cytology to determine the nature of the carcinoma: e.g. squamous cell.
- Radiology:
  - X-rays can demonstrate gross pathology.
  - CT/ MRI scanning reveals accurate images of disease and metastatic spread.
  - PET scan if recurrence, and/or following chemotherapy/radiotherapy.
- Endoscopy under general anaesthetic ± biopsy of any abnormal lesions; this may include laryngoscopy, pharyngoscopy and oesophagoscopy. The diagnosis may be determined using the international TNM classification (Box 12.17).

Assessment of a patient requiring surgery to the head and neck

The following activities of living specific to the needs of individuals suffering with head and neck disease who require surgery need to be assessed.

Breathing

Assessing the patient's normal respiratory function is essential, as head and neck disease and surgery involve the risk of acute airway obstruction. The patient may be experiencing breathing difficulties due to the effects of the tumour on laryngeal function and patency of the airway.

Maintaining a safe environment

Because of the rich blood supply to the head and neck, hae-morrhage and haematoma are potential postoperative risks. Assessing the patient's cardiovascular observations is performed preoperatively as a baseline. Some patients may be heavy drinkers or alcoholics: determining their weekly alcohol unit intake on initial assessment helps to prepare for any postoperative complications regarding alcohol withdrawal, and medication can be given in order to alleviate symptoms of withdrawal.

Controlling body temperature

The risk of postoperative infection requires assessment of the patient's temperature and ability to heal. Previous radiotherapy to the area can predispose to poor wound healing because of its effects on tissue integrity. Head and neck disease and major surgery can weaken the body's immune system, resulting in increased vulnerability to infections.

Assessing for early signs of infection, e.g. chest (pneumonia) and mouth (oral thrush), is therefore routine practice.

Eating and drinking

Often, patients are admitted having experienced dysphagia and weight loss for some time; they can be underweight and malnourished, so building up with fortified foods and drinks is required to maximize well-being for surgery. All patients are weighed, and this continues on a regular basis (three times per week) until discharge.

Preparing the patient for difficulties in eating and drinking during the postoperative phase is also undertaken. The admitting practitioner assesses the patient's understanding of the surgery and aftercare, in particular the need for prolonged 'nil by mouth' (approximately 7−14 days), enteral tube feeding, and the need for soft or puréed food once oral intake is permitted.

Box 12.17 **TNM classification**

Head and neck cancer diagnosis and prognosis use the tumour—node—metastases classification (Sobin et al, 2010) to describe:

- Tumour (T) — size of primary tumour.
- Nodes (N) — if regional lymph nodes have cancer in them.
- Metastases (M) — if cancer has spread to a different part of the body.

The UICC (International Union Against Cancer) TNM classification promotes a consensus of one global clinically relevant staging classification for cancer.

Elimination

Assessment of the patient's normal bladder and bowel functions is performed. Poor fluid and food intake prior to surgery may cause constipation. Preoperative urinalysis is performed to detect any abnormalities.

Communicating

Preoperatively, patients may complain of a hoarse voice (laryngeal disease), and discomfort or pain in the affected area can make speaking arduous. The speech therapist performs a thorough assessment of the patient preoperatively, and this includes an evaluation for appropriate methods of speech restoration.

Body image

Disfiguring disease and surgery of the head and neck often result in altered body image and low self-esteem. It is vitally important to prepare the patient as much as possible prior to surgery, and this includes an assessment of the patient's perception of disease and surgery, their effects on activities of living and the scarring involved.

Personal cleansing and dressing

As discussed previously, self-esteem is affected in patients with head and neck disease; the activity of cleansing and dressing is just as relevant. Any disfigurement may lead to a change in dress style, with the emphasis on covering up an unfortunate end-result.

Therefore, it is important to assess patients' style and views on presenting themselves, as well as their perceptions of postoperative recovery and appearance.

Working and social

Establishing the patient's occupation, social activities and home situation is essential for rehabilitation and discharge. For some, a long period of absence from work is required in order to allow for full treatment, which may include radiotherapy, and recovery. This could range between 2 and 12 months. Stopping work completely or changing occupation may be advised, as the surgery may irrevocably affect work performance, e.g. laryngectomy. Changes to an individual's lifestyle can be deeply distressing, both emotionally and financially. Assessing the need for social services is therefore indicated, and a referral can then be made.

Dying

Fears of dying can be overwhelming when dealing with a diagnosis of cancer or when facing major surgery and months of rehabilitation. The practitioner can explore these complex issues and provide realistic postoperative expectations, offering an empathetic and attentive approach when giving care. Head and neck cancer patients build very close and enduring bonds with their practitioners over prolonged hospital treatments.

Case study

The following case study of a patient undergoing a laryngectomy for squamous cell carcinoma of the larynx is presented to demonstrate aspects of care relevant to the field of head and neck surgery.

Mr Benedict Warren is admitted to the ward for a total laryngectomy the next day. He was diagnosed with cancer of the larynx following a laryngoscopy two weeks earlier.

Benedict is 63 years of age, married with children and grandchildren, and took retirement from banking three years ago.

Assessment

Box 12.18 details the assessment of Benedict upon admission for a laryngectomy.

Specific preoperative preparation

In the outpatient department, the following procedures will be performed:
- CT scanning.
- Blood tests, electrocardiogram (ECG) and chest X-ray.

Box 12.18 **Preoperative assessment of a patient undergoing laryngectomy**

Maintaining a safe environment

- Observation of vital signs is performed: pulse, 76 beats per minute and regular; blood pressure, 155/85 mmHg.
- Allergies: none known.
- Past medical history: atrial fibrillation diagnosed 2 years ago; dental clearance under general anaesthetic 1 year ago; 4 month history of hoarse voice; laryngoscopy 2 weeks ago diagnosing laryngeal carcinoma.
- Medication: digoxin 125 μg daily; occasional paracetamol for throat discomfort.
- Benedict is very anxious about surgery and his recovery; in particular, how he will cope with the laryngectomy stoma.

Breathing

- Respiration rate is 16 respirations per minute.
- Mild stridor (noisy breathing) noted.
- Oxygen saturation on air is 94%.
- Chest X-ray is satisfactory.
- Benedict smoked 20—30 cigarettes per day for 35 years and cut down to 10—15 per day since hoarseness of voice began; still has 5 cigarettes per day since diagnosis.

Controlling body temperature

- Benedict's temperature is 36.4°C.

Communicating

- Hoarseness of voice is apparent; Benedict's voice gets tired easily.
- Glasses are worn for reading.
- Normal hearing is present.
- Benedict states he is concerned that he will be unable to communicate after surgery, but he has come with a large pad of paper and pens. His son has made him a communication board to use while in hospital.
- Benedict and his wife have met the speech therapist and discussed voice rehabilitation; he is to be a candidate for Blom—Singer valve insertion, which he is pleased about.
- Benedict and his family have been reading the laryngectomy booklets, and he has brought them with him.

Eating and drinking

- Benedict manages a normal diet but avoids foods that require a lot of chewing, because of throat discomfort.
- Height is 1.84 m; weight is 82 kg.
- His appetite has become poor since diagnosis, due to apprehension.
- Benedict admits to being a heavy alcohol drinker (about 40 units per week) for many years but he has cut down to about 10 units per week, mainly wine, since diagnosis of his cardiac condition.

Personal cleansing and dressing

- Benedict dresses smartly. He requests to see the laryngectomy bibs and filters (devices worn over a laryngectomy stoma which protect the airway from airborne particles and help to humidify inhaled air). He takes a bath every night.

Mobility

- Benedict is independent.

Working and social

- Benedict retired from banking 3 years ago and enjoys a busy, varied home life. He and his wife holiday abroad twice a year and regularly visit his children and their families.
- Benedict's hobbies include gardening, golfing, socializing and amateur dramatics. He is saddened that he will no longer be able to perform on stage but hopes to continue with the drama club in a different way once radiotherapy after surgery is complete.

(Continued)

Box 12.18 (cont'd)

Body image

- Benedict is concerned that being dependent on staff will compromise his masculinity, and he states that he is 'not looking forward to the baby food'.

Sleeping

- Sleep has been disrupted by the hoarseness of voice and mild stridor, particularly in the past month. Since diagnosis, his sleep pattern is more erratic; he tends to manage 6 hours sleep, though wakes four or five times.

Elimination

- Benedict opens his bowels daily, and micturition is normal; urinalysis shows no abnormalities.
- Benedict knows that following a laryngectomy, regular bowel activity should be maintained, as the ability to close the glottis for straining is lost.

Dying

- Benedict feels confident about having an anaesthetic.
- He does state that, for the first time since his cardiac condition was diagnosed, he is fearful for the future.

- Meeting the speech therapist and discussing speech rehabilitation.
- Meeting a laryngectomy patient (if the patient requests).
- Preparation for surgery: i.e. discussion of surgery, altered anatomy, potential postoperative complications (difficulty in eating and drinking, and swelling), and the giving of information booklets.

Once admitted to the ward, psychological and physical preparations continue for the patient and family.

Postoperative care

The specific postoperative care for the activity of breathing is explored in the care plan (Box 12.19).

Postoperative care of patients who have had head and neck surgery

The following aims to clarify other specific potential problems for a patient having undergone a laryngectomy.

Maintaining a safe environment

Continuous observation of the patient's vital signs for signs of haemorrhage is indicated, as surgery involves an area containing a very rich blood supply. The risk of haematoma is also present for the same reason, and, in order to minimize this risk, two Redivac drains are inserted, one on each side of the neck, which drain blood and tissue fluid from the surgical site. Chapter 5 discusses care of surgical drains and wounds in more detail.

The patient who has undergone a laryngectomy tends to experience moderate pain and discomfort during the postoperative period. Often there are areas of numbness in the neck region due to the loss of more superficial nerves during surgical resection. A patient-controlled analgesia (PCA) system is used for the first 2–3 days, after which regular analgesics are given until no longer required. Chapter 8 discusses pain control in more detail.

Controlling body temperature

Prolonged 'nil by mouth' may precipitate oral fungal infection, i.e. thrush, so assessing the mouth for early signs and providing hourly mouth care in order to keep the oral mucosa moist and clean are necessary.

The laryngectomy stoma and neck incision wounds need constant assessment, and dressings to these areas are minimal. Often, a transparent vapour-permeable film dressing (e.g. OpSite) is applied over the stapled areas of the neck, with light gauze in place around the drains.

Eating and drinking

Most types of head and neck surgery, except salivary gland or neck lump excisions, require a prolonged period of 'nil by mouth' in order to allow the affected areas to heal. Enteral feeding aims to maintain the patient's nutritional status until an adequate oral diet is taken. Feeding tubes come in a variety of forms: nasogastric, percutaneous endoscopic gastrostomy (PEG), or jejunostomy. Once an oral diet is permitted, soft or puréed food is

Box 12.19 **Postoperative care of the activity of breathing for a patient having undergone a laryngectomy**

Benedict returns to the ward, orientated but drowsy. A tracheostomy tube (Shiley size 8, plain, cuffed and inflated) is in the laryngectomy stoma, secured with tapes; 40% humidified oxygen is in progress. Two surgical Redivac drains have been inserted, one on each side of the neck.

- *Problem*: Potential loss of clear airway and respiratory difficulty due to the effects of anaesthetic drugs, drowsiness, surgical swelling and the newly formed laryngectomy stoma.
- *Goal*: To maintain a clear airway and patent laryngectomy stoma. For Benedict to adapt to the laryngectomy stoma and to learn self-care.
- *Care*:
  - Ensure the oxygen and suction equipment function correctly, as Benedict relies upon them throughout his hospital stay.
  - Care for Benedict close to the nurses' station in clear view, in order to facilitate safe observation.
  - Benedict has lost the ability to speak, so provide alternative methods for communicating: call bell at hand always, pen and paper and communication picture board; encourage Benedict to mouth words and use gestures.

The first 72 hours

- Though it is a permanent structure, surgical swelling and secretions can occlude the laryngectomy stoma. To prevent this, ensure the tracheostomy tube remains *in situ*, well secured with tapes, until doctors instruct otherwise.
- Spare tracheostomy tubes (one the same type and size; the other, same type, one size smaller) and tracheal dilators should be kept at Benedict's bedside, as this enables a rapid change of tracheostomy tube if the tube becomes irreversibly blocked or displaced. Having a lower size at hand is safe practice in case the laryngectomy stoma shrinks.
- Benedict should be in an upright position with his head and neck well supported with pillows. These actions help to maintain a clear airway and to promote expectoration of secretions and surgical drainage; comfortable support reduces strain on the head, neck and surgical incisions.
- Benedict has permanently lost the ability to humidify and warm inhaled air, due to altered anatomy; alternative methods must be provided:
  - Ensure the prescribed oxygen always runs through a mechanical thermohumidifier.
  - Administer nebulized saline as prescribed.
  - Ensure a tracheostomy mask is used, as facemasks are not suitable for the neck region.
- These actions ensure inhaled oxygen is humidified and warmed, and that secretions remain loose, thus preventing tracheal irritation.
- Perform observations of respiratory status {1/4}-hourly for the first 2 hours and reduce regimen to 1–2-hourly overnight if condition is stable and observations are within normal limits. Frequency can be reduced thereafter to 4-hourly if Benedict is recovering well.
- Observations include those of:
  - Respiratory rate, depth, rhythm
  - Use of accessory muscles
  - Signs of cyanosis or pallor
  - % saturations of blood oxygen
  - Nature of tracheal secretions.
- Continually observe for accumulation of tracheal secretions, which will be apparent as any of the following signs:
  - Rhonchi (low-pitched gurgling)
  - Wheeze
  - Dyspnoea
  - Restlessness or anxiety
  - Poor air flow on expiration (detected by placing a hand close to the tracheostomy tube entrance)
  - Falling saturation levels of blood oxygen.
- If any of the above is noted, remove inner cannula of the tracheostomy tube and rinse away any secretions contained within, then dry and re-insert. Encourage Benedict to cough (impaired now due to loss of larynx) and perform deep breathing exercises in order to assist expectoration of secretions.
- If Benedict continues to show signs of respiratory difficulty, perform tracheal suctioning, following the recommended technique (see Box 12.15).

(Continued)

Box 12.19 (cont'd)

- Checking the inner cannula of Benedict's tracheostomy tube and any suctioning should be performed every 1–2 hours until the next morning because secretions can accumulate without obvious signs. Thereafter, this can be reduced to 2–4 hourly or as required.
- Maintain inflation of the tracheostomy tube cuff; this prevents aspiration of any secretions from the surgical site and from the tracheo-oesophageal puncture; monitor cuff pressure every 4 hours using the cuff manometer; overinflation of the cuff causes tracheal irritation and necrosis.
- Deflate cuff with a syringe only on doctor's instructions (usually after 2–3 days); secretions will have accumulated on top of the cuff; in order to prevent their aspiration, perform immediate suction.
- Maintain a stoma care chart, recording the following information:
  - Time of care given
  - Description of secretions
  - Episodes of checking and cleansing of inner tube and of suction
  - Episodes of checking cuff pressure.
- This chart facilitates evaluation of Benedict's progress, acts as an accurate reference for physiotherapists, doctors and other healthcare professionals, and ensures thorough record-keeping.
- The next morning, refer Benedict to the ward physiotherapist for assessment and input as required.

Days 3–7

- Perform care as already outlined but reduce the frequency of observations (to 6 hourly); laryngectomy stoma care and suction are given as required.
- Liaise with the doctors regarding the removal of Benedict's tracheostomy tube (once cuff is deflated), as prolonged use of the tube can cause tracheal irritation and mucosal breakdown.
- Upon the doctor's request, remove the tracheostomy tube and insert an appropriately sized stoma button (a small, tubular, plastic device) in order to support the stoma, prevent shrinkage and maintain airway.
- If the stoma button is prone to popping out, secure with neck tapes.
- Remove button as required in order to clean secretions; rinse it through, dry and re- insert.
- Continue to keep a spare tracheostomy tube and stoma button (of matching size) by Benedict's bedside, in case of sudden respiratory difficulty or occlusion of airway.
- Once Benedict's oxygen saturation levels appear within normal limits, tested when the oxygen is temporarily removed, and upon doctor's instructions, discontinue the humidified oxygen therapy, but continue to monitor oxygen saturations and respirations 6-hourly in order to detect respiratory insufficiency or difficulty.
- Continue to provide humidification by other means:
  - Regular saline nebulizers, which are particularly effective in loosening tenacious secretions
  - Saline-moistened gauze veils, which are secured with neck tapes and cover the laryngectomy stoma
  - Moistened laryngectomy bibs.
- Observe secretions for amount, viscosity and colour – blood-staining should have resolved.

Days 7 to discharge: the rehabilitation phase

- Begin to teach Benedict stoma care; step-by-step, instruct Benedict on how to clean the stoma with saline and gauze, how to cough and wipe away any secretions, and how to clean and insert the stoma button; adapt the teaching process to a pace that suits Benedict and his family, as this will enable better understanding and absorption of information.
- Supervise Benedict performing his own stoma care and give constructive feedback, including positive evaluation; reinforce the teaching process until Benedict is competent and self-caring.
- Include the family as much as possible during this time, as they will be feeling very apprehensive about Benedict's well-being and how to care for a laryngectomy stoma.
- If the stoma shows no evidence of shrinkage, and if the doctors instruct, remove the stoma button and leave the stoma exposed; the need for a button is indicated if the chin or neck flesh occludes the stoma, particularly more so at night when asleep.
- Remove stoma sutures as instructed (usually day 14); by then, the tracheal structure has healed in its new position.

Evaluation of care

Throughout, Benedict was cared for near to the nurses' station, and close observation of his condition was possible.

(Continued)

Box 12.19 (cont'd)

Safe and effective communication was achieved by Benedict writing things down, by using a picture board for the first day, as Benedict soon preferred other means, and by gesturing basic requests. Soon he was mouthing words and staff often easily understood these. Benedict kept hold of his call bell for the first 2 days, as he felt very anxious if it was out of sight. As his condition improved, Benedict became more relaxed and confident about communicating with staff and visitors. Oxygen and suctioning equipment were checked every shift; no faults were found, and they functioned correctly.

The first 72 hours

Benedict was very drowsy for the first 6 hours and was prone to slipping down the bed; two practitioners strategically placed pillows (behind the head, neck, torso and each arm), and an upright position was achieved.

The tracheostomy tube was secure; tapes were changed every shift to prevent soiling and hardening.

Forty per cent humidified oxygen was continuously maintained. Saturation levels of blood oxygen ranged between 96% and 99%; after 2 days, random tests of oxygen saturations on air were performed, but results fell below 90%, indicating that oxygen therapy was required in order to prevent hypoxia. His respiratory rate ranged between 14 and 20 rpm. Cleansing of the inner cannula of the tracheostomy tube and suctioning was performed every hour until the next morning — secretions were bloodstained and loose.

They then became more copious and viscous but remained bloodstained for the next 2 days. Inner cannula care and suctioning was required frequently, often every {1/2}–2 hours, in order to keep Benedict's airway patent. Saline nebulizers were prescribed and given every 4 hours; secretions appeared looser as a result. Benedict felt very anxious when secretions were building up, as he felt unable to breathe; he would use the call bell and gesture to the practitioners frequently for assistance. As the amount of secretions reduced, Benedict appeared to relax more.

On day 2, Benedict suddenly became acutely distressed: his respirations were 25 rpm, oxygen saturation was 88%, and there was minimal air flow felt by the tracheostomy opening. The inner tube was clear, so immediate suction was performed, and on the third attempt a large, sticky plug of accumulated bloodstained secretions was removed.

Benedict's respiratory status returned to normal, but he was very shaken by this episode. It was explained that mucous plugs could form from a combination of sputum, surgical secretions and under-humidification. Benedict was comforted and reassured that his laryngectomy stoma was functioning well and that mucous plugs were not uncommon.

Saline nebulizers were increased to 2–4 hourly in order to prevent under-humidification; this episode never occurred again. The cuff of the tracheostomy tube was checked every 4 hours in order to maintain safe pressure, and it was deflated, upon doctor's request, on day 3. A lot of stale bloodstained secretions were immediately suctioned out.

The physiotherapist assessed Benedict the next morning and found his lungs to be mildly consolidated. Twice-daily treatment was given for 3 days until his chest appeared clearer. Deep breathing and coughing exercises were taught, which helped Benedict to expectorate more efficiently.

Days 3–7

The nature of secretions had improved by day 5 and they were less viscous and clearer. The physiotherapist visited daily, mainly to check Benedict's progress. Benedict's suctioning needs were reduced to 3–4-hourly, as he was managing to expectorate more easily now into the inner cannula of the tracheostomy tube. Secretions were cleared more by cleansing the inner cannula than by performing suction. The intensity of humidification was reduced because the secretions were looser, and saline nebulizers were given 4–6-hourly.

The doctors instructed removal of the tracheostomy tube on day 5. The laryngectomy stoma was well formed and large; but if Benedict bent his head down, neck tissue, which was still swollen, occluded 50% of the stoma. A stoma button was inserted and secured with neck tapes, and this appeared to maintain stoma patency. Benedict had found the tracheostomy tube cumbersome and uncomfortable, so felt happier with the button *in situ*.

The button was removed every 2–4 hours, and any secretions were rinsed away.

Benedict's suctioning needs reduced as the week progressed, and by day 7 his secretions were minimal and suction was only required once or twice per shift.

Days 7 to discharge

Benedict and his family were keen to learn stoma care, so, once Benedict's chest secretions had become minimal, they were taught the basics. His family brought in a large tabletop mirror for Benedict to use when performing stoma care. Benedict needed to wear his glasses in order to visualize his stoma clearly. Benedict successfully managed to remove, clean, dry and re-insert the stoma button after only 2 days of instruction and supervision.

Benedict found the cleaning of his stoma more difficult, partly because his very large hands and fingers blocked his view and made it awkward to retrieve any secretions.

(Continued)

Box 12.19 (cont'd)

Benedict's wife offered to assist him, and she quickly learnt the techniques involved. Secretions would often dry and form crusts near the opening of the stoma, and she was able to use forceps to pick these away. Benedict remained enthusiastic and was determined to manage his own care so that he did not need to rely upon his wife. By his discharge, he had become more skillful and dexterous and was able to clean his stoma competently, though he left the picking of crusts to his wife.

By day 12, Benedict was wearing the stoma button only at night, when support was required while asleep. There appeared to be no evidence of stoma shrinkage during the day. However, Benedict and his family were advised to monitor stoma circumference once at home, as it could reduce over time, particularly while undergoing radiotherapy.

Radiotherapy causes local inflammation and swelling to the neck and stoma and can persist for weeks once treatment is complete. If any shrinkage is apparent, Benedict should wear the button all the time until side-effects settle.

By day 14, Benedict rarely required suctioning (once per day maximum), but the ward had requested that the district nurses provide a portable suction machine for home in case of emergency. The need for saline nebulizers (6-hourly) continued, as Benedict was prone to drying of secretions; again, the district nurses had arranged a nebulizer machine for home. Both these items of equipment were delivered prior to Benedict taking day and overnight leave before official discharge. Stoma sutures were removed on day 14; some sutures were deeply embedded, so, in order to make the procedure as comfortable as possible, surface anaesthetic cream (e.g. EMLA) was applied 1 hour prior to removal.

recommended, as the muscles involved in chewing and swallowing, including the tongue, are often greatly affected. The speech therapist can perform a swallowing assessment upon request and provide invaluable advice for improving any difficulties in swallowing. Chapter 6 discusses nutrition and enteral feeding in more detail.

Elimination

Postoperative enteral feeding can precipitate loose stools or diarrhoea, and, for some time after surgery, a urinary catheter may be *in situ* to facilitate micturition. Relying on commodes, bedpans or urinals can cause embarrassment to the patient, making this activity more awkward.

Communicating

Surgical removal of the larynx implies permanent loss of the ability to speak.

Postoperative rehabilitation by the speech therapist occurs over a long period of time and can be a slow, frustrating process for the patient. The electronic larynx and the Blom–Singer valve are examples of speech aids used. Preparations for the latter begin on the operating table with the formation of a tracheo-oesophageal puncture; this is a hole made in the tracheal wall which connects the trachea with the oesophagus, and which is large enough to initially house an enteral feeding tube (usually Ryles) and then the Blom–Singer valve itself. The speech therapist inserts the valve in the outpatient clinic, often weeks later, once radiotherapy and wound healing are complete. Until valve insertion occurs, the Ryles tube is used to keep the puncture site patent.

Body image

Some patients feel belittled by the presence of tube feeding and their dependency on staff to meet their daily needs. Tubes and equipment hinder the ability to attend to independence and self-care; subsequently, patients may feel depressed and suffer with low self-esteem. Once discharged home, maintaining intimate relationships can be awkward, and problems may arise. By providing thoughtful, and individualized care, both in hospital and at home with community support, one aims to alleviate these negative emotions. Chapter 7 discusses issues surrounding body image in more detail.

Discharge planning and education of patients who have had head and neck surgery

This commences in the preadmission clinic and continues throughout admission, as both the patient and family require a lot of support and preparation prior to discharge. For patients who have undergone laryngectomy or other major head and neck surgery, it is good practice to have a trial at home, either as day or weekend leave, in order to assess the patient's and family's ability to cope. Input from social services may be necessary, especially if the patient lives alone and requires assistance with the activities of washing, dressing, housework and shopping; any preparations required for this will have begun in the preoperative phase with the initial assessment, and postoperative home visits may be undertaken to assess the patient's needs.

Community nursing support is often required: district nurses can provide suctioning and nebulizing equipment if appropriate; supervision of stoma care and nutritional intake, including enteral feeding if this is continuing, can be maintained by community nurses; and although direct physical care may not be indicated, there is a need for psychological support and care, especially during the period of radiotherapy treatment.

Follow-up in the outpatient department ranges between 1 and 6 weeks. Radiotherapy treatment is often planned once the patient has settled back home and the wounds have healed.

Conclusion

This chapter has endeavoured to demonstrate the range of surgical procedures and patient care that represents the field of ear, nose and throat surgery. Recent surgical advances, including preservation of the hemilarynx, transoral laser surgery for pharyngeal and laryngeal malignancy, laser stapes surgery, bone-anchored hearing aids, and transnasal endoscopic sinus, neurological and ophthalmic surgery, all aim to provide the patient with the best result, using minimally invasive techniques that require an acute, shorter hospitalization and demand practitioners to provide excellent ENT care.

The ENT ward is a dynamic and challenging environment in which to practice, and has become an area of practice enriched with opportunities for professional development and fulfilment. Caring for a variety of individuals undergoing routine procedures and specialized complex surgery provides the practitioner with invaluable knowledge and skills, in particular concerning airway management, communication, nutrition and psychological care, which are of immense benefit in all healthcare settings.

SUMMARY OF KEY POINTS

- Having an understanding of relevant anatomy and physiology enables the practitioner to anticipate, plan and provide best practice.

(Continued)

(cont'd)

- A comprehensive assessment of the patient's physical and psychological status forms the basis on which to plan, implement and evaluate care.
- Clinical investigation of ENT disease encompasses patient history, audiometry, radiology, allergy testing, sleep studies, endoscopy and biopsy.
- Specific complications include the following:
  - ear surgery: further hearing loss, facial palsy or dizziness
  - nasal/sinus surgery: haemorrhage and infection
  - throat surgery: loss of a clear airway, dysphagia and reduced ability to communicate.
- Head and neck surgery encompasses a wide range of surgical techniques that aim to remove benign and malignant neoplasia and as far as possible restore function to the affected area.
- Specialized care is required for safe recovery and successful rehabilitation for the patient and their family.
- Discharge planning and patient education begins preoperatively in the outpatient clinic.
- A high standard of tracheostomy care is imperative; knowledge of altered anatomy, variety of tracheostomy tubes and the implications of breathing, eating, drinking and communicating with a stoma are vital.
- Written advice sheets are an invaluable patient education tool and should be given to most patients.

REFLECTIVE LEARNING POINTS

Having read this chapter, think about what you now know and what you still need to find out about. These questions may help:

- How can having ENT surgery have a bearing on a person's body image?
- ENT surgery affects the senses and ear surgery can impact on hearing and balance. What advice would the nurse offer the patient to ensure they are able to maintain a safe environment postoperatively?
- How can the nurse, when caring for people with cancer affecting the mouth, oral cavity, pharynx, larynx, salivary glands, or the nose and sinuses, ensure that care is patient-centred?

References

American Cancer Society. (2017). *Survival rates for laryngeal and hypopharyngeal cancers*. American Cancer Society. Available at: <www.cancer.org/cancer/laryngeal- and-hypopharyngeal-cancer/detection-diagnosis-staging/survival-rates.html>.

American Cancer Society. (2019). *About salivary gland cancer*. Atlanta: American Cancer Society. Available at: <www.cancer.org/cancer/salivary-gland-cancer/about.html>.

Behrbohm, H. (2015). *The nose - revision and reconstruction*. Stuttgart: Thieme.

Campbell, K. (2018). *Impedance audiometry*. Medscape. Available at: emedicine. medscape.com/article/1831254-overview.

Dhillon, R., & East, C. (2013). *An illustrated text: ear, nose and throat and head and neck surgery* (4th ed.). Edinburgh: Churchill Livingstone.

Freeman, S., & Kahwaji, C. (2018). Physiology, nasal. In S. Bolla (Ed.), *StatPearls [online]*. StatPearls Publishing. Available at: <www.ncbi. nlm.nih.gov/books/NBK526086/>.

Heidari, M., & Shahbaz, S. (2017). Nurses' awareness about principles of airway suctioning. *Journal of Clinical and Diagnostic Research, 11*(8), 17−19.

Holland, K. (2008). *Applying the Roper-Logan-Tierney model in practice* (2nd ed.). Edinburgh: Churchill Livingstone.

Lalwani, A. (2012). *Current diagnosis and treatment otolaryngology - head and neck surgery* (3rd ed.). Maidenhead: McGraw-Hill.

Luers, J., & Hüttenbrink, K.-B. (2016). Surgical anatomy and pathology of the middle ear. *Journal of Anatomy, 228*(2), 338−353.

Medina, J., & Vasan, N. (2018). *Cancer of the oral cavity, pharynx and larynx evidence-based decision making*. Geneva: Springer International Publishing.

Myatt, R. (2015). Nursing care of patients with a temporary tracheostomy. *Nursing Standard, 29*(26), 42−49.

Nursing and Midwifery Council. (2018). *The Code. Professional standards of practice and behaviour for nurses, midwives and nursing associates*. Available at: <www.nmc.org.uk/globalassets/sitedocuments/nmc-publications/nmc-code.pdf>

Pires, A., Fortuna, A., Alves, G., & Falcão, A. (2009). Intranasal drug delivery: how, why and what for? *Journal of Pharmacy and Pharmaceutical Sciences, 12*(3), 288−311.

Sobin, L., Gospodarowicz, M., & Wittekind, C. (2010). *TNM classification of malignant tumours* (7th ed.). Chichester: Wiley.

Tysome, J., & Kanegaonkar, R. (2017). *ENT: an introduction and practical guide* (2nd ed.). Florida: CRC Press-Taylor and Francis Group.

Van De Water, T. (2012). Historical aspects of inner ear anatomy and biology that underlie the design of hearing and balance prosthetic devices. *The Anatomical Record, 295*(11), 1741−1759.

Further reading

Bull, T., & Almeyda, J. (2009). *A color atlas of ENT diagnosis* (5th edn). London: Mosby-Wolfe.

Cascarini, L. (2011). *Oxford handbook of oral and maxillofacial surgery*. Oxford: Oxford University Press.

Dhillon, R., & East, C. (2013). *An illustrated text: ear, nose and throat and head and neck surgery* (4th ed.). Edinburgh: Churchill Livingstone.

Ludman, H. (2012). *ABC of ear, nose and throat*. London: BMJ Books.

Mitchell, D. (2015). *An introduction to oral and maxillofacial surgery*. Boca Raton: CRC Press, Taylor & Francis Group.

Munir, N. (2013). *Ear, nose and throat at a glance*. Chichester: Wiley-Blackwell.

Rogers, N. (2017). *Basic guide to oral and maxillofacial surgery*. Chichester: Wiley Blackwell.

Sami, A. S. (2017). *ENT made easy*. Banbury: Scion.

Scholes, M. (2015). *ENT secrets*. Philadelphia: Elsevier.

Scott, K. (2014). *Quick reference guide for otolaryngology: guide for APRNs, PAs, and other health care practitioners*. New York: Springer Publishing.

Relevant websites

American Cancer Society: www.cancer. org

British Medical Journals − Otolaryngology/ ENT: www.bmj.com/specialties/otolaryngology-ent

ENT UK: www.entuk.org

International Federation of Otorhino Laryngological Societies: www.ifos-world.org

National Institute on Deafness and Other Communication Disorders: www. nidcd.nih.gov

Royal College of Nursing − ENT and Maxillofacial Nursing: www.rcn.org.uk/get-involved/forums/ent-maxillofacial-nursing-forum

University of Cape Town − Professor Fagin: www.entdev.uct.ac.za

Chapter | **13** |

Patients requiring thyroid surgery

Deborah Robinson

KEY OBJECTIVES OF THE CHAPTER

At the end of the chapter the reader should be able to:
- describe the anatomy and physiology of the thyroid gland and related structures
- discuss the underlying conditions that require thyroid surgery
- explain the specific investigations required prior to thyroid surgery
- discuss specific issues related to nursing assessment
- discuss the relevant pre- and postoperative nursing care following surgery to the thyroid gland
- discuss the plan for a patient's discharge, including relevant patient education.

Areas to think about before reading the chapter

- What do you understand by the term myxoedema?
- Provide an overview of thyroid crisis.
- How many lobes does the thyroid have?

Introduction

People with a disorder of the thyroid gland may eventually require surgery, because of the effects on the body of an imbalance of the thyroid hormones, or due to malignancy. Indications of thyroid diseases include benign and malignant swellings, goitre, hypo/hyperthyroidism and inflammatory disorders. This chapter will explore issues related to the care of patients requiring thyroid surgery, recognizing issues related to the effect of an altered body image, and the potential complications that can occur.

Anatomy and physiology

The thyroid gland consists of two lobes, is highly vascular and lies either side of the trachea, and is situated in the anterior aspect of the neck, just below the larynx. The two lobes are joined by a band of tissue called the isthmus, which lies to the anterior surface of the trachea and is attached to trachea and cricoid cartilage by the ligament of Berry. The thyroid gland weighs approximately 20 g. The arterial blood supply to the gland comes from the superior and inferior thyroid arteries. The points at which these vessels enter the thyroid gland are important landmarks and are denoted as 'poles' of the thyroid. Venous drainage is through the superior, middle and inferior thyroid veins. The recurrent laryngeal nerves, a branch of the vagus nerve, supply the vocal cords, lie posterior to the thyroid gland and are responsible for innervating many of the intrinsic laryngeal muscles, as well as playing a vital role in voice production and airway maintenance. Lymphatic drainage is via the deep cervical chain (laterally) and to the pretracheal and mediastinal nodes (inferiorly).

The primary function of the thyroid gland is to produce three hormones: thyroxine, triiodothyronine and calcitonin. The lobes of the thyroid gland contain numerous follicles lined with epithelial cells. The follicles are filled with colloid, which is secreted from the epithelial cells. Thyroglobulin is a complex protein molecule that is also secreted from these epithelial cells. Iodine is an essential component for the synthesis of thyroxine and triiodothyronine. Production of the thyroid hormones is controlled by thyroid-stimulating hormone (TSH) from the anterior pituitary gland and by thyroid-releasing hormone (TRH) from the hypothalamus. The thyroid hormones thyroxine (T4) and triiodothyronine (T3) are stored in the form of thyroglobulin in the follicles prior to their release into the circulatory system (Marinelli, 2015). Thyroxine and triiodothyronine are essential for stimulating oxygen consumption of most cells within the body; regulating lipid and carbohydrate metabolism; normal growth and development; normal lactation; and the potentiation of the action of other hormones, e.g. insulin. Calcitonin is secreted by the parafollicular cells in response to an increase in blood calcium levels. It plays a part in reducing the calcium concentration in body fluids by promoting the excretion of calcium and phosphate in urine and movement into the bones.

The four parathyroid glands are attached to the posterior surface of the lateral lobes of the thyroid gland. The parathyroid glands secrete parathormone, a hormone that regulates the distribution and metabolism of calcium in the body. The blood concentration levels of calcium and phosphorus are regulated by its action on the intestine, bone and kidneys. It promotes the absorption of calcium in the intestine and the demineralization of bone and movement of calcium into the extracellular fluid. Undersecretion of the hormone can lead to low calcium levels, which will result in muscle spasm, e.g. tetany.

Disorders of the thyroid gland

Thyroid disorders tend to occur as a result of oversecretion of thyroid hormones, i.e. hyperthyroidism; undersecretion, i.e. hypothyroidism (myxoedema); or due to malignancy.

Goitre

Goitre refers to any enlargement of the thyroid gland and can occur in response to demand on the gland and includes benign or malignant nodules of the gland (Wilson & Giddens, 2009). A deficiency of iodine in the diet can also lead to the formation of a goitre.

A goitre presents as a mass in the neck which moves on swallowing. This is because the thyroid gland is attached to the larynx by fascia. The mass may be situated on one or both sides of the trachea. In some instances, the trachea may be displaced and compressed by the enlarged gland, which can lead to an alteration of tracheal, oesophageal and vocal function, and can compromise the patient's airway. On clinical examination, the doctor should be able to distinguish the shape and texture of the goitre. Goitres are often referred to as the following:

- smooth, non-toxic or physiological goitre
- nodular, non-toxic goitre
- smooth, toxic goitre (Graves' disease)
- toxic, nodular goitre (secondary thyrotoxicosis, known as Plummer's syndrome) (Franklin et al, 2012).

Hyperthyroidism

Hyperthyroidism, or thyrotoxicosis, can be caused by Graves' disease (an autoimmune disorder), toxic adenoma of the thyroid, and in multinodular goitres where the small thyroid nodules secrete excess thyroid hormone (Marinelli, 2015).

The prevalence of hyperthyroidism in females is 0.5–2% and is ten times more common in women than men (Franklin et al, 2012). The clinical features of hyperthyroidism vary between individuals (Table 13.1). Symptoms are characterized by an excess secretion of thyroid hormones and are due to increased catabolism, increased heat production, autonomic lability and increased sensitivity to catecholamines, and increased gastrointestinal activity.

Graves' disease can cause distressing symptoms of altered body image, because of the patient having a swollen neck, and the effect it has on the patient's eyes. This can range from the appearance of staring, to lid lag and lid retraction, and, in its severest form, exophthalmos. Exophthalmos (an abnormal protrusion of the eyeballs) and lid lag can result in corneal ulceration, which will cause visual disturbances, and in extreme cases can lead to papilloedema and an inability to move the eyeball (Lindholm & Laurberg, 2010).

Neoplasms of the thyroid gland

Neoplasms of the thyroid gland can be benign, e.g. an adenoma, or malignant. Malignant neoplasms of the thyroid can be divided into four groups – papillary, follicular, medullary and anaplastic. Thyroid cancer is the most

Table 13.1 Clinical features of hyperthyroidism (thyrotoxicosis)

Symptom	Problem
Weight loss	Muscle wasting Increased appetite Intolerance of heat Pyrexia Altered nutrition and metabolism
Tachycardia	Raised sleeping pulse Palpitations Angina Possible atrial fibrillation Increased blood pressure Cardiac failure Altered cardiovascular system
Shortness of breath	Altered respiratory activity
Moist, warm skin	Increased sweating Hair loss Retraction of eyelids Altered skin integrity
Weakness and fatigue	Tremor of hands Increased muscle tone and reflexes Shortness of breath on exertion Altered activity tolerance
Emotional lability	Increased anxiety Restlessness Increased irritability Insomnia Altered emotional and mental state
Diarrhoea	Increased gastrointestinal motility Altered bowel habits
Oligomenorrhoea or amenorrhoea	Low sex drive Impotence Altered sexuality

common malignant endocrine tumour and accounts for 90% of the cancers of the endocrine glands but constitutes 1% of all malignancies registered in the UK (Vanderpump, 2011). Thyroid cancer is the most common endocrine cancer and its incidence has continuously increased in the last three decades all over the world. This trend is present on every continent, where it could be argued that detection is possibly insufficient (Pellegriti et al, 2013). Aetiology of thyroid cancer is unknown, but risk factors include history of neck irradiation; Hashimoto's thyroiditis; family history of thyroid adenoma; Cowden's syndrome; familial adenomatous polyposis; familial thyroid cancer; and exposure to nuclear fallout (e.g. following the Chernobyl accident). The prognosis depends on the type and aggressiveness of the

tumour and the presence of metastases, as well as the patient's age and overall health. Following investigations and staging of the disease, a thyroidectomy will be undertaken (Franklin et al, 2012).

Conservative management of hyperthyroidism

Hyperthyroidism is initially treated conservatively by the use of a thionamide, e.g. carbimazole or propylthiouracil. These drugs suppress the formation of the thyroid hormones and hopefully produce a euthyroid state, i.e. a normally functioning thyroid gland, and are also used in the preparation of a patient prior to thyroid surgery. If the patient has cardiac symptoms, a beta-adrenergic blocking agent may be used to decrease the heart rate, e.g. propranolol.

Radioactive iodine therapy is an effective treatment for patients over the age of 45 years. It avoids the prolonged use of drugs or the need for surgery, although there is a risk of causing hypothyroidism in the patient (Milas, 2019). The patient swallows a solution of gamma-emitting radioactive sodium iodide, which destroys thyroid tissue and so reduces the production of the thyroid hormones T3 and T4.

The Nursing and Midwifery Council (2018) require nurses to be open and candid with all service users about all aspects of their care and treatment, including when any mistakes or harm have taken place. The nurse must explain the risks and provide the patient with an opportunity to ask questions and to seek clarification about their care.

Specific investigations of a patient with thyroid dysfunction

A variety of laboratory and other investigations are undertaken prior to surgery.

Blood tests

Serum levels of the following are measured to evaluate thyroid function, and to identify hyperthyroidism and malignancy:
- free thyroxine (FT4)
- free triiodothyronine (FT3)
- thyroid-stimulating hormone (TSH)
- thyroid antibodies
- thyroglobulin (Tg)

- thyroglobulin antibodies (TgAb)
- TSH-receptor antibodies (TSH-RAb)
- thyroid auto-antibodies
- calcitonin (Franklin et al, 2012).

Radioactive scanning procedures

This is useful in patients with a solitary autonomous toxic nodule or with toxic multinodular disease, but is of little value in the diagnosis of malignancy. The radioactive isotopes used are:
- ^{99m}technetium
- ^{131}iodine.

Other imaging procedures

These will identify any structural abnormalities within the thyroid gland:
- ultrasound
- duplex ultrasound scan
- computerized tomography (CT) scan
- magnetic resonance imaging (MRI)
- fluorescent scan (Okosieme et al, 2016).

Fine-needle biopsy

Fine-needle aspiration cytology (with or without ultrasound) allows an accurate diagnosis of the thyroid lesion to be determined, and should be used in the planning of surgery for patients with thyroid cancer.

Other investigations

These include the following:
- ECG — to detect atrial fibrillation
- cholesterol levels — to exclude hyperlipidaemia
- menstrual history — to identify abnormal menstrual cycle, fetal loss or subfertility
- a full blood count — to identify any abnormalities
- blood for typing and crossmatching (in case of haemorrhage peri- or postoperatively).

Nursing assessment of a patient requiring thyroid surgery

It is important to gain a comprehensive health history from the patient, as their health problems have often developed gradually over time and are often vague in nature. Knowledge of the effects of altered thyroid function enables the nurse to collect the relevant data and ask specific questions relating to the thyroid disorder. Using a model of nursing will also help to structure the assessment process (Box 13.1).

Box 13.1 Nursing assessment of Joanna Sweet

This assessment uses the Roper, Logan and Tierney model of nursing (Holland & Jenkins, 2019).

Joanna Sweet is a 30-year-old married woman with three young children aged 2, 4 and 7 years. She works as a presenter for the local television station, and her husband is a journalist. She developed hyperthyroidism and has been managed conservatively, but it is felt that surgery is now an option as the thyroid gland is causing Joanna much discomfort on eating and she is concerned by the appearance of her swollen neck. She is due for surgical removal of her thyroid gland as a short-stay patient in 2 weeks' time.

Maintaining a safe environment

Joanna is very anxious regarding the outcome of the surgery and is concerned as to the appearance of the scar, and whether people will be able to see it.

Observations of her vital signs are as follows:

- Pulse: 86 beats per minute; sleeping pulse: 78 beats per minute. She says that she has had palpitations in the past.
- Blood pressure: 138/80 mmHg.
  Drug therapy:
  - carbimazole 15 mg daily for the past 6 months
  - propranolol 20 mg three times a day
- Allergies: she is not allergic to anything that she knows of, and has had no problems with previous anaesthetics (she had an appendicectomy 10 years ago and drainage of a breast abscess 4 years ago).

Communicating

Joanna appears very anxious and asks lots of questions. She wears contact lenses as she is short-sighted.

(Continued)

Box 13.1 (cont'd)

Breathing

- Respiratory rate: 18 rpm; regular. Joanna used to smoke 10 cigarettes a day before she became pregnant with her first child.

Eating and drinking

Joanna weighs 58 kg and is 1.62 m tall. Her body mass index is 22. She says that her weight had dropped to 50 kg even though she was always eating. Her appetite has now returned to normal and she is nearly back to her normal weight. She enjoys a glass of wine with her evening meal, or when she and her husband have friends around.

Eliminating

She usually has her bowels open once to twice a day. Urinalysis shows no abnormalities.

Personal cleansing and dressing

Joanna is very conscious of her appearance and dresses very smartly. She likes to shower at least twice a day. She has a Waterlow score of 7.

Controlling body temperature

Joanna's temperature is 36.8°C.

Mobility

Joanna has no problems with this activity.

Working and playing

Joanna is a presenter for a daytime programme with a local television company. Her two youngest children attend nursery, and her eldest child attends school. She has found that her tolerance of people has altered and she gets irritated very easily. She and her husband enjoy entertaining.

Body image

Joanna takes pride in her appearance, and is very concerned as to how the scar will look after the surgery, and whether she will be able to conceal it from the viewers.

Sleeping

She usually sleeps 7 hours a night, but this varies, especially if she is stressed at work.

Dying

She expresses no fears about the anaesthetic.

Assessment of the patient's voice and trachea

A chest X-ray is taken to ensure that the enlarged thyroid gland is not constricting the trachea, nor causing it to deviate to one side. As there is a risk of the recurrent laryngeal nerves being damaged during the surgical procedure, it is essential that the vocal cords are assessed preoperatively. This is often undertaken in the outpatient department, where an indirect laryngoscopy is performed in order to assess the state of the vocal cords. Huang et al (2015) suggest the value of undertaking a comprehensive voice analysis pre- and postoperatively, as they found that other factors besides laryngeal nerve injury may alter the voice post-thyroidectomy.

Specific preoperative preparation

The patient will usually be admitted as a day case or short-stay patient (Bailey et al, 2019), and will have attended a pre-assessment clinic at least two weeks prior to surgery. The patient will have been taking a thionamide (e.g. carbimazole) preoperatively to create and maintain a euthyroid state, and may be taking a beta-blocker to reduce cardiac symptoms. Giving the patient sufficient preoperative information will assist in reducing their anxiety, and they will need to be made aware that they may have a sore throat postoperatively. The patient should be reassured that the surgical incision(s) will be in the natural folds of the neck and so should not be too noticeable. However, some surgeons may adopt a transaxillary or bilateral axillo-breast approach that would result in minimal visible scarring.

Surgical interventions

A variety of surgical techniques may be undertaken, depending on the type and position of the nodules in the thyroid gland, and many patients now undergo endoscopic or minimally invasive video-assisted thyroidectomy. The surgeon will always try to preserve a portion of the thyroid gland if possible, to allow continued production of the thyroid hormones, and in the hope of preventing problems with hypothyroidism postoperatively. It is also important to protect the parathyroid glands from damage or removal during the surgical procedure, as well as to prevent damage to the recurrent laryngeal nerves.

The more common surgical procedures are as follows.

- *Thyroid lobectomy*: one lobe of the thyroid gland is removed, including the isthmus.
- *Near-total lobectomy*: a total lobectomy leaving behind less than 1 g thyroid tissue, to protect the recurrent laryngeal nerve.
- *Near-total thyroidectomy*: complete removal of one thyroid lobe and a near-total lobectomy on the contralateral side. The advantage of this surgical procedure is that a small portion of the patient's thyroid gland is left intact, to allow thyroid hormone

production, reducing the need for replacement thyroid hormones postoperatively.

- *Total thyroidectomy*: both lobes and the isthmus of the thyroid gland are removed.

Endoscopic procedures

Endoscopic procedures and minimally invasive video-assisted thyroidectomy (MIVAT) are now undertaken in many centres (Radford et al, 2011; Marinelli, 2015), with the advantage of less postoperative pain and better cosmetic results. Radford et al (2011) found that, compared with conventional surgery, endoscopic thyroidectomy was associated with significantly less blood loss, and better cosmetic results. Radford et al (2011) identify that MIVAT is a favourable technique, with obvious benefits over the traditional surgery, and for small-volume thyroid disease that mainly affects a young female patient population, with lower complication rates and improved cosmesis.

Specific postoperative care

Postoperative care is the same as for any surgical patient, as has been briefly outlined in Chapter 2, and issues related to altered body image are outlined in Chapter 7. However, there are specific complications that can arise following this type of surgery, which need to be closely monitored in the immediate postoperative period. Post Anaesthetic Care Unit staff should observe the patient and be aware the patient could experience airway obstruction, haemorrhage, damage to the recurrent laryngeal nerves, thyrotoxic crisis and tetany (Marinelli, 2015). These will now be discussed and are also illustrated in a postoperative care plan (Box 13.2).

Box 13.2 **Postoperative care plan following a near-total thyroidectomy**

This care plan illustrates the specific nursing care of a patient following thyroid surgery using the Roper, Logan and Tierney model of nursing (Holland & Jenkins, 2019).

Joanna Sweet has returned to the ward following a near-total thyroidectomy for a benign nodule. She is conscious and is sitting in an upright position. She has an intravenous infusion *in situ*, but is able to take sips of water. The wound has been closed with a subcuticular non-absorbable suture and Steri-Strips, and is covered with a postoperative dressing.

Breathing

- *Problem:* Potential risk of respiratory difficulties due to anaesthesia, laryngeal spasm, damage to the recurrent laryngeal nerve, or the presence of a haematoma pressing on the trachea.
- *Goal:* Joanna is able to breathe normally.
- *Nursing actions and rationale for care:*
  - Joanna should be sitting in an upright position, with her neck well supported with pillows. Supporting her head and neck ensures that Joanna is comfortable. Sitting upright also assists her to cough and expectorate.

(Continued)

Box 13.2 (cont'd)

- Joanna may be prescribed oxygen therapy in the immediate postoperative period. Ensure it is given at the prescribed rate, and that Joanna's mouth is moistened.
- Observe Joanna's respirations for rate, depth and stridor, and note any complaints from her of a choking sensation, or signs of cyanosis or respiratory distress. A change in these observations may indicate laryngeal paralysis or compression of the trachea by a haematoma, both of which require prompt intervention.
- Encourage Joanna to take deep breaths and to cough and expectorate any sputum several times an hour. Deep breathing aids full chest expansion, and with expectorating any sputum, helps to reduce the risk of chest infection.
- *Evaluation*: Joanna's respiratory rate was 18–20 breaths per minute, and she showed no signs of respiratory problems. Oxygen therapy was discontinued after 2 hours. She was experiencing some discomfort coughing, but was able to expectorate any sputum.

Maintaining a safe environment

- *Problem:* Potential risk of haemorrhage.
- *Goal*: Early detection of possible haemorrhage.
- *Nursing actions and rationale for care*:
  - Ensure a stitch cutter is by her bed, in case the suture needs to be removed quickly, i.e. if a haematoma causes respiratory distress.
  - Observe Joanna's pulse and blood pressure {1/4}–{1/2}-hourly initially. An increase in pulse rate and a falling blood pressure can indicate haemorrhage and should be reported immediately.
  - Observe Joanna's respiratory state, as above, in order to detect any signs of respiratory distress, which may be caused by the formation of a haematoma around the trachea.
  - Observe the wound for signs of fresh bleeding, and check the side and back of Joanna's neck where blood may have collected.
  - If the presence of a haematoma is suspected, seek medical attention immediately, as aspiration may be required, or the suture may need to be removed to release the haematoma.
- *Evaluation*: Joanna's observations remained within normal limits. There was no sign of excessive bleeding.
- *Problem*: Potential risk of a thyroid crisis.
- *Goal*: Early detection of this potential complication of thyroid surgery.
- *Nursing actions and rationale for care*:
  - Observe Joanna's temperature, pulse, respirations and blood pressure at regular intervals. An increased temperature, pulse, respiratory rate or blood pressure could indicate a thyroid crisis.
  - Observe Joanna for complaints of feeling hot or having palpitations, which could indicate the onset of this potential complication.
  - Observe Joanna's mental state and monitor any periods of confusion or mania to detect signs of a thyroid crisis.
  - If any of these symptoms occur, seek medical advice immediately.
- *Evaluation*: Joanna showed no signs of developing a thyroid crisis. Her observations remained within normal limits and she had no episodes of palpitations. She was alert and oriented to time and place.
- *Problem*: Potential risk of tetany following surgery.
- *Goal*: Early detection of this potential problem.
- *Nursing actions and rationale for care*:
  - Monitor Joanna for any complaints of numbness or tingling in her fingers and toes, which may indicate hypocalcaemia.
  - Monitor Joanna for Trousseau's sign while taking her blood pressure, as seen by a contraction of her hand.
  - Tap the side of Joanna's face over the zygoma bone to monitor any facial muscle twitching, i.e. Chvostek's sign.
  - Observe Joanna for a change in the pitch of her voice, as this may indicate spasm of her vocal cords.
  - Monitor Joanna for any complaints of stomach cramps, as this may indicate tetany.
- *Evaluation*: Joanna showed no signs of developing tetany during her postoperative recovery.
- *Problem*: Joanna has a sore throat following surgery.
- *Goal*: To reduce her pain to an acceptable level.
- *Nursing actions and rationale for care*:
  - Assess Joanna's pain using a pain assessment tool.
  - Administer prescribed analgesics and monitor effectiveness after 30 minutes.
  - Ensure Joanna is in a comfortable position, with her head and neck well supported with pillows.

(Continued)

Box 13.2 (cont'd)

- *Evaluation*: Joanna initially complained of a sore throat, but this was effectively relieved with 25 mg diclofenac. The rest of the time her pain was relieved by taking 25 mg diclofenac and 1 g paracetamol every 6 hours.

Eating and drinking

- *Problem*: Joanna has difficulty in swallowing, because of a sore throat.
- *Goals*:
  - Joanna's hydration and nutritional state is maintained.
  - Joanna is eventually able to eat and drink normally.
- *Nursing actions and rationale for care:*
  - Monitor the intravenous infusion, to check it is running at the correct rate and is not running into the surrounding tissue. This is to ensure that Joanna does not become dehydrated and that the cannula remains within the vein.
  - Encourage Joanna to drink sips of water, and gradually increase this as she is able to tolerate it. Cool fluids are sometimes more suitable and better tolerated following thyroid surgery.
  - If Joanna feels nauseated following the anaesthetic, offer prescribed antiemetics and monitor effectiveness.
  - Once Joanna is taking sufficient oral fluids, the intravenous infusion can be discontinued.
  - Joanna's fluid intake and output should be measured and monitored on a fluid balance chart, until she is taking an adequate fluid intake, and is passing sufficient amounts of urine.
  - Joanna can eat a soft diet, once she feels able to.
- *Evaluation*: Joanna was able to drink a glass of water within 2 hours of returning to the ward, and had eaten a light breakfast before her discharge. Her intravenous infusion was discontinued after 8 hours, as she was able to drink adequately and did not feel nauseated. Joanna passed urine within 5 hours of returning to the ward and thereafter was passing sufficient quantities of urine.

Communicating

- *Problem*: Joanna has a hoarse voice following surgery.
- *Goals*:
  - To detect signs of recurrent laryngeal nerve damage.
  - To reassure Joanna that her voice should eventually return to normal.
- *Nursing actions and rationale for care:*
  - Observe Joanna for a loss of phonation or respiratory difficulties, as this may indicate damage to the recurrent laryngeal nerves.
  - Ensure Joanna has her vocal cords checked by the medical staff, to ensure that her cords are intact and have not been damaged during the surgery.
  - Reassure Joanna that her voice will eventually return to normal, as most hoarseness is usually a temporary situation.
- *Evaluation:* Prior to her discharge, her voice was beginning to return to normal.

Cleansing and dressing

- *Problem*: Joanna has a surgical wound on her neck.
- *Goals*:
  - The wound has healed when the suture is removed 5 days postoperatively.
  - There is no evidence of wound infection.
- *Nursing actions and rationale for care:*
  - Observe the wound dressing for signs of bleeding and report to the nurse in charge.
  - Theatre dressing is removed before discharge, and, if no exudate is present, the wound can be left exposed. If the wound is still exuding, apply a light sterile dressing, so as to protect the wound from microorganisms.
  - Observe the wound for signs of redness, heat, tenderness and swelling, as this could indicate infection.
  - Monitor Joanna's temperature 4-hourly, as a pyrexia may indicate infection.
- *Evaluation*: Joanna's temperature remained within normal limits. When the theatre dressing was removed, the wound was intact with no exudate present. However, Joanna felt very conscious of the wound, so a light gauze dressing was applied to it. As Joanna was discharged home after 23 hours, her suture was removed by the practice nurse after 5 days, when the wound edges were found to be united. Joanna was then encouraged to massage the scar with a gentle moisturizer daily, commencing 2 weeks after suture removal, so as to prevent contraction of the scar.

(Continued)

Box 13.2 (cont'd)

Body image

- *Problem*: Joanna is concerned with the appearance of the scar, as she works with the media.
- *Goal*: Joanna feels comfortable with her body image.
- *Nursing actions and rationale for care*:
  - Allow Joanna time to express her fears about her physical appearance.
  - Give Joanna some ideas as to how she may camouflage the scar initially, until she becomes happy with it, e.g. use of scarves.
  - Reassure Joanna that the scar should not be too noticeable, as it is in one of the natural folds of skin in her neck, and it will become flatter and paler as the healing process continues, and so will not be as evident.
  - Inform Joanna of the need to gently massage the scar with a light moisturizer from 2 weeks after the suture has been removed, as this should prevent contraction of the scar.
- *Evaluation*: Joanna was concerned as to how her colleagues would react to her scar, and she felt happier wearing a light gauze dressing covered with a scarf. She said that she had met other people who had had this type of surgery and that their scars had faded over time.

Potential problems following thyroid surgery

Obstructed airway

The patient's airway may become obstructed for a number of reasons:
- The trachea may have been damaged during surgery or compressed by a haematoma.
- The anaesthetic may have caused an increase in tracheal or bronchial secretions, or laryngospasm may occur because the trachea was irritated during intubation.
- A painful neck and sore throat may inhibit the patient's ability to expectorate any sputum.
- Damage to the recurrent laryngeal nerves during surgery can cause laryngeal paralysis, which will lead to respiratory difficulties, and may require an emergency tracheostomy. A loss of sensation above the vocal cords can lead to the patient aspirating any secretions.

Haemorrhage

The thyroid gland is a highly vascular organ, and although the risk of haemorrhage is rare, it should be closely observed for, as blood may collect in the area surrounding the trachea leading to respiratory difficulties, i.e. stridor and dyspnoea. This is an emergency situation and removal of the sutures/staples should be immediately undertaken in order to allow the haematoma to be released. Aspiration or surgical evacuation of the haematoma may be required if this has no effect on the patient's respiratory state.

The risk of haematoma formation is reduced if the surgeon can achieve good haemostasis during the surgical procedure. Marinelli (2015) suggests that the insertion of a drain is unnecessary in most patients undergoing uncomplicated thyroid surgery and suggests that a large haematoma can be drained by needle aspiration in the absence of a drain.

Recurrent laryngeal nerve damage

Damage to the superior laryngeal nerve will present as hoarseness, and the vocal cords may have a wrinkled appearance. Recurrent laryngeal nerve damage affects the patient's ability to speak. Damage to one side of the recurrent laryngeal nerve results in hoarseness and a paralysed vocal cord, while damage to both laryngeal nerves results in loss of speech and paralysed vocal cords, the latter causing respiratory problems. The damage may be temporary if due to swelling, i.e. laryngeal oedema, or permanent if the nerve is severed or damaged during surgery (Marinelli, 2015). The professional duty of candour requires nurses to be open and honest when things go wrong with their treatment or care which causes, or can cause, harm or distress.

Thyroid crisis

This may occur as a result of excessive amounts of thyroid hormones entering the circulation, causing an acute thyrotoxic state. It may be precipitated during surgery and is thought to be due to handling of the thyroid gland during the surgical procedure (Hampton, 2013), and is most likely to be seen 6–24 hours following surgery. The patient will become very breathless, feel very hot, complain of palpitations, and may also appear confused or manic. Due to the uncontrolled rise in metabolic rate, they will develop a hyperpyrexia, a noticeable tachycardia and become hypertensive. If this situation occurs, the patient should be given oxygen therapy, and prescribed sedatives and cool washes to reduce the hyperpyrexia, as well as having an intravenous infusion to correct dehydration and control hyperthermia. Intravenous beta-adrenoceptor blocking drugs (e.g. propranolol), anti-thyroid drugs (e.g. carbimazole) and glucocorticosteroids (e.g. hydrocortisone) will be given as an emergency treatment, as patients can die from cardiac failure.

Tetany

Damage or removal of the parathyroid glands during surgery can lead to a decrease in serum calcium concentrations — i.e. hypoparathyroidism causes hypocalcaemia — whereby the patient can develop tetany in the early days following surgery. This condition is commonly due to interference with the blood supply to the parathyroid glands, which occurs during surgery (Marinelli, 2015), or due to their inadvertent removal during a total thyroidectomy, and can be seen usually 24–72 hours postoperatively, although it can occur 1–3 hours postoperatively (Hughes & Marvell, 2011).

The patient may complain of numbness or tingling in the fingers and toes, and will also show evidence of carpopedal spasm, i.e. cramp in the hands and feet due to hypocalcaemia. Carpopedal spasm can be detected by observing for positive Trousseau's and Chvostek's signs (Hatfield, 2014). Trousseau's sign is where there is contraction of the hand induced by the application of a tourniquet around the upper arm, e.g. when taking the patient's blood pressure. A positive Chvostek's sign is seen by gently tapping the patient's face over the zygoma, which will produce spasm of the facial muscles. The patient's voice may become high-pitched and shrill, due to spasm of the vocal cords. Gastrointestinal cramps can also be associated with tetany. Initial treatment of tetany is with intravenous administration of calcium gluconate. If the parathyroid glands have been permanently damaged, the patient will need to receive oral calcium supplements.

Discharge planning and patient education

Most patients undergoing thyroid surgery only stay in hospital for a short period of time, so the amount of information they are given relating to their postoperative recovery is paramount if they are to make a full and successful recovery from surgery (see Chapter 9 for further information on discharge planning).

Patients are not always aware of how tired they will feel once they leave hospital; many anaesthetists give steroids as part of their anaesthetic technique. They need to be made aware of this, and also informed that this is quite normal following any kind of surgery, as it can take 2–3 months before they are fully recovered from the surgery.

Clear written and verbal information should be given to the patient regarding any potential complications, e.g. wound infection, tetany. The need to gently massage the scar(s) with a gentle moisturizer should be reinforced and should commence about two weeks following removal of the sutures/staples. Advice can also be given as to how to camouflage the neck scar(s) if required, e.g. by use of a scarf.

Six weeks after surgery, the patient will be required to attend the outpatient clinic. This is to enable the medical staff to ensure that wound healing is progressing and that the patient has no problems with their voice or swallowing. Bloods are taken for thyroid hormone levels, to ensure the patient is not becoming myxoedemic. If the patient is suffering from hypothyroidism (myxoedema), they will need to be prescribed replacement thyroxine therapy, and if they have had a total thyroidectomy, they will need thyroid replacement therapy for life.

Conclusion

Surgery to the thyroid gland is only undertaken in cases of malignancy, or when drug therapy has failed to control hyperthyroidism. A common problem facing patients undergoing thyroid surgery is the position of the scar following surgery, and how it may affect their body image, although with endoscopic surgery this problem is reduced. Postoperative nursing care is concerned with the early detection of specific potential complications, so that early intervention can be undertaken.

SUMMARY OF KEY POINTS

- Thyroidectomy is undertaken for either malignancy of the thyroid gland or uncontrolled hyperthyroidism.
- Patients should be in a euthyroid state prior to surgery.
- Preoperative assessment of the vocal cords is essential.
- Postoperative care relates to careful monitoring for potential complications, e.g. obstructed airway.
- Many patients have a sore throat postoperatively.
- Some patients may require replacement thyroxine therapy, depending on their thyroid hormone levels.

References

Bailey, C. R., Ahuja, M., Bartholomew, K., Bew, S., Forbes, L., Lipp, A., et al. (2019). *Guidelines for day-case surgery 2019*. Association of Anaesthetists and the British Association of Day Surgery. Available at: < https://anaesthetists. org/Portals/0/Images/Guidelines% 20cover%20images/ Guideline_day_case_surgery_2019.pdf? ver = 2019-05-05-075731-563 > .

Franklin, I. J., Dawson, P. M., & Rodway, A. D. (2012). *Essentials of clinical surgery* (2nd ed.). London: Elsevier Health Sciences.

Hampton, J. (2013). Thyroid gland disorder emergencies – thyroid storm and myxedema coma. *AACN Advanced Critical Care, 24*(3), 925–932..

Hatfield, A. (2014). *The complete recovery room book* (5th ed.). Oxford: Oxford University Press.

Holland, K., & Jenkins, J. (2019). Applying the Roper-Logan-Tierney model in practice *(eBook)*. Elsevier Health Sciences.

Huang, C.-F., Yeng, Y., Chen, K.-D., Yu, J.-K., Shih, C.-M., Huang, S.-M., et al.

(2015). The preoperative evaluation prevent the postoperative complications of thyroidectomy. *Annals of Medicine and Surgery, 4*(1), 5–10.

Hughes, S. J., & Marvell, A. (2011). *Oxford handbook of perioperative practice*. Oxford: Oxford University Press.

Lindholm, J., & Laurberg, P. (2010). Hyperthyroidism, exophthalmos, and goitre: historical notes on the orbitopathy. *Thyroid, 20*(3), 291–300. Available at: < https://doi.org/10.1089/ thy.2009.0340 > .

Marinelli, M. (2015). Thyroid and parathyroid surgery. In J. C. Rothrock (Ed.), *Alexander's care of the patient in surgery* (pp. 538–557). St Louis: Elsevier Mosby.

Milas, K.M. (2019). Radioactive iodine for hyperthyroidism. *EndocrineWeb*. Available at: < www.endocrineweb. com/conditions/hyperthyroidism/ radioactive-iodine-hyperthyroidism >

Nursing and Midwifery Council. (2018). The Code. Professional standards of practice and behaviour for nurses, midwives and nursing associates. Available

at: < www.nmc.org.uk/standards/ code/ >

Okosieme, O., Gilbert, J., Abraham, P., Boelaert, K., Dayan, C., Gurnell, M., et al. (2016). Management of primary hypothyroidism: statement by the British Thyroid Association Executive Committee. *Clinical Endocrinology, 84* (6), 799–808.

Pellegriti, G., Frasca, F., Regalbuto, C., Squatrito, S., & Vigneri, R. (2013). Worldwide increasing incidence of thyroid cancer: update on epidemiology and risk factors. *Journal of Cancer Epidemiology, 2013*, 965212.

Radford, P. D., Ferguson, M. S., Magill, J. C., Karthikesalingham, A. P., & Alusi, G. (2011). Meta-analysis of minimally invasive video-assisted thyroidectomy. *Laryngoscope: Head and Neck, 121*(8), 1675–1681.

Vanderpump, M. P. J. (2011). The epidemiology of thyroid disease. *British Medical Bulletin, 99*, 39–51.

Wilson, S. F., & Giddens, J. F. (2009). *Health assessment for nursing practice* (4th ed.). St Louis: Mosby.

Relevant website

British Thyroid Association: www.british-thyroid-association.org – A society for health professionals in the UK involved in the management of patients with thyroid disease.

Chapter | 14 |

Care of the patient requiring cardiac interventions and surgery

Louise Best and Kevin Barrett

KEY OBJECTIVES OF THE CHAPTER

At the end of this chapter the reader will be able to:

- describe the structure, function and blood flow through the heart
- identify the structural abnormalities that can affect the heart
- describe how to undertake a nursing assessment of the cardiac patient
- describe the procedure used for cardiac catheterization, its indications, and the nursing management required by patients before and after catheterization
- describe procedures used in the investigation and treatment of patients with cardiac arrhythmias
- identify the specific care required by patients needing temporary and permanent pacing and internal cardiac defibrillators
- discuss the nursing management of patients requiring open cardiac surgery
- identify the specific advice required by patients prior to discharge from hospital following cardiac investigations and therapy.

Areas to think about before reading the chapter

- Draw and label a diagram of the heart.
- What reason might there be for the considerable variation in mortality from coronary heart disease across the UK?
- What are the key causes of coronary heart disease?

Introduction

This chapter aims to give an overview of the principles of the care required by patients undergoing a range of invasive investigations and treatments for cardiovascular disease. The more invasive cardiac procedures are reviewed in detail to enhance understanding of what is involved for the patient, so that the nurse is able to tailor information to meet the individual's needs. Although this chapter describes accepted day-to-day clinical practice, this may differ to local policy and guidelines, and these must be taken into consideration.

Anatomy and physiology of the heart

The heart lies behind the sternum, with two-thirds in the left side of the chest. It is composed of three layers: the inner layer is the endocardium; the middle muscular layer is the myocardium; and the outer layer is the epicardium. The epicardial surface is surrounded by a protective, inelastic fibrous sac called the pericardium, which contains a small amount of lubricating serous fluid.

The heart has four chambers: an atrium and ventricle separated by a valve on both the right and left sides, with the atria and ventricles being separated by the intra-atrial and intraventricular septa. The heart can be thought of as a low-pressure and a high-pressure pump in series. Deoxygenated blood flows from the body via the inferior and superior vena cavae into the right atrium. Blood flow from the right atrium to the right ventricle mainly occurs passively (about 70%) while the heart is relaxed and not contracting. This phase is called diastole. When the heart contracts (systole), blood is propelled through the tricuspid valve into the right ventricle. When the ventricle contracts, the tricuspid valve closes and blood is expelled through the pulmonary valve into the pulmonary artery and into the pulmonary vascular system, where it is oxygenated in the lungs and carbon dioxide is removed. This is the low-pressure system.

From the lungs, oxygenated blood enters the left atrium via the pulmonary veins during diastole. Blood flows through the mitral valve into the left ventricle both passively and by contraction of the left atrium. When the ventricle contracts in systole, the mitral valve closes, the aortic valve opens and blood is ejected into the aorta. This is the high-pressure system, as high pressure is necessary to propel the blood through the body. For this reason, the left ventricle has greater muscle mass than the right ventricle. The blood then circulates around the body, becomes deoxygenated and returns once again to the right atrium via the vena cavae.

Contraction of the heart muscle (myocardium) needs to occur in a specific sequence for these events to occur. This is achieved by the specialized conducting system within the heart. This consists of the sinoatrial (SA) node, which is found at the junction of the superior vena cava with the right atrium, and is the cardiac pacemaker that determines the heart rate. Impulses pass across the atria to the atrioventricular (AV) node at the base of the right atrium and thence to either ventricle via the bundle of His. In the normal heart this is the only route that can be taken by electrical impulses passing from the atria to the ventricles. Impulses are then conducted by the right and left bundle branches to a network of Purkinje fibres which supply the respective ventricles. For practical purposes, events can be regarded as happening simultaneously on both sides of the heart, so that identical volumes of blood flow through both the right and left sides of the heart. Heart rate and strength of contraction are affected by the autonomic nervous system. The heart is richly innervated by sympathetic nerve fibres, which on stimulation increase both the heart rate and speed of electrical transmission via the conducting system. This

increases heart rate and strength of contraction. The vagus nerve of the parasympathetic nervous system also innervates the heart and has a broadly opposite effect — namely, slowing the heart rate on stimulation — and can therefore be considered as the heart's braking system.

Forward blood flow through the heart is maintained by the tricuspid and mitral valves, which prevent the blood flowing backwards from the ventricles to the atria, while the pulmonary and aortic valves prevent blood flowing backwards from the pulmonary artery and aorta into the right and left ventricles, respectively. Although these valves have similar functions, their structures differ. The tricuspid valve, positioned between the right atrium and ventricle, has three cusps, compared with two for the mitral valve, positioned between the left atrium and ventricle. The cusps are thin, strong and fibrous, and when opened are pushed against the ventricular wall to allow blood to flow through them. These valves are attached and stabilized within the heart by specialized parts of the cardiac muscle known as the papillary muscles, which are attached to the tricuspid and mitral valves via cords called chordae tendineae. The two semilunar valves positioned between the right ventricle and pulmonary artery (pulmonary valve) and the left ventricle and aorta (aortic valve) are anchored to the fibrous ring of the cardiac skeleton and do not have papillary muscles or chordae tendineae. Both the pulmonary and aortic valves have three cusps.

The myocardium receives its blood supply from the left and right coronary arteries. These arise from the aorta just above the aortic valve. The left main stem divides into the left anterior descending and circumflex branch. The left anterior descending artery supplies oxygenated blood to the intraventricular septum and the anterior wall of the left ventricle; the circumflex branch supplies the lateral wall of the left ventricle. The right coronary artery (RCA) supplies the inferior and posterior walls of the left and right ventricles. The myocardium receives its blood supply during the diastolic phase of the cardiac cycle. These vessels also supply the specialized conducting tissue with its oxygenated blood.

Basic pathophysiology of the heart

Any components of the heart can malfunction, either because of congenital abnormality or acquired disease. The heart can also be affected by conditions elsewhere in the body (Table 14.1).

Coronary heart disease is the most common cause of death in the UK, with 1 in 7 men and 1 in 12 women dying from the disease. Coronary heart disease causes

Table 14.1 Diseases affecting the heart, in relation to cardiac structure

	Myocardium	Pericardium	Coronary arteries	Valves	Conduction system
Congenital disease	Atrial/ventricular septal defects Hypertrophic obstructive myocardiopathies		Anatomical abnormalities Homozygous hypercholesterolaemia	Bicuspid atresia	Abnormal pathology Wolff–Parkinson–White syndrome Atrioventricular block
Acquired disease	Myocardial infarction Myocarditis Ventricular septal defect Cardiomyopathies	Pericarditis Tamponade Malignancy	Atherosclerosis Syndrome X	Rheumatic fever Infective Stenosis Regurgitation Papillary muscle rupture Chordae tendineae rupture Atrioventricular block Sick sinus syndrome AV nodal re-entrant tachycardia	Atrioventricular block Sick sinus syndrome AV nodal re-entrant tachycardia

around 66,000 deaths in the UK each year. The number of people dying from all-cause heart and circulatory disease in the UK in 2017 was 152,000 deaths (British Heart Foundation, 2018a). There is considerable variation in mortality from coronary heart disease across the UK. Death rates are highest in the north of England and Scotland and lowest in the south of England. Death rates are also higher in manual workers than in non-manual workers and are higher in certain ethnic groups. However, death rates from coronary heart disease have fallen considerably in the UK, with an approximate 40% reduction in the last 10 years. Although mortality rates are falling, the amount of morbidity is not falling. There are 2.3 million people in the UK living with coronary heart disease. There are also around 7 million people living with heart and circulatory disease, this is contributed to an ageing and growing population with improved survival rates from heart and circulatory events. In the 1960s more than 7 out of 10 myocardial infarctions in the UK were fatal. In 2018 at least 7 out of 10 people survived (British Heart Foundation, 2018a). In addition, there are just fewer than one million people in the UK living with heart failure (British Heart Foundation, 2018a).

A variety of factors such as smoking, diabetes, sedentary lifestyle, diets high in saturated fats and obesity eventually cause the lumen of the coronary arteries to narrow, causing angina and possible myocardial infarction. The general name for this condition is atherosclerosis. The disease process causing this is due to a variety of complex mechanisms responsible for the accumulation of fatty plaques within the vessel walls and calcification of the vessels; this causes narrowing of the arteries. If the fatty plaques become ulcerated, thrombosis occurs, which may lead to vessel occlusion. The formation of atherosclerosis is essentially an inflammatory process and is caused by a variety of risk factors (Shahawy & Libby, 2015). This disease process reduces the blood supply to the myocardium, causing ischaemic chest pain (angina) and, if the artery occludes completely, results in heart muscle death (myocardial *infarction*). A myocardial infarction can cause additional complications if the valves or conducting system are affected.

There are two main problems which can affect each heart valve:

- If they cannot close properly, they leak, which is called regurgitation.
- When they cannot open properly, they obstruct the flow of blood, and this narrowing is called stenosis.

The valves commonly affected by disease in adults are the aortic and mitral valves. Calcification of the valves due to repetitive mechanical stress can lead to stenosis and stiffening of the valve cusps, which partially obstructs blood flow, and so increases the workload of the heart. The process of degenerative aortic disease is an active process sharing some of the similarities and risk factors of atherosclerosis associated with coronary artery disease, such as hyperlipidaemia and inflammation (Natarajan & Prendergast, 2017). If this is not corrected early enough, it may eventually lead to heart failure. Myocardial infarction involving the papillary muscles or causing rupture of the chordae tendineae results in acute mitral regurgitation. This may require urgent surgical repair and/or replacement of the valve.

The conducting system is also affected by a number of conditions which can affect rhythm, resulting in heart rates

235

that can be dangerously fast or slow. Congenital abnormalities such as extra or anomalous conducting pathways (such as Wolff–Parkinson–White syndrome) provide an abnormal connection between the atria and ventricles, which allows the rapid transmission of impulses, causing tachycardia. Ageing, again, can cause fibrosis and calcification of the conducting tissue, which can produce rhythm abnormalities, including various degrees of heart block and slow heart rates. Conduction defects such as heart block may also be caused by coronary artery disease, as a result of occlusion of the artery that supplies blood to the conducting tissue.

Disease processes that affect the myocardium eventually interfere with the pumping action of the heart. This is a frequent cause of heart failure because the heart is no longer able to pump adequate amounts of blood to meet the body's oxygen demands. This may also lead to myocardial infarction.

Heart failure may also result from valve disease, hypertension, pericardial or infective heart disease, or cardiomyopathy. It is estimated that 920,000 people are living with the condition in the UK (British Heart Foundation, 2018a). The condition is serious with an improved survival from ischaemic heart disease, an ageing population and a rise in cardiovascular risk factors contributing to a sustained increase in prevalence (Taylor et al, 2019). The 5-year mortality rate is nearly 50%, which has showed no improvement, in contrast to cancer survival rates, which have doubled (Taylor et al, 2019). This illustrates the seriousness of a diagnosis of heart failure for the patient.

The cardiomyopathies are categorized as:

- dilated cardiomyopathy
- hypertrophic cardiomyopathy
- arrhythmogenic right ventricular cardiomyopathy or dysplasia
- restrictive cardiomyopathy.

Dilated cardiomyopathy is the most common and has numerous causes, including ischaemic heart disease, hypertension, valvular heart disease and infections; whatever the cause, it eventually results in congestive heart failure, which, when severe, may not respond to anti-failure drug therapy. Hypertrophic cardiomyopathy is thought to be genetically transmitted, resulting in thickening of the intraventricular septum, which eventually causes left ventricular obstruction and may result in sudden cardiac death from arrhythmias (Elliott et al, 2014). Arrhythmogenic right ventricular cardiomyopathy or dysplasia is also an inherited disease; it is characterized by fibrofatty replacement of the right ventricle outflow tract. It predisposes individuals to serious ventricular arrhythmias and sudden cardiac death and may eventually lead to right and then left ventricular failure (Corrado et al,

2017). Restrictive cardiomyopathy is the rarest form and has numerous causes; it results in restricted ventricular filling and reduced ventricular volume. It also causes end-stage heart failure and serious cardiac arrhythmias. Therapy for patients with cardiomyopathy is guided towards the alleviation of symptoms, anti-arrhythmic therapy, treating advancing heart failure, insertion of biventricular pacemakers, internal defibrillators and managing end-of-life heart failure.

Assessment and investigations

Patients with heart disease may require extensive assessment and investigations to diagnose and establish the extent of the disease and its effects on body function. Cardiac assessment should be specific and focused, and may also include risk factor assessment, and exploration of family and social history. The cardinal symptoms of cardiac disease should also be investigated: in particular, questions should be asked about chest pain, breathlessness, palpitations, dizziness, loss of consciousness and ankle oedema.

Cardinal symptoms of cardiac disease

Central chest pain is the most common presenting symptom in coronary heart disease and may also occur in valvular heart disease. It is characterized by radiation to the neck, arms, shoulder, jaw or back and is frequently described as a crushing or vice-like sensation which may come on at rest or after exercise. It may also be associated with other symptoms such as nausea, vomiting, and extreme anxiety. It should also be noted that patients with diabetes may not present with typical symptoms of chest pain and evidence of ischaemia may be painless (Junghans et al, 2015).

Heart disease may cause cardiac arrhythmias and therefore the patient should be asked if they have experienced the following symptoms: palpitations, dizziness or blackouts. These symptoms may be associated with both fast and slow arrhythmias, such as ventricular tachycardia, varying degrees of heart block and atrial fibrillation. These slow or rapid rhythms can result in decreased cardiac output and lowered blood pressure (hypotension), which can, if severe, lead to cardiogenic shock.

Patients with left-sided heart disease often experience breathlessness, either on exertion or at rest. They will often give a history of being unable to lie flat for any length of time, and of wakening from sleep with an episode of acute breathlessness. In addition, the patient should be asked if they have a productive cough and to describe what the sputum looks like. If the patient is expectorating large quantities of frothy, clear/pinkish sputum, this may indicate the presence of heart failure and pulmonary oedema.

The nurse should enquire whether the patient has noticed any ankle swelling, which indicates the presence of oedema and possible right-sided heart failure.

Past history

Previous clinical history is important for both diagnosis and risk stratification of patients. Questions should be asked about past and recent medical history, as many seemingly unrelated conditions can be the cause of the current cardiac complaint. Enquiries about diabetes mellitus should be made, as these patients have a substantially increased risk of coronary heart disease. This risk seems to be higher for women with type 2 diabetes mellitus, and these patients will often have other risk factors for coronary artery disease, such as hypertension and obesity (Norhammar & Schenck-Gustafsson, 2012). Hypertension, often referred to as the 'silent killer', causes heart failure, acute coronary syndrome and, if left untreated, is also linked to renal disease. A history of recent invasive treatment will be of particular importance in a patient with known valvular abnormalities, as it may cause infective endocarditis. The classic 'invasive treatment' is usually dental, with at-risk procedures involving the manipulation of the gingival region or perforation of the oral mucosa (Habib et al, 2015).

Social and family history

Many cardiac diseases have a familial or genetic component and tactful questioning may elicit this. It is recognized that there are up to 500 sudden arrhythmic deaths in young people each year and recent improvements in technology and clinical skills enable improved prevention, diagnosis and treatment for these at-risk patients. There are European guidelines available that gives explicit guidance on the investigation of any sudden unexplained death at a young age (Priori et al, 2015; Basso et al, 2017). Tactful enquiries as to the use of recreational drugs, including cigarettes and alcohol, should also be made, as these are all recognized risk factors for coronary heart disease.

Occupational and functional status

Occupation is important, as cardiac disease can also be caused by certain occupations, e.g. publicans may suffer with alcoholic cardiomyopathy, and organic solvents used in the dry cleaning industry are implicated in cardiac arrhythmias and cardiomyopathy. For medicolegal reasons, a diagnosis of cardiac disease can significantly limit, if not completely curtail, a career in the armed forces or police force, and limit the ability of an individual to hold a pilot license or public service vehicle license (PSV). In addition, the insertion of a cardiac internal defibrillator restricts individuals from driving a Category 1 or 2 vehicle (DVLA, 2019a).

Functional capacity should also be assessed, as patients may have deliberately reduced activities such as domestic duties, sporting or other hobbies to limit their symptoms (Innes et al, 2018). Enquiries regarding the patient's ability to climb stairs or walk uphill (particularly into cold winds) are particularly revealing, as in some cases coronary artery disease presents predominantly with breathlessness on exertion, associated with climbing inclines.

Risk factors

Cardiac risk factors can be divided into those which are modifiable and those which are non-modifiable. The predominant modifiable and non-modifiable risk factors are listed in Box 14.1.

Inquiry into these risk factors and also current drug therapy, including any recreational drugs and over-the-counter medications, should be recorded, as many treatments have cardiac side-effects. This will form a useful basis for any focused health education as part of the cardiac rehabilitation process. It is important to be non-judgemental regarding risk factors, as many patients are fully aware of the role of the risk factors in their current medical problem, and 'victim blaming' will only alienate

---

Box 14.1 Cardiac risk factors

Non-modifiable risk factors

Age
Gender
Ethnicity
Genetic predisposition
Hyperlipidaemia

Modifiable risk factors

Hypertension
Cigarette smoking
Diabetes
Obesity
Alcohol
Lack of exercise
High blood cholesterol levels

the patient and will not serve as a useful basis for a thera-peutic relationship.

Physical assessment

General observation of the patient can reveal useful infor-mation such as pallor, cyanosis, shortness of breath at rest and ankle oedema.

The pulse and blood pressure serve as useful tools to assess cardiac output. Measurements of the blood pressure and pulse rate determine whether they are within the nor-mal parameters of:

- pulse rate: 60–100 bpm
- systolic blood pressure: 100–140 mmHg
- diastolic blood pressure: 60–85 mmHg.

A pulse rate below 60 or above 100 bpm may compro-mise cardiac output, resulting in low blood pressure and insufficient perfusion of body tissues. The quality of the pulse should also be assessed by noting strength and rhythm. Some patients may have an irregularly irregular pulse that could be the result of atrial fibrillation, or an irregular pulse that may indicate ectopic beats.

Further circulatory assessment involves palpating the radial, brachial, femoral, popliteal, dorsalis pedis and pos-terior tibial pulses to determine their presence and strength. Capillary refill can be used as an indicator of arterial sufficiency, evaluated by applying firm digital pres-sure to the nail bed to produce blanching; on release of pressure, blood flow should return in less than 3 seconds. This information can be used for comparison of circula-tory status after cardiac catheterization.

Many cardiac abnormalities affect respiratory function and vice versa. A thorough respiratory assessment will establish the extent to which the respiratory system is affected. Respiratory assessment should include measure-ment of the respiratory rate and observation of the depth and rhythm of breathing, respiratory distress, speech pat-tern and the colour of mucous membranes (Smith & Rushton, 2015). Patients having difficulty with breathing frequently use their accessory muscles. This can be seen by observing for retraction of the skin on either side of the neck, just above the clavicles; if breathing difficulty is severe, the skin between the ribs retracts along with abdominal muscle movement. Patients should also be asked whether they experience any breathing difficulty, and which factors cause/ease any breathing problems. Oxygen saturation levels (SaO_2) can be measured with a pulse oximeter, and is a useful indicator of the amount of oxygen bound to the haemoglobin of the blood, which is normally in the range 95–99%. Central cyanosis is not usually detectable until the arterial oxygen tension falls below 8 kPa (kilopascal) and oxygen saturations fall below 80% (Olive, 2016). The nurse should also enquire whether the patient has a cough, and if sputum is

being expectorated, sputum colour, consistency and vol-ume should be noted and recorded.

A detailed history of the patient's smoking habits should be undertaken, including the following: type and quantity of cigarettes smoked; the period of time of being a smoker; and whether the patient has attempted to stop smoking in the past. This information will help in the formulation of a plan to help the patient give up smoking in the future.

Medical investigations

Some of these investigations are straightforward and, once explained, cause little discomfort for the patient. But the more invasive investigations such as cardiac catheteriza-tion can be uncomfortable and frightening and are associ-ated with a number of risks. The following gives an overview of these investigations, followed by a detailed account of the more invasive investigation of cardiac cath-eterization and the care required by the patient following this procedure.

Chest X-ray

This non-invasive investigation demands little of the patient other than being able to take a deep breath and hold it for a few seconds, long enough for a radiograph to be taken of the chest wall and its contents. This investiga-tion enables assessment of the lungs, heart and great ves-sels. No specific physical preparation is required, unless the patient is a woman within child-bearing age, in which case information will be required as to when she last menstru-ated, and whether there is any possibility of her being preg-nant, as there is a potential risk that radiation exposure during the radiography could affect the developing fetus.

Blood tests

Blood samples will be obtained for a number of tests: these include estimation of urea and electrolyte levels, which can give an indication of renal function; and full blood count, to assess for anaemia, polycythaemia and infection. Another useful marker of inflammation, which is typically raised in infections and autoimmune disease, is C-reactive protein (CRP) (Sproston & Ashworth, 2018). It has also been suggested that CRP is a strong predictive marker of increased cardiovascular risk (Sproston & Ashworth, 2018). Measurement of potassium is particu-larly important, since abnormally high or low levels may place the patient at risk of developing cardiac arrhythmias.

Clotting screening is necessary prior to any invasive investigation and treatment if the patient has been taking anticoagulant drugs. If clotting times are prolonged. the patient will be at risk of haemorrhage following any inva-sive procedure.

Serum cardiac markers are measured if there is suspicion of myocardial infarction. The myocardial-specific isoenzyme of creatinine kinase (CK-MB) and related proteins myoglobin and troponin (troponin T and I) usually remain within the cell; however, if the cell is stressed or damaged, they are released into the circulation. The cardiac troponins are the best markers for definitive diagnosis and are also used to risk stratify patients with chest pain. Normal values for these markers can be obtained through individual hospital laboratories (Bodor, 2016).

Electrocardiography

The 12-lead ECG records electrical activity generated by the heart by recording current from leads placed at specific points on the body surface. Different leads look at different areas of the heart, from different directions. The resulting lead patterns give specific information about different anatomical locations of the heart and in particular about conduction disturbances, myocardial perfusion and chamber enlargement. The interpretation of the ECG requires a basic understanding of the physiology underlying the waveforms and an understanding of the 'view' ECG leads have of the heart. The interpretation of the ECG is out of the remit of this book but seeking the help of a knowledgeable senior is always helpful, and many useful ECG textbooks are available for the novice ECG interpreter (Sampson & McGrath 2015a,b).

Care should be taken to ensure a good-quality tracing, to accurately label the ECG with time and date of the recording and to note the presence and type of chest pain and any other contextual factors.

Ambulatory electrocardiography

Ambulatory ECG recording is used to determine whether a patient's symptoms are due to an intermittent arrhythmia or to myocardial ischaemia. Also referred to as Holter monitoring, this involves the patient wearing a small tape-recording unit which is attached to three ECG electrodes placed on the patient's chest wall. The tape recorder continuously records the patient's ECG for a period of 24–48 hours. The patient is able to activate an event marker that will indicate on the tape when symptoms have been experienced, which can be correlated with the recorded ECG.

Echocardiogram

Transthoracic echocardiography is a non-invasive test which enables the cardiac anatomy and function to be assessed by producing images of the heart from recorded sound waves. The sound waves are recorded from the heart by moving a transducer over the anterior chest wall. Transthoracic echocardiography can identify structural changes of the heart. It can measure the size of the heart chambers, providing information about enlargement or constriction of the ventricle, as well as detecting such abnormalities as the presence of tumours or excess fluid within the pericardial sac (which, if impairing the function of the heart, is known as cardiac tamponade). It is also used to evaluate the functioning of the valves. The test is painless, lasting about 45 minutes, and on completion the patient can resume normal activity.

By comparison, transoesophageal echocardiography is more invasive and therefore associated with some risks. This involves introducing the transducer into the oesophagus, which provides a more direct view of the heart. This test is useful in identifying mitral regurgitation or prolapsed valve, and a dissecting aortic aneurysm. The patient should give informed consent before the procedure, as the procedure involves sedation, fasting and the application of an anaesthetic to the throat to assist insertion of the probe. The patient should therefore be recovered in the normal manner and carefully observed for potential arrhythmias during the recovery period.

Exercise stress (tolerance) test

This is usually performed on a treadmill or bicycle. It employs a continuous 12-lead ECG and blood pressure recordings, and is an invaluable test to reveal cardiac symptoms or ECG changes which may not occur at rest. The test is also used to assess prognosis in patients with known cardiac disease and to evaluate treatments. It is not without risks and should always be performed by trained personnel, with resuscitation equipment nearby (Society for Cardiological Science and Technology, 2011). A significant proportion of patients cannot perform an exercise test and in these cases an imaging technique such as perfusion scintigraphy may be utilized instead.

Nuclear scans

Nuclear scanning is an evolving area of medicine and enables the assessment of myocardial perfusion, viability and ventricular function. Single-photon emission computerized tomography (SPECT) involves the intravenous injection of a radioactive substance such as technetium-99 or thallium-201. The substance is taken up by the heart, which is then visualized using a gamma-camera. The radioactive substances enable either myocardial damage (hot-spot detection) or hypoperfusion (cold-spot detection) to be demonstrated. The techniques may be combined with exercise testing for a more accurate method of assessment. Technetium is the increasingly favoured agent used due to its superior image quality.

Cardiac magnetic resonance imaging

Cardiac magnetic resonance imaging (MRI) is a non-invasive test increasingly being used to diagnose and give information on specific heart conditions. MRI is available in most UK hospitals and the number of scans performed has grown at a rate of 15–20% per year (British Heart Foundation, 2019a). It uses a powerful magnetic field, radio waves and a computer to produce detailed pictures of the structures within and around the heart. It enables the evaluation of the anatomy and function of the heart, including heart valves, coronary arteries, ventricles and pericardium, and can aid in the treatment and planning of cardiovascular interventions.

Computerized tomography coronary angiogram

Computerized tomography coronary angiogram (CTA) is a test that looks at the arteries that supply the blood to the heart. It requires the injection of contrast and the CTA scan helps to diagnose and evaluate blood vessel disease or related conditions, such as aneurysms and carotid artery disease, severity of coronary artery disease and congenital abnormalities.

Cardiac catheterization

This investigative procedure confirms and evaluates the extent of heart disease. The procedure involves gaining access to the heart via major blood vessels. Access to the left side of the heart is commonly achieved by catheterizing either the femoral or radial artery with the brachial artery being used in some situations. Right heart catheterization is performed via the venous route, usually the femoral vein, although the subclavian or jugular veins may also be used. The procedure is performed under local anaesthesia.

Information regarding cardiac function is gained by measuring intracardiac pressures, while X-ray visualization of the heart's pumping action and blood flow within the coronary arteries, aorta and pulmonary artery is achieved by injecting a radio-opaque dye during X-ray fluoroscopy. This enables visualization of any abnormalities within the chambers of the heart, as well as stenosis or occlusion in the coronary and pulmonary arteries.

Cardiac catheterization is used to confirm, treat and evaluate the progression of the following disorders:
- coronary artery disease
- valve disease
- ventricular dysfunction
- pulmonary and aortic artery disease/disorders
- atrial and ventricular wall defects
- electrical conduction abnormalities.

Catheterization procedure

Both the femoral and radial approaches involve introducing a needle into the artery, followed by threading a long, thin guidewire via the needle into the artery. The needle is removed, leaving the wire, over which an introducer sheath is inserted (Fig. 14.1). During this part of the procedure the patient will experience some discomfort, usually a feeling of pressure over the groin or wrist as the introducer sheath is inserted into the artery, and perhaps mild discomfort as the catheter is advanced along the artery. The patient's blood pressure and ECG are monitored closely throughout the procedure for any arrhythmias and ischaemic changes.

The introducer sheath allows for repeated access to the artery and heart with different catheters. Within the sheath is a valve that prevents blood loss when the catheter is removed. A catheter can then be threaded up the descending aorta and the tip gently manipulated across the aortic valve into the left ventricle. Radio-opaque dye is injected rapidly into the ventricle (ventriculogram) so that its pumping action can be observed and recorded during X-ray fluoroscopy (Fig. 14.2). This will also identify the presence of abnormalities such as a ventricular aneurysm, valvular regurgitation, or leakage via holes in the septal wall of the heart (atrial or ventricular septal defects).

During the ventriculogram the patient will experience a 'hot flushing' sensation, which may also include a feeling of urinary incontinence. This lasts for a few seconds and is due to the vasodilatory effects of the injected dye. The ventriculogram is followed by manipulating a different catheter into the opening of the coronary artery (Fig. 14.3). Once in position, a small amount of radio-opaque dye is injected into the coronary artery (Fig. 14.4). This will allow the arteries to be visualized by X-ray fluoroscopy and will show any irregularities within the artery, such as areas of stenosis or occlusion. During this part of the procedure, patients do not experience a hot flushing sensation; however, some patients do experience angina, due to partial obstruction of the coronary artery by the catheter and displacement of blood by the dye. The angina usually lasts for a few seconds only, but it is important that the patient informs the staff about the pain so that it can be monitored and treated with a vasodilator such as glyceryl trinitrate (GTN).

The average length of the procedure is between 15 and 30 minutes. On completion, the arterial introducer sheath is removed, and firm pressure is applied 1 cm superior and 1 cm medially to the femoral puncture site to prevent bleeding and promote haemostasis. Various measures are employed to achieve this; one method is to apply digital pressure for 10–20 minutes (depending on sheath size) following arterial sheath removal. Various devices can also be used to promote haemostasis from the femoral artery site, such as pneumatic devices (FemoStop), suturing and

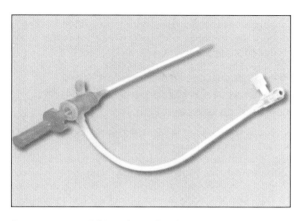

Figure 14.1 Arterial introducer sheath.

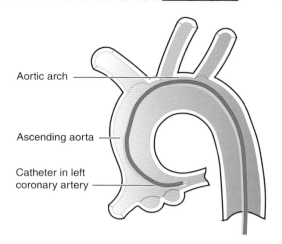

Figure 14.3 Diagram of a left Judkins-shaped catheter positioned in the ostia of the left coronary artery.

Aortic arch

Ascending aorta

Catheter in left coronary artery

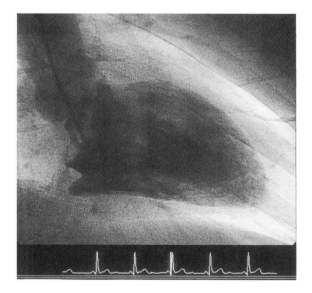

Figure 14.2 Ventriculogram of the left ventricle during cardiac catheterization.

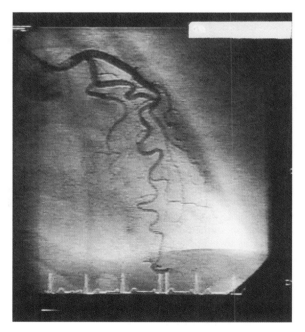

Figure 14.4 An angiogram of the left coronary artery system.

clip devices (Perclose and StarClose), and biodegradable devices which involve implanting a collagen seal into the arterial puncture site (Angio-Seal) or a dressing device (Clo-Sur PAD) (Saleem & Baril, 2019). Although suture and biodegradable devices seal the puncture site rapidly and enable earlier mobilization than does digital compression, the patient continues to require monitoring for complications, as there is an increased risk of haematoma, pseudoaneurysm and arterial occlusion with these devices (Di Loreto & Sampson, 2018). However, on patient comfort, Kandarpa et al (2016) find that closure devices are more preferable than manual compression, however each

device comes with its own potential for complications. Understanding of the device's indications, instructions for use and patient selection criteria is imperative for the success of the device and minimizes complications (Bontrager & Abraham, 2017).

Haemostasis from the radial artery site can be achieved with digital pressure, or with various devices such as a pneumatic compression device (TR band). Radial artery procedures are now widely accepted and are associated with reduced vascular access complications, earlier patient mobilization, and, as a consequence, shorter hospital admission stay (Manda & Baradhi, 2018).

Catheterization via the brachial artery differs in that a small skin incision is made over the artery in the antecubital fossa to expose the artery. On completion of the procedure, the arteriotomy is sutured, followed by suturing of the skin incision. Otherwise, the procedure is the same as that described for the femoral approach. Once haemostasis is achieved, the patient is transferred to the ward for further assessment and care.

Electrophysiology studies

Electrophysiology studies (EP) are used for patients with symptomatic arrhythmias to assess the conduction system of the heart – namely, the sinoatrial node, atrioventricular node and the Purkinje system. These studies are performed using right heart catheterization procedures similar to those described in the section on cardiac pacing. They are used to identify (and treat) the mechanism of an arrhythmia and the location of the anatomical abnormality (Lee & Linker, 2014). Conditions investigated in this way include supraventricular tachycardias such as those caused by Wolff–Parkinson–White syndrome, atrial flutter and fibrillation, ventricular tachycardias or bradyarrhythmias, and syncope suspected to be cardiac in origin (Gillingham, 2018). This procedure is used to obtain information about the electrical activity from within the heart, by recording and mapping intracardiac signals during normal sinus rhythm and during the induction of the patient's arrhythmia (Lee & Linker, 2014). The electrical signals of the cardiac conducting system are recorded by electrodes, which can also pace the heart. EP studies will often lead to a decision about the possibility of a catheter ablation being carried out to treat the underlying cause of the patient's condition and symptoms (Gillingham, 2018).

These studies can be lengthy, taking up to 4 hours to complete. The patient is usually conscious but may be lightly sedated during the study. Patients frequently find the procedure uncomfortable because of having to lie still for lengthy periods of time. In addition, patients frequently experience symptoms of their induced arrhythmia, which may be frightening and associated with symptoms such as dizziness, chest pain and palpitations.

Pre- and post-procedural care is similar to that for catheterization, except that patients may need to discontinue antiarrhythmic therapy some time before the study. Cessation of drug therapy leaves the patient without prophylactic protection against arrhythmias. This can cause some patients much anxiety during the period leading up to the study, as it may take many weeks before the body is cleared of some of the drugs.

Pre-procedure assessment and preparation of the patient prior to cardiac catheterization

It should be documented whether the patient is aware of any allergies to contrast medium or iodine. Although rare, some patients are allergic to the iodine contained in the contrast medium, which may cause symptoms of allergy, anaphylaxis and, rarely, death. Women aged between 15–50 years should be asked when they last menstruated and whether there is any possibility of them being pregnant, since the small dose of radiation from the X-rays could affect the developing fetus.

To enable the patient to give informed consent, the procedure should be explained and consent obtained by the medical staff. The Nursing and Midwifery Council (NMC) (2018) point out that in order to act in the best interests of patients at all times it is important to ensure that properly informed consent is gained and that this is documented before carrying out any action. The Royal College of Nursing (2017) provides guidance on the principles of consent for nurses including professional accountability and information to guide practice.

Assessment of the patient's level of anxiety can be used as a gauge to establish the depth of information required about the procedure. This could be in the form of verbal and non-verbal cues, such as posture, tone of voice and facial expressions. Recording baseline observations provides a basis for post-procedure comparison. Assessment includes measuring blood pressure, pulse, ECG, temperature and respiratory rate. The rate and volume of pedal pulses for the femoral approach and/or radial and ulnar pulses for the brachial approach should be assessed. These pulses can sometimes be difficult to find after catheterization, so a small pen mark with the patient's permission can indicate their exact position. The colour and temperature of all limbs should be documented, noting the pulse strength and capillary refill times, as these can be useful indicators of arterial sufficiency following the procedure.

Body weight should be recorded, since the dose of many drugs is calculated according to weight: e.g. heparin, which is commonly given during catheterization.

It is necessary to ensure that blood results regarding the patient's coagulation status and blood chemistry are available prior to catheterization, and that medical staff are informed of any abnormalities. A prolonged prothrombin time may result in bleeding after catheter insertion, whereas abnormal electrolytes may cause cardiac arrhythmias during or after the procedure. Patients at risk of developing contrast-induced nephropathy and those with preexisting renal impairment, diabetes or anaemia, or of advanced age should be risk-assessed and may need to have pre-hydration and their medication managed prior to the procedure (Mullasari & Victor, 2014). Patients taking metformin are advised to stop taking it 48 hours prior to and 48 hours post procedure; this is due to the risk of lactic acidosis when receiving contrast (Young, 2014).

Studies suggest that early education for patients waiting for elective cardiac catheterization may have a positive impact on patients' quality of life and perceived anxiety (Roberts-Collins et al, 2017; Haddad et al, 2017).

The patient should be fasted for a minimum of 2−3 hours according to local policy, as fasting will reduce gastric contents and the risk of inhaling vomit during the procedure, and will reduce this risk in the event of complications requiring emergency surgery. Longer fasting periods cause patient discomfort and dehydration, which can increase the difficulty of gaining venous access.

Management of the patient following cardiac catheterization

The main goals of care after catheterization are early detection of complications and to enhance patient comfort and safety. While cardiac catheterization remains the 'gold standard' in assessing coronary anatomy and cardiac function, it does carry a low but definite complication rate of <1% and mortality rate of 0.05% (Manda & Baradhi, 2018).

Whatever the method used for promoting haemostasis, the patient will require regular assessment of vital signs, distal pulses and the skin puncture site for haemorrhage and haematoma formation.

Assessment for impaired circulation of the affected limb includes palpation of the radial and ulnar pulses if the radial or brachial approach was used, and the dorsalis pedis and posterior tibial pulses in the foot if the femoral approach was used. These pulses should be assessed every 15 minutes for the first hour (or according to local policy). Presence or absence of the pulse should be assessed, as well as strength and rate. Colour, warmth and sensation of the limb distal to the arterial puncture site should also be assessed regularly according to local policy, and Doppler ultrasound may be useful when a pulse is weak or difficult to palpate. A cool, pulseless, pale limb with loss of sensation indicates poor or absent circulation due to interruption of blood flow by arterial occlusion. Capillary refill should be assessed and should be less than 3 seconds.

The introducer site, which may be covered with a clear dressing, should also be observed regularly for signs of bleeding and/or haematoma formation. If either is evident, a sterile dressing and firm pressure should be applied a few centimetres above the puncture site for approximately 15 minutes or until haemostasis is achieved. Occasionally, large haematomas require surgical evacuation, although most are reabsorbed over a period of time.

Providing the patient has not had any arrhythmias during the procedure, continuous ECG monitoring may not be necessary. If arrhythmias or myocardial ischaemia have been a problem, the patient's ECG is continuously monitored for further signs of arrhythmias, ischaemic changes and infarction. Vital signs should be recorded every 15 minutes for the first hour (depending on local policy) and reduced thereafter. Assessment should be carried out for symptoms such as shortness of breath, chest pain, back pain, access site pain and pain in the extremity, which should be identified and treated promptly. The patient should be monitored for changes in neurology, for example, decreased consciousness or limb/facial weakness, which may be caused by a stroke or a sedative effect. Vagus nerve stimulation may result in a decrease in pulse rate and myocardial contractility and vasodilatation, causing bradycardia and hypotension. If the heart rate is below 60 beats per minute and associated with hypotension, the immediate goal of care is to increase venous return and therefore blood pressure by placing the patient in a supine position with the lower limbs elevated. If bradycardia persists, the patient may be given atropine, which increases the heart rate and subsequently the blood pressure by inhibiting vagal stimulation (Bernelli, 2015). Intravenous fluids may be given to increase intravascular volume and therefore blood pressure. Atropine may cause angina in some susceptible patients because of the increase in heart rate and subsequent increase in myocardial oxygen demand, but the need for atropine usually outweighs this complication.

Patients may experience discomfort from the needle puncture or incision site, as well as ischaemic pain due to angina. The patient's level of pain and discomfort should be assessed regularly using a pain scale. Prescribed analgesics should be given as required and their effects evaluated. Pain that is unresolved should be investigated further, as angina unrelieved by vasodilators may indicate myocardial infarction, which requires urgent medical intervention. Pain experienced in the affected limb may indicate haematoma formation, or reduced or occluded blood supply, all of which require immediate attention and appropriate intervention.

Providing the patient is neither nauseated nor drowsy, oral fluids and diet can be recommenced; if the patient's fluid intake is not restricted, an oral fluid intake of 2.5 L in 24 hours should be encouraged to counteract dehydration due to the diuretic effect of the contrast medium. Increasing fluid intake also increases renal excretion of the contrast medium, which can be toxic to the renal tubules and can cause acute renal failure. Adequate hydration, before and after the procedure, is particularly important for any patient with impaired renal function (Mullasari & Victor, 2014).

Bedrest and immobilization are required for patients after catheterization of the femoral artery, to ensure that haemostasis has been achieved and to minimize haematoma formation. During the period of bedrest, the patient should be advised to keep the affected limb straight and relaxed with minimal movement until haemostasis is established. Duration of bedrest following cardiac catheterization relies on local practice, but need be no longer than 2–4 hours, depending on the type of vascular closure device used. Shorter duration of bedrest improves patient comfort and independence. Gentle mobilization can be commenced after the prescribed period of bedrest, providing there are no signs of bleeding or haematoma.

Preparation for discharge

The majority of patients admitted for these investigations have the procedure performed as a day case. Patients should be given appropriate advice before their discharge home, and should be advised to minimize their physical activity and to rest for 24 hours following the procedure. DVLA driving restrictions apply and patients should be given this advice on discharge. They should be advised not to lift heavy objects for 72 hours, to prevent bleeding from the arterial puncture site. If bleeding should occur, the patient or their carer should be advised to apply firm pressure to the puncture site for 15 minutes. If bleeding is not controlled, they should contact their general practitioner or a telephone advice number given by the hospital or clinic. If severe bleeding occurs, they should lie flat, ask someone to apply pressure and if it does not stop they should call the emergency services. Patients should similarly contact their GP or the hospital if the puncture site becomes red, painful or swollen, which is indicative of infection.

Patients should be advised of the results of their angiography and given further advice about lifestyle modification, management of risk factors and pharmacological therapy. Undergoing cardiac catheterization can be a difficult and anxious time for many patients. Enhancing knowledge and understanding about the procedure and self-care afterwards should reduce anxiety (Carroll et al, 2016).

Therapeutic catheterization

Patients requiring percutaneous coronary intervention and stent implantation or valvuloplasty should be prepared as for cardiac catheterization.

Percutaneous coronary intervention and stent implantation

Percutaneous coronary intervention (PCI) is a treatment for angina which eliminates or delays the need for coronary artery bypass grafts.

The aim of the procedure is to dilate the stenosed or narrowed segment(s) of the coronary artery or, if the artery is completely occluded by thrombus and atheroma, to reopen the artery. Angioplasty and stent implantation widens the diseased vessel lumen and improves blood flow, thus eliminating or reducing the symptoms of angina.

The procedure is similar to cardiac catheterization but differs in that a fine guidewire is introduced into a guiding catheter positioned in the opening of the affected coronary artery. The atraumatic wire is gently advanced into the artery and manipulated across the stenosed or occluded segment. Once the wire is in place, a tiny balloon measuring anything between 1.25 and 4 mm in diameter and between 10 and 30 mm in length (depending on the size of the artery and length of diseased segment) is threaded over the guidewire until it is positioned across the stenosed segment. Once the balloon is in place, it is inflated with a mixture of contrast medium and saline. Inflation of the balloon compresses the atheroma, which may also crack, thus widening the vessel lumen; however, a side-effect of this is local dissection of the arterial medial layer (Khan, 2018a). Widening of the vessel improves blood flow to the myocardium, with cessation or reduction of angina. Nearly all PCI procedures in practice employ a combination of balloon angioplasty and stent implantation (Khan, 2018a).

Stents are tiny tubes made of a wire mesh which, when expanded by a balloon within them, remain expanded and hold the artery open once the balloon has been deflated and withdrawn (Fig. 14.5). Stents provide structural support for the vessel wall by resisting elastic recoil and hold back any dissected tissue which could otherwise cause the artery to occlude immediately. Although stents have dramatically improved the angiographic results and halved the need for reintervention (Buccheri et al, 2016), they are associated with tissue hyperplasia, leading to in-stent restenosis. This becomes clinically apparent usually within 6 months after the procedure, with repeat revascularization required due to the reoccurrence of ischaemic symptoms and an increased morbidity and mortality (Khan, 2018a). In an attempt to overcome in-stent restenosis, stents that are coated with a drug that inhibits tissue proliferation into the stent lumen are available. These are referred to as drug-eluting stents and are recommended for use dependent upon the anatomy of the target lesion. The National Institute for Health and Care Excellence (NICE) recommends drug-eluding stents for use in patients in whom the lesion is longer than 15 mm or if the target artery has less than a 3-mm calibre (NICE, 2008). These stents have evolved and there are now second-generation stents which have a reported lower rate of stent thrombosis due to improvements in the design (Khan, 2018b).

The stent comes pre-mounted on a balloon catheter and is introduced into the coronary artery (Fig. 14.6A).

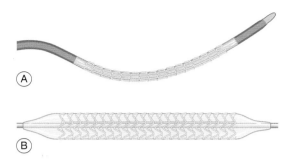

Figure 14.5 (A) A stent crimped onto a coronary angioplasty balloon. (B) A stent expanded by the balloon.

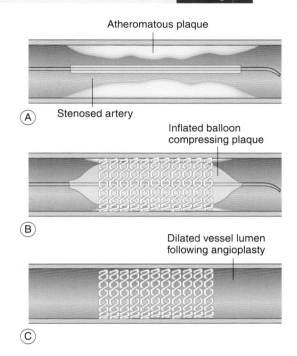

Figure 14.6 Percutaneous transluminal coronary angioplasty and insertion of an intracoronary stent. (A) Diagrammatic representation of a stenosed artery with a stent mounted on a balloon catheter within the artery lumen. (B) Angioplasty balloon inflated, expanding the stent within the artery wall. (C) Balloon removed, leaving behind the stent to maintain an open vessel lumen to improve blood flow.

When the balloon is inflated, the stent expands and is embedded into the artery wall (Fig. 14.6B); the balloon is deflated and removed, leaving the stent behind (Fig. 14.6C). The stent remains in the artery for life to provide structural support, keeping the arterial lumen open. The patient remains conscious but sedated throughout the procedure, which can take as little as 20 minutes (although a complex procedure can take longer). During balloon inflation, patients often experience moderate to severe angina caused by total occlusion of blood flow. Pain lasts while the balloon is inflated (Fig. 14.7), usually 15–60 seconds, and subsides on deflation. This is managed with vasodilating drugs such as glyceryl trinitrate. However, if the pain is severe, an opioid such as diamorphine may be given intravenously.

Pre-procedure preparation

Preparation of the patient is the same as that for cardiac catheterization.

To reduce the incidence of thrombus formation within the stent, patients undergoing percutaneous coronary intervention are prescribed a pre-treatment regimen of aspirin and clopidogrel, which inhibits platelet aggregation; in addition, thrombotic complications can be treated with glycoprotein IIb/IIIa receptor antagonists, which may be introduced before or during the procedure when *in situ* thrombus is present. Prasugrel can be used as an alternative to clopidogrel and has been found to have a significant benefit over clopidogrel with respect to cardiovascular events without an increase in bleeding (Young, 2014). It is also recommended by NICE as possible treatment for adults with acute coronary syndrome that are having PCI (NICE, 2014a). Ticagrelor is also another treatment option that has been found to improve outcomes compared to clopidogrel (NICE, 2014a). However, prasugrel and ticagrelor are reserved for selected high-risk patients undergoing complex PCI procedures (Neumann et al, 2018).

Unfractionated heparin is traditionally used during PCI procedures. Bivalirudin is an alternative anticoagulant to glycoprotein IIb/IIIa receptor antagonists and heparin, which may reduce the risk of bleeding in the perioperative period (Young, 2014). It is recommended for use if the patient is at risk of heparin-induced thrombocytopenia (Neumann et al, 2018).

The procedure should be explained, and consent obtained from the patient. As additional procedures such as emergency coronary artery bypass surgery may be required, patients must also consent to this. The patient and their family must be informed of these potential complications, and the implications of these understood by them (Neumann et al, 2018).

Post-procedure care and assessment

Assessment of vital signs and management post procedure are similar to those for cardiac catheterization, except that the removal of the arterial introducer sheath

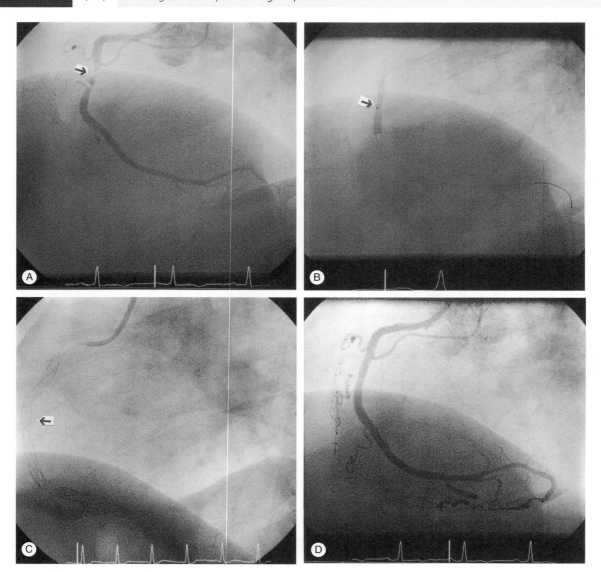

Figure 14.7 A sequence of radiographs showing (A) right coronary artery with stenosed segment (arrow); (B) angioplasty balloon inflated within the stenosed vessel; (C) a long stent within the vessel wall; (D) angiogram of the right coronary artery after angioplasty and stent implant.

from the femoral artery is delayed until the anticoagulant effects of heparin have worn off. Reversal of heparin is monitored by measuring activated clotting time (ACT), and the sheath is removed when this is <150 seconds (Kern et al, 2018). However, sheath removal may be done immediately after the percutaneous coronary intervention if a closure technique such as collagen implant or a suture device is used to seal the artery puncture site.

The patient should be placed in a supine position and instructed not to bend the leg at the hip, as this can cause kinking of the sheath, occlusion of the femoral artery or bleeding at the sheath site. To alter the patient's position, a 'log roll' procedure should be used. The sheath site should be observed regularly for bleeding and distal pulses assessed according to local guidelines. The temperature and colour of the affected limb should be assessed as above for signs of circulatory insufficiency, indicated by a cool, pale, pulseless limb.

The patient is continuously monitored by ECG to detect arrhythmias and waveform changes such as ST elevation or depression, which are indicative of cardiac ischaemia. Vital signs such as pulse, blood pressure and circulation are frequently monitored in the early post-procedure period, as described on page 243.

Any procedure that breaches the body's protective skin barrier requires strict asepsis when the arterial sheath is removed. The sheath is removed by a doctor or nurse deemed competent in sheath removal, once ACT is <150 seconds. Haemostasis is achieved by applying firm pressure over the sheath site with digital compression or with a femoral artery compression device such as the FemoStop for 20–30 minutes. Some patients may continue to require the FemoStop for a prolonged period due to anticoagulation, but at a reduced pressure. Analgesics should be given prior to sheath removal, to enhance comfort while firm groin pressure is required. Patients are able to mobilize 2–3 hours after sheath removal, providing there is no bleeding and their vital signs are stable (according to local policy).

There are a number of potential complications that can occur at varying times in both the immediate and late post-procedure period, including the following:

- *Tamponade* should be suspected if there is a change in the patient's haemodynamic status, such as a falling blood pressure and rising heart rate. The patient will require urgent bedside echocardiography if tamponade is suspected and this will require drainage (Young, 2014).
- *Retroperitoneal bleeding* due to bleeding from the posterior wall of the artery (a potentially serious complication). This manifests within 24–48 hours post-procedure with hypotension, back, flank or abdominal pain, and skin discoloration.
- *Femoral neuropathy* due to excessive pressure from the haemostasis device (early complication).
- *Stent thrombosis or coronary vessel occlusion* (early/delayed complication). Coronary artery spasm and occlusion can occur at any time after the procedure. Spasm and restenosis are more common after PCI when a stent has not been used. The patient should be monitored for chest pain and ischaemic ECG changes.
- *Pseudoaneurysm* due to damaged or ruptured vessel wall, resulting in bleeding into the surrounding tissue, and indicated by an enlarging, painful haematoma and widespread bruising (Stone et al, 2014).

In view of these complications, the nurse's role is to monitor the patient closely to detect these early and minimize their effects.

Following stent implantation, patients are prescribed clopidogrel and aspirin for their antiplatelet effects. Following elective stenting, dual antiplatelet therapy (DAPT) is recommended for approximately 6 months irrespective of stent type following PCI. It may be increased up to 12 months in specific clinical scenarios (Neumann et al, 2018). These drugs prevent stent thrombosis while protective endothelial tissue grows over the stent. It is essential that the patient has a good understanding of and is concordant with this drug therapy, as poor concordance may result in thrombosis and occlusion of the vessel, causing myocardial infarction or death. Once endothelialization is complete, the risk of thrombosis reduces and clopidogrel can be stopped, although aspirin is continued for life.

Care of the puncture site is much the same as that described in the cardiac catheterization section (see p. 243).

Primary percutaneous coronary intervention

Patients presenting with an acute ST-segment elevation myocardial infarction (STEMI) require myocardial reperfusion therapy as an emergency. This may be achieved by fibrinolytic (thrombolytic) therapy or by primary percutaneous coronary intervention (P-PCI). The procedure is similar to that described above and requires rapid access to the facilities of a cardiac catheterization laboratory with appropriately trained personnel. Following PCI and stenting for STEMI or non-ST-segment elevated myocardial infarction (NSTEMI) the patient should receive aspirin and a P2Y12-inhibitor for 12 months irrespective of stent type, if there is no excessive bleeding risk (Neumann et al, 2018). The patient will continue aspirin for the rest of their life.

Patient education

The patient should be provided with information on the management of chest pain, which could be caused by an in-stent thrombosis or stent restenosis. The patient should be advised on the use of glyceryl trinitrate (GTN) spray and informed to contact the emergency services if they feel unwell irrespective of GTN, or the chest pain lasts longer than 10 minutes.

The patient should be advised that they should not stop taking their aspirin and clopidogrel. The patient's cardiologist should be contacted if there are bleeding concerns. There is a risk of stent thrombosis if these drugs are discontinued.

The patient should be provided with information on the management of bleeding. They should avoid hot baths and showers for 48 hours and avoid heavy lifting for up to 72 hours to prevent the risk of bleeding.

The DVLA advises that the patient should not drive for 1 week following a successful PCI. If it was not successful this is increased to at least 4 weeks (DVLA, 2019b).

Dietary advice is pertinent to any patient with a history of atherosclerosis. A reduction in salt, sugar and saturated fat is recommended. Saturated fats should be replaced by polyunsaturated and monounsaturated fats, while an increased intake of fibre in the form of fresh fruit and vegetables, and replacement of fatty red meat with fish and chicken, should be advised (Piepoli et al, 2016).

Cardiac rehabilitation is an important part of the patient's treatment plan and should be recommended to all patients who undergo PCI procedures. It includes health education, advice on reducing cardiovascular risk, physical activity and stress management (Dalal et al, 2015). Cardiac rehabilitation programmes are also recommended by NICE, Department of Health, British Association for Cardiovascular Prevention and Rehabilitation (BACPR), and within wider European guidelines (Dalal et al, 2015).

Cardiac treatments

The following therapies involve catheterization of the right side of the heart via the venous system. Veins commonly used are the cephalic, subclavian, jugular and femoral veins. Electrodes may be inserted for:
- temporary or permanent pacing
- an implantable cardioverter defibrillator (ICD)
- ablation of intracardiac conduction pathways
- mitral valvuloplasty.

Cardiac pacing

Cardiac pacemakers are battery-powered devices that electrically stimulate the heart to contract when the patient's heart rate is abnormally slow – this is termed 'capture'. Pacemakers have two major functions: to sense the cardiac rhythm and to pace the heart. If the rhythm slows, the pacemaker will sense this and pace the heart at a pre-programmed rate. If the rhythm is faster than the pro-grammed rate, the pacemaker is inhibited until the heart rate slows again. This is known as demand pacing and maintains a stable heart rate. Biventricular pacing involves insertion of an additional pacing wire into the coronary sinus at the base of the right atrium. This acts as the left ventricular pacing lead, which aims to improve cardiac output, quality of life, and reduced hospital admissions in patients with chronic heart failure and left bundle branch block (Eftekhari et al, 2017).

Temporary pacemakers consist of a battery outside the body (the 'pacing box'), which is attached to an electrode positioned within the right atrium and/or right ventricle of the heart. Permanent pacemaker batteries are implanted under the skin of the chest wall (Fig. 14.8). The indications

for cardiac pacing and anti-arrhythmia devices have been reviewed (Brignole et al, 2013) and include:
- support for the conduction system following cardiac surgery, transcatheter aortic valve implantation (TAVI), and heart transplantation (usually temporary but may require permanent pacing)
- following myocardial infarction complicated by permanent atrioventricular block (usually temporary but may require permanent pacing)
- prophylaxis during general anaesthesia for patients with slow heart rates or asymptomatic atrioventricular block (usually temporary)
- conduction disturbances resulting in sinus arrest and ventricular standstill; bradycardia associated with a low cardiac output (usually a permanent system is required)
- overdrive pacing for tachyarrhythmias (permanent pacemakers with antitachycardia functions)
- when a permanent pacing system has failed or become infected (temporary)
- for cardiac resynchronization in some patients with heart failure (NICE, 2014b).

Cardiac pacing is usually done under local anaesthesia, and involves introducing a pacing electrode (wire) via the cephalic or subclavian vein into the right ventricle for single-chamber pacing, or into both the right atrium and ventricle for dual-chamber pacing. The heart can then be electrically stimulated to contract by an external temporary or

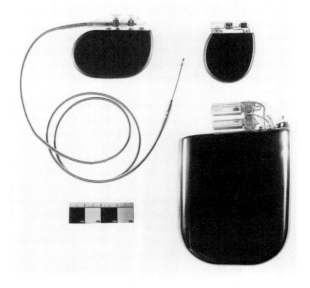

Figure 14.8 Implantable permanent pacemakers and pacing electrode. The larger device is an implantable cardioverter defibrillator with pacing functions.

permanently implanted pacemaker. An electrical impulse is initiated by the pacemaker, via the pacing electrode, which stimulates the heart muscle to depolarize and contract.

Preparation for cardiac pacing

As well as being a post-cardiac surgery manoeuvre, temporary pacing is often performed as an emergency procedure (Pitcher & Nolan, 2015) with little time to prepare the patient psychologically, whereas permanent pacing is usually performed electively, allowing adequate time for patient preparation.

The patient should not eat for 4–6 hours prior to the procedure but may be able to take oral fluids up until 2 hours before (according to local policy) (Fawcett & Thomas, 2018), as dehydration and subsequent collapse of the veins causes difficulty in cannulation for insertion of the pacing electrode. Blood pressure, pulse, temperature, respiratory rate and 12-lead ECG are recorded.

Informed consent should be obtained by the medical staff, although this may not be possible during an emergency. The patient's understanding of the procedure and their need for information should be ascertained. An explanation of why pacing is required and what to expect during and immediately after the procedure should be given, and the patient reassured that the procedure is not unduly painful.

Postoperative care and assessment

Caring for the patient following temporary or permanent pacing is similar, except that with temporary pacing the pacing box is external and will require intermittent checks to ensure correct functioning (Reade, 2007). The ECG is monitored for rhythm, rate and presence of pacemaker-induced beats, which are preceded by an artefact called the pacing spike. The pacing spike either appears before the P wave in atrial pacing or before the QRS complex in ventricular pacing. Patients with temporary pacemakers require the dressing to be inspected to ensure that it is secure and clean, and that the pacing electrode is taped to prevent movement and accidental removal. It is important to check that the electrode is securely attached to the pacing box, which is positioned safely to prevent it falling. The pacemaker settings, such as rate, pacing mode and energy output, should be recorded in the patient's nursing notes. Vital signs should be monitored closely for the first hour (or according to local policy), because although complications are uncommon, they can be serious (Iig, 2014); thus, it is important that they are detected early on and treated. Complications that can occur with temporary or permanent pacing, or following electrophysiology studies or ablation, include:

- *Pneumothorax/haemothorax* (1–3%): frequently asymptomatic, caused by air or blood entering the pleural space during subclavian vein cannulation.

Respiratory status is monitored for dyspnoea, increased resting respiratory rate, unequal chest movement, tachycardia, hypotension and reduced oxygen saturation. Diagnosis is confirmed by a chest X-ray, which will show the absence of lung markings in the lung field. If symptomatic, treatment with an intercostal chest drain may be required.

- *Cardiac perforation:* caused by the electrode penetrating the heart during the procedure. It is often asymptomatic and resolved by repositioning the electrode. Rarely, this can result in the serious complication of cardiac tamponade, wherein blood leaks into the pericardial space, gradually inhibiting the ability of blood to fill the ventricles during diastole (Jenson et al, 2017). Blood, trapped in the pericardial space, compresses and progressively reduces the size of the ventricles, compromising ventricular filling and cardiac output, resulting in hypotension and tachycardia. This emergency is managed by inserting a needle through the chest wall into the pericardial space to aspirate the blood and relieve the tamponade (pericardiocentesis), or may even require sternotomy or thoracotomy (Vanezis et al, 2017).

- *Pacemaker pocket haematoma:* caused by inadequate haemostasis within the pocket or by backflow from around the pacing electrode in the vein. Haematomas frequently resolve without the need for intervention and are slowly absorbed; however, the pocket should be monitored for pain and haematoma formation, as pocket haematoma has been recorded at 5.2% of insertions, resulting in prolonged hospital stay for some patients (Palmer, 2014).

- *Infection:* 1%–6% of pacemaker systems become infected and may require removal and replacement. Infection causes appreciable morbidity and mortality. Strict asepsis during and after pacemaker implantation is essential to prevent this; if infection does occur, early detection and antibiotic treatment are important.

Pacemaker dysfunction

The ECG should be monitored for pacing failure – either failure to sense or failure to capture (Palmer, 2014; Mulpuru et al, 2017), as indicated by the following:

- *Oversensing:* pacemaker senses and is inhibited from pacing by non-cardiac signals such as skeletal muscle contraction. These extra signals switch the pacemaker off, causing an absence of pacing, with the heart rate dropping below the set demand rate of the pacemaker. To remedy this fault, it may be necessary to decrease the sensitivity level of the pacemaker or remove any ungrounded electrical equipment which may be interfering with the pacemaker.

- *Undersensing:* pacemaker is unable to sense the patient's underlying rhythm and so paces regardless, which may initiate ventricular tachycardia if a pacing stimulus coincides with the vulnerable phase of the heart's relative refractory period. Undersensing may be caused by the following:

- loose connections (temporary pacemaker), requiring tightening of the lead connections
- loss of electrode contact with the myocardium, or lead fracture, requiring repositioning or replacement of the lead (temporary or permanent pacemaker)
- low battery, necessitating pacemaker replacement
- pacemaker sensitivity levels set too low.
- *Failure to capture*: pacemaker fails to capture or pace the heart, indicated by a pacing spike that is not followed immediately by a QRS complex. Possible causes for this fault are similar to those causing under- or oversensing.

The threshold of temporary pacemakers should be checked daily. The threshold is a measure of the minimum amount of energy required to pace or depolarize the heart continuously (Reade, 2007). It is normal for the threshold to rise slightly during pacing. This is due to inflammation resulting from the repetitive electrical stimulation of the heart by the pacemaker, although some metabolic disturbances such as acidosis and hyperkalaemia will also increase the threshold. It will also rise if the electrode has moved or become displaced within the ventricle.

Threshold is measured by a cardiac technician or nurse deemed competent in performing the procedure. A continuous pacing rhythm must be present; to achieve this it may be necessary to increase the pacing rate above the patient's intrinsic heart rate. Caution should be exercised if the patient's intrinsic rate is high, as pacing at a higher rate may cause ventricular tachycardia or fibrillation. Once a pacing rhythm is detected on the ECG monitor, the voltage output switch is slowly reduced until the pacing rhythm is interrupted (Reade, 2007); this is the pacing threshold. The pacing output should then be reset to a level two to three times greater than the threshold. This allows for subsequent threshold increases, and the pacing rate to be reduced to the prescribed level. If the pacing threshold has increased dramatically, medical staff should be informed, since the pacing electrode may require repositioning to prevent pacing failure.

Patient education

Generally, patients recover quickly from pacemaker insertion and experience an improvement in physical activity and confidence due to cessation of pre-pacing symptoms (British Heart Foundation, 2018b). Patients with permanent pacemakers need to be provided with information about their pacemaker prior to discharge home. It is essential that the patient understands the need to regularly attend pacemaker clinic appointments, where pacemaker functions can be checked using non-invasive techniques.

Some alteration in lifestyle may be required, and the patient is given the following information:

- Patients should be advised not to undertake vigorous exercise for 4–6 weeks following implantation of the pacemaker. Patients can resume sexual activity but are advised to avoid positions that place pressure on their arms and chest for 4 weeks after insertion. This prevents dislodgement of the pacing electrode from the heart (British Heart Foundation, 2018b). After this period, scar tissue develops and holds the electrode firmly within the heart.
- Pacemaker manufacturers provide patient information sheets with advice about electrical equipment to be avoided, e.g. mobile phones should be held on the opposite side to the pacemaker and shop alarm systems and security systems at airports may be activated by the metal components in the pacemaker (British Heart Foundation, 2018b).
- Patients with pacemakers should not, generally, have MRI scans. However, some of the new models are able to withstand MRI scanning. The patient should be informed of this and have it documented on their pacemaker ID card (British Heart Foundation, 2018b).
- The patient is advised to seek medical advice if the original symptoms return, so that the pacemaker function can be checked.
- The patient should be given information on how to recognize signs of wound infection, and actions to take in the event of this.
- The patient should be encouraged to always carry a pacemaker identification card.
- Pacemakers have a life span of 6–10 years (British Heart Foundation, 2018b), so patients should be aware that the pacemaker will eventually need to be replaced because of a flat battery.
- The DVLA must be notified if a patient has had a pacemaker inserted. Patients should not drive a vehicle until after their first pacemaker check (usually 1 week after insertion), which will ensure that it is functioning correctly (DVLA, 2019c). This is providing that there is no other disqualifying condition (DVLA, 2019c).

Patients should be reassured that pacemakers are very reliable and encouraged to resume their pre-pacing lifestyle. Useful patient information about pacing and cardiac procedures can be obtained from the British Cardiology Society website.

Implantable cardioverter defibrillator

Implantable cardioverter defibrillators (ICDs) were introduced in the late 1980s. These devices have numerous functions, as described below, but are essentially used for patients at risk of sudden cardiac death due to malignant ventricular cardiac arrhythmias. In the UK, 50,000–70,000 sudden cardiac deaths occur annually and this represents the single most significant cause of death from coronary heart disease (NICE, 2014c). ICDs act in a similar way to pacemakers in sensing cardiac rhythms, triggering antitachycardia pacing, providing bursts of pacing impulses and, if necessary, delivering high-energy defibrillation to revert ventricular fibrillation. A summary of the current guidelines is given in Table 14.2.

The ICD looks very similar to a pacemaker except that it is larger and heavier, weighing about 75 g rather than about 30 g (British Heart Foundation, 2019b) (see Fig. 14.8); it is implanted in the same way as a pacemaker.

The ICD has a number of functions: it is able to detect life-threatening tachyarrhythmias and terminate these by either overdrive pacing, cardioversion or defibrillation. When the ICD detects a fast rhythm, it will attempt to slow it down by initiating a short burst of rapid pacing that may interrupt the tachycardia, thus slowing the rate. If this is unsuccessful, the ICD either will cardiovert the rhythm with a low-energy shock or, if the rhythm degenerates into ventricular fibrillation, will defibrillate the heart with a higher-energy shock. The ICD is also able to pace the heart in the event of the recovering rhythm being too slow (Bryant et al, 2016).

Specific pre- and post-implant care

Physical preparation and post-implant care of the patient are the same as for pacemaker implantation. Patients will be reviewed after 2–4 weeks to check the insertion site, and thereafter for device analysis every 3–6 months (Mansour & Khairy, 2014) The patient will require a very high level of psychological preparation and support before and after the procedure. The ICD does not cure the patient's arrhythmia, it merely controls it. The shocks emitted from the ICD are sudden and painful, whatever the energy level of the shock. The shocks can bring into sharp focus the fact that the patient has probably just experienced a life-threatening arrhythmia. Some patients may even lose consciousness prior to the shock, due to interruption of cardiac output as a result of the tachyarrhythmia. The ICD battery lasts about 4–8 years and the patient should be advised that the battery will not be allowed to run out and it may bleep or vibrate to warn that it needs to be changed (British Heart Foundation, 2019b). The latest ICDs can also be followed up from home with a home monitor. This allows the hospital team to monitor the ICD closely without the patient having to attend hospital, but it does not replace follow-up appointments. This is new technology and not available to all ICDs (British Heart Foundation, 2019b).

Patient education and support

A number of issues should be discussed with patients to help them adjust to living with an ICD (Pedersen et al, 2016). These include giving the patient the opportunity to talk about the meaning of the shocks, which will involve honest discussion regarding the seriousness of the arrhythmia. The patient must be prepared for the fact that the

---

Table 14.2 Indications for implantable cardioverter defibrillators

Secondary prevention (in absence of a treatable cause)	Primary prevention
Cardiac arrest due to ventricular tachycardia or ventricular fibrillation	A history of previous (no more than 4 weeks) myocardial infarction **OR:** Left ventricular dysfunction with a left ventricular ejection fraction of <35% **and** QRS duration of ≥120 milliseconds
Spontaneous sustained ventricular tachycardia, causing syncope or haemodynamic compromise	Familial cardiac conditions causing sudden cardiac death, such as long QT syndrome, hypertrophic cardiomyopathy, Brugada syndrome or arrhythmogenic right ventricular dysplasia (ARVD), or having undergone surgical repair of congenital heart disease
Sustained ventricular tachycardia, without syncope or cardiac arrest and who have an associated reduction in ejection fraction (left ventricular ejection fraction of <35%) but their symptoms are no worse than class III of the New York Heart Association (NYHA) functional classification of heart failure.	

Source: NICE (2014).

shocks may be painful and sudden, and have been described by some patients as like being kicked in the chest by a horse. Both patient and relatives need to be reassured that the shock will not be felt by anyone else touching the patient during the shock.

Patients with heavy goods vehicle or public service vehicle licences lose these automatically (DVLA, 2019c); the patient will not be able to drive because of the risk of losing consciousness during activation of the ICD. For drivers of other vehicles, the regulations are somewhat complex, but generally they may not drive for 6 months following the implantation, and subsequently they must be free from any intervention from the device for 6 months before resuming driving (DVLA, 2019c).

Considerable time may need to be spent with both the patient and relatives, both of whom need help to understand the implications of having an ICD (Humphreys et al, 2018) and assistance to regain confidence in the patient's ability to resume the normal activities of living. Anxiety is very common following ICD implantation, affecting up to 87% of patients, and depression is reported in up to 20–35% of patients (Clarke, 2015). Psychological support is identified as an essential need from the patient's own perspective (Clarke, 2015). Some patients, however, are reported to be so frightened by the prospect of receiving a shock that their quality of life is actually profoundly inhibited (Clarke, 2015).

Many centres which insert ICDs now offer considerable support for their patients through patient-led support groups and cardiac rehabilitation; national organizations also offer such support, e.g. the Cardiomyopathy Association.

Implantable loop recorders

Implantable loop recorders (ILRs) are small electronic devices that are planted subcutaneously to monitor the patient for arrythmias that could be the cause of unexplained syncope, unexplained palpitations, and detection of paroxysmal atrial fibrillation. They can be programmed to detect pre-specified arrythmias and can also be manually activated to record when the patient experiences symptoms (Gilmore & Anderson, 2016). They allow for an accurate detection, diagnosis and access to treatment such as pacemakers, ICDs and anticoagulation for atrial fibrillation (Eftekhari et al, 2017).

Cardiac ablation

When abnormal conducting tissue is discovered during electrophysiology studies, cardiac ablation may be considered; this involves the destruction of the abnormal conducting tissue.

A variety of conduction abnormalities causing symptomatic and potentially life-threatening tachyarrhythmias are indications for this procedure (Katritsis et al, 2017).

- *Wolff–Parkinson–White syndrome (WPW)*, which is a congenital abnormality where the atria and ventricles are connected by abnormal conducting muscle fibres, known as accessory pathways. Impulses can travel along these pathways very rapidly, causing tachycardia. There is a >95% success rate for this procedure, particularly for Wolff–Parkinson–White syndrome and atrioventricular nodal re-entrant tachycardia (Sternick et al, 2017).
- *Atrioventricular nodal re-entrant tachycardia (AVNRT)* occurs when there are slow- and fast-conducting pathways in the AV node or perinodal tissue. Impulses normally travel via the fast pathway. If the patient has a premature atrial ectopic, this conducted impulse may find the fast pathway blocked, or refractory to further stimulation, and so is conducted via the slow pathway. If the fast pathway has recovered sufficiently, the impulse can then return via this route to re-excite the atrium, causing a re-entrant tachycardia. This type of tachycardia can be treated by partially destroying the AV node (Katritsis et al, 2016).
- *Atrial fibrillation (sustained and paroxysmal)* that is symptomatic despite antiarrhythmic medication. The pulmonary vein is isolated, and ablation performed to the left and right atrium to stop the pathway that supports re-entry waves that sustain atrial fibrillation (Ramrakha & Hill, 2012). The patient may require a transoesophageal echo to ensure there is no thrombus in the left atrial appendage of left atrium prior to the procedure (Ramrakha & Hill, 2012).
- *Atrial flutter and ventricular tachycardia* may also be treated by ablation.

Ablation of the abnormal conduction pathway is carried out most commonly by using radiofrequency electric current. Radiofrequency ablation delivers an electrical current directly to the abnormal endocardial tissue via the catheter; the interface between the catheter and the endocardium is heated to temperatures over 50°C until focal cell death occurs (Ramrakha & Hill, 2012). This results in the disappearance of electrical activity in the ablated tissue. Alternatively, cryoablation techniques destroy the tissue by freezing it to −70°C (Ramrakha & Hill, 2012). During the procedure, the patient should not experience pain, but may well sense the passing of the catheters through their blood vessels, as well as the discomfort of having to lie still for prolonged periods. The patient will therefore require reassurance and support throughout their treatment.

The procedure is carried out under local anaesthesia, and the patient will be given both sedation and analgesics during this often lengthy and potentially uncomfortable procedure. Catheters can be positioned in the heart from the femoral, subclavian or jugular veins, or from the femoral artery. These catheters are removed after the procedure while the patient is still in the catheterization laboratory. Haemostasis is achieved through the application of firm pressure over the insertion sites, as described in the section on pages 240–241.

Pre-procedure preparation

Physical preparation of the patient is the same as that for pacemaker insertion, although psychological preparation should be tailored to helping the patient understand the treatment and likely sensations that will be experienced during the ablation. There is a 1% risk of complete heart block for patients with atrioventricular nodal re-entrant tachycardia (Asirvatham & Stevenson, 2015), which would result in the need for a permanent pacemaker.

Post-procedure management

On return to the ward, the patient should be monitored for early detection of the original arrhythmia (Thanavaro, 2019). Vital signs should be monitored closely in the immediate post-procedure period for complications such as pneumothorax and tamponade associated with catheter insertion although complications are currently found in less than 4% of ablation patients (Thanavaro, 2019). Vascular puncture sites should be observed for bleeding and haematoma formation. If the artery was cannulated during the procedure, perfusion of the affected limb should also be monitored as described on page 243.

Providing the patient is well and has not had any complications, discharge from hospital usually occurs the following day. Prior to discharge, the patient should be given advice about puncture site management and educated about relevant drug therapy. Patients who receive clear, instructive and relevant information tailored to their individual needs are more likely to adapt better to any constraints of their illness, and are in a position to make informed choices.

Mitral valvuloplasty

Mitral valve stenosis is a progressive disease which is usually fatal without some form of intervention that will enlarge the valve orifice enough to allow adequate cardiac output. Stenosis occurs when the valve cusps thicken and there is fusion of the commissures, which interferes with normal valve opening and closing. This disease process frequently occurs as a result of a previous episode of rheumatic heart disease (Ancona & Pinto, 2019)

Percutaneous balloon mitral valvuloplasty (PBMV) is the treatment of choice for the majority of patients with symptomatic mitral stenosis (Baumgartner et al, 2017). The preparations for valvuloplasty are similar to those for cardiac catheterization. The patient remains conscious,

although sedated, throughout the procedure. Although the mitral valve is in the left side of the heart, an Inoue balloon catheter is introduced into the right side, over a pre-positioned guidewire, via the femoral vein (Fig. 14.9). Access to the left atrium and ventricle is obtained by puncturing the atrial septum from inside the heart with a transseptal needle. This part of the procedure is usually well tolerated by the patient. Alternatively, retrograde arterial approaches into the left atrium are also possible but there is high risk of arterial damage (Sanati & Firoozi, 2017). Once the balloon is positioned within the valve opening, it is inflated with diluted contrast medium, which separates the fused commissures of the stenosed valve.

On completion of the procedure, the balloon and other catheters are removed, and the vascular introducer sheaths are removed once the anticoagulant effects of heparin have reversed. Nursing management of the introducer site varies between manual techniques and those employing vascular closure devices. The patient should avoid moving the affected limb, to assist haemostasis, and should remain on bedrest until haemostasis has been achieved and vital signs are stable. Pre- and post-procedure care is similar to the care described for patients undergoing

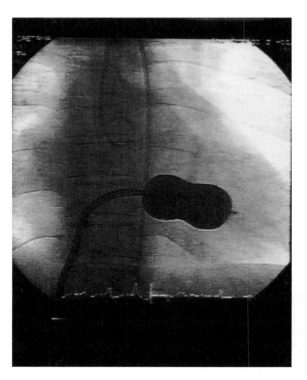

Figure 14.9 An X-ray of an inflated valvuloplasty balloon dilating a stenosed mitral valve.

cardiac catheterization. However, the patient should be closely monitored for the first few hours for any arrhythmias, and for signs of tamponade caused by compression of the heart's chambers by fluid in the pericardial space (Jenson et al, 2017). This may occur if the guidewire or catheter punctures the myocardial wall and causes blood to leak into the pericardial space. This results in hypotension, low cardiac output, tachycardia and tachypnoea, and requires immediate medical intervention to prevent irreversible shock and death. Patients are discharged home the following day, providing there have been no postprocedure complications, which include systemic emboli and bleeding. Damage to the valve resulting in severe regurgitation is rare but could require mitral valve replacement surgically (Sanati & Firoozi, 2017). Balloon valvuloplasty can also be carried out in patients with aortic valve stenosis, but with less success, and typically would be for patients for whom aortic valve replacement is unsuitable or for assessment prior to transcatheter aortic valve implantation (Keeble et al, 2016).

Transcatheter aortic valve implantation

Calcification of the aortic valve is the most common cause of aortic stenosis in the ageing population. A buildup of calcium within the layers of the valve leaflets develops and restricts the leaflets from moving, which can obstruct the left ventricle during systole (Carpenter, 2019).

Transcatheter aortic valve implantation (TAVI) may be offered to symptomatic patients not suitable for surgery due to risk factors such as old age, severe comorbidities and left ventricular dysfunction (Carpenter, 2019). TAVI was first developed in 2004 as a less invasive procedure than aortic valve surgery for high-risk patients that develop symptomatic aortic valve stenosis (AS) (Khosravi & Wendler, 2018). Patients who are put forward for the TAVI procedure should also expect to live for more than one year (Baumgartner et al, 2017). Access is gained commonly via both femoral arteries (but subclavian, transaortic, and transapical approaches are used) and a xenograft prosthetic valve (porcine or bovine) is placed in the aortic valve via a catheter or a balloon which will push the native diseased valve out of the way (Carpenter, 2019). The new graft is mounted on a frame, so it does not require sutures to remain in place.

The patient will need cardiac monitoring post-procedure due to the risk of developing heart block (Carpenter, 2019). The patient's vital signs will need to be monitored closely for the risk of deterioration, which will require immediate intervention. The access sites will need to be monitored for complications as described in postoperative management of cardiac catheterization on page 243. Pacing wires may be placed during the procedure and should be removed only when indicated. Neurological function should be closely monitored for signs of stroke, as patients are at increased risk post-TAVI (Carpenter, 2019). If there are no complications, the patient can normally sit out of bed the next day and the nurse should ensure that pain relief is given (British Heart Foundation, 2019c). Currently dual antiplatelet therapy with aspirin and clopidogrel for up to 6 months is the recommended treatment after TAVI (Magkoutis et al, 2016).

Open cardiac surgery

Cardiac surgery is required for a number of disorders that cannot be controlled or treated by conservative management. Coronary artery disease and valvular disease are the most common conditions requiring open cardiac surgery. A proportion of patients will require heart transplantation due to end-stage heart failure where other treatments are no longer effective in controlling the condition.

Prior to cardiac surgery, patients have usually undergone a series of investigations and treatments, as discussed above. The patient and their family typically attend a preadmission clinic 2—4 weeks prior to admission, so that the appropriate blood tests and other investigations can be carried out. Preoperative education is given on either an individual or a group discussion basis. Not surprisingly, patients are often very anxious prior to cardiac surgery and it is often difficult to balance the need to explain the procedure against the risk of unduly alarming them. Physical preparation for surgery is as for any surgery (see Chapter 2). Psychological preparation for surgery plays an important role postoperatively, as anxiety and pain may be reduced.

Coronary artery bypass surgery

A number of patients do not get symptomatic relief from percutaneous coronary interventions, or have extensive coronary artery disease, and may require coronary artery bypass grafting (CABG). A small number of patients require this surgery urgently, either due to acute deterioration or following complications from cardiac catheterization or percutaneous transluminal coronary angioplasty. This is a major procedure and postoperative care in the intensive care unit may be required; however, stable patients are increasingly extubated early and 'fast tracked' back to high dependency areas, so reducing the pressure on intensive care beds (Bainbridge & Cheng, 2017).

The traditional procedure involves exposing the heart through a median sternotomy and placing the patient on cardiopulmonary bypass, which takes over the function of the heart and lungs during surgery. This is followed by excision of a portion of a donor vessel, which is then anastomosed to the aorta and distally to the coronary artery below the obstruction, thus re-establishing blood flow via the graft.

The most common donor grafts used to include the long saphenous vein or the radial artery. An alternative technique is to use the internal mammary artery. In this case, the artery is only detached distally and the free end anastomosed to the coronary artery below the blockage. Use of the internal mammary artery is the 'gold standard' graft for bypassing the left anterior descending (LAD) coronary artery in patients undergoing CABG and is used in over 95% of patients worldwide (Squiers & Mack, 2018). The internal mammary artery is used because it remains patent for a longer time than other grafts; this appears to be due to its resistance to atheroma formation. Bilateral internal mammary artery grafts are also being used in carefully selected individuals (Squiers & Mack, 2018). The use of the internal mammary artery is not without risk, however, as its use may lead to delayed sternal healing because the internal mammary artery supplies the chest wall and much of the area incised to access the heart. Respiratory complications may be more common, due to the concomitant increase in pain associated with this procedure and thus a reluctance to deep breathe.

Recovery from surgery takes longer than that from percutaneous techniques; as well as the sternal wound, there may also be wounds in the thigh, leg, and/or wrist if the saphenous vein and/or radial artery have been used. If the saphenous vein has been used, the thigh/leg wound may take longer to heal than the sternal wound for a number of reasons; these include anaemia, oedema and reduced blood supply to the lower limb because of the presence of peripheral vascular disease. Furthermore, saphenous vein grafts are known to have a 50% occlusion rate by the tenth year when used for revascularization (McKavanagh et al, 2017). Arterial grafts such as the left internal mammary artery (LIMA) and radial arterial grafts are reported to have a 90% patency rate at 10 years (Bachar & Manna, 2019).

Newer approaches

Recent years have seen discussions regarding the safety of the conventional approach of full sternotomy, cardiopulmonary bypass and induced cardiac arrest — cardioplegia. There is particular concern about the manipulation of the aorta when the patient is first put on cardiopulmonary bypass, as it increases the risk of microemboli in the general circulation. In addition, cardiopulmonary bypass may cause a total inflammatory response, due to contact of the blood with the artificial surfaces of the cardiopulmonary bypass circuit (Kraft et al, 2015). As a result, cardiopulmonary bypass may be responsible for causing many of the postoperative complications: myocardial dysfunction, respiratory failure, acute kidney injury (AKI), neurological

dysfunction, and bleeding disorders (Kraft et al, 2015). Consequently, less interventional surgery such as minimally invasive coronary artery surgery using a mini-thoracotomy incision has been developed (Langer & Argenziano, 2016). This reduces the risks associated with sternotomy and cardiopulmonary bypass, which is experiencing increasing patient demand (Langer & Argenziano, 2016) and has been identified as being advantageous to the increasing population of elderly (over 75 years old) cardiac surgery patients (Barsoum et al, 2014). Off-pump or beating heart surgery, using a device known as an octopus to stabilize and immobilize a portion of heart tissue during graft anastomosis, is an alternative approach to this problem, with a reduced associated incidence of atrial fibrillation, stroke, renal failure and chest infections (Head et al, 2017).

Valve replacement

Patients undergoing valve replacement surgery will benefit from an improvement in their symptoms. However, valve replacement poses a new set of potential complications related to the valve prothesis and they all carry limitations for the patient. Types of prosthetic valve used are mechanical valves, animal valves (xenografts), or valves from a cadaver (homografts) (Fig. 14.10).

An example of a mechanical heart valve is the St Jude bileaflet valve (Fig. 14.10B). Mechanical valves are at risk of thrombosis and therefore obstruction, which could lead to a disabling or fatal stroke. This means that the patient has to take anticoagulants for the rest of their life. Thromboembolism and anticoagulant-related bleeding present the majority of complications experienced by prosthetic valve replacement patients (Baumgartner et al, 2017). Infection is another significant problem. However, if neither of these complications occur, mechanical valves are very durable, lasting for many years.

Animal valves (also known as bioprosthetic valves) are commonly harvested from a pig (porcine) or a cow (bovine), e.g. a Carpentier—Edwards Magna Ease valve, which can be treated with glutaraldehyde for human use (Fig. 14.10C). Cadaver valves are used less commonly due to the lack of availability (NHS Blood and Transplant, 2019).

It is important that the patient is involved in the decision-making process, as for some patients it may not be feasible to accept a xenograft or homograft for religious, moral or ethical reasons, while other patients may not manage with long-term anticoagulation. The choice between a mechanical or a bioprosthetic valve is normally determined by estimating the risk of anticoagulant-related bleeding and thromboembolism with a mechanical valve versus the structural deterioration with a bioprosthesis and by considering the patient's lifestyle and preferences. Bioprostheses may be considered in patients whose life

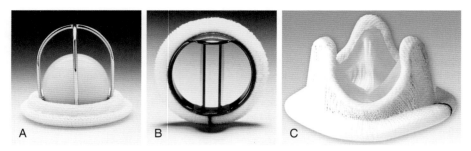

Figure 14.10 Examples of prosthetic valve. (A) Starr—Edwards caged ball valve. (B) St Jude medical bileaflet valve. (C) Carpentier—Edwards Magna valve (xenograft). ((From deWit, S.C., Stromberg, H.K., Vreeland Dallred, C. (2017). *Medical-Surgical Nursing: Concepts and Practice* (3rd edn.). Elsevier Inc, with permission.))

expectancy is lower than the presumed durability of the valve (Baumgartner et al, 2017). One result of the number of patients undergoing successful valve replacement and an ageing population is that more 'redo' replacements are now being performed.

Patients with a prosthetic valve may require future replacement because of the valve developing faults. All patients with prosthetic valves need to take precautions against infection. Prophylactic antibiotics must be taken prior to any invasive surgical or dental procedure (Baumgartner et al, 2017). There is also a risk of developing infective endocarditis, particularly in the first 3 months after surgery, which can damage the anastomosis, causing life-threatening valve failure — although the incidence is reported as being 1—6% (Karchmer et al, 2019).

Postoperative management following open heart surgery

Patients undergoing cardiac surgery were traditionally considered as being critically ill and remained in the intensive care unit for 24—48 hours postoperatively. This has now been reduced to only a few hours or an overnight stay, before being transferred back to a high-dependency area within a ward where close monitoring can be continued. The Enhanced Recovery After Surgery (ERAS) programme is developing rapidly within cardiac surgery as a result of advances in surgical and anaesthetic techniques and the need to streamline cardiac services, with the increased demand for cardiac surgery (Li et al, 2018). It encourages patients to play an active role in preparing for surgery and their recovery. The key principles of the ERAS programme include patient education, optimization pre- and postoperatively, medical optimization, early extubation, nausea and vomiting control, good pain control, encouraged nutritional intake, minimal invasive procedures, and early mobilization (McConnell et al, 2018). The ERAS programme also provides the patient with daily goals they should strive to work towards.

Most patients following the ERAS programme will have been identified at the preassessment clinic. Factors taken into account include the patient being fit preoperatively with a lower preoperative risk. As well as the preoperative risk, the length of operation, maintenance of haemodynamic stability and early extubation must be considered (Ljungqvist et al, 2017).

This group of patients spend less time in intensive care and return to the ward as soon as they are haemodynamically stable. Blood loss from chest drains should also be minimal, with minimal oxygen requirement, and maintaining satisfactory arterial blood gases and oxygen saturation levels. Once the patient is transferred back to the ward, the continuing goals of care in the postoperative period are to maintain adequate spontaneous ventilation, oxygenation and haemodynamic stability, which will in part be achieved if the patient is comfortable, pain-free and mobilizing.

Cardiac rhythm disturbances

ECG monitoring is required for early detection of atrial/ventricular arrhythmias; atrial fibrillation is one of the commonest arrhythmias, occurring in approximately 35% of surgical patients postoperatively (Greenberg et al, 2017). Arrhythmias are common due to electrolyte derangement resulting from cardiopulmonary bypass and the induced hypothermia as part of the procedure. Rhythm disturbances can compromise blood pressure, so appropriate drug therapy will be prescribed. The patient may develop dysrhythmias during or after surgical manipulation, which can also affect blood pressure and require temporary cardiac pacing via the epicardial pacing electrodes which are inserted during surgery (Ley & Koulakis, 2015).

Fluid balance disturbances

The central venous pressure (CVP) is monitored for pressure increases (indicating hypervolaemia) or decreases (indicating hypovolaemia). Central venous pressure is also an indicator of right ventricular function, with raised pressure indicating some degree of impairment. Frequent blood pressure monitoring is required. Hypotension may indicate vasodilatation due to elevated core temperature, or hypovolaemia due to blood loss or inadequate fluid replacement. Nurses frequently manage fluid balance using integrated care pathways that detail which medications or intravenous infusions should be given to optimize the patient's fluid balance (Hardin & Kaplow, 2019).

Hypertensive episodes (systolic pressure >140 mmHg) may cause rupture or blood leakage at the graft suture lines or may 'drive' a small bleed from an anastomosis. Prevention of these complications requires treatment with an intravenous vasodilator such as glyceryl trinitrate, which is titrated against the patient's blood pressure to maintain normotension. Hypertensive episodes may be caused by pain and therefore require effective analgesia. Anxiety may be reduced by the nurse reassuring the patient and perhaps involving relatives in the patient's care; if these measures fail, anxiolytic treatment may be required.

Chest drains are inserted at the time of surgery into the pleural, mediastinal and pericardial spaces; these must be closely monitored and blood loss recorded (see Chapter 15). Low suction — about 5 kPa — is commonly applied to the chest drains to encourage drainage.

In the immediate postoperative period, measurement of drainage will be carried out regularly, and if excessive (≥100 mL/h), although most cardiac units will have their own local policies, indicating an active bleed, it should be reported to medical staff. If there is no or very little drainage and the patient is haemodynamically unstable, a high index of suspicion should be assumed that there may be collections in the pericardial or pleural spaces, requiring further investigation.

If drainage does not diminish, it may indicate complications such as rupture of the suture line or a clotting disorder due to anticoagulants given during cardiopulmonary bypass and requires immediate medical management. It is important that a cause for the bleeding, either coagulation or surgical bleeding, is established. Bleeding that arises form coagulation issues includes residual heparin effects, clotting factor deficiencies, platelet dysfunction and extensive fibrinolysis (Brand et al, 2018). Point of care testing (thromboelastography) is useful for directing treatment to cryoprecipitate, protamine or other coagulation factors; it is also useful in establishing if there may be a surgical cause of bleeding.

Surgical bleeding in the absence of a coagulation cause is associated with a larger blood loss and requires surgical re-exploration (Brand et al, 2018). Common sites for postoperative bleeding include anastomosis sites, cardiopulmonary artery bypass sites, side branches of grafts, and sternal wire sites.

Once drainage has been minimal (≤10—25 mL/h) for typically three consecutive readings or within 24 hours and there are no air leaks noted, the drains can normally be removed. The pericardial drain will normally be removed after pacing wire removal, if used. Chest drains can be a source of pain, and nursing care should ensure that the drains neither restrict patient mobility nor pull on the patient's skin.

Pain management

In the immediate postoperative period, pain will be controlled with non-opioid and opioid analgesics, normally delivered intravenously until the patient is awake. Many patients will also benefit from controlling their own pain with a patient-controlled analgesia (PCA) pump (Zubrzycki et al, 2018). Pain must be well controlled to enhance patient comfort, prevent episodes of hypertension and enable the patient to breathe deeply and expectorate, thus preventing lung infection and alveolar collapse. Painful procedures, such as removal of chest drains, may require additional boluses of opioids or nitrous oxide and oxygen (Entonox). The need for opioids diminishes over time, but effective pain control remains a priority to enable the patient to regain mobility and thus prevent the many complications associated with immobility, such as deep vein thrombosis and chest infection.

Delirium

Approximately 26—52% of patients experience psychological disturbance in the early postoperative period. It was previously poorly defined as post-cardiotomy psychosis or post-pump psychosis, however it now comes under a common definition of post-cardiac surgery delirium (Kotfis et al, 2018). Delirium is defined as a change or fluctuation in a patient's behaviour that may affect cognitive function, perception, physical function and social behaviour (NICE, 2019).

A patient with delirium may experience:

- Hyperactive delirium: restlessness, agitation and aggression
- Hypoactive delirium: withdrawn, quiet and sleepy
- Mixed delirium: includes both hyperactive and hypoactive signs and symptoms, and the patient may fluctuate between both.

This results in behavioural disturbance, manifestations of which range from confusion and disorientation to visual and auditory hallucinations. Nursing patients with post-cardiac surgery delirium can be challenging, posing a threat to the patient's safety, since the patient may be aggressive and uncooperative with treatment. This condition is also very alarming for the patients themselves and their relatives, who may observe behaviour that is uncharacteristic of their loved one.

Delirium is usually temporary, however it is important to rule out or manage any underlying causes, such as dehydration, constipation, hypoxia, infection, pain, poor nutrition, sleep deprivation and sensory impairment. The nurse should ensure that there is effective communication and reorientation with the patient and provide reassurance to the patient and their family (NICE, 2019). The distressed patient who is at risk of harm may require antipsychotic medication in the short term.

Surgical wounds

Sternal and leg wounds should be observed for signs of infection and impaired healing. Dressings are typically removed on day 3 or 4 after surgery; if the wounds are clean and dry, they can be left exposed. If the wound is oozing or open, it should be managed aseptically and covered with an appropriate dressing. Wounds are generally closed with a soluble suture material, which does not need to be removed, although loose ends of the suture may need to be trimmed close to the skin.

Newer wound therapies have been developed in preventing the risk of surgical site infections (SSIs). Single-use negative wound therapy systems such as a PICO dressing may be applied to high-risk patients with closed surgical wounds and low exudate levels. High-risk patients include those with diabetes, renal dialysis, poor physical status, and high BMI (NICE, 2018). High-risk patients may also benefit from a post-thorax sternum support vest, designed to take the stress off the sternal wires and prevent the two halves of the sternum moving, minimizing sternal complications (Caimmi et al, 2016). The post-thorax vest will need to be worn day and night for usually 6 weeks postoperatively until the sternum has healed. Women should be advised to wear a soft, non-underwired, front fastening bra day and night following surgery. The weight and movement of their breasts may pull on the sternal wound, which can compromise and place a strain on the surgical wound.

Neurological events

Neurological complications such as stroke or behavioural changes may be seen postoperatively. Stroke occurs in approximately 6% of patients, with a higher incidence in the elderly (Raffa et al, 2019). These events are due to disruption of the atheromatous plaque, with the release of debris, when the aorta is clamped during surgery. Frequent neurological assessment of the patient in the early postoperative period will detect any neurological disturbance and enable early investigation for brain injury (NICE, 2017).

Respiratory complications

The patient should be monitored closely in the immediate postoperative phase for breathing difficulties due to pneumothorax, atelectasis, pleural effusions and hypoventilation due to pain (Miskovic & Lumb, 2017). The patient's lungs are also vulnerable to areas of collapse (atelectasis), where the lung has not fully expanded after being collapsed during surgery and having undergone a period of mechanical ventilation postoperatively.

Respiratory assessment involves monitoring and recording respiratory depth and rate for hypoventilation or hyperventilation, and pulse oximetry for reduction of oxygen saturation indicated by a saturation level (SaO_2) of $\leq 94\%$. Humidified oxygen should be given to maintain SaO_2 levels at $\geq 94\%$. A focus on optimal positioning, comfortable coughing to expectorate phlegm and early mobilization is the basis of supportive and prophylactic care for respiratory function.

Body temperature should be monitored 4-hourly for elevation $\geq 37°C$, which may indicate the presence of infection. The most likely sources in a cardiac surgical patient are the lungs, surgical wounds, urinary tract, and central lines (Rhee & Sax, 2014).

Nutrition and hydration

Patients are encouraged to start postoperative oral intake as soon as possible along with early feeding and mobilization (Maes et al, 2019). There has been a move away from maintenance fluid therapy in the cardiac surgical patient and has moved towards targeted fluid therapy to reduce the incidence of fluid overload and hemodilution.

Patients frequently experience a loss of appetite postoperatively and need to be encouraged to start eating as soon as possible, to facilitate wound healing and to regain strength. Regaining a normal dietary pattern may take time and will need to be built up slowly with small, light nutritious meals.

Elimination

The majority of patients will have a urinary catheter for up to 24 hours postoperatively. This enables urinary output and renal function to be monitored. Urinary output should be measured and recorded hourly. If output is less than 0.5 mL/kg/h, it may indicate that the patient is hypovolaemic and/or the kidneys are poorly perfused due to hypotension, which will require immediate medical attention to prevent acute renal failure.

A high standard of urinary catheter hygiene, maintenance of a closed system (NICE, 2014d), and high fluid intake will help to reduce the risk of catheter-related infection. Patients with a prosthetic heart valve who develop a urinary tract infection may be at risk of developing infective valvular endocarditis (Cahill et al, 2017). Providing the patient makes an uncomplicated recovery, the catheter may be removed earlier than 24 hours to reduce this risk.

Mobilization

Patients are usually exhausted after cardiac surgery and have to contend with pain and bruising from sternal and leg wounds. Gentle mobilization is encouraged the day after surgery, providing the patient's condition is stable. This will start with getting out of bed with assistance and sitting in a chair, followed by gradually increasing activity from walking around the bed area to longer excursions around the ward. Active limb exercises help to prevent deep vein thrombosis, along with early mobilization, which also helps in the prevention of chest infection and pressure ulcers, and increases the patient's self-esteem and enhances recovery from surgery.

Preparation for discharge

Providing the patient has had an uncomplicated recovery, they are discharged home on/about the fourth or fifth postoperative day, which may be earlier if they are completing the ERAS programme. Prior to discharge, the patient will require the following information and will normally be seen by the rehabilitation team on discharge:

- Nutritional information should be given to optimize wound healing, maintain ideal body weight and reduce cholesterol levels if elevated. Patients should be taught about healthy eating, avoiding foods high in sugar and saturated fats. They should also eat plenty of fresh fruit, vegetables, cereals, pulses, fish and lean meat. Foods high in saturated fats should be eaten in moderation or avoided completely. Salt intake is associated with hypertension and should also be reduced to at least 5 g daily (Piepoli et al, 2016). Simple measures such as not adding salt to food can help to reduce intake.
- If the patient has a leg wound, advice should be given about contacting their general practitioner if the wound becomes red, painful or swollen. The patient should also be told that ankle swelling at the end of the day is not uncommon. This can be minimized by elevating the leg, wearing a support stocking, and avoiding crossed legs when sitting.
- Sternal wounds tend to heal quicker than the leg wounds but still require observation for signs of infection and poor healing. Although the incidence of sternal wound infection is low, the risk of infection is increased in those who have a tracheotomy. This is due to the proximity of the tracheotomy to the sternal wound and associated risk of contamination from respiratory pathogens. When the internal mammary artery has been used in revascularization, the blood supply to the sternum may have been interrupted during dissection and this may cause delayed sternal

healing (Squiers & Mack, 2018). If a post-thorax vest is worn, advice should be given on wearing day and night and how to wash and care for the garment. Advice should also be given on washing/showering and protecting their wounds.

- The patient should be informed that chest discomfort may take a few weeks to settle. It is tempting for the patient to sit in a hunched position, which may worsen aches and stiffness and reduce air entry to the lungs. It is important that the patient protects their breastbone to aid healing, lifting heavy weights should be avoided for up to 12 weeks after surgery. This will include restrictions on pushing and pulling through their arms. When travelling in a car they are advised to wear a seatbelt, and this may be more comfortable by using a small pillow between the chest and the seatbelt.
- Some patients may develop chest pain a number of days to weeks after surgery, because of post-pericardiotomy syndrome. This is an inflammatory condition of the pericardium which causes fever, pain, dyspnoea, and a pericardial or pleural friction rub. This syndrome usually responds to analgesics, anti-inflammatory agents and diuretics (Sasse & Eriksson, 2017).
- Physical activity should be positively encouraged because this may reduce blood pressure, cholesterol levels and body weight. This will normally be reintroduced in conjunction with the rehabilitation team. Patients should be encouraged to exercise at least five days a week, but preferably daily for a period of 30 minutes (Piepoli et al, 2016). Exercise does not need to be complex or competitive; a daily walk is sufficient to gain health benefits.
- There are no restrictions on having sex and advice should be given on returning to sexual activity once they feel confident to do so. It is important that they find a comfortable position that protects their wound and does not place stress on their chest or restrict their breathing.
- Patients who have had valve replacements require additional verbal and written information about protecting their prosthetic valve from infective endocarditis which will result in valve damage or death. Dental infections can affect the valve, so it is important that the patient understands the importance of oral hygiene and visiting a dentist regularly. Prophylactic antibiotics are required prior to any dental treatment, including scaling and polishing, and other surgical procedures (Baumgartner et al, 2017).
- Patients with mechanical prosthetic valves will require anticoagulation for life to prevent valve thrombosis and embolism. Effective education and information are required to enhance understanding of and concordance with drug therapy.

Heart transplantation

A number of patients will deteriorate so much that conventional therapies are no longer effective in controlling their heart failure. The most common heart conditions causing end-stage heart failure are dilated cardiomyopathy (46%), coronary heart disease (21%) and congenital heart disease (5%) (NHS Blood and Transplant, 2018a).

These patients are severely limited physically, often requiring continuous oxygen therapy and a 'cocktail' of drugs, and these measures may only maintain life for about a year. Many patients in the UK require heart transplants, but due to a limited supply of donor organs, fewer than 200 transplants occurred in 2017/2018 (NHS Blood and Transplant, 2018a). All transplant activity will be coordinated through the UK Transplant Support Service Authority (www.organdonation.nhs.uk). Unfortunately, some patients suitable for transplantation will die before a suitable heart becomes available. In 2017−2018, however, heart transplantation activity increased by 10% (NHS Blood and Transplant, 2018b).

Before being selected for transplantation, patients undergo a rigorous selection procedure (NHS Blood and Transplant, 2018c), which aims to establish whether all other treatment options have been exhausted. Secondly, it must be established that the patient does not meet any of the contraindication criteria, including any pre-existing conditions such as renal failure that may increase the risk of the transplanted heart failing and being rejected, or malignancy that would make transplantation futile (NHS Blood and Transplant, 2018c). Those not selected for transplantation may require a great deal of emotional support to help them accept this disappointment and come to terms with their impending death. Survival after transplant has improved over the years because of an improvement in the management of rejection and infection. The one-year survival rate is now 83% (NHS Blood and Transplant, 2018a).

Patients deemed suitable for transplantation may have to wait anything from a few days to over a year before a suitable heart becomes available. During this time the patient will require both physical support to maintain optimum health before surgery and psychological support to help them come to terms with issues surrounding being the recipient of a donor heart. Additionally, the period of waiting is unpredictable, and patients and families benefit from and require ongoing emotional and psychological support from nurses (McDermott et al, 2010).

Immediate postoperative care is similar to that for any patient undergoing cardiac surgery, except that, because the patient is receiving immunosuppressant drugs, signs of infection may be masked. Essentially, the postoperative management can be detailed as control of primary graft dysfunction, control of allograft rejection, minimizing side-effects of immunosuppression, and coping with the transplantation procedure itself (Bhagra et al, 2018).

Any transplanted tissue will be rejected by the body's immune system in the absence of immunosuppressant therapy. When rejection occurs, the transplanted tissue is attacked by the immune cells (Bhagra et al, 2018) and thus begins to fail. Drugs that suppress this immune response will have to be taken for life. Immunosuppressive drugs also curb the body's ability to fight infection, which causes an added burden for the patient, potentially leaving them vulnerable to serious infections that increase morbidity and mortality. The drugs also have a number of other side-effects, which may reduce patient concordance over time.

Typical anti-rejection therapy revolves around the following drugs: corticosteroids, azathioprine, ciclosporin A, FK506 (tacrolimus), cyclophosphamide and mycophenolate mofetil (Koomalsingh & Kobashigawa, 2018). Steroids may be prescribed for a limited period only, but the other drugs will be taken for life. There are a number of side-effects of these drugs, resulting in altered fat distribution across the shoulders, causing a hump, and in the face, causing a rounded appearance or 'moon face'. Corticosteroids also reduce bone density, leading to osteoporosis, so increasing the risk of fractures. Side-effects of these drugs can be unpleasant and may affect patient concordance, especially if the patient is an adolescent, when altered body image may be perceived as being important.

Azathioprine is a cytotoxic agent which suppresses the bone marrow, with inhibition of lymphocyte production, thus reducing the number of immune cells responsible for rejection. Because all cells made by the marrow are suppressed, however, patients may become anaemic, and higher doses are associated with renal dysfunction (Rang et al, 2016).

Ciclosporin (cyclosporine) suppresses T-cell production and activation − cells which are responsible for the destruction of transplanted tissue − although ciclosporin is less toxic to bone marrow cells (Adams et al, 2016). The drug can also alter appearance, increasing body hair growth and gum hypertrophy for example (Rang et al, 2016), which may affect patient concordance with this drug. The overall aim of drug therapy is to maintain a fine balance between preventing rejection and not suppressing the immune system too much so that the patient is unable to fight infection. In spite of immunosuppressant therapy, patients still experience episodes of acute rejection, which places the heart at risk of being destroyed by their own immune system. Episodes of acute rejection are difficult to diagnose because there are few reliable clinical signs to indicate its presence, so endomyocardial biopsy will need to be performed regularly (Asher, 2017). This involves the insertion of a bioptome catheter into the right ventricle via the subclavian or jugular vein, so that small samples of heart tissue can be removed for histological examination.

Acute rejection episodes decline with time and the patient's immune system develops some tolerance to the transplanted tissue. However, the majority of patients experience chronic rejection, which is manifested by a diffuse form of coronary artery disease which gradually narrows the coronary arteries, causing the myocardium to become ischaemic. Coronary artery disease is the main cause of death in those surviving more than one year after transplantation, but, because the donor heart is denervated as a result of surgery, the majority of patients do not experience angina. Additionally, long-term immunosuppressive therapy (azathioprine being particularly implicated) is associated with an increased risk of malignancy, such as cutaneous tumours (Inman et al, 2018).

Second to rejection, the main risk for transplant patients is infection — the current leading infections resulting in mortality are bacterial pneumonia and fungal infections (Stehlik et al, 2018). If the intraoperative period has been uneventful, patients may be extubated and their haemodynamics maintained with low-level inotropic support and diuretics (Pettit & Kydd, 2018).

Patients who have undergone transplant are required to attend regular hospital appointments to monitor organ function. This involves a range of tests, from simple blood tests, echocardiography and ECG, to the more invasive endomyocardial biopsies which initially may be as frequent as monthly and then every 4–6 months for the next 2–5 years. Monitoring chronic rejection may require annual cardiac catheterization and coronary angiography, to monitor for the development of coronary artery disease (Koomalsingh & Kobashigawa, 2018).

Thorough health education enables patients to adjust to lifestyle changes required to keep their hearts healthy; they need to understand that good hygiene in both personal care and food preparation is required to prevent infection. In addition to this, the patient needs to know how to monitor themselves for signs of infection, so that early antibiotic therapy can be given. The patient must be shown how to take their temperature; this should be done twice a day and recorded. If abnormalities indicating infection or a possible rejection episode are detected, patients must consult their general practitioner or return to hospital. Furthermore, the patient may have to cope with alterations in body image, induced by anti-rejection therapy. Patients also need to be fully educated in what they can do for themselves to maintain a healthy heart. This should centre on healthy eating, aimed at preventing weight gain, which increases the heart's workload, and maintaining blood cholesterol at normal levels to slow down the disease process that causes coronary atherosclerosis and subsequent myocardial infarction: accelerated atherosclerosis is the major cause of death for recipients surviving more than one year (Chih et al, 2016). Healthy eating involves avoiding foods high in saturated fats, sugar and calories, and eating foods such as fresh fruit,

vegetables, white meat and oily fish (Piepoli et al, 2016). Transplant patients should be encouraged to exercise regularly; however, heart rate is usually increased by stimulation of the sympathetic nervous system and, because the transplanted heart is non-innervated, it has to rely on the slower release of catecholamines to increase heart rate and blood pressure with exercise (Grupper et al, 2018). Conversely, it takes longer for the heart rate to fall after exercise, since it takes about 15 minutes for the catecholamines to be broken down and for their effect to be reduced. Consequently, any exercise programme should involve a 10–15-minute warm-up and cool-down period.

Conclusion

Cardiac surgery and interventional procedures are common treatments for conditions involving specific structures such as the coronary arteries, valves or the conduction system. Heart transplantation is the definitive option when other treatments are no longer effective; however, the number of patients receiving heart transplants is limited by the availability of donor hearts.

SUMMARY OF KEY POINTS

- Nursing cardiac patients requires an extensive knowledge of the heart's function and the effects of its dysfunction on the body.
- The nurse needs to be able to carry out a comprehensive assessment to establish the effects of heart disease on the individual's physical and psychological function and well-being.
- Cardiac care is constantly changing as knowledge of heart disease progresses and innovative therapies develop. This requires the nurse to be an informed and knowledgeable practitioner.

REFLECTIVE LEARNING POINTS

Having read this chapter, think about what you now know and what you still need to find out about. These questions may help:
- What strategies can the nurse use to help reduce anxiety that may be associated with cardiac interventions?
- What information should be offered to a patient with an internal cardiac pacemaker when travelling through electronic security systems?
- How might you advise a patient with regard to the resumption of sexual activity post implantation of a pacemaker?

References

Adams, M., Holland, N., & Urban, C. (2016). *Pharmacology for nurses: a pathophysiologic approach* (5th ed.). New York: Pearson.

Ancona, R., & Pinto, S. (2019). Mitral valve incompetence: epidemiology and causes. *E-Journal of Cardiology Practice*, *16*(11). Available from: < www.escardio.org/Journals/E-Journal-of-Cardiology-Practice/Volume-16/Mitral-valve-incompetence-epidemiology-and-causes >.

Asher, A. (2017). A review of endomyocardial biopsy and current practice in England: out of date or underutilised? *British Journal of Cardiology*, *24*, 108−112.

Asirvatham, S., & Stevenson, W. (2015). Atrioventricular nodal block with atrioventricular nodal reentrant tachycardia ablation. *Circulation: Arrhythmia and Electrophysiology*, *8*(3), 745−747.

Bachar, B., & Manna, B. (2019). Coronary artery bypass graft. *StatPearls* [Internet]. Available from: < www.ncbi.nlm.nih.gov/books/NBK507836/ >

Bainbridge, D., & Cheng, D. (2017). Current evidence on fast track cardiac recovery management. *European Heart Journal Supplements*, *19*(suppl A), A3−A7.

Barsoum, E., Azab, B., Shah, N., Patel, N., Shariff, M., Lafferty, J., et al. (2014). Long-term mortality in minimally invasive compared with sternotomy coronary artery bypass surgery in the geriatric population (75 years and older patients). *European Journal of Cardio-Thoracic Surgery*, *47*(5), 862−867.

Basso, C., Aguilera, B., Banner, J., et al; Association for European Cardiovascular Pathology. (2017). Guidelines for autopsy investigation of sudden cardiac death: 2017 update from the Association for European Cardiovascular Pathology. *Virchows Archiv*, *471*(6), 691−705.

Baumgartner, H., Falk, V., Bax, J. J., et al. (2017). 2017 ESC/EACTS Guidelines for the Management of Valvular Heart Disease. *European Heart Journal*, *38*, 2739−2791.

Bernelli, C. (2015). Pharmacotherapy in the cardiac catheterization laboratory. *Cardiovascular Pharmacology: Open Access*, *04*(03).

Bhagra, S., Pettit, S., & Parameshwar, J. (2018). Cardiac transplantation: indications, eligibility and current outcomes. *Heart*, *105*(3), 252−260.

Bodor, G. (2016). Biochemical markers of myocardial damage. *The Journal of the International Federation of Clinical Chemistry and Laboratory Medicine*, *27*(2), 95−111.

Bontrager, M., & Abraham, S. (2017). Comparison of complications after transfemoral coronary angiography between mechanical and manual closure techniques. *Cogent Medicine*, *4*(1).

Brand, J., McDonald, A., & Dunning, J. (2018). Management of cardiac arrest following cardiac surgery. *BJA Education*, *18*(1), 16−22.

Brignole, M., Auricchio, A., Baron-Esquivias, G., Bordachar, P., & Boriani, G. (2013). 2013 ESC Guidelines on cardiac pacing and cardiac resynchronization therapy. The Task Force on cardiac pacing and resynchronization therapy of the European Society of Cardiology (ESC). Developed in collaboration with the European Heart Rhythm Association (EHRA). *European Heart Journal*, *34*(29), 2281−2329.

British Heart Foundation. (2018a). *Heart and circulatory diseases statistics 2018*. Available at: < www.bhf.org.uk/what-we-do/our-research/heart-statistics/heart-statistics-publications/cardiovascular-disease-statistics-2018 >

British Heart Foundation. (2018b). *Pacemaker*. Available at: < www.bhf.org.uk/informationsupport/publications/treatments-for-heart-conditions/pacemakers >

British Heart Foundation. (2019a). *What is an MRI scan?* Available at: < www.bhf.org.uk/informationsupport/heart-matters-magazine/medical/tests/cardiac-mri >

British Heart Foundation. (2019b). *Implantable cardioverter defibrillators (ICDs).* Available at: < www.bhf.org.uk/informationsupport/publications/heart-conditions/implantable-cardioverter-defibrillators >

British Heart Foundation. (2019c). *TAVI*. Available at: < www.bhf.org.uk/informationsupport/treatments/tavi >

Bryant, H., Roberts, P., & Diprose, P. (2016). Perioperative management of patients with cardiac implantable electronic devices. *BJA Education*, *16*(11), 388−396.

Buccheri, D., Piraino, D., Andolina, G., & Cortese, B. (2016). Understanding and managing in-stent restenosis: a review of clinical data, from pathogenesis to treatment. *Journal of Thoracic Disease*, *8*(10), E1150−E1162.

Cahill, T., Baddour, L., Habib, G., Hoen, B., Salaun, E., Pettersson, G., et al. (2017). Challenges in Infective Endocarditis. *Journal of the American College of Cardiology*, *69*(3), 325−344.

Caimmi, P., Sabbatini, M., Kapetanakis, E., Cantone, S., Ferraz, M., Cannas, M., et al. (2016). A randomized trial to assess the contribution of a novel thorax support vest (corset) in preventing mechanical complications of median sternotomy. *Cardiology and Therapy*, *6*(1), 41−51.

Carpenter, S. (2019). The nursing aspects of a transcatheter aortic valve implantation patient's pathway. *British Journal of Cardiac Nursing*, *14*(4), 1−11.

Carroll, D., Malecki-Ketchell, A., & Astin, F. (2016). Non-pharmacological interventions to reduce psychological distress in patients undergoing diagnostic cardiac catheterization: a rapid review. *European Journal of Cardiovascular Nursing*, *16*(2), 92−103.

Chih, S., Chong, A., Mielniczuk, L., Bhatt, D., & Beanlands, R. (2016). Allograft vasculopathy: the Achilles' heel of heart transplantation. *Journal of the American College of Cardiology*, *68*(1), 80−91.

Clarke, S. (2015). Shock therapy: psychological impact and patient support. *British Journal of Cardiac Nursing*, *10*(3), 116−123.

Corrado, D., Link, M., & Calkins, H. (2017). Arrhythmogenic right ventricular cardiomyopathy. *The New England Journal of Medicine*, *376*, 61−72.

Dalal, H., Doherty, P., & Taylor, R. (2015). Cardiac rehabilitation. *BMJ*, *351*, h5000.

Di Loreto, F., & Sampson, M. (2018). Evidence to practice: use of Angio-Seal following PCI. *British Journal of Cardiac Nursing*, *13*(1), 20−28.

DVLA. (2019a). *Heart attacks, angioplasty, and driving*. Available at: < www.gov.uk/heart-attacks-and-driving >

DVLA. (2019b). *Assessing fitness to drive: a guide for medical professionals*. Available from: < www.gov.uk/guidance/assessing-fitness-to-drive-a-guide-for-medical-professionals >

DVLA. (2019c). *Cardiovascular disorders: assessing fitness to drive*. Available from: www.gov.uk/guidance/cardiovascular-disorders-assessing-fitness-to-drive#pacemaker-implant–including-box-change

Eftekhari, H., Hayat, S., Dhangal, T., & Osman, F. (2017). Cardiac pacing and devices: history, technologies and current innovations. *British Journal of Cardiac Nursing*, 12(6), 280–289.

Elliott, P., Anastasakis, A., Borger, M. A., et al. (2014). 2014 ESC Guidelines on diagnosis and management of hypertrophic cardiomyopathy. *European Heart Journal*, 35(39), 2733–2779.

Fawcett, W., & Thomas, M. (2018). Preoperative fasting in adults and children: clinical practice and guidelines. *Anaesthesia*, 74(1), 83–88.

Gillingham, I. (2018). The electrophysiology study. *British Journal of Cardiac Nursing*, 13(5), 220–228.

Gilmore, M., & Anderson, M. (2016). An update on the use of implantable loop recorders. *British Journal of Cardiac Nursing*, 11(1), 21–29.

Greenberg, J., Lancaster, T., Schuessler, R., & Melby, S. (2017). Postoperative atrial fibrillation following cardiac surgery: a persistent complication. *European Journal of Cardio-Thoracic Surgery*, 52(4), 665–672.

Grupper, A., Gewirtz, H., & Kushwaha, S. (2018). Reinnervation post-heart transplantation. *European Heart Journal*, 39, 1799–1806.

Habib, G., Lancellotti, P., & Iung, B. (2015). 2015 ESC Guidelines for the management of infective endocarditis. *European Heart Journal*, 36(44), 3075–3128.

Haddad, N., Saleh, M., & Eshah, N. (2017). Cardiac catheterisation and patients' anxiety levels. *British Journal of Cardiac Nursing*, 12(7), 353–358.

Hardin, S., & Kaplow, R. (2019). *Cardiac surgery essentials for critical care nursing* (3rd ed.). Burlington, MA: Jones and Bartlett Learning.

Head, S., Milojevic, M., Taggart, D., & Puskas, J. (2017). Current practice of state-of-the-art surgical coronary revascularization. *Circulation*, 136(14), 1331–1345.

Humphreys, N., Lowe, R., Rance, J., & Bennett, P. (2018). Living with an implantable cardioverter defibrillator: partners' experiences. *British Journal of Cardiac Nursing*, 13(6), 279–285.

Ilg, K. (2014). Cardiac pacemakers and implantable defibrillators. In B. Nallamothu, & T. Baman (Eds.), *Inpatient cardiovascular medicine*. New Jersey: John Wiley & Sons Inc.

Inman, G., Wang, J., Nagano, A., et al. (2018). The genomic landscape of cutaneous SCC reveals drivers and a novel azathioprine associated mutational signature. *Nature Communications*, 9(1), 3667.

Innes, A., Dover, A., & Fairhurst, K. (2018). *Macleod's clinical examination* (14th ed.). London: Elsevier.

Jenson, J., Poulsen, S., & Molgaard, H. (2017). Cardiac tamponade: a clinical challenge. *E-Journal of cardiology practice*, 15(17). Available at: < www.escardio.org/Journals/E-Journal-of-Cardiology-Practice/Volume-15/Cardiac-tamponade-a-clinical-challenge >.

Junghans, C., Sekhri, N., Zaman, M., Hemingway, H., Feder, G., & Timmis, A. (2015). Atypical chest pain in diabetic patients with suspected stable angina: impact on diagnosis and coronary outcomes. *European Heart Journal - Quality of Care and Clinical Outcomes*, 1(1), 37–43.

Kandarpa, K., Machan, L., & Durham, J. (2016). *Handbook of interventional radiologic procedures* (5th ed.). Philadelphia: Wolters Kluwer.

Karchmer, A., Chu, V., Calderwood, S., & Baron, E. (2019). *Prosthetic valve endocarditis: Epidemiology, clinical manifestations, and diagnosis*. Available at: < www.uptodate.com/contents/prosthetic-valve-endocarditis-epidemiology-clinical-manifestations-and-diagnosis >

Katritsis, D., Boriani, G., Cosio, F. G., et al. (2017). European Heart Rhythm Association (EHRA) consensus document on the management of supraventricular arrhythmias, endorsed by Heart Rhythm Society (HRS), Asia-Pacific Heart Rhythm Society (APHRS), and Sociedad Latinoamericana de Estimulación Cardiaca y Electrofisiologia (SOLAECE). *EP Europace*, 19(3), 465–511.

Katritsis, D., Zografos, T., Katritsis, G., Giazitzoglou, E., Vachliotis, V., Paxinos, G., et al. (2016). Catheter ablation vs. antiarrhythmic drug therapy in patients with symptomatic atrioventricular nodal re-entrant tachycardia: a randomized, controlled trial. *Europace*, 19, 602–606.

Keeble, T., Khokhar, A., Akhtar, M., Mathur, A., Weerackody, R., & Kennon, S. (2016). Percutaneous balloon aortic valvuloplasty in the era of transcatheter aortic valve implantation: a narrative review. *Open Heart*, 3(2), e000421.

Kern, M., Seto, A., & Forsberg, M. (2018). Vascular access. In M. Kern, P. Sorajja, & M. Lim (Eds.), *The interventional cardiac catheterization handbook* (4th edn). Philadelphia: Elsevier.

Khan, N. (2018a). Coronary artery stents: part 1. *British Journal of Cardiac Nursing*, 13(4), 168–172.

Khan, N. (2018b). Coronary artery stents: part 2. *British Journal of Cardiac Nursing*, 13(5), 229–234.

Khosravi, A., & Wendler, O. (2018). TAVI 2018: from guidelines to practice. *e-Journal of Cardiology Practice*, 15(29). Available at: < www.escardio.org/Journals/E-Journal-of-Cardiology-Practice/Volume-15/TAVI-2018-from-guidelines-to-practice > .

Koomalsingh, K., & Kobashigawa, J. (2018). The future of cardiac transplantation. *Annals of Cardiothoracic Surgery*, 7(1), 135–142.

Kotfis, K., Szylińska, A., Listewnik, M., Strzelbicka, M., Brykczyński, M., Rotter, I., et al. (2018). Early delirium after cardiac surgery: an analysis of incidence and risk factors in elderly ≥ 65 years) and very elderly ≥ 80 years) patients. *Clinical Interventions in Aging*, 13, 1061–1070.

Kraft, F., Schmidt, C., Van Aken, H., & Zarbock, A. (2015). Inflammatory response and extracorporeal circulation. *Best Practice & Research Clinical Anaesthesiology*, 29(2), 113–123.

Langer, N., & Argenziano, M. (2016). Minimally invasive cardiovascular surgery: incisions and approaches. *Methodist DeBakey Cardiovascular Journal*, 12(1), 4–9.

Lee, D., & Linker, N. (2014). Electrophysiology study in patients with tachycardia. *British Journal of Cardiac Nursing*, 9(1), 25–29.

Ley, S., & Koulakis, D. (2015). Temporary pacing after cardiac surgery. *AACN Advanced Critical Care*, 26(3), 275–280.

Li, M., Zhang, J., Gan, T. J., et al. (2018). Enhanced recovery after surgery pathway for patients undergoing cardiac surgery: a randomized clinical trial. *European Journal of Cardio-Thoracic Surgery*, 54(3), 491–497.

Ljungqvist, O., Scott, M., & Fearon, K. (2017). Enhanced recovery after surgery. *JAMA Surgery*, 152(3), 292.

Maes, S., Meuwissen, A., Diltoer, M., Nguyen, D., La Meir, M., Wise, R., et al. (2019). Impact of maintenance, resuscitation and unintended fluid therapy on global fluid load after elective coronary artery bypass surgery. *Journal of Critical Care, 49*, 129–135.

Magkoutis, N., Fradi, S., Azmoun, A., Ramadan, R., Ben Ouanes, S., Vavuranakis, M., et al. (2016). Antiplatelet therapy in TAVI: current clinical practice and recommendations. *Current Pharmaceutical Design, 22*(13), 1888–1895.

Manda, Y., & Baradhi, K. (2018). *Cardiac catheterization, risks and complications.* Available at: www.ncbi.nlm.nih.gov/books/NBK531461/

Mansour, F., & Khairy, P. (2014). ICD Follow-up and troubleshooting. In K. Ellenbogen, & K. Kaszala (Eds.), *Cardiac pacing and ICDs* (6th ed.). Chichester: John Wiley & Sons Ltd.

McConnell, G., Woltz, P., Bradford, W., Ledford, J., & Williams, J. (2018). Enhanced recovery after cardiac surgery program to improve patient outcomes. *Nursing, 48*(11), 24–31.

McDermott, A., Hardy, J., & McCurry, M. (2010). Emotional impact on patients and families on the heart transplant waiting list. *British Journal of Cardiac Nursing, 5*(6), 280–284.

McKavanagh, P., Yanagawa, B., Zawadowski, G., & Cheema, A. (2017). Management and prevention of saphenous vein graft failure: a review. *Cardiology and Therapy, 6*(2), 203–223.

Miskovic, A., & Lumb, A. (2017). Postoperative pulmonary complications. *British Journal of Anaesthesia, 18* (3), 317–334.

Mullasari, A., & Victor, S. (2014). Update on contrast induced nephropathy. *e-Journal of Cardiology Practice, 13*(4). Available at: < www.escardio.org/Journals/E-Journal-of-Cardiology-Practice/Volume-13/Update-on-contrast-induced-nephropathy > .

Mulpuru, S., Madhavan, M., McLeod, D., Cha, Y., & Friedman, P. (2017). Cardiac pacemakers: function, troubleshooting, and management. *Journal of the American College of Cardiology, 69* (2), 189–210.

Natarajan, D., & Prendergast, B. (2017). Aortic stenosis – pathogenesis, prediction of progression, and percutaneous intervention. *Journal of the Royal College of Physicians of Edinburgh, 47*(2), 172–175.

National Institute for Health and Care Excellence (NICE). (2008). *Drug-eluting stents for the treatment of coronary artery disease.* Technology appraisal guidance [TA152]. Available at: < www.nice.org.uk/guidance/ta152/chapter/1-Guidance >

National Institute for Health and Care Excellence (NICE). (2014a). *Prasugrel with percutaneous coronary intervention for treating acute coronary syndromes (review of technology appraisal guidance 182).* Available at: < www.nice.org.uk/guidance/ta317/documents/prasugrel-with-percutaneous-coronary-intervention-for-treating-acute-coronary-syndrome-review-of-ta182-final-appraisal-document2 >

National Institute for Health and Care Excellence (NICE). (2014b). *Implantable cardioverter defibrillators and cardiac resynchronisation therapy for arrhythmias and heart failure.* Technology appraisal guidance [TA314]. Available at: < www.nice.org.uk/guidance/ta314/chapter/2-Clinical-need-and-practice >

National Institute for Health and Care Excellence (NICE). (2014c). *Implantable cardioverter defibrillators and cardiac resynchronisation therapy for arrhythmias and heart failure.* Technology appraisal guidance [TA314]. Available at: www.nice.org.uk/guidance/ta314

National Institute of Health and Care Excellence (NICE). (2014d). *Infection prevention and control.* Quality standard [QS61]. Available at: www.nice.org.uk/guidance/qs61/chapter/Quality-statement-4-Urinary-catheters

National Institute of Health and Care Excellence (NICE). (2017). *Stroke and transient ischaemic attack in over 16s: diagnosis and initial management.* Clinical guideline [CG68]. Available at: < www.nice.org.uk/guidance/cg68/chapter/1-Guidance#rapid-recognition-of-symptoms-and-diagnosis >

National Institute for Health and Care Excellence (NICE). (2018). *PICO negative pressure wound therapy for closed surgical incision wounds.* Medtech innovation briefing [MIB149]. Available at: < www.nice.org.uk/advice/mib149/chapter/The-technology >

National Institute for Health and Care Excellence (NICE). (2019). *Delirium: prevention, diagnosis and management.* Clinical guideline [CG103]. Available at: < www.nice.org.uk/guidance/cg103/chapter/1-Guidance >

Neumann, F., Sousa-Uva, M., Ahlsson, A., et al. (2018). 2018 ESC/EACTS Guidelines on myocardial revascularization. *European Heart Journal, 40*(2), 87–165.

NHS Blood and Transplant. (2018a). *Annual report on cardiothoracic organ transplantation: Report for 2017/2018.* [Online] NHS Blood and Transplant & NHS England.

NHS Blood and Transplant. (2018b). *Organ donation and transplantation: Activity report 2017/18.* [Online] NHS Blood and Transplant.

NHS Blood and Transplant. (2018c). *Heart transplantation: Selection criteria and recipient registration.* [Online] NHS Blood and Transplant.

NHS Blood and Transplant. (2019). *NHS Blood and Transplant warns of a shortage of heart valve donors.* Available at: < www.nhsbt.nhs.uk/news/nhs-blood-and-transplant-warns-of-a-shortage-of-heart-valve-donors/ >

Norhammar, A., & Schenck-Gustafsson, K. (2012). Type 2 diabetes and cardiovascular disease in women. *Diabetologia, 56*(1), 1–9.

Nursing and Midwifery Council. (2018). *The Code. Professional standards of practice and behaviour for nurses, midwives and nursing associates.* Available at: < www.nmc.org.uk/globalassets/sitedocuments/nmc-publications/nmc-code.pdf >

Olive, S. (2016). Using pulse oximetry to assess oxygen levels. *Nursing Times, 112* (16), 12–13.

Palmer, S. (2014). Post-implantation pacemaker complications: the nurse's role in management. *British Journal of Cardiac Nursing, 9*(12), 592–598.

Pedersen, S., Knudsen, C., Dilling, K., Sandgaard, N., & Johansen, J. (2016). Living with an implantable cardioverter defibrillator: patients' preferences and needs for information provision and care options. *Europace, 2016*, euw109.

Pettit, S., & Kydd, A. (2018). Heart transplantation. In K. Valchanov, N. Jones, & C. Hogue (Eds.), *Cardiothoracic critical care* (2nd ed.). Cambridge: Cambridge University Press.

Piepoli, M., Hoes, A., Agewall, S., Albus, C., Brotons, C., Catapano, A., et al. (2016). 2016 european guidelines on cardiovascular disease prevention in clinical practice. *European Heart Journal,, 37*, 2315–2381.

Pitcher, D. & Nolan, J. (2015). *Peri-arrest arrhythmias.* Available at: < www.resus.org.uk/resuscitation-guidelines/peri-arrest-arrhythmias/ >

Priori, S., Blomström-Lundqvist, C., Mazzanti, A., Blom, N., Borggrefe, M., Camm, J., et al. (2015). 2015 ESC Guidelines for the management of patients with ventricular arrhythmias and the prevention of sudden cardiac death. *European Heart Journal*, *36*(41), 2793–2867.

Raffa, G., Agnello, F., Occhipinti, G., Miraglia, R., Lo Re, V., Marrone, G., et al. (2019). Neurological complications after cardiac surgery: a retrospective case-control study of risk factors and outcome. *Journal of Cardiothoracic Surgery*, *14*(1).

Ramrakha, P., & Hill, J. (2012). *Oxford handbook of cardiology* (2nd ed.). Oxford: Oxford University Press.

Rang, H., Ritter, M., Flower, J., & Henderson, G. (2016). *Rang and Dale's pharmacology* (8th ed.). London: Elsevier Ltd.

Reade, M. (2007). Temporary epicardial pacing after cardiac surgery: a practical review . Part 1: General considerations in the management of epicardial pacing. *Anaesthesia*, *62*(3), 264–271.

Rhee, C., & Sax, P. (2014). Evaluation of fever and infections in cardiac surgery patients. *Seminars in Cardiothoracic and Vascular Anesthesia*, *19*(2), 143–153.

Roberts-Collins, C., Anderson, C., MacCallam, J., Randle-Phillips, C., & Medley, A. (2017). Cardiac catheterisation and the promotion of positive coping and self-management. *British Journal of Cardiac Nursing*, *12*(7), 342–351.

Royal College of Nursing. (2017). *Principles of consent: Guidance for nursing staff*. London: Royal College of Nursing.

Saleem, T., & Baril, D. (2019). Vascular access closure devices. *StatPearls*. Available at: <www.ncbi.nlm.nih.gov/books/NBK470233/>

Sampson, M., & McGrath, A. (2015a). Understanding the ECG Part 2: ECG basics. *British Journal of Cardiac Nursing*, *10*(12), 588–594.

Sampson, M., & McGrath, A. (2015b). Understanding the ECG. Part 1: Anatomy and physiology. *British Journal of Cardiac Nursing*, *10*(11), 548–554.

Sanati, H., & Firoozi, A. (2017). Percutaneous balloon mitral valvuloplasty. *Interventional Cardiology*, *2017*, 100–116. [Online]. Available at: <www.intechopen.com/books/interventional-cardiology/percutaneous-balloon-mitral-valvuloplasty>.

Sasse, T., & Eriksson, U. (2017). Post-cardiac injury syndrome: aetiology, diagnosis, and treatment. *e-Journal of Cardiology Practice*, *15*(21). Available at: <www.escardio.org/Journals/E-Journal-of-Cardiology-Practice/Volume-15/Post-cardiac-injury-syndrome-aetiology-diagnosis-and-treatment>.

Shahawy, S., & Libby, P. (2015). Atherosclerosis. In L. Lilly (Ed.), *Pathophysiology of heart disease: A collaborative project of medical students and faculty* (6th ed.). Philadelphia: Wolters Kluwer.

Smith, J., & Rushton, M. (2015). How to perform respiratory assessment. *Nursing Standard*, *30*(7) 34–36.

Society for Cardiological Science and Technology (SCST). (2011). *Clinical guidance by Consensus: Recommendations for clinical exercise tolerence tests. Updated 2011*. Available at: <www.scst.org.uk/resources/ETT_consensus_March_2008.pdf>

Sproston, N., & Ashworth, J. (2018). Role of C-reactive protein at sites of inflammation and infection. *Frontiers in Immunology*, *9*, 754.

Squiers, J., & Mack, M. (2018). Coronary artery bypass grafting—fifty years of quality initiatives since Favaloro. *Annals of Cardiothoracic Surgery*, *7*(4), 516–520.

Stehlik, J., Kobashigawa, J., Hunt, S., Reichenspurner, H., & Kirklin, J. (2018). Honoring 50 years of clinical heart transplantation in Circulation: in-depth state-of-the-art review. *Circulation*, *137*(1), 71–87.

Sternick, E., Faustino, M., Correa, F., Pisani, C., & Scanavacca, M. (2017). Percutaneous catheter ablation of epicardial accessory pathways. *Arrhythmia & Electrophysiology Review*, *6*(2), 80.

Stone, P., Campbell, J., & AbuRahma, A. (2014). Femoral pseudoaneurysms after percutaneous access. *Journal of Vascular Surgery*, *60*(5), 1359–1366.

Taylor, C., Ordóñez-Mena, J., Roalfe, A., Lay-Flurrie, S., Jones, N., Marshall, T., et al. (2019). Trends in survival after a diagnosis of heart failure in the United Kingdom 2000-2017: Population based cohort study. *BMJ*, *2019*, l223.

Thanavaro, J. (2019). Catheter ablation for atrial fibrillation. *The Journal for Nurse Practitioners*, *15*(1), 19–25.e1.

Vanezis, A., Prasad, R., & Andrews, R. (2017). Pacemaker leads and cardiac perforation. *JRSM Open*, *8*(3), 205427041668143.

Young, S. (2014). Coronary angioplasty: Patient management and nursing care. *British Journal of Cardiac Nursing*, *9*(9), 430–435.

Zubrzycki, M., Liebold, A., Skrabal, C., Reinelt, H., Ziegler, M., Perdas, E., et al. (2018). Assessment and pathophysiology of pain in cardiac surgery. *Journal of Pain Research*, *11*, 1599–1611.

Relevant websites

British Cardiology Society: www.bcs.com

Cardiomyopathy UK: www.cardiomyopathy.org/

Society for Cardiothoracic Surgery in Great Britain and Ireland: scts.org

Chapter | **15** |

Care of the patient requiring thoracic surgery

Madhini Sivasubramanian

KEY OBJECTIVES OF THE CHAPTER

Upon completion of this chapter, the reader should:

- have revised the anatomy and physiology of the respiratory system and the fundamental principles of breathing
- have an understanding of the disease processes that require patients to undergo investigative and operative procedures related to the chest
- understand the principles of respiratory assessment
- understand the rationale for the nursing care of postoperative thoracic surgical patients, and associated research, including the management of chest drains
- be able to plan for the patient's discharge with the inclusion of appropriate patient education.

Areas to think about before reading the chapter

- Draw and label a diagram of the lungs.
- When assessing respiratory function, what factors must the nurse take into account?
- What is the difference between apnoea and dyspnoea?

Introduction

One in five of the UK population suffer from lung disease, with 550,000 new diagnoses happening each year (British Lung Foundation, 2016). Lung disease, or respiratory disease, can encompass a number of lung conditions including asthma, bronchiectasis, chronic obstructive pulmonary disease (COPD), cystic fibrosis, idiopathic pulmonary fibrosis (IPF), lung cancer, mesothelioma, obstructive sleep apnoea, pneumonia/lower respiratory tract infections, respiratory tuberculosis and sarcoidosis. It continues to be a major factor in health inequalities – those living in the most deprived areas of the country are more than twice as likely to develop lung cancer and COPD than those living elsewhere.

Around 2% of the UK population live with diagnosed COPD, an umbrella term for chronic bronchitis and emphysema. This makes it the second most common lung disease in the UK following asthma, with research suggesting that prevalence is on the rise (British Thoracic Society, 2017). COPD causes 115,000 emergency admissions per year, 24,000 deaths per year and 16,000 deaths within 90 days of admission (NHS England, 2014). It is the fifth biggest killer disease in the UK, with numbers of deaths from COPD increasing with age, as the lungs become more obstructed over time (NICE, 2019).

Thoracic surgery is generally dominated by treatment of malignant disease, concerned with conditions of the lungs, chest wall, esophagus and diaphragm. Significant changes to patient demographics in the last 20 years have meant that the subspecialty operates on an increasingly infirm and ageing population. It is essential for healthcare professionals working within the specialty of thoracic surgery to understand the anatomy and the physiology of the respiratory system, the relationships between the structures of the ribs, pleura, lungs, chest wall and diaphragm, together with the associated structures of the mediastinum. An appreciation of the mechanics and regulation of breathing is also important when considering changes in respiratory pattern.

This chapter begins with an overview of respiratory anatomy and physiology. This is followed by an examination of respiratory disorders requiring surgical intervention, the care required by patients undergoing surgical intervention and the associated nursing care.

An overview of the respiratory system and the mechanics of breathing

The primary function of the respiratory system is the efficient transfer of oxygen from the atmosphere, through the respiratory tract to the alveoli within the lungs, and the elimination of carbon dioxide in the opposite direction. This function is facilitated by the process of breathing. Breathing can be described as an automatic, rhythmic process, which is centrally regulated within the brainstem and results in contraction and relaxation of the skeletal muscles of the diaphragm, ribcage and abdomen, with the consequent movement of gas in and out of the pulmonary alveoli.

Respiration is the overall process (which includes breathing) of controlled oxidation of carbohydrates and fat, to generate energy within all cells of the body, and the production of carbon dioxide as a waste product.

This section will consider the structure and function of the respiratory system and the manner in which ventilation and gaseous diffusion takes place.

Structure and function

The thorax contains two lungs, each consisting of airways, an extensive blood supply and elastic connective tissue. The right lung consists of three lobes and the left lung has two. A division of the left upper lobe, called the lingula, arguably corresponds to the right middle lobe. The airways, which are the conducting passages for airflow into and out of the lungs,

commence with the nose and mouth and include the pharynx and larynx (see Chapter 12 for details of anatomy and physiology). The trachea is the beginning of the lower respiratory tract and commences below the larynx and continues into the mediastinum, where it divides into the right and left main bronchi. The adult trachea averages 2–2.5 cm in diameter, and ranges from 10 to 12 cm in length. The trachea remains patent through the support of 16–20 C-shaped cartilaginous rings. Posteriorly, situated directly behind the trachea, a thin muscle extends between the open ends of the cartilage, which stretches to allow the passage of food down the oesophagus. A bolus of food passing down the oesophagus temporarily decreases the lumen of the trachea.

At the point of tracheal bifurcation into the right and left main bronchi, there is a sharp dividing cartilage known as the carina. The carina helps to divide airflow to the right and left sides, minimizing turbulence. The right main bronchus angles off the midline at roughly 20–30 degrees, with the left main bronchus deflecting at a sharper angle of 45–55 degrees. The consequence of this difference is that objects inhaled or aspirated in an upright position tend to follow the straighter course into the right main bronchus. In the supine position, aspirated or inhaled objects go into the dependent segments of the lung.

Functionally, the lungs can be divided into two zones: the conducting airways and the respiratory zone. The conducting airways (the volume of which is referred to as anatomical dead space) do not contain alveoli, and therefore do not participate in gaseous exchange. Gaseous exchange takes place in the alveolar-containing regions of the lung, called the respiratory zone, which accounts for most of the lung volume.

The conducting airways

The right and left main bronchi subdivide into lobar and then segmental bronchi. Terminal bronchioles, the smallest airways without alveoli, are the product of smaller subdivisions. These airways become progressively narrower, shorter and more numerous as they penetrate the lung. The terminal bronchioles subdivide further into respiratory bronchioles, which contain some alveoli within their walls, and therefore enter the respiratory zone.

By convention, the conducting airways can be broadly categorized into two distinct types: cartilaginous bronchi and membranous bronchioles. The trachea, main bronchi and subsequent divisions of the bronchi contain supporting cartilaginous plates within their walls. These cartilaginous plates maintain patency in the large airways thus enabling the bronchi to dilate or constrict independently of lung volume. As the bronchi progressively subdivide, the cartilage gradually disappears. In airways of ≤1 mm, i.e. terminal bronchioles and further subdivisions, the cartilage disappears completely.

Additionally, the bronchi are characterized by a pseudostratified columnar epithelium on spiral bands of smooth muscle and ciliated, mucus-producing epithelium. The 'mucociliary escalator' is a significant function of the respiratory system, trapping dust and other inhaled particles in the mucus, which along with scavenging macrophages are swept up to the larynx by the cilia and coughed out, swallowed or removed by nose blowing. This mechanism may contribute to airway obstruction when patients are unable to cough adequately to clear secretions, either because of tracheal intubation, poor cough reflex, or pain following thoracic surgery.

The respiratory zone

The respiratory bronchioles contain some alveoli within their walls and subdivide finally into the alveolar ducts, which are completely lined with alveoli. These airways, lined with a simple cuboidal epithelium, contain no cartilage within their walls. An important functional difference between the bronchi and the bronchioles is that the latter are embedded directly into the connective tissue framework of the lungs, and, with no cartilage support, their diameter is dependent on lung volume.

The alveoli are thin-walled sacs, each approximately 0.3 mm in diameter and covered in a network of fine capillaries. The surface tension of the thin film of liquid within the alveoli would tend to cause inward collapse of the air space, but this is prevented by a secretion from the cells lining the alveoli. The secretion contains surfactant, which lowers the surface tension, thereby preventing alveolar collapse. Collapse of these small air spaces remains a potential problem, and frequently occurs in respiratory disease.

Pleura

The shape of the lungs conforms to that of the thoracic cavity, through a balancing of tensions within the thorax, held in balance by the pleura. The pleura is a double membrane: the visceral pleura covers the surface of the lung and doubles back as the parietal pleura, which covers the internal surface of the chest wall. The visceral pleura is devoid of a sensory nerve supply, whilst the parietal pleura receives innervation from the intercostal and phrenic nerves, providing pain and sensation properties.

The two pleura function as one unit due to the small volume of pleural fluid existing between the two layers. This fluid acts as a lubricant to permit the sliding of one layer across the other during respiratory movements, but does not allow the pleura to be pulled apart (rather as two plates of glass with a small drop of water between them cannot be separated except by sliding apart). The pleura, acting together, permit the transfer of movement from the respiratory muscles of the chest wall to the lungs, facilitating the variations of intrathoracic pressure, which are vital for respiratory function.

The tendency of the lungs to pull away from the chest wall and collapse is due to the natural elasticity of the pulmonary connective tissue, and the surface tension in the fluid lining the alveoli. The negative intrapleural pressure balances these tensions throughout the entire respiratory cycle. The negative intrapleural pressure is a consequence of the external forces on the pleura in the form of the inward pull of the lungs away from the chest wall, and outward movements of the chest wall.

Removal of inhaled particles

Filtration of inspired air is accomplished by large hairs within the nose and by the nasal mucosal membrane, which traps inhaled particulate matter. The direction of the inspired airstream changes abruptly at the nasopharynx, causing particulate matter to land on the back wall of the pharynx. The tonsils and adenoids located nearby provide the immunological defence against biologically active inspired material. Smaller inhaled particles may reach the lower airways, some of them lodging in the mucous epithelium, and are removed via the mucociliary escalator, or by reflex coughing or sneezing. Some small particles remain suspended as aerosols and are simply exhaled. Alveoli are not ciliated, and particles that deposit there are engulfed by macrophages, and removed from the lung via the lymphatic system or the blood flow.

Nasal breathing is the normal mechanism for air entry because of the additional pulmonary defence mechanisms it provides. Mouth breathing is necessary during colds (when the nasal passages are congested) and when large volumes of air need to be moved in and out, e.g. during exertion. Mouth breathing is a basic physiological response to dyspnoea, since the nasal turbinates create twice the resistance to airflow through the nose, compared with airflow through the mouth. Oral breathing bypasses the protective mechanisms of the nose, thereby allowing unwarmed, unfiltered, dry air to enter the tracheobronchial tree.

Inspiration and expiration

The rate and depth of respiration is a complex activity regulated by the respiratory centre in the medulla oblongata within the brainstem. Breathing is regulated to some extent through voluntary (behavioural) control, where breathing may be temporarily suspended or altered. The main regulation is through metabolic (automatic) control. Voluntary control of breathing allows ancillary actions related to breathing to occur, e.g. talking, singing, swallowing, straining, sneezing and coughing. Metabolic control serves the basic body requirements for oxygen.

The respiratory centre receives sensory input from many sources, including chemoreceptors and proprioceptors. Chemoreceptors are receptors that respond to changes in the chemical composition of blood or other fluid. Central chemoreceptors are found on the brainstem surface surrounded by brain extracellular fluid. They are sensitive to changes in hydrogen ion concentration (pH), where an increase, i.e. a fall in pH, stimulates ventilation. Carbon dioxide dissolved in cerebrospinal fluid causes a fall in pH, and is a powerful stimulus to respiration. Peripheral chemoreceptors are located in the carotid bodies at the bifurcation of the common carotid arteries, and in the aortic bodies above and below the aortic arch. The peripheral chemoreceptors respond to decreases in arterial oxygen concentrations (PaO_2) and increases in arterial carbon dioxide levels ($PaCO_2$). These receptors are responsible for the increase in ventilation that occurs in response to arterial hypoxaemia. A fall in oxygen concentration is a stimulus to respiration, but only a weak one. It becomes more important in chronic obstructive pulmonary disease where there is tolerance to an established rise in levels of carbon dioxide.

The rhythmicity of respiration is controlled by the pneumotaxic centre in the pons, responding to impulses from the proprioceptors, or lung stretch receptors, which are believed to lie within the smooth muscle of the bronchi and possibly the bronchioles. They respond to distension of the lung, which dilates and stretches the airways and alveoli, with the effect of inhibiting further inspiratory activity. The opposite response is also seen, i.e. deflation of the lungs tends to initiate inspiratory activity. The stretch receptors help to prevent overinflation of the lung, and, in the presence of airway narrowing or slow inspiration, their delayed activation allows inspiration to last longer until an adequate tidal volume is achieved.

Irritant receptors are thought to lie between epithelial airway cells, and are stimulated by noxious gases, cigarette smoke, inhaled dusts and cold air. They are similar to receptors found within the nose, nasopharynx, larynx and trachea. Various responses may be initiated, such as sneezing, coughing and bronchoconstriction. It is possible that these receptors play a role in the bronchoconstriction of asthma, as a result of their response to released histamine.

The mechanics of breathing

Gas flows from a region of higher pressure to one of lower pressure. When the total pressure in the alveoli is equal to atmospheric pressure, there is no airflow. For inspiration to occur, alveolar pressure must be less than atmospheric pressure, and the reverse for expiration. There are two ways of creating the pressure difference necessary for inspiration to occur: alveolar pressure can be lowered, as in natural breathing, or airway pressure can be raised, as in positive pressure ventilation by mechanical ventilators.

Inspiration is the active phase of breathing, during which time the diaphragm and external intercostal muscles contract. The contraction of the diaphragm forces the abdominal contents downwards, and the contraction of the intercostal muscles produces elevation of the ribs. This results in expansion of the thoracic cavity and lowering of the pressure in the pleural space surrounding the lungs. As the pressure falls in the pleural space, the distensible lungs expand passively, causing the required pressure drop within the alveolar ducts and air spaces. As the pressure decreases, air flows down the airways into the alveolar spaces until the pressures are equalized, marking the end of the inspiratory phase.

During expiration, which is generally the passive phase, the diaphragm and intercostal muscles relax, allowing the elastic recoil of the lungs to occur, which increases the alveolar pressure, and gas flows out of the lungs. During exercise and voluntary hyperventilation, expiration may become active rather than passive. The significant muscles of expiration are the muscles of the abdominal wall, including the rectus abdominis, the internal and external oblique muscles and the transversus abdominis. When these muscles contract, intra-abdominal pressure is raised, and the diaphragm is pushed up.

Other muscles which may be used to assist respiration are the accessory muscles in the neck and shoulders, the scalene muscles which elevate the first two ribs, and the sternomastoid muscles which raise the sternum. There is very little or no activity in these muscles during quiet breathing, but during exercise or laboured breathing they may contract vigorously.

The exchange of carbon dioxide and oxygen between alveolar air and the pulmonary capillaries occurs by a simple process of diffusion from areas of high concentration to areas of relatively low concentration. The large surface area of the lungs provided by the alveoli is estimated to be $50-100$ m^2 and, with the extremely thin blood–gas barriers of the alveolar membrane and capillary membrane, create the ideal environment for gaseous diffusion to occur. Carbon dioxide is highly soluble and diffuses much more rapidly than oxygen across the membranes.

Blood gas concentration

Oxygen is carried in the blood in two forms: dissolved and in combination with haemoglobin. The amount of dissolved oxygen is proportional to the partial pressure of oxygen, but is insufficient alone to meet the demands for oxygen by the tissues. Oxygen transported in combination with haemoglobin, i.e. oxyhaemoglobin, is the significant mode of oxygen carriage, and ensures that the dissolved oxygen within the plasma can be continuously replenished, for uptake by the tissues. Oxygen forms an easily reversible combination with haemoglobin and will

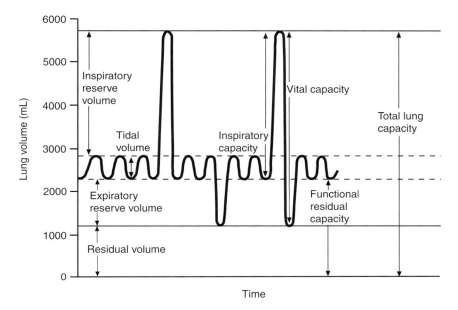

Figure 15.1 Lung volumes. (From Foss (1989).)

combine with or separate from the haemoglobin depending on the relative partial pressures of the surrounding plasma. Differences within the amino acid chains within the haemoglobin can produce variants of haemoglobin with diminished oxygen-carrying capacity, e.g. haemoglobin S or sickle cell.

Oxygen saturation is defined as the ratio of the concentration of oxyhaemoglobin to the concentration of desaturated (or reduced) haemoglobin and is expressed as a percentage. Normal haemoglobin levels are approximately 15 g haemoglobin/100 mL of blood and the normal oxygen saturation level of arterial blood is 97% when all the haemoglobin is carrying oxygen to full capacity. The oxygen saturation of venous blood is about 75%, reflecting the uptake of oxygen by the tissues, and a large reserve of remaining oxygen. Arterial blood gas analysis measures the PaO_2, where the normal range is 11.5–13.5 kilopascals (abbreviated to kPa).

Lung volumes

For the purposes of measurement and description, the total volume of air in the lungs is divided into volumes and capacities, where a capacity is considered to be the combination of two or more volumes (Fig. 15.1). While breathing at rest, the volume of air moved in and out, i.e. tidal volume, TV or VT, approximates to 500 mL. The volume of air remaining in the lungs at the end of tidal expiration is the functional residual capacity (FRC), which is composed of the expiratory reserve volume (ERV) and the

volume of air remaining in the lungs at the end of full expiration, called the residual volume (RV). The ERV is required when increases in breathing are needed, e.g. during exercise. From knowledge of the FRC, other volumes may be assumed. The inspiratory capacity (IC) is the maximum volume that can be inspired and consists of the tidal volume and the inspiratory reserve volume (IRV). The latter, like the ERV, is the additional volume available during exercise, or other increased levels of breathing.

At maximum inspiration, the total volume of air is the total lung capacity (TLC). The RV, the TLC and the FRC cannot be measured directly without complex equipment. However, the vital capacity can be efficiently measured, and indicates the difference in volume between the TLC and the RV. In considering these facts, it is obvious that the lungs have large reserve volumes and capacity for increased ventilation. The consequences of lung resection, therefore, may not greatly limit respiratory function if the remaining lung tissue is healthy and the reserve capacity can be utilized.

Respiratory assessment

Respiratory assessment is a vital part of the care of patients undergoing thoracic surgery. The purpose is to gain a clinical impression of the respiratory function or dysfunction and severity of symptoms, to confirm the need for medical interventions and to highlight subject areas for subsequent patient education.

Assessment of breathing

Rate, depth and quality determine the pattern of breathing. Respiratory rate is calculated by counting the number of chest movements per minute. One rise and fall of the chest is one full respiratory cycle. The normal respiratory rate at rest is 12–18 breaths per minute (in adults); it is faster in infants and children. The ratio of pulse rate to respiration is approximately 5:1. The depth of respiration is the volume of air moving in and out with each breath, i.e. the tidal volume (≈ 500 mL). The quality of breathing is compared with normal relaxed breathing, which is effortless, automatic, regular and almost silent.

Breathing patterns

Hyperpnoea
Hyperpnoea is an increased depth and rate of respiration. It can be a normal physiological response, e.g. during exercise to meet the metabolic demand of tissues.

Tachypnoea
Tachypnoea is an increased respiratory rate and refers to rapid, shallow breathing. It can be seen in fever as the body tries to rid itself of excess heat. Respirations increase by approximately seven breaths per minute for every 1°C rise in temperature. Respiratory rate also rises in pneumonia, obstructive pulmonary diseases, respiratory insufficiency, and lesions in the respiratory centre of the brainstem.

Bradypnoea
Bradypnoea is a decreased but regular respiratory rate, e.g. caused by depression of the respiratory centre in a response to opioid drugs or a brain tumour.

Dyspnoea
Dyspnoea is difficult and laboured breathing. Dilated nostrils are often apparent, and the entire chest wall and shoulder girdle are raised and lowered in an exaggerated manner. Dyspnoea is a subjective complaint, being an unpleasant awareness of inappropriate effort required for breathing and can be caused by obstruction to airflow.

Orthopnoea
Orthopnoea is breathlessness which occurs when a patient is lying flat. The condition is relieved by adopting a more upright position; the number of pillows required may give a rough indication of the degree of dyspnoea experienced.

Hypoventilation
Hypoventilation is an alteration in the pattern of respiration, which becomes irregular or slow and shallow in depth, as a result of drugs, carbon dioxide narcosis or anaesthetic agents.

Hyperventilation
Hyperventilation is an increase in the rate and depth of respiration, e.g. in fear, anxiety, hysterical states, hepatic coma, midbrain lesions of the brainstem, and acid–base imbalance such as diabetic ketoacidosis (Kussmaul's respiration).

Cheyne–Stokes respiration
Cheyne–Stokes respiration is a cyclical pattern in which respirations gradually increase in rate and depth and then decrease over a cycle of 30–45 seconds. Periods of apnoea (20 seconds) alternate with these cycles. This type of breathing pattern is associated with increased intracranial pressure, severe congestive heart failure, renal failure, meningitis and drug overdose. It is also commonly associated with the dying patient.

Apnoea
Apnoea is the total absence of respirations. It may be periodic or cyclical.

Respiratory noise heard without the aid of a stethoscope

Additional information about respiratory status can be determined by listening to the breathing of the patient. Descriptions of respiratory noise heard without the aid of a stethoscope are given below.

Stertorous
These noisy, snoring-type respirations, usually caused by excessive secretions in the trachea or bronchi, are commonly heard in the unconscious patient.

Stridor
Stridor is a loud, harsh, high-pitched sound on inspiration, usually caused by laryngeal obstruction and the resulting disrupted airflow. It tends to be louder and harsher than a wheeze.

Wheeze
A wheeze is a high- or low-pitched sound mainly heard on expiration. Wheezes are generated by the vibration of the walls of narrowed airways as air travels at high velocity through them. The diameter of the airway may be reduced by bronchospasm, mucosal oedema or by foreign objects. The pitch of the wheeze is unrelated to the length of the airway but is directly related to the degree of airway compression, i.e. the tighter the airway, the higher the pitch.

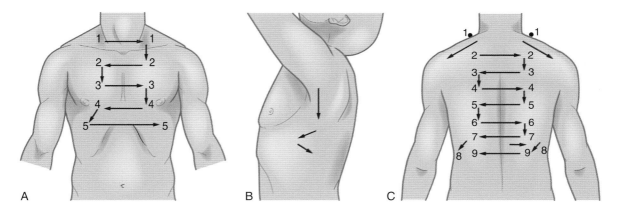

Figure 15.2 Chest auscultation. The numbers represent the order in which to listen. (From Lewis, S.L., et al. (2017). Medical Surgical Nursing: Assessment and Management of Clinical Problems (10th edn.). Elsevier Inc.)

Respiratory auscultation

Respiratory auscultation is heard with the aid of a stethoscope (Fig. 15.2).

Rales/crackles

Rales or crackles are discontinuous noises that can be differentiated into fine, medium or coarse crackles. The sound is like the crackling of tissue paper at the end of the stethoscope. It is believed that crackles are moist sounds produced by excess liquid in the airways, and are significant in pneumonia, pulmonary fibrosis and congestive cardiac failure.

Pleural rub

Pleural rub is characterized by a low-pitched rough grating sound heard in both inspiration and expiration, caused by inflammation of the pleural surfaces. The pleural rub is associated with breathing but unaffected by coughing.

Additional observations

Additional observations may contribute further to the assessment of respiratory status.

Cyanosis

Cyanosis is a bluish discoloration of the skin caused by a relative decrease in oxygen saturation within the capillaries of the skin. Generally, cyanosis is said to occur when more than 5 g of deoxygenated haemoglobin is present per 100 mL of blood, i.e. when the haemoglobin level is within normal limits. Patients who are anaemic do not appear cyanotic unless they are severely hypoxaemic, and polycythaemic patients require considerably lower percentages of deoxygenated haemoglobin to display cyanosis. Cyanosis, when present in fingers, toes and ear lobes, i.e. peripheral cyanosis, is usually related to circulatory problems, such as heart failure. Central cyanosis is present when the patient's more central regions are affected, e.g. the tongue and lips, and the trunk. This is related to a lack of oxygenation of arterial blood through the pulmonary system. Acute cyanosis can happen as a result of asphyxiation or choking.

Clubbing of the digits

Clubbing of the digits is a significant manifestation within chronic cardiopulmonary disease, although the mechanism is unknown. It is identified most commonly in patients who have bronchogenic carcinoma, chronic obstructive pulmonary disease or cystic fibrosis. It is characterized by a painless enlargement of the terminal phalanges of the fingers and toes, and a widening and deepening of the nail bed.

Cough

Coughing is the most common symptom in patients with pulmonary disease, particularly within the lower respiratory tract, and can be initiated by inflammatory, mechanical or thermal stimulation of the receptors located in the pharynx, larynx, trachea, large bronchi and even the lung and visceral pleura.

The character of a cough should be evaluated using the descriptions in Table 15.1, and assessed in terms of relationship to time, patient's position and environmental exposure. Coughs of recent onset suggest probable infection and those most noticeable on wakening suggest bronchitis or a suppurative lung disease. Nocturnal paroxysms of coughing may be indicative of asthma or left-sided heart failure. Coughs that worsen on lying down may be due to bronchiectasis or a postnasal drip from sinusitis, and those associated with food intake

Table 15.1 Evaluation of cough

Evaluation of cough	Possible causes/indications
Throat clearing	Postnasal drip
Dry and hacking	May be due to nervousness, viral infections, bronchogenic carcinoma or congestive cardiac failure
Loud and harsh	Irritation in the upper airway
Wheezing	Associated with bronchospasm
Severe, or changing in character or with position	May be bronchogenic carcinoma
Loose	Indicates problems in peripheral bronchi and lung parenchyma
Painful	May indicate pleural involvement, or chest wall disease

Table 15.2 Types of cough

Type of cough	Description of cough
Effective	Strong enough to clear the airway
Inadequate	Audible but too weak to move the secretions
Productive	Mucus expelled as a result of the cough
Dry	Moisture or secretions not produced
Barking	Like a seal bark, indicative of a problem in the upper airways, e.g. croup, laryngotracheal bronchitis
Brassy/hoarse	Harsh, dry cough, associated with upper airway disorders, e.g. laryngitis, laryngotracheal bronchitis
Hacking	Frequent brief periods of coughing or clearing the throat. The cough may be dry, as a result of smoking, a viral infection or postnasal drip

Source: Adapted from Wilkins, R., Krider, S., Sheldon, R. (1995). Clinical Assessment in Respiratory Care (3rd edn.). London: Mosby.

to aspiration of food into the trachea. A worsening cough is the most common presenting symptom of bronchial cancer. Cough also occurs for psychological reasons. Types and descriptions of coughs are shown in Table 15.2.

Sputum

Sputum is the substance expelled from the tracheobronchial tree, pharynx, mouth, sinuses and nose. The term phlegm refers strictly to secretions from the lungs and tracheobronchial tree; phlegm may contain mucus, cellular debris, microorganisms, blood, pus and inhaled particulate matter. Normal secretions of up to 100 mL are produced daily, removed by the mucociliary escalator and swallowed unnoticed. Sputum may be described as thin, thick, viscous (i.e. gelatinous), tenacious (i.e. extremely sticky), frothy, mucoid or mucopurulent. Other observations of sputum include colour, odour and quantity (Table 15.3).

Haemoptysis

Haemoptysis is the expectoration of blood, ranging from sputum containing flecks of blood to expectoration of large amounts of frank blood. The source of blood may be from the mouth, nose, airways or lung tissue. Careful questioning may help to differentiate haemoptysis from haematemesis. Massive bleeding can occur with pulmonary tuberculosis, lung abscesses, pulmonary embolism and pulmonary infarction, bronchiectasis and bronchogenic carcinoma. Haemoptysis can also occur following lung surgery, lung biopsy or bronchoscopy, and so the patient should be warned of these possibilities.

Chest pain

Thoracic pain is associated with a number of cardiac and pulmonary disorders. Careful assessment of precipitating

Table 15.3 Description of sputum

Description of sputum	Possible causes/indications
Clear or mucoid	Viral infection, chronic bronchitis, postnasal drip
Yellow or green	Primary or secondary bacterial infections
Rusty	May indicate bacterial pneumonia
Malodorous	Due to lung abscess, infection from anaerobic organisms
Frothy and pink	Acute pulmonary oedema

Source: Adapted from Kumar and Clark (2005).

factors, type and quality of pain, and the location and duration of the pain is required to distinguish between them.

Chest pain of pulmonary origin involves the chest wall and parietal pleura, the major airways, diaphragm and mediastinum. Pain arising from the chest wall is well localized and very sharp, increasing with deep breaths and coughing. It is often referred to as pleuritic pain because of the similarity to the pain experienced with pleurisy. Pleuritic pain is a knife-like pain in the chest, particularly associated with a deep intake of breath. Pain associated with neoplasms of the lungs or major bronchi is less well defined, being less localized and dull. Diaphragmatic pain is experienced as referred pain in the shoulders.

Common disorders requiring surgical intervention

Conditions affecting the pleura

Recurrent pneumothorax

Pneumothorax is a condition in which air enters the pleural space for a variety of reasons and causes collapse of the underlying lung. Air entry into the pleural space disrupts the surface tension of the fluid film that holds the two pleurae together, with loss of negative intrapleural pressure. The two pleurae separate and no longer function as one unit. The underlying lung collapses, since the elastic recoil forces of the lung are now greater than the intrapleural pressure. Small pneumothoraces may go unnoticed. Pain may accompany the occurrence of the pneumothorax, particularly if parietal pleural irritation also occurs, due to the innervation of the parietal pleura. With a large pneumothorax the patient appears acutely dyspnoeic, tachypnoeic and tachycardic, with reduced chest movement on the affected side. The diagnosis is confirmed by chest X-ray.

Pneumothoraces can be broadly categorized into three main types: spontaneous, traumatic and tension.

Spontaneous pneumothorax

Spontaneous pneumothorax can occur without (primary) or with (secondary) pulmonary pathology. Primary pneumothorax commonly occurs in tall, thin, young men. Possible explanations include the rupture of alveoli or bullae, which disrupts the visceral pleura (bullae are air cavities within the lung tissue which are created when alveoli rupture). Secondary pneumothorax can be a consequence of chronic lung disease, e.g. severe asthma, emphysema or cystic fibrosis, and also arises from the rupture of alveoli or bullae.

Traumatic pneumothorax

Traumatic pneumothorax occurs when air enters from outside the chest wall, e.g. following chest wall trauma such as stab wounds or fractured ribs. Thoracentesis, pleural biopsy or the insertion of a central venous catheter or pacemaker can likewise result in pleural rupture. Thoracic surgery itself creates a pneumothorax because of the necessity of entering the pleural cavity to reach the lung tissue. Positive pressure ventilation, particularly when positive end-expiratory pressure is used, can cause a pneumothorax since it involves raised airway pressure throughout the entire respiratory cycle. Rupture of the oesophagus can also allow air to enter the pleural space.

Tension pneumothorax

Tension pneumothorax is a serious and potentially fatal condition, caused by air entering the pleural space on inspiration, which cannot escape during expiration, resulting in progressive compression of the underlying lung. If left untreated, a tracheal and mediastinal shift towards the unaffected lung can occur, compromising both the ventilation of that lung and venous return to the heart, resulting in shock and potential death.

Treatment

Small pneumothoraces usually resolve spontaneously because the air is reabsorbed from the pleural space. Larger pneumothoraces may require the insertion of an underwater seal chest drain, or Heimlich valve, to facilitate air drainage and consequently the resolution of the surface tension within the pleural spaces as the lung re-expands. Recurrence of spontaneous pneumothoraces may result in consideration for surgical intervention, i.e. pleurodesis or pleurectomy.

Pleural effusion

Pleural effusion is an abnormal accumulation of fluid in the pleural space because of changes in hydrostatic pressure. Causes of pleural effusion include malignant disease, infection, congestive heart failure, hypoprotein states, atelectasis and following radiotherapy.

The size of the effusion will influence the patient's presenting symptoms, i.e. the degree of dyspnoea experienced (ranging from mild to severe) and the degree of pain experienced (chest or referred shoulder pain). The pulmonary symptoms result from the space-occupying effects of the fluid within the pleural space and may include cough, fever, sweats and sputum production. A fluid volume of 300 mL or more can be seen on X-ray, along with a mediastinal shift, depending on the volume of fluid collection.

Thoracentesis

Thoracentesis will provide a definitive diagnosis, and small effusions may be effectively drained in this way. Larger or recurrent effusions may require the insertion of a chest drain, since repeated thoracentesis can cause loculation, whereby the fluid collects in multiple pockets caused by adhesions from repeated aspiration attempts. Palliative surgery, such as pleurodesis, may be required in malignant disease where repeated collections of fluid are problematic, thus preventing further accumulations.

Empyema

Pleural empyema, i.e. pyothorax, is a collection of infected or purulent fluid within the pleural space. It represents the end stage of a pathological process starting with a contaminated pleural effusion following bacterial pneumonia, the rupture of a lung abscess into the pleural space, or from a subphrenic abscess. Bronchopleural fistulae, traumatic penetration of the pleura and the necessity for prolonged use of chest drains can likewise result in infection. Empyema classically starts as an infection of low-viscosity pleural effusion with an underlying lung that is fully expansible. The progression of the empyema will eventually reduce lung capacity because of increasing viscosity of the fluid and the development of a thick, fibrous walled cavity surrounding the infected fluid.

Patients with empyema can experience pleural pain and fever. Initial treatment of the empyema may be conservative, with attempts to drain the empyema using chest drains and antibiotics. Chronic, cavitated empyema requires surgical intervention because drainage alone will not prevent recurrence of a collection of infected fluid within the cavity. The surgical procedure includes decortication and drainage of the fluid.

Malignant disease of the pleura

Primary malignancy of the pleura is rare and is associated with exposure to asbestos. Of the primary pleural tumours that do occur, most are mesotheliomas, of which there are two types:
- *pleural fibroma*: a localized fibrous mesothelioma which may be treated by surgical excision
- *diffuse malignant mesothelioma*: a thick fibrous sheet producing rapidly occurring high-volume pleural effusions; it carries a poor prognosis and surgery is purely palliative in an attempt to prevent further effusion forming.

Malignant disease of the lung

Bronchogenic carcinoma refers to a malignant tumour of the lung arising within the wall or epithelial lining of the bronchus. The lung is also a common site for metastatic spread from cancer elsewhere within the body.

Lung cancer is one of the top three prevalent forms of cancer, with approximately 46,000 cases diagnosed a year in the UK, with 79% of these being preventable. The extraordinary rise in the incidence of lung cancer in the 20th century is attributed to cigarette smoking. Although previously much more common in men, figures are reaching parity as 46% of individuals with lung cancer are female. Almost 36,000 individuals die every year in the UK as a result of lung cancer, and overall, only 5% of lung cancer patients survive for 10 or more years after diagnosis (Cancer Research UK, 2015).

Histological types of lung cancer

Detailed by the 2015 WHO classification of lung tumours, the six most important histologically unique lung cancers are as follows:
- Squamous cell carcinoma: a form of non-small-cell type lung cancer, it most commonly arises in central lung fields, in the epithelium of large bronchi. There are three main subtypes – keratinizing, non-keratinizing and basaloid squamous cell carcinoma (Travis et al, 2015).
- Adenocarcinoma: a form of non-small-cell type lung cancer, it arises peripherally, in glandular tissue. Its pattern of differentiation may be one of the following: lepidic, acinar, papillary, micropapillary, or solid (Travis et al, 2015).
- Large cell: a form of non-small-cell type lung cancer, it arises peripherally, from lung epithelial cells. Often diagnosed in

Table 15.4 Descriptors of T-staging

T-stage	Tumour size and descriptors
Tx	Cannot be assessed, not visualized on imaging
T0	No evidence of primary tumour
Tis	Carcinoma *in situ*
T1a	Tumour <1 cm
T1b	1 cm < tumour ≤ 2 cm
T1c	2 cm < tumour ≤ 3 cm
T2	• Within main bronchus • Invasion of visceral pleura • Obstructive atelectasis • Local invasion of diaphragm
T2a	3 cm < tumour ≤ 4 cm
T2b	4 cm < tumour ≤ 5 cm
T3	5 cm < tumour ≤ 7 cm • Local invasion of chest wall, parietal pericardium, phrenic nerve • Satellite nodule (same lobe)
T4	7 cm < tumour • Invasion to mediastinum, trachea, heart/great vessels, oesophagus, cerebra, carina, recurrent laryngeal nerve • Satellite nodule (different lobe, same lung)

Source: Adapted from Lim et al (2018).

the absence of histopathological features of other, more specific forms of lung cancer (Travis et al, 2015).

- Neuroendocrine: consisting of small cell lung carcinomas and large cell neuroendocrine carcinomas, these carcinoid tumours originate in neuroendocrine cells. Generally, carcinoid patients have a superior prognosis partially due to the slow growth of the tumour, and do not display the same smoking-related association as is seen with most other lung cancers (Travis et al, 2015).
- Sarcomatoid: a general term for a collection of very rare forms of lung cancer including, but not limited to, pleomorphic carcinoma, carcinosarcoma, and pulmonary blastoma (Travis et al, 2015).
- NUT: a carcinoma associate with chromosomal rearrangement in the *NUT* gene (Travis et al, 2015).

The poor survival rates of patients with lung cancer are due to its insidious development, with symptoms becoming evident only later in the progress of the disease. Occasionally, the presence of a tumour is detected early as part of X-ray screening for routine medical examinations. These patients may feel fit and well and have difficulty accepting that such a diagnosis has been made.

An international coding system for stage grouping is used in the diagnosis of lung cancer, which enables the medical team to optimize therapeutic interventions. Three factors are considered:

- T = tumour size
- N = nodal involvement
- M = possible metastatic spread

Descriptors of staging can be seen in Tables 15.4 to 15.7.

Specific investigations required prior to surgery

Many investigative procedures are dependent upon patient cooperation for their success, with the evident need for clear explanations and informed consent. The period of investigation is one of extreme anxiety for the patient, because of the uncertainty about diagnosis, treatment and possible outcomes. Many of these investigations are performed with the outcome of malignancy as a possibility.

Chest X-ray

Chest X-ray can be used to detect, and observe the progression of, alterations within the lungs caused by disease

Table 15.5 Descriptors of N-staging

N-stage	Nodal descriptor
Nx	Regional lymph nodes cannot be assessed
N0	No regional lymph node metastasis
N1	Metastasis in ipsilateral peribronchial and/or hilar lymph node and intrapulmonary node, including involvement by direct extension
N2	Metastasis in ipsilateral mediastinal and/or subcarinal lymph nodes
N3	Metastasis in contralateral mediastinal, contralateral hilar, ipsilateral, or contralateral scalene, or supraclavicular lymph node(s)

Source: Adapted from Lim et al (2018).

Table 15.6 Descriptors of M-staging

M-stage	Metastatic descriptor
M0	No distant metastasis
M1a	Separate tumour nodule(s) in a contralateral lobe; pleural nodules or malignant pleural or pericardial effusion
M1b	Single extrathoracic metastasis or involvement of a single distant (non-regional) node
M1c	Multiple extrathoracic metastases in one or several organs

Source: Adapted from Lim et al (2018).

Table 15.7 Overall stage groupings based on T-, N- and M-staging

	N0	N1	N2	N3
T1a	IA1	IIB	IIIA	IIIB
T1b	IA2	IIB	IIIA	IIIB
T1c	IA3	IIB	IIIA	IIIB
T2a	IB	IIB	IIIA	IIIB
T2b	IIA	IIB	IIIA	IIIB
T3	IIB	IIIS	IIIB	IIIC
T4	IIIA	IIIA	IIIB	IIIC
M1a	IVA	IVA	IVA	IVA
M1b	IVA	IVA	IVA	IVA
M1c	IVB	IVB	IVB	IVB

Source: Adapted from Lim et al (2018).

processes; determine the position of chest drains and central venous lines; and evaluate the effectiveness of treatment. Chest X-rays do not allow definitive diagnoses to be formed except in the case of pneumothorax.

Standard chest X-rays are taken in two directions.

- *Posteroanterior (PA) view:* the patient stands in front of the film and is X-rayed from behind. As the heart is in the anterior half of the chest, this view produces less cardiac magnification. The patient stands with their hands on their hips so that the scapulae are displaced to the sides of the chest and do not overlap the lung fields.
- *Lateral view:* generally, a left lateral film is taken, where the patient stands with their left side against the film. This view provides less cardiac magnification and a sharper image of the left lower lobe, which is partially obscured on the posteroanterior view by cardiac shadow. Similarly, a right lateral film will produce sharper images of a right-sided lesion.

Portable films are required in the immediate post-operative phase or while the patient is critically ill. A portable film is taken with the film behind the patient and is therefore an anteroposterior view. Interpretation of the film requires skill due to the shadows superimposed by sheets, nightclothes and any tubes, etc. The scapulae may also be evident.

Chest X-rays are usually taken with the patient maintaining full inspiration. Expiratory films may be helpful when detecting small pneumothoraces, because the lung volume is reduced while the volume of pleural air remains the same but occupies a greater percentage of the thoracic volume.

Computerized tomography

Computerized tomography (CT) scanning is invaluable in the investigation of pulmonary disorders because the clarity of the images is superior to that of those produced by conventional radiography. The non-invasive cross-sectional views create images that will confirm chest wall invasion by tumour involvement, metastatic spread or small metastatic nodes.

Positron emission tomography

Positron emission tomography (PET) is a nuclear medicine technique that measures biochemical and metabolic activity of cells following the injection of a positron-emitting isotope. PET scanning is useful in the detection and staging of malignant cells.

Magnetic resonance imaging

Magnetic resonance imaging (MRI) is a non-invasive procedure in which hydrogen atoms in the patient's body are aligned by a magnetic field. Radio waves passed through the body are absorbed by the hydrogen atoms and their subsequent movement causes a detectable change in the magnetic field. Different tissue types have differing concentration of hydrogen, which is how an image can be constructed.

Lung (pulmonary) function tests

Lung function tests are a means of assessing the functional status of the lungs. Measurements can determine tidal volumes, rates of gas flow, and the stiffness, i.e. compliance, of the lungs and chest wall. The diffusion characteristics of gas movement across the alveolar–capillary membrane can also be demonstrated.

Lung function tests are not a diagnostic tool. They are, however, of value in distinguishing between a restrictive defect within the lungs, e.g. pleural effusion or rib fractures, and an obstructive defect, e.g. asthma or emphysema. The importance of lung function testing in the context of surgery lies within the assessment of the degree of pulmonary involvement in the diseased lungs, and the assessment of pulmonary function prior to anaesthesia.

The primary tool in lung function tests is the spirometer, which is designed to measure lung volumes and gas flows. Spirometry is now also performed with small, portable, hand-held devices. The tracings from spirometry show the ratio of volume of air expired in one second (FEV_1) compared to the total volume of expired air (FVC). Normal lung function would show an FEV_1/FVC ratio of 75–80%. A ratio of less than 70% is found in patients with airflow obstruction. In restrictive disorders, the FVC is reduced but the FEV_1 is normal, which may show a ratio of over 80% (Kumar & Clark, 2005).

Peak expiratory flow rate (PEFR), commonly known as peak flow, is also used to determine functional status of the lungs, since it measures the maximum expiratory flow rate during forced expiration following full inspiration. It correlates closely with the FEV_1 described above and provides a readily available measure of lung function through a peak flow meter.

Oxygen saturations

Non-invasive assessment of oxygen saturation can be performed by pulse oximetry. This technique measures the absorption of selected wavelengths of light passed through a finger, toe or earlobe. As blood loses oxygen in the capillary beds, it becomes less permeable to red light. The oximeter measures the differences in light absorption and converts the value to a percentage, representing the level of oxygen saturation of the haemoglobin. False readings may be obtained when patients have received intravascular dyes, in patients with sickle cell anaemia, or if the patient is wearing nail polish (Jubran, 2015).

Sputum examination

Respiratory secretions may be sent for bacteriological or cytological examination to ensure appropriate treatment is prescribed. Cytological examination is appropriate if malignancy is suspected, because malignant cells may be shed into the airways. However, a negative result is not necessarily indicative of a diagnosis of non-malignancy.

Arterial blood gas analysis

Arterial blood gas analysis provides precise information concerning the acid–base balance and the level of oxygen and carbon dioxide present in arterial blood. Accurate interpretation of the results requires knowledge of the patient's total clinical picture, including treatments. Arterial blood is used for the sample, as it contains levels of oxygen and carbon dioxide that are determined by the lungs. Venous blood does not reflect lung function.

The arterial samples are commonly obtained from the radial artery, the femoral artery and occasionally the brachial artery. Alternatively, arterial samples may be taken from an arterial line if the patient has one. Normal gas measurements of arterial blood are shown in Table 15.8.

Table 15.8 Arterial blood gas measurements

Parameter	Range
pH	7.35–7.45
PO_2	11.5–13.5 kPa
PCO_2	4.5–6.0 kPa
HCO_3	25–30 mmol/L
Saturation	95–99%
Base excess	−2 to +2

Source: Hatchett & Thompson (2008).

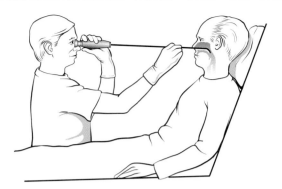

Figure 15.3 Fibreoptic bronchoscopy (pernasal). The patient adopts a sitting position. The bronchoscope is passed directly backwards through the nose, into the nasopharynx. (From Stradling (1991).)

Bronchoscopy

Bronchoscopy provides an endoscopic view of the tracheobronchial tree and is performed using either a flexible fibreoptic or a rigid bronchoscope. A bronchoscopy can be diagnostic or therapeutic, i.e. for alleviation of stenosis or removal of a foreign body, and is performed under a local or general anaesthetic.

The procedure involves the passage of a bronchoscope through the larynx and the trachea into the major airway branches. The bronchial walls can be visualized; biopsies, brushings and aspirate taken for examination; and non-surgical interventions applied. The patient is placed in a recumbent or upright position, supported with pillows. The bronchoscope is then advanced into the trachea either through the nose or the mouth (Fig. 15.3). Six hours of fasting is required prior to the procedure, to reduce the risk of aspiration should the patient vomit.

Rigid bronchoscopy

This is a palliative procedure usually performed under general anaesthesia for the relief of airway obstruction within the trachea and main bronchi. Rigid bronchoscopies are also performed for biopsies and for the retrieval of inhaled foreign objects. Stenting, laser ablation, and bronchial brachytherapy, a delivery of high doses of radiation over a short period of time without damaging healthy tissue, can be implemented via this route.

Fibreoptic (flexible) bronchoscopy

The larynx and upper airway are anaesthetized prior to the insertion of the bronchoscope, so the patient is required to fast. The patient is placed in a recumbent or upright position, supported with pillows. The bronchoscope is advanced into the trachea through either the nose or mouth in order to visualize the upper airways and airways distal to the main bronchial tree.

Potential complications following bronchoscopy

Complications following bronchoscopy are rare. However, pneumothorax, haemorrhage, and/or transient fever may occur (Vachani et al, 2012).

Post-procedure care includes maintenance of the airway and observation for laryngeal spasm (which usually resolves spontaneously but may require a high concentration of humidified oxygen until it does). Fasting is required following local anaesthetic until the effects have worn off. The gag reflex can be tested with sips of water, and this should precede free drinking and eating. Fluids can be taken approximately 2 hours post-procedure because topical anaesthetic is sprayed into the throat. It is common for sputum to be bloodstained following a bronchoscopy, especially if biopsies have been taken.

Transthoracic/percutaneous needle biopsy

This investigation is used when peripheral lung lesions are present, particularly unresectable lesions, in order to determine the choice of treatment, i.e. chemotherapy or radical radiotherapy. A biopsy needle is inserted into the lungs to gain aspirate for cytology or tissue samples for histology. Pneumothoraces can be a complication of either procedure. A chest X-ray is performed following the procedure and the patient may need to stay in hospital overnight.

Contraindications for this procedure include coagulopathies, multiple emphysematous bullae, haemoptysis or air embolus. An open lung biopsy under a general anaesthetic may be required when transthoracic/percutaneous or bronchoscopy methods have been unsuccessful. The biopsy will therefore need to be obtained via a small thoracotomy

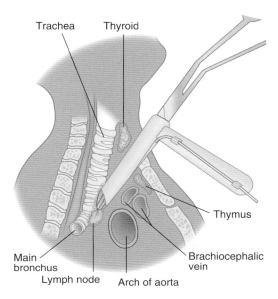

Trachea   Thyroid

Thymus

Main bronchus
Lymph node   Arch of aorta

Brachiocephalic vein

Figure 15.4 Mediastinoscopy. Diagram of a mediastinoscope in position, anterior to the trachea, allowing biopsy of a lymph node in the region of the main carina. (Reproduced from Crompton (1987), with permission of Blackwell Science Ltd.)

incision (Margereson & Riley, 2003). The procedure may be performed with a view to proceeding with resectional surgery, following confirmation of histology by examination of a frozen section.

Mediastinoscopy and mediastinotomy

This is a diagnostic technique to establish the histology of enlarged mediastinal lymph nodes found by chest X-ray or imaging. The approach is via an incision midway between the bottom of the sternal notch and the cricoid cartilage, allowing the examination of the mediastinum and obtaining a biopsy. The mediastinoscope is passed through the incision into the tract made by finger dissection through the pretracheal fascia (Fig. 15.4). Complications of the procedure include haemorrhage, hoarseness due to damage of the recurrent laryngeal nerve, and pneumothorax.

Anterior mediastinotomy is an alternative approach used to reach nodes that are inaccessible by mediastinoscopy. Nodes around the aortic arch to the left of the tracheal bifurcation and anterior mediastinal nodes on either side of the chest can be accessed via this route. The incision is made over the second cartilage/intercostal space and may involve opening of the pleura in order to inspect the hilum.

Thoracoscopy

A rigid thoracoscope is inserted into the pleural space, unless pleural adhesions are present to obstruct the passage or view of the thoracoscope. Access is gained via the intercostal spaces. Other procedures can also be performed through the thoracoscope, e.g. pleurodesis by poudrage (using powder), biopsy or pleurectomy. A chest drain is usually inserted following the procedure, to reinflate the lung.

Preoperative care

The psychological stress of patients awaiting surgery is well documented in the literature (see Chapter 4). However, the specific needs of patients awaiting thoracic surgery are not well defined. It is known that patients who are in good physical health, but who require admission for surgery, have higher levels of anxiety than those who are ill on admission (Livingstone et al, 1993). This is of particular relevance to thoracic patients, since those waiting for surgery for conditions such as persistent pneumothorax, or those who have been found to have a malignancy on a routine medical examination, often feel well when admitted electively. The patient will also be anxious about the possibility of malignancy and whether their condition is operable, because the surgeon cannot guarantee that resection is possible until surgery is underway. In these circumstances, the patients fear that they will recover from the anaesthetic to learn that the surgeon has been unable to proceed. Patients will often attend a preadmission clinic so that a comprehensive nursing assessment taking into account any personal, social, medical, psychological, spiritual or cultural needs can be undertaken. It also provides an opportunity for both patients and their relatives to discuss the implications of surgery, as well as allow the patient to undergo other preoperative investigations.

Assessment of the patient prior to surgery may include some or all of the investigations described earlier, some of which may have occurred in the outpatient setting. Occasionally, investigations such as chest X-rays may be repeated to observe for disease progression. The preoperative phase will also include the recording of a 12-lead electrocardiogram (ECG) to assess fitness for general anaesthesia, and blood testing for haemoglobin levels, clotting screen and crossmatching. Usually 2 units of blood will be requested to be made available for the surgery and immediate postoperative period.

During the preoperative phase, a physiotherapist will assess the patient and discuss the breathing exercises that need to be performed postoperatively. Other multidisciplinary personnel may need to be involved, e.g. the dietitian if the patient is undernourished or has lost weight through disease progression. The Nursing and Midwifery Council (2018) note that the nurse must work in partnership not only with the patient but with other health and social care professionals to make sure that the care that is delivered is safe and effective. The patient will be required to fast preoperatively, according to the protocol of the unit, and to undergo skin preparation which may include bathing and removal of hair from the operation site.

Thoracic surgical procedures

Although surgery offers hopeful outcomes in many types of lung cancer, only up to 30% of cases may be eligible for resection. Despite this, 60–80% of surgical patients operated on during stage 1 disease reach 5 years of survival. The overall 5-year survival rate of patients post-surgery is 37% for squamous cell carcinoma, and 27% for adenocarcinoma (Tobias & Hochhauser, 2014).

Thoracotomy

Thoracotomy is the normal surgical approach to the lungs and pleura, although exposure of the anterior mediastinum may be made via a median sternotomy. This latter approach may also be utilized when there are bilateral pulmonary lesions, or to perform bilateral pleural surgery.

Thoracotomy incisions, approximately 20–22 cm long, are made along the line of the fifth intercostal space, with the underlying chest muscles being incised in layers. Thoracotomy approaches may be made in several ways but commonly are either an anterolateral incision, which is situated more to the front of the chest, or a posterolateral incision, which is placed more towards the back and is seen as the gold standard for access to the thorax. The patient is positioned into the lateral decubitus position. The thoracic cavity may also be accessed via an axillary incision.

Following the incision, access to the thoracic organs is facilitated through the spreading of the ribs and entry of the pleura is accomplished. The patient is ventilated throughout the procedure with a double-lumen endotracheal tube, which enables the anaesthetist to ventilate selectively through the right or left main bronchus. While the surgery is in progress, the operated lung is deflated and the patient is ventilated entirely through the other lung. Prior to closing the chest, the affected lung is reventilated and inflated, allowing the surgeon to check the security of any suture lines and to test their ability to withstand the pressure changes occurring throughout the respiratory cycle, and one or two intercostal drains are then inserted.

The thoracotomy approach allows several surgical procedures to be performed and these are detailed below.

Pulmonary resection

Resectional surgery is performed to remove malignant or infected portions of the lung. Resectional surgery usually follows the anatomical divisions of the lungs and may involve:
- removal of a whole lung: pneumonectomy
- removal of one or two lobes of a lung: lobectomy
- removal of a segment of a lung: segmentectomy
- removal of lung tissue without reference to anatomical divisions: wedge resection (Margereson & Riley, 2003).

The extent of the resection depends upon the size, location and cell type of the tumour. A tumour which does not cross a fissure within the lung, and is located within one lobe, may be treated by lobectomy or possibly segmentectomy. Tumours which cross the fissures and affect more than one lobe will require more extensive resection. Tumours which affect the hilum of the lung may require pneumonectomy since removal of the entire tumour may not be otherwise possible.

Pulmonary function may demand a more limited resection than is desirable, in order to conserve adequate lung function following surgery. This would be particularly relevant in patients with limited lung function due to asthma or emphysema.

Resectional surgery may also be performed using bronchoplastic procedures, which aim to preserve lung tissue while removing a diseased section of the bronchus. The free ends of the bronchus are then anastomosed together. An example of this type of surgery is a sleeve resection, where an upper lobe is removed with a sleeve of main bronchus, and the remaining lower lobe is then anastomosed by its bronchus to the trachea.

Segmentectomy

Segmentectomy is indicated for patients with limited pulmonary reserve. Also known as a segmental resection, a section of a lobe of the lung is removed and involves a blunt dissection and resection of the bronchopulmonary segment. Chest drains are inserted following the procedure, to aid lung reinflation and drainage of haemoserous fluid.

Lobectomy

Lobectomy is the removal of a lobe of the lung because of benign/malignant tumours.

Pneumonectomy

Pneumonectomy is the removal of one lung because of a primary carcinoma or infection.

The pneumonectomy space

Changes occur in the pneumonectomy space following resection of the whole lung. The space is reduced, by diaphragmatic elevation, to less than that previously occupied by lung tissue. In the immediate postoperative period, the space is filled with air (during the final stages of surgery centrality of the mediastinum is ensured by regulation of the volume of gas in the space). Occasionally, patients develop dyspnoea and deteriorating oxygen saturation levels following surgery and a chest X-ray may reveal deviation of the trachea and mediastinum, usually away from the space, compromising existing lung function. Correction can be achieved through removal of a volume of air or blood from the space and a repeat chest X-ray to check tracheal alignment.

Bleeding into the space occurs within the first 36 hours following surgery, producing a visible fluid level above the diaphragm on chest X-ray. In some centres, the volume of fluid accumulating within the space may be regulated for the first 24 hours with a chest drain, which is kept clamped, but released for 1 minute every hour. This procedure allows fluid to accumulate slowly and any increase in the rate of blood loss to be observed. The volume of gas within the space gradually lessens, as firstly the carbon dioxide and then the oxygen within the air is reabsorbed. Over the ensuing days, the fluid volume is increased by an inflammatory exudate, and it gradually changes in nature from a fluid state to become a more solid substance by changes within the fibrin content. The final changes in the space occur slowly, involving the reabsorption of nitrogen and the development of a negative pressure with a slight shift in the centrality of the mediastinum. This promotes the formation and accumulation of a low-protein fluid, effectively filling the remainder of the space (Merritt et al, 2011).

The space remaining following lobectomy is much smaller. Filling of this space is achieved by elevation of the diaphragm and expansion of the remaining lobes of the lung.

Pleural surgery

Indications for pleural surgery are spontaneous and recurrent pneumothoraces.

Pleurectomy

Pleurectomy involves stripping the parietal pleura away from the apex and posterolateral surface of the lung via a small posterolateral thoracotomy incision or a less-invasive keyhole approach using video-assisted thoracoscopic surgery (VATS) (Petrella & Spaggiari, 2016). Complete pleurectomy is impossible since the parietal pleura cannot be stripped from the diaphragm. The ensuing inflammatory response, as a result of stripping of the pleura, causes adhesion of the visceral pleura (with underlying lung) to the chest wall. Where parietal pleura remains, adhesion is achieved by mechanical abrasion to produce the required inflammatory response. The surgery is completed with the insertion of chest drains.

Pleurodesis

Pleurodesis involves stimulating an inflammatory response to promote adhesion of the pleurae. This can be done either chemically, for example through the instillation of iodized talc, i.e. chemical pleurodesis, or it can be done surgically, by mechanical abrasion of the pleural surfaces with video assistance (VATS) or thoracotomy incision, i.e. surgical pleurodesis. This procedure is useful in preventing the recurrent pleural effusions associated with malignant disease, as well as recurrent pneumothorax. One or two chest drains are inserted at the close of the procedure.

Procedures involving the pleura are very painful and careful attention to pain control is required following surgery, to ensure that the patient can breathe easily. Unresolved pain will cause the patient to minimize breathing, so compromising lung expansion.

Thoracoscopy

Advances in thoracoscopic techniques have resulted in the use of telescopes and video-assisted devices that project magnified images onto video-recording monitors, enabling the surgeon to perform pulmonary and mediastinal resections, biopsies, thymectomies, and drainage of pericardial and pleural effusions. In many cases, thoracoscopic procedures have replaced the need for thoracotomy, with consequent benefits of greatly reduced incisions, i.e. two to four small puncture sites of 5−7 mm instead of a thoracotomy incision, less pain and less restricted muscle activity in the shoulder (that results from dissection through muscle in thoracotomies).

Thoracoscopic procedures still necessitate the insertion of chest drains at surgery, but these seldom remain in place for longer than 2 days.

Drainage of empyema and decortication

This technique involves the removal of the thick fibrous crust from the surface of the lung and the chest wall, via a small posterolateral thoracotomy incision, in order to allow the underlying lung to re-expand. The surgery often causes a large blood loss, which may continue following surgery. Chest drains will be inserted to monitor the severity of blood loss following the procedure.

Some patients may not tolerate decortication, so open drainage may be considered. This option necessitates a rib resection to facilitate the insertion of a large-bore chest drain. The drain is cut short and the end inserted into a stoma bag for drainage. It may be left in place for long periods of time, as necessary. This drain differs from other intercostal drains in that an underwater seal is not required. The empyema cavity is sealed by the fibrous coating with no connection to the pleural space. An open drain is therefore possible without the danger of pneumothorax.

Lung volume reduction

This procedure is performed via a median sternotomy to allow the excision of 25–30% of volume from each lung in an attempt to improve elastic recoil and reduce respiratory workload as a result of severe empyema.

Thymectomy

The thymus gland lies retrosternally within the mediastinum (see Fig. 15.4), and enlargement of the gland may cause respiratory embarrassment due to exerted pressure. Tumours of the thymus may be benign (e.g. cysts or teratomas) or malignant (e.g. carcinoma or sarcoma). The prognosis following surgical resection is directly related to the aggressiveness of the lesion and the associated systemic disorder. Pathological changes within the thymus gland are often observed in patients with myasthenia gravis, an autoimmune disorder of neuromuscular transmission characterized by weakness and fatigue of voluntary muscles. In these cases, thymectomy may influence the clinical course of the disorder. Thymectomy is usually performed via a median sternotomy and a chest drain is inserted postoperatively.

Lung transplantation

Lung transplants have been successfully completed for over two decades and account for 54% of the patients waiting for a cardiothoracic transplantation. In the UK in March 2018, there were 338 people on the active lung transplant waiting list (NHS Blood and Transplant, 2019). Initially, lung transplantation was limited to patients with pulmonary vascular disease, but it is also an option for end-stage parenchymal lung disease. Indications for this include chronic obstructive pulmonary disease, interstitial pulmonary fibrosis and cystic fibrosis (Whitson & Hayes Jr, 2014). Single lung transplantation is performed via a posterolateral thoracotomy, with the anastomosis being made at the level of the main bronchus (Gust et al, 2018). Immunosuppressive medication will need to be taken to suppress any graft rejection.

Internationally, adult lung transplant patients between 1990 and 2014 had a median survival of 5.8 years, though survival at 1 year gave a median survival of 8.0 years.

The survival rates are as follows: 3 months – 89%; 1 year – 80%; 3 years – 65%; 5 years – 54%; and, 10 years – 32% (Yusen et al, 2016).

Postoperative care

The priorities of nursing care following thoracic surgery are broadly similar, irrespective of the type of surgery that the patient has undergone, i.e. assessment and maintenance of respiratory and haemodynamic status and provision of adequate pain control. Table 15.9 illustrates the postoperative care for a patient following thoracic surgery.

Potential complications following thoracic surgery

Respiratory failure

Respiratory failure is the inability to maintain adequate gaseous exchange. Causes include surgically induced haemopneumothorax, pneumonia, atelectasis and occasionally the administration of opioids for pain relief. This will be indicated by shortness of breath, reduced respiration rate, decreased oxygen saturation levels, abnormal arterial blood gases, reduced lung expansion, respiratory sounds and cyanosis. Patient management should include upright positioning, use of prescribed oxygen therapy titrated against oxygen saturation levels and provision of reassurance.

Haemorrhage

Blood loss can become more apparent following surgery when blood pressure stabilizes and small vessels begin to bleed, having been previously prevented from doing so either by vasoconstriction or by hypotension. More serious bleeding can occur from larger vessels such as the pulmonary artery or vein, and will require further surgery to repair the defect. Management of haemorrhage includes oxygen and fluid administration and correction of any coagulation problems by either returning to theatre or drug administration, depending on the cause of bleeding.

Sputum retention

Sputum retention is the accumulation of secretions in the lower tracheobronchial tree. It can be detected as airway obstruction with hypoxia and respiratory acidosis due to retained carbon dioxide and inadequate oxygenation. The nursing management includes administration of humidified oxygen or nebulized saline and bronchodilators; bronchoscopy to remove the plug of sputum; or mini-tracheotomy to permit airway suction.

Table 15.9 Postoperative care following thoracic surgery

Nursing priorities	Rationale
Haemodynamic monitoring	
Following surgery, the patient will need to be closely observed and monitored	To observe the postoperative recovery of the patient
Assessment of temperature, pulse, blood pressure and respiratory rate are performed initially half-hourly and reduced in frequency as the patient becomes stable	To assess for any haemodynamic changes that may indicate bleeding, shock, respiratory distress or infection
A chest X-ray may be required within a few hours of surgery	To observe for centrality of the mediastinum and reinflation of the lung
Following pneumonectomy, cardiac monitoring may be required	Possibility of cardiac dysrhythmias following pneumonectomy if the pericardium has been opened
Respiratory assessment	
Careful observation of oxygen saturations is required, either by continuous monitoring or at the time of other vital signs measurement	To ensure that the patient is receiving oxygen at an adequate percentage, particularly if pneumonectomy or other resection has been performed
Some routine arterial blood gas samples may be taken in the early postoperative stages	To monitor all respiratory parameters, including PO_2 and PCO_2
Oxygen, set at the prescribed rate, and using a delivery system that humidifies and permits precise oxygen percentages, should be utilized	Humidification facilitates expectoration of sputum by maintaining the moisture within the secretions
Pain control	
Careful attention to the patient's experience of pain is required, to minimize the pain as far as possible	Patients who are in pain will be reluctant to breathe deeply and cough, increasing their risk of chest infection. They will also be reluctant to move around in bed, increasing the risk of pressure ulcers and deep vein thrombosis
Several methods of pain control are available: patient-controlled analgesia (PCA) is becoming increasingly popular following thoracic surgery, and is an effective method of pain control if the patient is adequately prepared preoperatively in its use. PCA utilizes opioid analgesics and commonly an antiemetic. Use of any opioids necessitates careful respiratory monitoring	PCA facilitates patient involvement, allowing them a degree of control over their pain. Careful preoperative teaching is required, as the patient may not wish to be bothered to learn following surgery. Opioid analgesics can cause depression of the respiratory centre
Some centres use epidural analgesia, again an effective means of pain control, but this may hinder mobility of the patient	The patient is generally on bedrest until the epidural catheter has been removed. Some urinary retention may also be observed, due to reduced sensation
Continuous intravenous infusion of opioid analgesics	An effective delivery system; controlled by the nurse
Pain control needs to be continually reviewed, particularly as intravenous forms are changed to oral preparations	Continuous assessment is necessary to ensure that the patient's pain is effectively managed
Pain levels may be significantly reduced following removal of the chest drain	The chest drain is a significant factor in the pain experienced by the patient

(Continued)

Table 15.9 Postoperative care following thoracic surgery—cont'd

Nursing priorities	Rationale
Fluid balance	
Maintenance of crystalloid fluid will be prescribed	To prevent dehydration of the patient, and to replace any small-volume blood loss
Fluid balance will need to be maintained in accordance with: • blood loss • blood pressure • urine output • central venous pressure (CVP)	Larger-volume blood loss will need to be replaced with plasma expanders or blood, to sustain blood pressure and to maintain the oxygen-carrying capacity of the blood To maintain a blood pressure that sustains systemic perfusion Low urine output may indicate a dehydrated state In the absence of urine output, a CVP measurement will indicate whether the patient is dehydrated and needs fluids, or whether the patient is volume overloaded and needs diuretics to stimulate renal function
The patient will be able to commence small volumes of fluid and progress to a light diet when able, unless any oesophageal surgery has been performed, or an anaesthetic spray applied to the throat	To encourage drinking and eating as tolerated by the patient. Oesophageal surgery will require the patient to be nil by mouth to allow anastomoses to heal. Anaesthetic throat spray can cause the patient to aspirate while swallowing
Chest drain	
Most thoracic procedures will result in one or two chest drains being inserted	Chest drains facilitate lung re-expansion by the drainage of blood and air from the pleural space
The chest drains will be connected to an underwater seal drainage unit	The underwater seal acts as a one-way valve, permitting air draining from the chest to bubble through the water, but it cannot return to the chest
A low vacuum suction may be applied	A low vacuum encourages drainage from the chest, and therefore re-expansion of the lung
Blood loss into the drainage bottle should be recorded at least hourly for the first 24–48 hours	To monitor the rate of blood loss, and to ensure large losses are replaced
Observe the drain for swinging of the fluid level within the tube	Swinging corresponds to pressure changes within the lungs during respirations but may be absent if the drain becomes blocked, or if suction is applied. The fluid will move towards the patient on inspiration and away from the patient on expiration. This movement may be masked in the presence of suction. If the patient is ventilated by positive pressure ventilation, the pattern will be reversed, i.e. moves away from the patient during inspiration
Observe the drain for bubbling	Bubbling corresponds to the drainage of air from the chest during expiration and coughing. It signifies a patent drain. Bubbling may be vigorous, particularly if suction is applied, and may be continuous with suction. In the absence of suction, bubbling will be associated with expiratory activity and coughing. Both bubbling and swinging may diminish as the lung becomes fully inflated

(Continued)

Table 15.9 Postoperative care following thoracic surgery—cont'd

Nursing priorities	Rationale
Ensure that the chest drain bottle remains lower than chest level	Facilitates drainage of fluid from the chest. Prevents siphoning of fluid back into the pleural space
See text for differences in the care of pneumonectomy drains	
Chest physiotherapy	
The aim of physiotherapy is to promote deep breathing, coughing and mobility	This will help to facilitate re-expansion of the lung
Initially, the patient is encouraged to sit upright	To facilitate optimum lung expansion
The physiotherapist, who was involved preoperatively, sees the patient soon after surgery	To encourage the patient to take deep breaths and cough, to ensure the operated lung is quickly restored to full expansion and to remove any retained secretions. This will also help to prevent a chest infection
Between the physiotherapist's visits the nursing staff will continue to encourage deep breaths and coughs	
As the postoperative course progresses, the physiotherapist will be involved in helping the patient to mobilize	Mobility, as exercise, is an effective means of encouraging good lung expansion
Mobility	
Pressure area relief must be provided while the patient is in bed	Thoracic patients tend to predominantly sit upright, causing a lot of pressure on the skin of their sacrum
The patient is encouraged to sit out of bed on day 1 following surgery	Early mobilization is encouraged to prevent complications of bedrest
Progressive mobilization is encouraged on the following days, particularly once the chest drains are removed. The patient is encouraged to begin mobilizing to the bathroom initially, and then to go for longer walks. The patient will be observed climbing a flight of stairs prior to discharge	Increased mobility promotes lung expansion and improves exercise tolerance
Mobility of the affected shoulder is encouraged through exercises provided by the physiotherapist	To restore normal range of movement and to prevent a frozen shoulder
Wound care	
Theatre dressings are observed regularly in the early postoperative phase	To observe for bleeding from the incision
Theatre dressings are left intact for 48 hours (or according to unit protocol)	To prevent wound infection
Wound observation and care according to unit protocol	The wound should be regularly observed for signs of exudate or infection
Removal of staples/sutures according to protocol	The staples/sutures are commonly removed prior to discharge, or arrangements made with the community team to remove them following discharge

Chest infections

Chest infections can occur in patients who are unable to mobilize effectively or cannot tolerate physiotherapy due to poor pain tolerance. They are more common if the patient was a smoker prior to surgery. Effective pain relief to permit mobilization and breathing exercises is vital to prevent this occurring.

Cardiac arrhythmias

Atrial fibrillation (AF) remains the most common medical complication after thoracic surgery, with an incidence ranging from 10% to 20% after pulmonary lobectomy, and as much as 40% after pneumonectomy (Onaitis et al, 2010, cited by Andrea et al, 2012). The use of oral or intravenous antiarrhythmic medication may be considered should the patient become compromised.

Bronchopleural fistula

A bronchopleural fistula is a communication between the airways and the pleura following surgery and may be due to problems at the time of surgery involving disease of the bronchial stump, or stump breakdown at a later stage due to lack of healing or infection. It can occur following lobectomy, but is more common following pneumonectomy. The symptoms include the expectoration of pneumonectomy space fluid and the potential for contamination of the remaining lung with infected fluid. Small fistulae may heal spontaneously but may require the insertion of a chest drain to prevent movement of fluid into the airways. Surgery to the bronchial stump may include excision of infected or necrotic tissue and repair with pericardial or intercostal tissue.

Surgical emphysema

Surgical emphysema may be a consequence of a bronchopleural fistula, but not exclusively so; it can also accompany a pneumothorax. Surgical emphysema indicates the presence of air in the subcutaneous tissues, particularly in the neck, chest wall and head. If the air leak in the chest is extensive, the surgical emphysema can be very debilitating, including complete closure of the eyelids through swelling, with consequent temporary blindness for the patient and requirements for skilled nursing care. The subcutaneous air usually reabsorbs spontaneously when effective chest drainage is established.

Nursing management of intercostal chest drains

Intercostal (chest) drainage is required following surgery, to facilitate the drainage of air and blood from the chest and to allow the lung to re-expand fully. Some nursing observations of the drain are noted in Table 15.9.

Chest drains are attached to a sterile water chamber, providing a one-way valve. This allows air removal in expiration (column of water falls or bubbling may occur) and prevention of air re-entry on inspiration (column of water rises) (Fig. 15.5). External suction can be added to the system to provide a greater negative pressure draw to assist in the expansion of the lung.

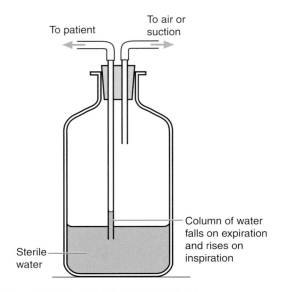

Figure 15.5 Intercostal chest drainage bottle.

To patient
To air or suction
Column of water falls on expiration and rises on inspiration
Sterile water

Clamping of the drains should be avoided because air will build up within the thoracic cavity, creating an increase in positive pressure and thus increasing the potential for a tension pneumothorax. The stripping or milking of drains is an extremely controversial issue and is strongly discouraged because of the associated increase in intrathoracic pressure and risk of pneumothorax.

Patients whose drains become disconnected are best treated by swift reconnection of the tubing, and, secondly, coughing to dispel any air. A subsequent chest X-ray to assess for a change in condition should be undertaken.

Removal of the chest drain should only be considered when the lung has reinflated or the drainage has stopped. A modified Valsalva manoeuvre is employed while the drain is being withdrawn, i.e. the patient takes a full inspiration and holds their breath in order to diminish the risk of air entry into the pleura. Analgesics will be required prior to removal of the drain. The purse-string suture ensures skin closure as the drain is removed. The suture is removed approximately 2–5 days later, or according to unit protocol. A small dressing is usually sufficient to absorb any local blood loss and can be removed the following day. Any obvious air leaks should be referred immediately to the medical team. Application of paraffin gauze (thought to prevent air leaks through the skin) is unnecessary. Originally, routine chest X-rays are advised following drain removal, however recent studies have shown that omission of this in patients following cardiothoracic surgery is safe and should only be performed when clinically indicated (Sepehripour et al, 2012).

Specific health education/patient teaching and preparation for discharge

Many people who have undergone pulmonary resection for lung cancer regard the surgery as curative and expect a fairly rapid return to good health. Those who have had a pneumonectomy may find that initially they are quite short of breath due to reduced lung capacity, and, if unprepared for this fact, may become quite disheartened. Careful preparation of each patient for discharge should include realistic expectations of exercise tolerance and how this may be improved. The physiotherapist will be closely involved in this aspect of discharge.

Patients preparing for discharge will require advice on a number of issues, including pain control, wound care, resumption of sexual activity, diet and sports. The advice will need to be tailored according to the patient's age, surgery and pre-surgery fitness, as well as being specific to the individual unit policies.

The majority of patients will not return to work until they have been seen by the surgeon, i.e. 6–8 weeks postoperatively. Similarly, patients will be advised not to drive until after the appointment, and they need to inform their insurance company of their surgery.

Advice about smoking cessation may also be pertinent. Specific advice may be sought by some patients concerning permission to fly, and individual airlines will be able to give advice. It is difficult to be prescriptive concerning health education since each patient has differing needs and levels of understanding, but attempts should be made to offer individualistic health education as appropriate.

Conclusion

Thoracic surgery is a rapidly expanding specialty, challenging the nurse working within this field. It is therefore essential that nurses should fully understand the anatomy and physiology of the respiratory system and associated surgical procedures.

SUMMARY OF KEY POINTS

- Knowledge of the normal physiology of the lungs is essential to an understanding of the altered physiology consequent to disease or surgery.
- Breathing is normally an automatic, rhythmic process that continues without conscious effort. Respiratory disease or thoracic surgery can disrupt this process to one of painful effort.
- Respiratory assessment is fundamental to the nursing care of respiratory patients undergoing surgery.
- Knowledge of the disease processes that alter respiratory anatomy and function will be important in assessing the resultant symptoms affecting the patient.
- Understanding of the investigative procedures that precede thoracic surgery is vital in order to prepare patients physically and psychologically. Sensory and procedural information are both important.
- The role of the nurse in the preoperative phase is essential in recording a comprehensive nursing assessment, taking account of personal, social, medical, psychological, spiritual and cultural needs.
- Thoracic surgical procedures are very painful and require skilled nursing care to alleviate pain and maintain optimum respiratory effort.
- Knowledge of postoperative nursing care and potential complications are vital to the safe recovery of the patient.
- Specific health education and health promotion opportunities should be actively sought in order to ensure that the patient is fully informed to their satisfaction throughout the perioperative period.

REFLECTIVE LEARNING POINTS

Having read this chapter, think about what you now know & what you still need to find out about. These questions may help:

- How is oximetry performed?
- Describe the TNM staging system in relation to lung cancer.
- How can the nurse assist the patient who is experiencing dyspnoea?

References

British Lung Foundation. (2016). The battle for breath – the impact of lung disease in the UK. Available at: <www.blf.org.uk/policy/the-battle-for-breath-2016>

British Thoracic Society. (2017). *Literature review: the economic costs of lung disease and the effectiveness of policy and service interventions.* London: British Thoracic Society.

Cancer Research UK. (2015). *Lung cancer mortality statistics.* [Online] Available at: <www.cancerresearchuk.org/health-professional/cancer-statistics/statistics-by-cancer-type/lung-cancer/mortality#-heading-Zero>

Crompton, G. (1987). *Diagnosis and management of respiratory diseases* (2nd ed.). London: Blackwell Scientific.

Foss, M. (1989). *Thoracic surgery*. London: Austen Cornish.

Gust, L., D'Journo, X.-B., Briodue, G., et al. (2018). Single-lung and double-lung transplantation: technique and tips. *Journal of Thoracic Disease, 10*(4), 2508–2518.

Hatchett, R., & Thompson, T. (2008). *Cardiac nursing – a comprehensive guide* (2nd ed.). London: Churchill Livingstone.

Jubran, A. (2015). Pulse oximetry. *Critical Care, 16*(19), 272.

Kumar, P., & Clark, M. (2005). *Clinical medicine* (6th ed.). London: W.B. Saunders.

Lim, W., Ridge, C. A., Nicholson, A. G., & Mirsadraee, S. (2018). The 8th lung cancer TNM classification and clinical staging system: review of the changes and clinical implications. *Quantitative Imaging in Medicine and Surgery, 8*(7), 709–718.

Livingstone, J. I., Harvey, M., Kitchen, N., et al. (1993). Role of pre-admission clinic in a general surgical unit: a six month audit. *Annals of the Royal College of Surgeons of England, 75*(3), 211–212.

Margereson, C., & Riley, J. (2003). *Cardiothoracic surgical nursing. Current trends in adult care*. London: Blackwell Science.

Merritt, R. E., Reznik, S. I., DaSilva, M. C., Sugarbaker, D. J., Whyte, R. I., Donahue, D. M., et al. (2011). Benign emptying of the postpneumonectomy space. *The Annals of Thoracic Surgery, 92*, 1076–1081.

NHS Blood and Transplant. (2019). *Organ donation and transplantation – activity figures or the UK as at April 2019*. Available at: nhsbtdbe.blob.core.windows.net/umbraco-assets-corp/15720/annual_stats.pdf

NHS England. (2014). *Overview of potential to reduce lives lost from Chronic Obstructive Pulmonary Disease (COPD)*. Available at: <www.england.nhs.uk/wp-content/uploads/2014/02/rm-fs-6.pdf>

National Institute for Health and Care Excellence (NICE). (2019). *Chronic obstructive pulmonary disease*. Available at: cks.nice.org.uk/chronic-obstructive-pulmonary-disease#!topicSummary

Nursing and Midwifery Council. (2018). *The code. Professional standards of practice and behaviour for nurses, midwives and nursing associates*. Available at: <www.nmc.org.uk/standards/code/>

Onaitis, M., D'Amico, T., Zhao, Y., O'Brien, S., & Harpole, D. (2010). Risk factors for atrial fibrillation after lung cancer surgery: analysis of the Society of Thoracic Surgeons general thoracic surgery database. *The Annals of Thoracic Surgery, 90*, 368–374.

Petrella, F., & Spaggiari, L. (2016). The smaller the better: a new concept in thoracic surgery? *The Lancet Oncology, 17*(6), 699–700.

Sepehripour, A. H., Farid, S., & Shah, R. (2012). Is routine chest radiography indicated following chest drain removal after cardiothoracic surgery? *Interactive Cardiovascular and Thoracic Surgery, 14*(6), 834–838.

Stradling, P. (1991). *Diagnostic bronchoscopy: a teaching manual*. Edinburgh: Churchill Livingstone.

Tobias, J. S., & Hochhauser, D. (2014). *Cancer and its management*. New Jersey: John Wiley & Sons.

Travis, W. D., Brambilla, E., Nicholson, A. G., et al. (2015). The 2015 World Health Organization Classification of Lung Tumors: Impact of Genetic, Clinical and Radiologic Advances Since the 2004 Classification. *Journal of Thoracic Oncology, 10*(9), 1243–1260.

Vachani, A., Haas, A. R., & Sterman, D. H. (2012). Bronchoscopy. In S. G. Spiro, G. A. Silvestri, & A. Agustí (Eds.), *Clinical Respiratory Medicine* (pp. 154–173). Philadelphia: Saunders.

Whitson, B. A., & Hayes, D., Jr (2014). Indications and outcomes in adult lung transplantation. *Journal of Thoracic Disease, 6*(8), 1018–1023.

Yusen, R. D., Edwards, L. B., Dipchand, A. I., et al. (2016). The Registry of the International Society for Heart and Lung Transplantation: Thirty-third Adult Lung and Heart–Lung Transplant Report—2016; Focus Theme: Primary Diagnostic Indications for Transplant. *The Journal of Heart and Lung Transplantation, 35*(10), 1170–1184.

Further reading

Finkelmeier, B. A. (2000). *Cardiothoracic surgical nursing* (2nd ed.). Philadelphia: Lippincott.

Scanlon, C., Spearman, C., & Sheldon, R. (1995). *Egan's fundamental principles of respiratory care* (6th ed.). London: Mosby.

West, J. (1990). *Respiratory physiology – The essentials* (5th ed.). London: Williams & Wilkins.

Wilkins, R., Krider, S., & Sheldon, R. (1995). *Clinical assessment in respiratory care* (3rd edn). London: Mosby.

Relevant website

The European Society for Cardiovascular Surgery: escvs.com

Chapter 16

Patients requiring upper gastrointestinal surgery

Jay Macleod (with a contribution by Nuala Davison)

KEY OBJECTIVES OF THE CHAPTER

At the end of the chapter the reader should be able to:
- describe the essential anatomy and physiology of the upper gastrointestinal system
- briefly explain specific investigations
- briefly explain causes, conditions and surgical interventions
- give examples of assessment procedures for patients undergoing upper gastrointestinal surgery
- highlight specific pre- and postoperative management
- give a case study example and evidence-based care planning
- assist in the education and discharge planning of patients.

Areas to think about before reading the chapter

- What is the key purpose of preoperative fasting?
- Provide an overview of policy and practice in the place where you work regarding preoperative fasting.

(Continued)

(cont'd)

- Describe the procedure for the insertion of a nasogastric tube in the conscious patient.

Introduction

This chapter will provide information for nurses who are caring for patients on a surgical ward that specializes in upper gastrointestinal surgery. It will focus on surgical interventions that are carried out when all other methods of treatment have been ineffective, or are indeed inappropriate. This chapter will also include endoscopic practice, and both diagnostic and therapeutic procedures will be outlined.

It must also be remembered that there are many different techniques and practices in the field of gastroenterology. Therefore, surgical procedures may have slightly different names, according to their origin. It is important to use this book in conjunction with current evidence-based practice and research.

Each organ will be addressed in distinct sections of this chapter, and the associated anatomy and physiology will be discussed, followed by details of specific nursing assessment. However, the specific investigations will be addressed together at the beginning of the chapter in order to avoid repetition.

Nursing assessment refers to the collecting of data, reviewing or analysing the data, and identifying problems and making a nursing diagnosis. It is essential that a comprehensive history is taken from the patient or their family to serve as a baseline for assessment. Assessment can be completed through interviewing, i.e. asking questions related to the patient's condition, observation for any non-verbal indications of discomfort or distress, and measuring through use of tools of assessment, e.g. pain assessment chart. It is a continuous process and needs to be frequently reviewed. For the purpose of this chapter the framework is based on the Roper, Logan and Tierney model of nursing, as described in Williams (2015), as this remains best practice in the ward environment. The generalized pre- and postoperative management remains the same as for any patient undergoing upper abdominal surgery, and only specific problems will be highlighted following the discussion of the disease or organ dysfunction.

Overview of the anatomy and physiology of the digestive system

The digestive system refers to the organs, structures and complementary glands of the digestive canal that together are involved in the breaking down of food constituents into smaller components for absorption and final utilization by the cells. The digestive system, therefore, consists of the gastrointestinal tract, which is a continuous musculomembranous tube lined with mucous membrane, which is approximately 9 m long. This tube extends continuously through the body cavity from the mouth to the anus, and includes the mouth, pharynx, oesophagus, stomach, small intestine, large intestine, rectum and anus.

There are four basic activities that take place in the digestive system:
- ingestion – taking the food into the body (eating)
- peristalsis – movement of the food along the gastrointestinal tract
- absorption of nutrients into the cells for use
- defecation – the elimination of waste products.

Two methods of digestion are employed: chemical and mechanical digestion. Chemical digestion is where large carbohydrates, proteins and lipid substances are broken down by chemical reactions. Ancillary organs which produce and store digestive enzymes are involved in this process. These include the salivary glands, liver, gall bladder and pancreas, and are external to the digestive tract. Mechanical digestion is where the food is physically moved, e.g. chewing, and mixing or churning the contents in the stomach with the digestive enzymes.

Investigations

There are many investigative procedures that a patient may undergo in order to diagnose the disorder and enable the surgical team to plan the relevant course of action or surgical intervention (Table 16.1). It is often a process of elimination by considering differential diagnoses.

Table 16.1 Investigations of the gastrointestinal or biliary tract undertaken prior to surgical intervention

Investigation	Surgery
Abdominal X-rays	GI tract/biliary tract
Fluoroscope	GI tract/biliary tract
CT scan	GI tract/biliary tract
Barium meal	Upper GI tract
Barium swallow	Upper GI tract
Cholecystogram	Biliary tract
Cholangiogram	Biliary tract
Cholangiography	Biliary tract
Oesophagogastroduodenoscopy (OGD)	Upper GI tract
Endoscopic retrograde cholangiopancreatography (ERCP)	Biliary tract
Percutaneous transhepatic cholangiography (PTC)	Biliary tract
Ultrasound	GI tract/biliary tract
Endoscopic ultrasound	Upper GI tract

The patient requires a full explanation of the proposed investigation, in order to make an informed decision about whether to go ahead with the test or not. Patients will be required to give verbal and, often, written consent. Informed consent will involve a discussion with the patient, outlining what the test will look at specifically, the risks involved, and the potential outcomes of the test and, indeed, not having the test at all. The Nursing and Midwifery Council (NMC) (2018) and Department of Health (DoH) (2009) explain the issues with regards to consent. The most common investigations are briefly described in Table 16.1.

Abdominal X-rays

Under normal circumstances, dense material may be penetrated by X-rays, which give an outline of the organs under investigation. When investigating the soft tissue and organs of the abdominal cavity, it is often necessary to use a contrast medium such as barium sulphate to highlight the spaces and cavities in the gastrointestinal tract. X-rays use ionizing radiation and therefore carry a degree of risk, particularly during rapid cell division.

Nursing issues

The most at-risk patients are female patients of reproductive capacity, as there is an increased possibility of affecting a fetus through pelvic X-rays. Consequently, any abdominal radiography should be carefully monitored and only carried out if absolutely essential. A 28-day rule applies to all radiological examinations for female patients of reproductive age if there is any chance that they could be pregnant and their period is overdue (RCR, 2013). The older 10-day rule can still apply, requiring the examination to be carried out within 10 days following the first day of the last menstrual period, for high-dose examinations. There may be some exceptions to this rule for those women who have undergone tubal ligation, are not menstruating or are not sexually active. Abdominal X-rays are useful in detecting gallstones (approximately 10% of gallstones are radio-opaque) and abdominal fluid levels.

CAT (computerized axial tomography) scan/ CT scan

This provides a computerized picture of a part of the body, which is achieved by combining fine X-rays, often with a contrast medium. 'Slices' of the abdomen are produced and are useful for detecting irregular anatomy, including tumours.

Barium studies

A radio-opaque contrast medium called barium sulphate is used for radiological studies of the gastrointestinal tract. It is a fine, milky contrast medium that is taken orally, to allow detection of small alterations in the stomach.

Barium swallow and barium meal

This test is usually undertaken to highlight the oesophagus, stomach and upper intestinal tract, therefore assisting in detecting any exacerbation of oesophagitis, dysphagia, gastric or duodenal ulcers, or the presence of abnormalities such as hiatus hernia, strictures, obstruction or fistulae.

Nursing issues

It is advisable for the patient not to have anything to eat or drink for a period of 6–8 hours prior to the investigation, as the examination is more successful if the stomach is empty.

Cholecystogram

A cholecystogram is an X-ray showing the gall bladder following the introduction of a radio-opaque contrast medium containing iodine. This may be introduced by ingestion or injection, and the technique is usually undertaken to detect gallstones or biliary obstruction, or to assess the ability of the gall bladder to fill and empty. Alternative investigative methods, such as ultrasonography and computed tomography (CT) scans, are now widely used instead.

Cholangiogram or cholangiography

The radio-opaque contrast medium is injected directly into the biliary tract or intravenously. The procedure is carried out during biliary surgery to detect any abnormalities or blockages, as it allows the bile ducts to be viewed on X-ray film. A cholangiogram can also be performed postoperatively in order to check the patency of the common bile duct following exploratory surgery and removal of any residual gallstones (sometimes the common bile duct can become oedematous and inflamed). The contrast medium is introduced through the indwelling T-tube inserted during the surgical procedure.

Nursing issues

The postoperative cholangiogram should be carried out and results reviewed by the surgical team prior to the removal of the T-tube. The nursing role will be discussed later in this chapter.

Endoscopy

The cavities or interior of the gastrointestinal tract can be investigated through the use of an endoscope, which is a luminous fibreoptic instrument that can be inserted through a natural orifice for viewing cavities and internal organs, then relaying them to a television screen. The fibreoptic endoscope is often used to reach areas previously inaccessible with other instruments, as it has greater flexibility. Instruments can also be passed through the special tube of the endoscope to obtain biopsies or perform other procedures such as polypectomy.

Oesophagogastroduodenoscopy

For examination of the upper gastrointestinal tract, it is necessary to wait for the stomach to be empty, for visualization and prevention of aspiration. Oesophagogastroduodenoscopy (OGD) is usually performed to detect and diagnose ulcers and tumours. It is also used to establish the cause of upper gastrointestinal bleeding and to obtain biopsy samples.

Nursing issues
It is necessary for the patient to have nothing orally for approximately 6 hours prior to these procedures, in order to ensure that the stomach is empty. During the procedure, an anaesthetic spray is often used to anaesthetize the throat. Therefore, following the procedure, it is usual to wait for throat sensation to return to normal prior to drinking. This takes approximately 1 hour, after which the patient may eat or drink normally. Sometimes, fluids are withheld following an oesophageal dilatation until X-rays have been taken, in order to rule out any damage or trauma caused by the procedure.

Endoscopic retrograde cholangiopancreatography

Endoscopic retrograde cholangiopancreatography (ERCP) views the biliary tree endoscopically. It can be purely diagnostic or also used for therapeutic purposes. The endoscope with a fine catheter is passed via the oesophagus, stomach and duodenum to the duodenal papilla. There, the pancreatic and common bile ducts are injected with the contrast medium introduced through the ampulla of Vater. Any irregularities will be viewed on the screen, and biopsies and cytology specimens may be taken. The investigation is usually performed to aid diagnosis of obstructive jaundice, chronic pancreatitis or pancreatic carcinoma, or biliary colic, and can also facilitate the removal of gallstones.

Nursing issues
The patient should be nil by mouth for at least 6 hours prior to the procedure. An anaesthetic throat spray may be used, as may sedation. Following the procedure, the effects of the anaesthetics may last for up to an hour, leaving the patient unable to eat or drink during that time. Observations should include blood pressure and pulse for indications of bleeding or perforation. This procedure may be contraindicated in patients with cardiac and respiratory disorders (Eykyn, 2014).

Percutaneous transhepatic cholangiography

In percutaneous transhepatic cholangiography (PTC), heavily concentrated contrast medium dye is injected straight into the biliary tree, enabling all parts of the biliary system to be viewed. This is done through a needle and catheter introduced transcutaneously under ultrasound guidance. It is particularly useful for investigating persistent symptoms related to the biliary system of those patients who have already undergone a cholecystectomy or gastrectomy and cannot have an ERCP.

Nursing issues
As in ERCP.

Ultrasound

High-frequency sound waves are transmitted by the ultrasound probe and echoes are received from various organs, outlining them. It is safe, as it is non-invasive and does not use ionizing radiation. It is used in gastroenterology to investigate and detect abnormalities of the biliary system, pancreas, liver and spleen.

Nursing issues
If the ultrasound is carried out for investigation of the gall bladder or pancreas, it may be necessary for the patient to stop eating for up to 8 hours and drink clear fluids only prior to the procedure in order that there is no food or fluid covering the area to be examined. It will also ensure that the gall bladder will be fully enlarged due to the retention of bile.

Upper gastrointestinal disorders

Mouth

Anatomy and physiology

This chapter will not discuss disorders of the mouth but will highlight the importance of a healthy mouth in the role of digestion. The mouth contains structures that are involved in the preparation of food for passage through the gastrointestinal tract. These structures are the tongue, teeth, hard and soft palates, and salivary glands. The act of biting and chewing requires the ability of the extrinsic muscles of the tongue to move the food from side to side, and the intrinsic muscles of the tongue to alter the shape of the food for swallowing. This act of chewing is also variable according to the dental pattern and shape of the mouth of the individual and the type of food ingested.

The formation and assisted passage of the bolus requires the secretion of saliva from the parotid, submandibular and sublingual salivary glands, which secrete mucus and amylase. The flow of saliva is dependent on the stimulus initiated from taste and pressure in the mouth. Saliva is also responsible for keeping the mouth clean and removing food particles through keeping it moistened (Tortora & Derrikson, 2014).

It is therefore important that individuals have moistened, clean mouths and regular dental check-ups to assist and facilitate the function of chewing, forming and swallowing the bolus of food.

Oesophagus

Anatomy and physiology

The oesophagus, sometimes called the gullet, is approximately 24 cm long, and is a muscular canal which is collapsible. It runs from the base of the pharynx, behind the trachea, through the opening between the thoracic cavity and abdominal cavity, terminating at the lower oesophageal sphincter of the stomach. It comprises four layers:

- The tunica adventitia (outer layer).
- The muscularis – longitudinal and circular muscles that aid propulsion of food via the action of peristalsis. These muscles graduate from voluntary or striated muscles at the upper, pharyngo-oesophageal sphincter to involuntary or smooth muscles at the cardiac sphincter.
- The submucosal layer, containing blood vessels and tissue.
- The mucosal layer, which aids passage of the food bolus along the oesophagus through the secretion of mucus from special glands.

The function of the oesophagus is to transport the food bolus along the canal by the involuntary action of peristalsis (contractions and waves). The whole process takes 1–8 seconds, depending on the consistency of the food bolus. The pharyngo-oesophageal and gastro-oesophageal sphincters control the flow of the bolus by relaxing, so as to allow the passage of the food through, and contracting, to prevent backflow of contents.

Oesophageal dysfunction

Dysfunction refers to any condition that disrupts or affects the normal function of the oesophagus, resulting in uncomfortable symptoms. Symptoms may include acute pain (odynophagia) and difficulty in swallowing (dysphagia), obstruction of food, and feeling the passage of liquids when swallowing, and often the patient will be able to point to the locality of the problem. Some of the conditions, causes and interventions are shown in Table 16.2 and are described below.

Oesophageal diverticulum

Oesophageal diverticulum refers to a weakness in the muscle wall of the oesophagus where a pouch of mucosa and submucosa can slip through, causing a protrusion. Diagnosis is through barium swallow and X-rays.

Table 16.2 Oesophageal dysfunction – causes and surgical interventions

Cause	Intervention
Oesophageal diverticulum	Oesophagomyotomy
Oesophageal trauma/perforation	Gastroscopy/ oesophagogastroduodenoscopy/ reconstructive surgery
Oesophageal achalasia	Oesophagomyotomy or dilatation
Oesophageal stricture	Dilatation, insertion of a stent
Oesophagitis	Dilatation, oesophagogastrostomy, fundoplication, vagotomy and pyloroplasty
Oesophageal cancer	Oesophagectomy, insertion of a stent

Gastroscopy or passing of a nasogastric tube is not undertaken, as there is an increased risk of perforation.

Intervention. Intervention is by removal of the pouch surgically. Because of its position, care must be taken to avoid damaging the adjacent vessels, and often a myotomy (a cut in the muscle) is performed to reduce the risk of spasticity to the muscle.

Oesophageal trauma and/or perforation

External trauma can be caused by stab, bullet or crush wounds. Internal trauma can be caused by swallowing foreign bodies, puncture from sharp objects or following an investigative procedure. Examples of these are metallic objects, dentures, fish bones and medical instruments. Other trauma effects can be through the ingestion of poisonous substances, or continuous unrelieved strain caused by vomiting, resulting in mucosal trauma (Mallory–Weiss tear) or full-thickness rupture of the oesophagus.

Intervention. Oesophagoscopy is commonly undertaken with removal of the foreign body or dilatation. In severely traumatized cases, a gastrostomy is created for the insertion of a feeding tube to allow the traumatized area of the oesophagus and oedema to subside. Antibiotics may be prescribed following a perforated oesophagus, as there is an increased risk of infection.

Oesophageal achalasia

Oesophageal achalasia is a neuromuscular change that causes benign spasm of the lower oesophageal sphincter, sometimes with marked dilatation of the oesophagus. The lower oesophageal sphincter fails to respond and relax in order to facilitate swallowing. This results in the patient feeling that food is stuck in the gullet. Food is often regurgitated, and oesophageal distension occurs. There is a danger of spillover of food from the oesophagus into the trachea, causing respiratory aspiration. Diagnosis is through OGD and barium swallow.

Intervention. The aim would be to dilate the lower oesophageal sphincter using a balloon under pressure, inserted under X-ray or endoscopic guidance. There is a risk of perforation in a small percentage of the procedures. A surgical oesophagomyotomy, i.e. division of the muscle wall, may be performed if dilatation fails.

Oesophageal varices

Oesophageal varices are enlarged, swollen, engorged vessels at the base of the oesophagus that are at risk of rupturing, causing a torrential haemorrhage, which can be life-threatening.

Intervention. The aim of treatment is to stop the haemorrhage. This is done endoscopically by injecting the varices with adrenaline (epinephrine), or by placing a band around the bleeding vessel. In an emergency situation a Sengstaken–Blakemore tube is inserted to block the gastro-oesophageal junction to stop bleeding.

Oesophageal stricture

Oesophageal stricture may be caused by intensive and prolonged radiotherapy; through external pressure on the oesophagus by an enlarged adjacent organ or tumour; cancer of the oesophagus; or ingestion of caustic substances. The commonest cause of oesophageal stricture, however, is an inflammatory stricture caused by acid reflux (see below). Diagnosis involves a specific comprehensive history of any recent changes in swallowing, and investigations include endoscopy and biopsy.

Intervention. Intervention is by treatment of the underlying cause and may include dilatation of the lumen of the oesophagus and possibly the insertion of a stent.

Oesophagitis

The mucosal lining of the oesophagus becomes inflamed following an acute or chronic episode of infection, e.g. fungal; irritation, which includes malignancy, chemical ingestion or prolonged use of a nasogastric tube; complications following gastric/duodenal surgery; or trauma, caused by repeated vomiting, reflux, bending, coughing, stooping or straining. Investigations include a specific history, oesophagoscopy and/or biopsy (Kumar et al, 2014).

Intervention. Intervention is by treatment of the underlying cause and may involve medical treatment or dilatation, oesophagogastrostomy, fundoplication, vagotomy and pyloroplasty.

Oesophageal cancer

This is the 14th most common type of cancer in the UK, with around 9100 new cases each year. Approximately 5%

of the total cancer deaths in the UK are caused by oesophageal cancer (Cancer Research UK, 2016a). Incidence of oesophageal cancer is more common in people over the age of 85, and is more common in men than in women. The 5-year survival rate is 15% and 10-year survival rate is 12%.

There are two main types of oesophageal carcinoma.

- *Squamous cell carcinoma* accounts for half of the diagnosed cases, and develops in the squamous cells which form the lining of the oesophagus.
- *Adenocarcinoma* begins in the gland cells that make the mucus in the lining of the oesophagus, and is usually found in the lower third of the oesophagus. It may infiltrate adjacent structures up and down the oesophagus, is insidious in its onset and does not cause symptoms in the early stages. Symptoms may include involvement of the vocal cords, i.e. hoarseness, dysphagia leading to total blockage in some cases, anorexia with weight loss, pain, regurgitation of undigested food, persistent cough or clearing of the throat, halitosis or foul-smelling breath and haemoptysis. The tumour may eventually invade other adjacent structures, such as the bronchi, trachea, pericardium and great blood vessels, with metastases in the lymph nodes and liver. Around 1–5% of patients with Barrett's oesophagus, a condition where the lower oesophagus has ulcerative benign lesions in the columnar epithelium, will develop this type of cancer (Cancer Research UK, 2016a). It is therefore important that the individual undergoes regular gastroscopy surveillance.

Oesphageal carcinomas are thought to be associated with obesity, an increased consumption of alcohol (drinking more than 14 units per week), smoking or using tobacco, and rare medical conditions such as achalasia (Cancer Research UK, 2016a).

Investigations. Investigations include a specific history as outlined in assessment, barium swallow, OGD, biopsy, endoscopic ultrasound and CAT scan. A bronchoscopy may also be performed to rule out any tracheal involvement.

Endoscopic ultrasound. Endoscopic ultrasound (EUS) has revolutionized the staging of oesophageal cancers. The patient undergoes a gastroscopy, but a fibreoptic tube is inserted that uses sound waves, instead of the camera, to size the tumour, establish its relation to adjacent structures and assess the lymph nodes.

Intervention. Surgical intervention is undertaken if the tumour is considered curative, i.e. partial or total oesophagectomy, or palliative intervention may include the insertion of a self-expanding metallic stent. Treatment may also involve chemotherapy, or laser treatment (photodynamic therapy or PDT). Radiotherapy may be effective with an early-stage carcinoma, or as a palliative measure in the advanced stages. If the patient is severely dysphagic, a feeding jejunostomy may be created to meet nutritional needs.

Insertion of a stent. When the carcinoma is severely advanced or involves adjacent organs and tissues, palliative intervention may be the option of choice. An expanding stent is passed to ensure that the oesophagus remains patent (Fig. 16.1).

Surgical intervention. Surgical intervention is by an oesophagectomy, where part or all of the oesophagus is removed. The surgical approach may be through the thorax and abdomen, abdomen alone or thorax alone, leaving the stomach positioned in the thoracic cavity. Radiotherapy and chemotherapy can also be used in conjunction with an oesophagectomy, either prior to or following surgical intervention.

Oesophageal surgery – specific preoperative assessment

Eating and drinking is clearly one of the problems for a patient undergoing an oesophagectomy and should be discussed in detail as part of the specific preoperative assessment. Questions should be asked and documented in relation to the specific history to identify changes in appetite, increasing dysphagia, substernal pain, regurgitation, vomiting, severe weight loss, increased anxiety, metastatic gland enlargement in the neck, haematemesis and, finally, melaena or anaemia. Examples of questions are: 'How long have you had difficulty in swallowing?' 'Does it affect all foods or just fluids?' 'Do you regurgitate the food?' 'How

long does it take you to swallow the food?' 'Where does the food stick?' 'Does it cause pain?' 'If so, whereabouts?' 'Is it getting worse or better?' As a result of the appropriate questions being asked, specific problems are identified, as shown in Box 16.1.

Specific postoperative nursing interventions

Maintaining a safe environment

Immediate assessment is made of the patient following the A, B, C, D and E structure in order to prevent further

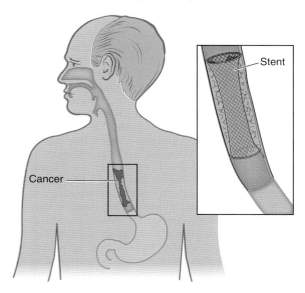

Figure 16.1 Oesophageal stent.

> **Box 16.1 Specific issues related to eating and drinking**
>
> - Nutritional deficit – due to alteration in appetite as a result of nausea, anorexia, regurgitation, dysphagia or pain on ingesting food.
> - Increased weight loss – following alteration in appetite/pathology.
> - Potential risk of malnutrition – following decrease in nutritional status/pathology.
>
> *Specific objective* will be to ensure that adequate nutritional levels are maintained and that the patient is well nourished prior to surgical intervention. Any associated pain and discomfort is relieved or removed.
>
> **Nursing intervention and rationale**
>
> - Assess the ability of the patient to retain food and fluids. Document food, calorie and fluid intake on the appropriate charts along with weight charts. This will help to monitor nutritional intake and any weight fluctuation, and identify need for further intervention.
> - Facilitate passage of food by offering drinks along with food intake; sometimes, soda water will help to clear the blockage and dislodge any food that is trapped. Small, frequent, light meals should be offered that are easy to swallow. All meals should be offered in a conducive environment.
> - It may be necessary to give liquidized nutritional intake with vitamin supplements and high-protein fluid drinks, or totally replace enteral nutritional intake with parenteral feeding in order to provide the nutritional requirements.
> - It is advisable to involve the dietitian and/or the nutritional specialist nurse to provide additional educational input, thus preventing further complications or problems following the introduction of special diets.
> - Initiate appropriate referral to dietitian and possibly gastroenterologists.
> - Maintain food chart/nutritional documentation to monitor patients' requirements.

complications arising of hypovolaemic shock, postoperative atelectasis and unrelieved pain (Hatfield, 2014).

Breathing

Specific postoperative assessment should consider the respiratory needs and possible management of a closed chest drain. This drainage system is positioned in the pleural cavity and may or may not be on suction to ensure that the lungs remain inflated. The water should be deep enough to cover the drainage tube in the drainage bottle and has the function of acting as a valve to prevent air from re-entering the pleural cavity. Circulatory needs require the monitoring of vital signs to identify if the patient is at risk of hypovolaemic shock. Encourage movement by passive and active exercises to prevent thromboembolic complications.

Eating and drinking

It is important that postoperative nutritional and fluid needs are met by a regimen of fluid replacement and volume expanders intravenously, including total parenteral nutritional (TPN) replacement and/or supplements. Often, a jejunostomy tube is inserted at operation for postoperative feeding, before the patient is allowed to ingest food some days later when the anastomosis has healed.

Personal cleansing and dressing

There is a high risk of wound infection; therefore, careful monitoring of the wound for signs of clinical infection, i.e. redness, swelling, heat, pain and exudate, should be undertaken. Comfort needs include assistance with hygiene and creating a safe environment.

Elimination

Monitor for urinary retention, which is related to the neuroendocrine response to stress, anaesthesia and recumbent position.

Additional specific potential complications

These complications include anastomotic leakage, malnutrition, pneumothorax, aspiration pneumonia, wound infection, blocked stent, fistula development, poor prognosis and associated high levels of anxiety.

Stomach

Anatomy and physiology

The anatomy of the stomach is consistent with the rest of the digestive system tract, but it has the specific function of accommodating and digesting the food following ingestion. This is achieved by its shape and modification to receive food and become a reservoir when full. The contraction and churning of the stomach contents is aided by the muscular lining of smooth oblique, circular and longitudinal muscles. The upper part of the stomach wall is thought to be thinner, with little contractile ability; the pylorus is thicker, with an increased contractile function. The passage of food from the oesophagus, stomach and duodenum is controlled by neuromuscular control and sphincter activity.

The mucosa has the ability to secrete enzymes through gastric glands that are present in the columnar epithelium in the mucosa. These cells are known as zymogenic and secrete pepsinogen; parietal cells secrete hydrochloric acid; and mucous cells are responsible for secreting mucus and the intrinsic factor.

Secretion of gastric juices and hydrochloric acid is stimulated by the hormone gastrin from the pyloric mucosa. Gastrin is stimulated by protein foods in the stomach and is released into the bloodstream to reach the gastric glands. Water and glucose are absorbed by the stomach wall along with some drugs and alcohol. The normal pH of the stomach is $1.2-3.0$ and is maintained by the secretion of hydrochloric acid (Tortora & Derrikson, 2014).

Pathology

Hiatus hernia

There is a herniation of the stomach through an opening in the diaphragm into the thoracic cavity. In patients who are symptomatic, gastro-oesophageal reflux is displayed, in which the acid contents backflow into the oesophagus, causing inflammation. It generally affects people over 50 years old. Muscular weakness and diaphragmatic abnormalities cause the herniation to occur, and these may result from increased intra-abdominal pressure, e.g. because of pregnancy, obesity, malignancy, trauma or persistent coughing/sneezing.

Sliding hiatus hernia. Sliding hiatus hernia is the most common type of hiatus hernia. The upper stomach and gastro-oesophageal junction are moved upwards and slide in and out of the thorax. Diagnosis is through radiological studies and fluoroscopy. Clinical manifestations are classically heartburn, regurgitation and dysphagia. Contemporary surgical management, if the patient is symptomatic, is a laparoscopic Nissen fundoplication, although open procedures are still practised by some surgeons.

Para-oesophageal hiatus hernia. All or part of the stomach pushes through the diaphragm opening next to the gastro-oesophageal junction. Investigations are the same as for a sliding hiatus hernia. Clinical manifestations often present with fullness after eating, or chest discomfort, haemorrhage, obstruction, and pain as a result of strangulation of the hernia, which is aggravated when lying flat. Reflux does not usually occur, and a small percentage of the patients who have this type of hiatus hernia are asymptomatic.

Surgical intervention. Anterior gastropexy can be performed, where the weak portion of the stomach is placed in its normal position and anchored to the abdominal wall.

Gastric dysfunction

Reduced absorption occurs, leading to an accumulation of fluid; reversed peristalsis, causing vomiting; and failure of the mucus to act as a barrier.

Peptic ulceration

Peptic ulceration refers to erosion and ulceration of the mucosa of the stomach or duodenum. It is thought that most of these ulcers are due to infection caused by *Helicobacter pylori*, the use of NSAIDs, and/or increased acid secretion (Tortora & Derrikson, 2014). These ulcers, which can be gastric, duodenal or stress ulcers, are diagnosed by gastroscopy, barium studies and a breath test for *H. pylori*.

Gastric ulceration. Peptic ulceration occurs in the prepyloric area of the stomach. It is particularly associated with a familial tendency, stress, alcohol consumption, smoking and ulcerogenic drugs. Aspirin, phenylbutazone and other non-steroidal anti-inflammatory drugs (NSAIDs) predispose to gastric ulcers because they inhibit prostaglandin synthesis. Prostaglandins contribute to the protective effect whereby the mucosa resists damage from gastric juices and hydrochloric acid. Steroids and chemotherapy drugs have similar effects. Other factors that have an influence on the mucosal layer, causing damage, are intestinal reflux, and hypersecretion of hydrochloric acid, which produces gastritis.

Clinical manifestations are mainly associated with burning pain in the epigastric region that occurs approximately 45−90 minutes following a meal, and this is often relieved by vomiting. Food does not help and may increase the pain. Other manifestations can include persistent belching, haematemesis, and the patient may appear malnourished. Gastric ulcers have the added complication of a higher mortality associated with complications of bleeding. Very few of these ulcers are malignant, and most malignant gastric ulcers occur in the antrum body.

Intervention. Treatment is by blocking acid secretion using proton pump inhibitors, as well as eradication of *H. pylori* using combination antibiotics. The vast majority of patients never require surgery, which until 20 years ago was the only treatment available. Surgery is now only required for complications such as bleeding, perforation or cancer (Table 16.3).

Duodenal ulcer. A duodenal ulcer is located in the first 1−2 cm of the duodenum and is the result of excessive gastric acid release and *H. pylori*. It is often seen in the age group between 45 and 64 years and is twice as common in men than in women (nidirect, 2019).

Table 16.3 Peptic ulceration – conditions and surgical intervention

Condition	Intervention
Gastric ulceration	Partial gastrectomy Total gastrectomy Oesophagogastrectomy
Duodenal ulceration	Truncal vagotomy Highly selective vagotomy Antrectomy Pyloroplasty

Clinical manifestations are again associated with pain, which presents in the mid-epigastric region 2−3 hours following the intake of food and often during the early hours of the morning between 0100−0200 h. It is often described as back pain, or heartburn. This pain may be relieved by the intake of food, particularly milk or antacids. Duodenal ulcers are rarely malignant but have for many years been associated with the ingestion of caffeine, stress, alcohol abuse, cirrhosis, chronic pancreatitis, chronic renal failure and smoking. Investigation and diagnosis is by gastroscopy, blood tests in order to correct any anaemia, and a general physical examination. Gastric function tests, to detect the presence or absence of hydrochloric acid and hypersecretion, are occasionally undertaken.

Intervention. Treatment is again by the use of proton pump inhibitors such as omeprazole and lansoprazole and other new preparations, which are extremely potent suppressors of acid secretion, as well as combination antibiotics, to eradicate *H. pylori*. Surgery is reserved for acute complications such as bleeding and perforation, as previously discussed. On very rare occasions when medical treatment fails and there is recurrent symptomatic ulceration despite maximum medical treatment, then elective surgery can be considered (see Table 16.3).

Stress ulcer. Stress ulcer may result following infection, shock, burns or severe trauma, and can occur either in the stomach or duodenum. It is thought to be associated with increased pepsin, acid and ischaemia of the stomach wall. Its onset is rapid, initially within the first 48 hours, and it may be very extensive by the fifth to sixth day. As long as the stressful circumstances remain, the ulcers will spread. The patient is generally treated symptomatically with antacids.

Acute complications

- *Haemorrhage* is a common complication of peptic ulceration and occurs most commonly in the distal stomach and proximal duodenum. Haemorrhage is characterized by melaena but is also often life threatening. It must be corrected by replacing lost fluids, giving blood or blood derivatives, e.g. plasma.

Adrenaline (epinephrine) or fibrin/thrombin can be injected at endoscopy to stop the bleeding.

> *Surgical intervention* may be necessary for bleeding that is not responsive to endoscopic treatment or for heavy bleeding.

• *Perforation* and subsequent peritonitis has a sudden onset, sometimes without prior warning. It is a surgical emergency, and surgery should be performed as soon as the patient's condition allows it. Upper abdominal pain is experienced, which may be referred to the right shoulder. The abdomen is distended and rigid. The patient may rapidly become shocked.

> *Surgical intervention* is by oversewing of the perforation, with intravenous antibiotic therapy to treat bacterial peritonitis.

• *Obstruction* results when scarring and stenosis occur in the pyloric sphincter. The patient feels full and becomes nauseated and vomits. Decompression is initially required and can be achieved by removing the stomach contents via nasogastric tube aspiration.

> *Surgical intervention*: gastroenterostomy is a palliative operation for pyloric obstruction (Fig. 16.2). Vagotomy and antrectomy involve severing the vagus nerve and removing the antrum of the stomach. This will help to reduce hypersecretion of hydrochloric acid if treatment with proton pump inhibitors fails. These patients may require TPN if severe weight loss has occurred.

Gastric cancer

In the UK, gastric or stomach cancer is now the seventeenth most common cancer in adults, the number of

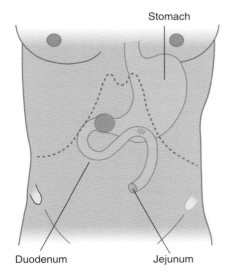

Figure 16.2 Gastroenterostomy.

people being diagnosed falling in the last 10 years, with over 6700 new cases diagnosed in 2015. It is more common in men than in women, with half of all cases being in people over 75 years (Cancer Research UK, 2016b).

Predisposing factors include the following:

• *Dietary*: eating a lot of salted, cured and smoked foods is suggested to increase an individual's risk.
• *Infection*: H. pylori is a common bacterial infection of the stomach. It is diagnosed on gastroscopy and biopsy, and a simple course of antibiotics often eradicates it. If left untreated, it increases the individual's risk of developing gastric cancer by up to five times.
• *Previous stomach surgery* is suggested to increase the risk of stomach cancer, due to reduced acid production.
• *Pernicious anaemia* is also a predisposing factor, in that the stomach does not produce enough gastric enzymes to take up vitamin B_{12}. However, vitamin B_{12} levels can be topped up with regular 3-monthly injections of hydroxocobalamin.

Prognosis is poor, as many tumours are asymptomatic and therefore present late, often with metastases. Those situated in the lesser curvature do not cause gastric function disorder, while some tumours that occur in the cardiac or pyloric orifice display symptoms caused by disturbed gastric motility. Only 15% of people with stomach cancer survive for 10 years or more (Cancer Research UK, 2016b).

Because of the asymptomatic nature of the disease in its early stage, there has been speculation as to the advantage of a screening programme for all patients over 40 years old who present with dyspepsia. However, dyspepsia is a very common disorder and affects a large proportion of the general population, whereas gastric cancer is relatively uncommon.

Clinical presentation includes dyspepsia over 4 weeks, anorexia, nausea, vomiting or haematemesis, hoarseness, epigastric discomfort, abdominal distension, pain, weight loss, blood in stool and iron deficiency anaemia.

Diagnosis can be made through investigating occult bloods, while OGD/gastroscopy is the gold standard investigation which allows biopsies and histological confirmation. CT scan and laparoscopy are carried out to stage the disease and determine resectability.

Intervention. A partial or total gastrectomy may be performed (Figs. 16.3 and 16.4). Total gastrectomy is often associated with a high morbidity and mortality.

Pre- and postoperative care of patients with gastric cancer

Specific preoperative assessment

Patients with gastric cancer may have many problems that require nursing intervention. Anxiety related to the

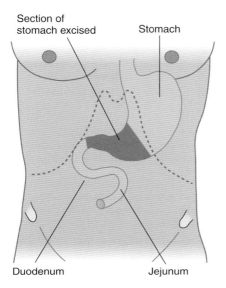
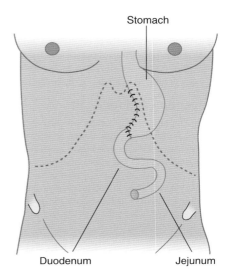

Figure 16.3 Gastroduodenostomy – Billroth I.

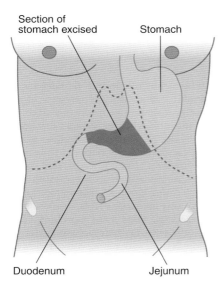
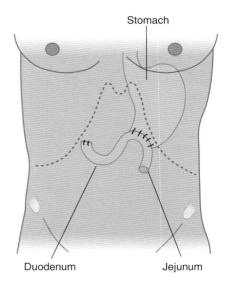

Figure 16.4 Partial gastrectomy – Billroth II.

impending surgical procedure is common in most surgical patients, but is made more threatening by the possible diagnosis of cancer and poor prognosis. Other specific problems associated with gastric cancer are nutritional deficiency related to anorexia; subsequent weight loss; and pain. The management of pain pre- and postoperatively in gastric cancer surgery is paramount, and questions should be focused on the nature of the pain, location, pattern, duration, intensity and reaction to the pain, in order to plan nursing care effectively (Box 16.2).

Specific postoperative nursing interventions

Maintaining a safe environment. Immediately postoperatively, the patient should be placed in the semi-recumbent position for comfort and to help with breathing.

Box 16.2 Specific issues related to pain

- Pain related to abnormal presence of epithelial cells in tumour formation, sometimes causing pressure on nerves and other organs.
- Pain related to presence of metastases or ascites.

Specific objective will be to ensure that pain is relieved and aim for the optimum state of being pain-free.

Nursing intervention and rationale

- Use a pain assessment chart to monitor for the possible indicators of pain: e.g. restlessness, irritability, verbalization and withdrawal. Verbal reports may not always be accurate, because of the effects of the disease process and medication.
- Analyse the information on the assessment chart to indicate pain characteristics. This will aid in the differential diagnosis of pain, therefore ensuring that the appropriate intervention is implemented.
- Discuss with the patient the purpose of pain control and that the aim is to strive for a pain-free state. This will ensure that patients understand why they should report any increase in pain sensation before the pain becomes severe.
- Use a variety of non-pharmacological strategies to relieve the pain: positioning, cutaneous stimulation and massage with oils. Due to the multiple factors that cause and exacerbate pain, a combination of methods of relieving pain may be more effective than a single approach.
- Behavioural pain-relieving strategies may include distraction, relaxation and imagery. These strategies enable patients to divert their attention from the pain and may stimulate endorphin release through having a sense of control and relaxed muscles.
- Liaise with the medical staff to discuss and determine an effective method and dose of analgesics. These may include opioids, non-opioids and adjunctives.
- Discuss impending surgery and the method of controlling pain postoperatively. Ensure that patients have time to ask questions related to the surgery and postoperative management. This will provide patients with as much information as they require, to ensure that they understand what is expected of them.
- Initiate appropriate referral to the specialist pain service/nurse specialist for monitoring and advice.

Breathing and communicating. To avoid pulmonary complications, analgesics should be given which will encourage deep breathing and productive coughing. This will result in increased oxygen and carbon dioxide interchange, therefore providing adequate oxygen content for circulation. Adequate analgesics will prevent shallow breathing and allow for physiotherapy.

Eating and drinking. A nasogastric or nasojejunal tube may be *in situ*. Irritation or bleeding from the position of the nasogastric tube on the mucosa should be avoided by observing and checking the position of the tube and giving nasal and mouth care. Drainage contents should also be monitored. Oral fluids are often withheld, in order to protect the anastomosis. There may be a risk of dehydration; therefore, fluid intake will need to be monitored and replaced by an intravenous infusion. This will compensate for loss in drainage and vomit, as well as maintaining normal hydration needs. Accurate recording is required, and the nasogastric tube is removed once it is felt that the anastomosis has healed. Often a contrast X-ray is performed prior to removal of the nasogastric or nasojejunal tube. Oral fluids are gradually increased as tolerated, but, again, strict observation should be made for signs of abdominal distension and pain.

There is also an increased risk of malnutrition and/or starvation. Once eating is re-established, dietary needs should be met by offering small bland and frequent meals and drinks. It may also be necessary to replace vitamin B_{12}, and give vitamin supplements, since following resection of the stomach it is possible that the absorption of vitamins will be affected, including the production of intrinsic factor, which is important for the absorption of cyanocobalamin (vitamin B_{12}). The patient should be observed for any evidence of regurgitation, which may be caused by eating too much, eating too fast or as a result of oedema along the anastomosis.

Occasionally, when there is prolonged ileus or complications, it may be necessary to commence parenteral feeding support for 5–6 days postoperatively, commencing normal eating when bowel function returns and the patient feels hungry.

Mobilizing. The patient may have limited mobility because of the disease process, the surgery, pain on movement and the effects of anaesthesia. Mobility should be encouraged by giving sufficient analgesics, and monitoring for the side-effects of low blood pressure and dizziness. The goal is to increase mobility daily as the individual is able.

Personal cleansing and dressing. There may be a risk of wound infection, so it is important to observe for signs of such. The amount and type of wound drainage should be monitored. The dressing should be changed as necessary. The dressing may be removed, and the wound left exposed around the third day. Sutures/staples are removed after approximately 7–10 days.

Additional specific complications

These may include shock, haemorrhage, pulmonary complications and the following:

Steatorrhoea. Unabsorbed fat in the stools results from rapid gastric emptying, where the pancreatic and biliary secretions have not had the opportunity to break down and digest the gastric contents.

Dumping syndrome. Dumping syndrome is where vasomotor and gastric symptoms occur after meals, usually after about 10–90 minutes. If the stomach has been anastomosed to the jejunum, the contents may pass through too quickly; therefore, full absorption may not occur. This has implications for the absorption of carbohydrates and electrolytes, as they need to be diluted before absorption can occur. If fluids are taken at mealtimes, this will also encourage the stomach to empty too quickly, giving rise to the symptoms of dizziness, faintness, weakness, sweating, pain and fullness. These symptoms occur as a result of rapid distension of the jejunal loop anastomosed to the stomach, caused by the hypertonic solution of intestinal contents drawing the extracellular fluid into the intestinal contents for dilution.

Gastritis. Because of the removal of the pylorus, its function as a barrier to reflux of duodenal contents is impaired – likewise for the oesophagus when the cardiac sphincter is involved. Vitamin B_{12} deficiency, leading to anaemia, can occur on occasions.

Education and discharge planning

For the patient who is undergoing surgery for an upper gastrointestinal disorder, it is important that the condition is fully addressed and that the patient is fully informed of all procedures and investigations that they are expected to undergo. The procedures and results should be explained in appropriate language that facilitates the asking of questions. The adjustment period is very important for the patient, who is required to alter their lifestyle as a result of surgical intervention or palliative management. A multidisciplinary approach that involves health professionals, the patient, and close family and friends will assist in the planning of aftercare and rehabilitation. If the disorder has not been cured, it may be necessary for the patient to have nutritional advice on how to adjust their diet to meet altered nutritional needs; information so as to identify any complications; appropriate contact numbers for specialist support; and advice on how to control and manage their pain and how to manage specialized equipment, i.e. gastrostomy tube or parenteral feeding. In advanced disease, early referral to the palliative care team is a prerequisite before the patient is discharged back into the community. This ensures that adequate care and support is in place, which can help prevent and/or anticipate some of the distressing symptoms produced by advanced gastric cancer.

Gall bladder

Anatomy and physiology

The gall bladder, a small muscular pouch or sac, is tucked underneath the liver, and is attached to the liver by connective tissue and to the common bile duct via the cystic duct. Its inner walls are similar in construction to the mucous membrane of the stomach. Bile is secreted from the liver into the hepatic duct continuously, but the majority of bile is concentrated and stored in the gall bladder. Bile is then secreted into the duodenum in response to the ingestion of food under neuroendocrine control. Concentrated bile may become saturated with cholesterol and form crystals, which mark the beginning of gallstones.

Bile flow is stimulated by vagus nerve activity. When foods are released into the duodenum, the sensory receptors are stimulated, causing reflex activity in the vagus. Acetylcholine is released and the gall bladder muscle contracts. At the same time the duodenal mucosa produces the hormone cholecystokinin, which stimulates the gall bladder to contract and eject the stored bile into the digestive system in order to assist with the emulsification of fats.

Bile consists of water, conjugated bile salts (i.e. sodium glycocholate, sodium glycochenodeoxycholate, sodium taurocholate and sodium taurochenodeoxycholate) derived from cholesterol, bile pigments (i.e. bilirubin and biliverdin), and a number of lipids. It is a dark yellow/green substance that has a bitter taste. It has a pH of 7.6–8.6 and approximately 800–1000 mL is secreted daily. It has the dual function of aiding digestion of fats by emulsifying them, and aids excretion through stimulating peristalsis. When erythrocytes are broken down, iron, globin and bilirubin are released. The iron and globin are recycled, but some of the bilirubin is excreted into the bile ducts. It is eventually broken down in the small intestine, giving colour to the faeces, and assisting in the synthesis of vitamin K.

Incidence of gall bladder disease

Suggested predisposing factors for developing gall bladder disease are ethnic background, female gender, increasing age, or genetics, along with obesity, a sedentary lifestyle and rapid weight loss (Stinton & Shaffer, 2012).

Clinical presentation

Many patients have a history of biliary discomfort, colic and intolerance to fatty foods, but have not sought medical advice. Gall bladder disease can induce symptoms ranging from mild discomfort following a fatty meal, to the patient who presents to their doctor with acute nausea, vomiting and severe pain. The pain is situated in the right hypochondrium, often radiating to the right shoulder. It is severe and intense and can be spasmodic, easing when stones have been passed from the gall bladder to the common bile duct. If the pain remains untreated and persistent vomiting occurs, shock can ensue. Pyrexia may be present due to infection. Jaundice can be present as a result of the gallstones obstructing the common bile duct (Box 16.3).

Conservative and symptomatic management

Many patients in this acute stage are admitted to the surgical ward for symptomatic control prior to surgical intervention. Previously it was common practice to avoid surgery until the inflammation had subsided, often for a period of up to 6 weeks. However, research is showing that there is an improved outcome with early laparoscopic surgery, carried out within 48 hours of an admission for cholecystitis (Ozkardes et al, 2014).

Nursing issues. The patient is given regular analgesics for the severe pain. There is a risk of peritonitis following perforation of the gall bladder; therefore, pain levels and vital signs are monitored and appropriate interventions implemented. Patients are allowed fluids but may be prevented from eating solids, particularly if nauseated and vomiting. A nasogastric tube may be passed for persistent vomiting. Fluids are replaced by intravenous infusion, and fluid and electrolyte balance is carefully monitored.

Box 16.3 **Gall bladder disease**

- *Cholelithiasis*: presence of gallstones in the gall bladder or common bile duct. *Intervention*: dissolution of stones, ERCP — with or without sphincterotomy, cholecystectomy, choledocholithotomy, exploration of common bile duct, and percutaneous removal of gallstones
- *Cholecystolithiasis*: gallstones in the gall bladder. *Intervention*: open cholecystectomy, or laparoscopic cholecystectomy
- *Choledocholithiasis*: gallstones in the common bile duct. *Intervention*: dissolution of stones, ERCP, choledocholithotomy, cholecystectomy with exploration of common bile duct
- *Cholangitis*: inflammation of bile ducts. *Intervention*: conservative and symptomatic management
- *Cholecystitis*: inflammation of the gall bladder. *Intervention*: conservative and symptomatic management, or surgery

---

Antibiotic therapy is commenced to reduce the inflammation of the gall bladder associated with the infection.

Investigations include abdominal X-rays, ultrasound examination, and ERCP or endoscopic ultrasound if there is jaundice or cholangitis.

Laparoscopic cholecystectomy

A laparoscope is introduced into the abdomen under general anaesthesia. Carbon dioxide is used to inflate the abdomen to give clear vision. Three more small incisions are made to facilitate the manipulation of instruments. The gall bladder is then dissected and removed via the umbilicus. There are a number of advantages to this procedure. The patient is able to mobilize more fully at an earlier stage in their recovery, thus preventing the possibility of complications. Surgical disfiguration is limited, and any drains are removed within 24 hours. This procedure is less painful; therefore, there is a reduced need for opioid analgesics, although there is some discomfort experienced following the introduction of carbon dioxide.

However, in up to 5–10% of cases the procedure is not possible laparoscopically and an open cholecystectomy is performed. Laparoscopic cholecystectomy is the gold standard of care for symptomatic gallstones. However, it is associated with a higher incidence of bile duct injury, a catastrophic complication associated with significant perioperative morbidity and mortality. The early and accurate diagnosis of bile duct injury is very important as it can result in severe complications (Renz et al, 2017).

Specific postoperative management

Nursing management is consistent with normal recovery from a general anaesthetic. Analgesics are required for any discomfort associated with the procedure and inflation with carbon dioxide. Oral fluids can be commenced when the patient has fully recovered from the anaesthetic, and diet taken usually the following day. Normal discharge is within 24 hours, although increasingly the procedure is being carried out as a day case. Sutures will then need to be removed after a week by the practice nurse.

Surgical interventions

Cholecystoduodenostomy

This is a surgical procedure for obstructive jaundice, arising from a stricture of the bile duct caused by congenital factors, inflammation, previous surgery or inoperable tumours of the pancreas or local lymph nodes. The gall bladder is anastomosed to the duodenum, bypassing the common bile duct, ampulla of Vater and sphincter of Oddi (Fig. 16.5). This allows the bile to flow directly into the duodenum.

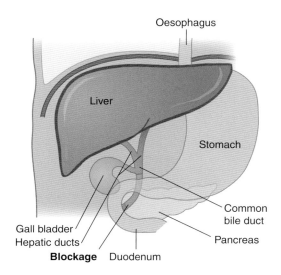

Figure 16.5 Cholecystoduodenostomy.

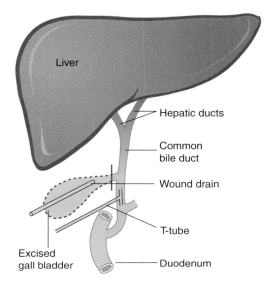

Figure 16.6 Cholecystectomy (exploration of common bile duct).

Choledochostomy (exploration of the common bile duct)

This technique allows the removal of stones from the bile duct, and insertion of a T-tube to allow drainage from the bile duct and a precautionary wound drain to the gall bladder bed (Fig. 16.6).

Cholecystectomy and exploration of the common bile duct

This is the removal of the gall bladder followed by an explorative procedure in the common bile duct and is usually performed to remove gallstones. A T-tube drain is inserted to ensure the common bile duct remains patent for the safe passage of bile (see Fig. 16.6). This tube is then removed approximately 2 weeks postoperatively, following a postoperative cholangiogram. A precautionary wound drain is often inserted to the gall bladder bed. This procedure can be performed laparoscopically or as an open procedure.

Principles of a T-tube. During the operation, a cholangiogram is performed to detect gallstones in the common bile duct. If stones are identified, then the surgeon will usually explore the common bile duct and remove the stones or gravel. Following this procedure, the common bile duct is susceptible to leakage, inflammation and oedema; therefore, a T-tube is inserted to maintain the patency of the duct. The function of this T-tube is to allow safe drainage of bile, approximately 300−450 mL during the first day, which gradually decreases as the oedema subsides.

A postoperative cholangiogram is performed approximately 8−10 days following the cholecystectomy. Depending on the

surgeon, some T-tubes are clamped prior to the postoperative cholangiogram. Particular attention should be paid to any complaints of pain associated with the clamping of the tube. If this arises, then the clamp should be removed immediately and the surgical team informed.

The results are viewed by the surgeon, and if they indicate that the oedema has subsided and there are no stones present and no leakage of bile, then the T-tube is removed by the nursing staff. It is usual to give the patient analgesics at least 30 minutes prior to the removal of the T-tube. After removal it is important to monitor the patient for a sudden drop in blood pressure, or rise in pulse, and for evidence of pain, as this may indicate that the patient has developed biliary peritonitis caused by seepage of bile into the peritoneal space.

Cholecystojejunostomy

This is a palliative surgical procedure for obstructive jaundice due to a tumour of the pancreas. The gall bladder is anastomosed to the jejunum, bypassing the common bile duct, ampulla of Vater and sphincter of Oddi (Fig. 16.7). A precautionary drain may be inserted to the area of anastomosis.

Pancreatectomy (Whipple's operation)

This procedure is for carcinoma of the head of pancreas. The duodenum and part of the pancreas are resected, and the common bile duct and pancreatic ducts are joined to the jejunum (Fig. 16.8). There are many variations of this procedure.

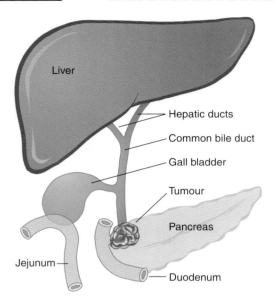

Figure 16.7 Cholecystojejunostomy.

Pre- and postoperative care of patients undergoing biliary surgery

Specific preoperative assessment

The patient who requires surgery for biliary dysfunction has many problems that require nursing intervention. The specific problems are associated with the risk of peritonitis due to possible perforation of the gall bladder; haemorrhage associated with reduced vitamin K production and absorption following obstructive jaundice; wound infection following the obstruction or dislodgement of the T-tube; and postoperative chest infection due to the pain associated with the high abdominal incision preventing deep breathing and coughing. However, with the advent of laparoscopic cholecystectomy, more that 90% of these operations are being carried out using minimally invasive techniques, which therefore reduces the need for a subcostal incision. The specific problems associated with breathing are detailed in Box 16.4.

Specific postoperative nursing interventions

Maintaining a safe environment. It is important to monitor vital signs for possible shock; the abdomen for signs of distension; and level of pain, including location and character. These all indicate the possibility of peritonitis, perforation and/or haemorrhage. Early detection will ensure that immediate action can be implemented, i.e. fluid replacement and/or emergency surgery.

Communication. Pain has already been mentioned in detail in the section on gastric surgery and in relation to breathing following biliary surgery. However, the

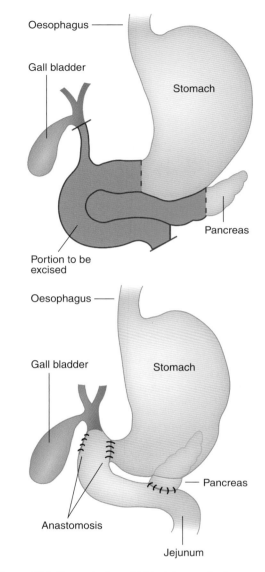

Figure 16.8 Pancreatectomy (Whipple's operation).

management of pain also has important implications for mobilization and the prevention of deep vein thrombosis.

Eating and drinking. Eating and drinking can usually be commenced immediately postoperatively following a laparoscopic cholecystectomy, and at 24 hours following an open procedure.

Personal cleansing and dressing. Wound management has been discussed in previous nursing interventions, although there is a risk of infection associated with the T-tube drain. Any signs of clinical infection, redness,

> Box 16.4 **Specific issues related to breathing**
>
> - Inadequate air exchange – due to reduced ventilation of the lungs.
> - Reduced ventilation of the lungs – due to frequent, shallow respirations.
> - Shallow respirations – due to the risk of associated pain when expanding the lungs.
> - Potential risk of chest infection – due to the difficulty in expectorating sputum and limited mobility.
> - Difficulty in expectorating sputum – due to the tenacity of the lung secretions and a lack of strength to expectorate.
>
> *Specific objective* will be to maintain optimal air exchange (lung expansion) and prevent chest infection.
>
> **Nursing intervention and rationale**
>
> - Accurate recordings and monitoring should be carried out postoperatively to establish the depth and frequency of respirations, along with oxygen saturation levels.
> - Deep breathing (diaphragmatic) should be taught to the patient prior to surgery and encouraged postoperatively. This will allow full lung expansion and prevent consolidation of lung secretions. Involve the physiotherapist, especially if the patient has had respiratory problems identified prior to surgery.
> - Ensure the patient's pain is assessed and analgesics are administered prior to intensive deep breathing exercises or physiotherapy and mobilization.
> - Instruct the patient in supporting their abdominal wound prior to coughing and expectorating sputum, thereby reducing any stress or pulling on the incision line.
> - Encourage a good fluid intake, which will have the effect of reducing the tenacity of the lung secretions and facilitating expectoration of sputum.
> - Mobilize as soon as the patient's condition allows, as this encourages deeper respirations, therefore ensuring that the lungs are adequately ventilated.
> - Initiate appropriate referral to physiotherapist, for mobility and check.

swelling, heat, pain, purulent drainage or odour should be documented and reported, as this will ensure that systemic antibiotic therapy is introduced if required.

Signs of T-tube obstruction should be observed for, by noting any change in skin colour (jaundice), pale stools, dark yellow urine, nausea and vomiting, and reduced amount of drainage in the bile bag. Any of these signs can indicate that the passage of bile is obstructed, causing pressure within the common bile duct and sometimes the liver and portal system. The skin surrounding the T-tube should be observed for any redness and excoriation, and protected with a small keyhole dressing, as bile contents, when leaking around the tube, can cause skin irritation and pain.

Additional specific complications

It should be remembered that the elderly have an increased risk of morbidity and mortality when undergoing surgery of the biliary tract in an emergency, due to an increased risk of complications associated with the cardiovascular system.

Education and discharge planning

As previously stated in this chapter, it is important that the patient who undergoes surgery should be fully educated and aware of the implications of the surgery. The patient who has had a cholecystectomy may have

symptoms that are associated with the free passage of bile. The gall bladder is no longer there to be used as a reservoir, so the bile will be continually secreted. This may mean that when fatty foods are eaten the patient may feel nauseated and may develop post-cholecystectomy diarrhoea. The patient should also be aware of the need to report any further pain, nausea or change in skin colour, as this may indicate further biliary obstruction.

Bariatric surgery (by Nuala Davison)

Worldwide obesity has tripled since 1975. According to the World Health Organisation (WHO) in 2016 more than 1.9 billion adults aged 18 years and older were overweight. Of these, over 650 million were obese. In the UK, NHS data shows 10,660 hospital admissions directly attributable to obesity in 2017/18 and a further 710,000 admissions where obesity was a factor (NHS Digital, 2019).

Obesity is a major risk factor for cardiovascular disease and other chronic diseases such as hypertension, type 2 diabetes, and dyslipidaemia. A reduction in these risk factors has been shown after bariatric surgery (Beamish et al, 2016). Bariatric surgery has been shown to be a safe and efficient method of weight loss. In general, bariatric procedures are performed using laparoscopic surgery rather than open procedures. All primary bariatric procedures are performed under general anaesthetic.

The degree of obesity of an individual is assessed by calculating their Body Mass Index (BMI). People are defined as being overweight if they have a BMI equal to or greater than 25 kg/m² and obese if their BMI is greater than 30 kg/m².

$$BMI\ (kg/m^2) = weight\ (kg)/height\ (m^2)$$

In the UK, eligibility for bariatric surgery is guided by criteria set by the National Institute for Health and Care Excellence (NICE), but whether an individual is able to access bariatric surgery is influenced by funding criteria set by the individual's local CCG (Clinical Commissioning Group) – these criteria may vary from area to area.

In general, an individual will be deemed eligible for surgery if they meet the following criteria:

- A BMI of 40 kg/m² or more, or between 35 kg/m² and 40 kg/m² associated with other significant disease (for example, type 2 diabetes, obstructive sleep apnoea, ischaemic heart disease or uncontrolled high blood pressure) that could be improved with weight loss.
- Evidence that all appropriate and available non-surgical measures have been adequately tried but have failed to achieve or maintain adequate, clinically beneficial weight loss for at least 6 months; this would include weight loss medications and diets.
- The person has been receiving or will receive intensive management in a specialist obesity service; in the UK this will usually mean attendance at a Tier 3 specialist weight management programme for a period of between 12 and 24 months (this will include input from an obesity physician, specialist nurses, dietitians, psychology/psychiatry and exercise specialists).
- The person is generally fit for anaesthesia and surgery.
- Commitment to the need for long-term follow-up.
- Obesity surgery is also recommended as a first-line option (instead of lifestyle interventions or drug treatment) for adults with a BMI of more than 50 kg/m² in whom surgical intervention is considered appropriate.

In 2017/18 there were 6627 hospital admissions with a primary diagnosis of obesity with a main or secondary procedure of bariatric surgery (NHS Digital, 2019).

Types of surgery

Bariatric surgery achieves and maintains weight loss through a variety of mechanisms but will only reach its full potential when accompanied by behavioural changes from the patient. The most common types of surgery currently undertaken in the UK are gastric bypass, sleeve gastrectomy, adjustable gastric banding, and gastric balloon insertion. Biliopancreatic diversion and duodenal switch are far less common.

The main mechanisms of action are:

- *Restriction of food intake* (gastric banding, sleeve gastrectomy and gastric balloon)
- *Malabsorption* – reducing the amount of small intestine where food is absorbed (biliopancreatic diversion and duodenal switch)
- *A combination of restriction and malabsorption* (Roux-en-Y gastric bypass).

Adjustable gastric banding

In this procedure a silicone band is placed around the upper part of the stomach near the oesophageal junction creating a small stomach pouch (Fig. 16.9). The band induces a feeling of satiety and slows the transit of food to the area of the stomach below the band (Burton & Brown, 2011). The band can be adjusted (tightened or loosened) by injecting saline through a subcutaneous port if the band is not providing enough restriction or too much restriction. Most foods can be eaten although some patients find certain foods, such as white bread and red meat, hard to swallow. This gives a slow gradual weight loss.

Sleeve gastrectomy

The outer part of the stomach is removed to leave a narrow tube-shaped stomach (Fig. 16.10). The size of the stomach is reduced by 70–80%. Appetite is reduced and patients experience early satiety from a smaller portion of food due to the small stomach size. It is can be performed

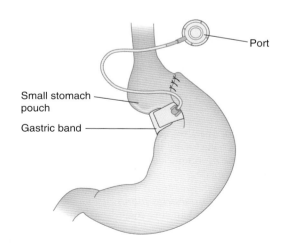

Small stomach pouch

Gastric band

Port

Figure 16.9 Adjustable gastric banding.

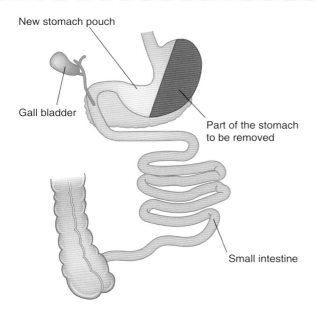

Figure 16.10 Sleeve gastrectomy.

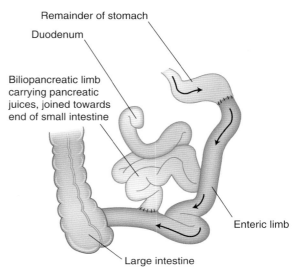

Figure 16.11 Biliopancreatic diversion and duodenal switch.

as a standalone procedure or as the first stage of two-stage gastric bypass for super-obese individuals. If weight loss stops, a second procedure such as gastric bypass or duodenal switch may be performed. Patients will need to take lifelong vitamin and mineral supplements following the procedure.

Biliopancreatic diversion and duodenal switch (BPD/DS)

These procedures are the least commonly performed bariatric surgeries; they give greater weight loss than other procedures but are more complex and technically challenging surgeries.

These procedures involve reducing stomach size (restricting portion sizes) and shortening the length of functional intestine where absorption occurs (malabsorption). Food passes from the stomach into the alimentary limb. In both procedures a length of duodenum (biliopancreatic limb) is anastomosed to the alimentary limb to allow transit of bile and pancreatic juice (Fig. 16.11). The two limbs join to form the common limb where digestion and absorption of nutrients take place — the length of this limb can vary according to the procedure used. Shortening the length of intestine where absorption occurs can put the patient at risk of iron, calcium, vitamin and protein malabsorption. The patient is required to take vitamin and mineral supplements for life and have regular blood tests. Rapid weight loss is expected after BPD/DS and can lead to formation of

gallstones. Sucandy et al (2015) found this occurring in 22.7% of patients post-BPD/DS.

Gastric bypass

In this procedure weight loss is achieved through the creation of a small upper stomach pouch (restricting intake) and a shortening of the functional intestine (mild malabsorption). The small stomach pouch is connected to the lower part of the small intestine (Roux limb) (Fig. 16.12). Pancreatic juices and bile travel from the bypassed portion of the stomach and duodenum and mix via anastomosis to the Roux limb, thereby creating a common channel. The amount of malabsorption is less than with the biliopancreatic diversion/duodenal switch although iron or vitamin B_{12} deficiencies are a risk and vitamin and mineral supplements should be taken for life along with regular blood tests. Dumping syndrome can occur in patients following gastric bypass surgery when large amounts of carbohydrates or fats are consumed. Symptoms include diarrhoea, dizziness, tremor, sweating, and nausea. Avoidance of food triggers will lessen the symptoms.

Gastric balloon

The gastric balloon is a temporary weight-loss device that can be used for short-term weight loss or for initial weight loss in super-obese patients where laparoscopic surgery is deemed too technically challenging. The balloon is placed endoscopically, usually under general anaesthetic (Fig. 16.13). The balloon will fill the stomach meaning the patient will feel fuller from a smaller portion than prior to the procedure. The

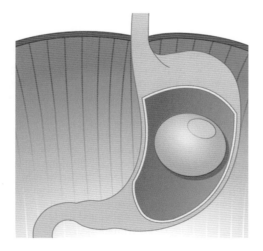

Figure 16.12 Gastric bypass.

Oesophagus

Small stomach pouch

'Short' intestinal Roux limb

Pylorus

Duodenum

Bypassed portion of stomach

Figure 16.13 Gastric balloon.

balloon is filled with saline and methylene blue dye so that any rupture of the balloon would be identified by the patient passing blue/green urine. The balloon can come in a variety of sizes and can stay for differing lengths of time according to the manufacturer – this will usually be between 6 and 12 months.

In most cases further surgery will be planned for after the balloon removal to prevent weight regain.

Specific preoperative care

A multidisciplinary approach is essential to ensure the patient is fully evaluated, medically stabilized, and receives the education needed to make lifestyle changes necessary for surgery to be successful (Still, 2007). The team should include representatives from nursing, surgery, medicine (endocrinology, cardiology, gastroenterology, respiratory), psychology, dietetics and anaesthetics. The type of surgery a patient receives can depend on co-morbidities, dietary habits, psychological disorders such as binge-eating behaviour, age, type of obesity and the patient's preference.

Specific postoperative care

Care of patients following bariatric surgery should be carried out in an environment adapted for this speciality. Provision of equipment with adequate safe working loads for the patient population is essential. This should include seating (outpatient and inpatient areas), scales, beds, examination couches, toilets/commodes, wheelchairs, operating tables, hoists and mobility aids. Appropriately sized gowns should be provided.

Postoperative vital signs monitoring should be carried out with the appropriate equipment (large-sized blood-pressure cuffs). Attention should be paid to signs of sepsis, which can signal an anastomotic leak. Anastomotic leaks can present a potentially fatal complication following sleeve gastrectomy, gastric bypass and BPD/DS. Signs of a leak can include tachycardia, respiratory distress, left shoulder pain, abdominal pain and anxiety (Dunham, 2012). A return to theatre is usually indicated for a leak.

Pulmonary embolism (PE) risk has reduced in recent years due to the use of prolonged VTE (venous thrombo-embolic episode) prophylaxis (Montravers et al, 2015). All patients should be given anti-embolic prophylaxis (e.g. Clexane/enoxaparin), wear anti-embolic stockings, and be encouraged to mobilize as soon as possible to minimize risk of deep vein thrombosis or PE.

Patients on diabetic medication should have regular blood glucose monitoring in the postoperative phase until nutritious fluids are commenced. They should be seen by a member of the local endocrinology/diabetes team. Insulin and antihypertensive medication requirements can drop significantly post-surgery and should be reviewed. Medication should be given in regular release formulas rather than sustained release in patients who have undergone malabsorptive procedures (Still, 2007).

The introduction of fluids and food depends on the type of surgery performed. Patients should be well educated by the dietitian prior to surgery, with a follow-up visit soon after. Patients undergoing procedures involving stapling of the stomach (gastric bypass, sleeve gastrectomy and BPD/DS) will require checks for staple leaks prior to commencing any oral intake either in radiology or with the use of methylene blue administered orally and monitored via drain output. Typically, most patients will graduate from sips of fluids, to free smooth fluids, to a puréed diet, to a normal diet albeit with smaller portions over a period of 6–8 weeks. Nausea and vomiting should be managed with antiemetic medication and intravenous fluids until adequate oral intake is achieved.

Special attention needs to be paid to skin care following surgery. Frequent repositioning and monitoring of pressure areas, use of appropriate pressure-relieving mattresses and control of moisture between skin folds are essential (Hatfield, 2014). Surgical wounds should be closely monitored, especially in diabetic patients.

Nurses caring for patients undergoing bariatric surgery need to recognize with sensitivity the specific needs of their client group (NMC, 2018). Weight stigma can lead to discriminatory practice such as denial of employment and healthcare deprivation (Turner et al, 2011). A thorough understanding of the causes of obesity and the specific physical and psychological effects it can have on the individual is essential to provide quality nursing care.

Specific discharge education

The success of bariatric surgery is dependent on the patient making changes to their diet and lifestyle. The dietitian will provide written dietary advice for the patient to follow in the first six weeks after surgery and beyond.

Arrangements should be made with district or practice nurses for removal of sutures if necessary. Patients should be discharged with two weeks' supply of VTE prophylaxis and should be supplied with a sharps bin and educated on self-administration. Patients should be given the initial supply of their multivitamin and mineral supplements with instructions given in their discharge summary for ongoing requirements. Contact numbers for the dietitians and clinical nurse specialist should be supplied. Reinforcement should be given to the patient about the need for them to attend long-term follow-up appointments.

Long-term complications specific to the procedures

Gastric band

Long-term complications can include food intolerance, gastro-oesophageal reflux disease (GORD), leakage, band erosion, port site infection and oesophageal dilatation. Some of these can be managed in the outpatient department

but some, such as band slippage, migration, and port site complications, will require further surgery.

Sleeve gastrectomy

Complications include staple line leak, narrowing of the sleeve/stenosis, GORD, oesophagitis, and chronic nausea (Rogula et al, 2018).

Biliopancreatic diversion/duodenal switch

Complications include staple line leak, small bowel obstruction, pancreatitis, gallstones, vitamin and mineral deficiencies, protein malnutrition, increased gas and bloating, and malodorous gas and stools (Rogula et al, 2018). Lifelong monitoring of patients is essential to avoid vitamin and mineral deficiencies.

Gastric bypass

Complications include staple line leak, marginal ulcer at the join between the stomach pouch and jejunum), strictures (narrowing at the join between the stomach pouch and jejunum), gastrogastric fistula (a channel between the pouch and gastric remnant) (Rogula et al, 2018), dumping syndrome and reactive hypoglycaemia. Careful monitoring of bloods is required to assess for vitamin and mineral deficiencies.

SUMMARY OF KEY POINTS

- This chapter has described the pathophysiology of the organs of the upper gastrointestinal tract. Diagrams have been used to facilitate understanding, and the dysfunction of the organs and surgical interventions have also been discussed.
- Aetiology and epidemiological data, where appropriate, have been included, but it must be remembered that, as medical intervention progresses and research is undertaken, these statistics may alter.
- Some guidance has been offered to assist the nurse to use a problem-solving approach in assessment, planning care, setting goals and initiating intervention for those patients who undergo surgery for a variety of disorders of the upper gastrointestinal tract.
- Finally, patient education and preparation for discharge has been highlighted, suggesting that it is necessary to focus on the importance of health promotion. Patient education plays an important part in preventing complications from arising, and in dealing with the implications of failed surgery that may require further intervention.

REFLECTIVE LEARNING POINTS

Having read this chapter, think about what you now know and what you still need to find out about. These questions may help:

• What key areas would the nurse need to address preoperatively with the patient to help them deal with

(Continued)

(cont'd)

the anxiety of impending upper gastrointestinal tract surgery?
• How might the nurse manage nausea and vomiting?
• What do you need to know prior to administering a blood transfusion?

References

Beamish, A. J., Olbers, T., Kelly, A. S., & Inge, T. H. (2016). Cardiovascular effects of bariatric surgery. *Nature Reviews Cardiology, 13* 730–743.

Burton, P. R., & Brown, W. A. (2011). The mechanism of weight loss with laparoscopic adjustable gastric banding: induction of satiety not restriction. *The International Journal of Obesity, 35*(3), S26–30.

Cancer Research UK. (2016a). *Oesophageal cancer statistics.* Available at: <www.cancerresearchuk.org/health-professional/cancer-statistics/statistics-by-cancer-type/oesophageal-cancer#heading-Two>

Cancer Research UK. (2016b). *About stomach cancer.* Available at: <www.cancerresearchuk.org/about-cancer/stomach-cancer/about-stomach-cancer>

Department of Health (DoH). (2009). *Reference guide to consent for examination or treatment* (2nd ed.). Available at: <www.gov.uk/government/publications/reference-guide-to-consent-for-examination-or-treatment-second-edition>

Dunham, M. (2012). Increasing incidence of the biliopancreatic diversion with duodenal switch as a surgical weight loss option; implications for nursing care. *Bariatric Nursing and Surgical and Patient Care, 7*(2).

Eykyn, F. (2014). Endoscopic retrograde cholangiopancreatography (ERCP) performed under propofol sedation. *Gastrointestinal Nursing, 11*(10), 44–48.

Hatfield, A. (2014). *The complete recovery room book* (5th ed.). Oxford: Oxford University Press.

Kumar, M., Sweis, R., & Wong, T. (2014). Eosinophilic oesophagitis: investigations and management. *Postgraduate Medical Journal, 90,* 273–281.

Montravers, P., Ribeiro-Parenti, L., & Welsch, C. (2015). What's new in postoperative intensive care after bariatric surgery? *Intensive Care Medicine, 41,* 1114–1117.

NHS Digital. (2019). *Statistics on obesity, physical activity and diet, England.* Available at: <digital.nhs.uk/data-and-information/publications/statistical/statistics-on-obesity-physical-activity-and-diet/statistics-on-obesity-physical-activity-and-diet-england-2019 >

nidirect. (2019) *Stomach ulcer and duodenal ulcer.* Available at: <https://www.nidirect.gov.uk/conditions/stomach-ulcer-and-duodenal-ulcer>

Nursing and Midwifery Council. (2018). *The Code. Professional standards of practice and behaviour for nurses, midwives and nursing associates.* <www.nmc.org.uk/globalassets/sitedocuments/nmc-publications/nmc-code.pdf>

Ozkardes, A. B., Tokac, M., Dumlu, E. G., Bozkurt, B., Ciftci, A. B., Yetisir, F., et al. (2014). Early versus delayed laparoscopic cholecystectomy for acute cholecyctitis: a prospective, randomized study. *International Surgery, 99*(1), 56–61.

Renz, B. W., Bosch, F., & Angele, M. K. (2017). Bile duct injury after cholecystectomy: surgical therapy. *Visceral Medicine, 33*(3), 184–190.

Rogula, T. G., Schauer, P. R., & Fouse, T. (2018). *Prevention and management of complications in bariatric surgery.* Oxford: Oxford University Press.

Royal College of Radiologists (RCR). (2013). *Radiation and the Early Fetus.* London: Royal College of Radiologists. Available at: <www.rcr.ac.uk/system/files/publication/field_publication_files/BFCR%2813%294_radiation.pdf>.

Still, C. (2007). Before and after surgery the team approach to management. *Supplement to OGB Management, 19*(4), 15–21.

Stinton, L. M., & Shaffer, E. A. (2012). Epidemiology of gallbladder disease Cholelithiasis and cancer. *Gut Liver, 6* (2), 172–187.

Sucandy, I., Abulfaraj, M., Naglak, M., & Antanavicius, G. (2015). Risk of biliary events after selective cholecystectomy during bioliopancreatic diversion with duodenal switch. *Obesity Surgery, 26* (3), 531–537.

Tortora, G. J., & Derrikson, B. (2014). *Principles of anatomy and physiology* (14th edn). New Jersey: Wiley.

Turner, R. N., Wildschut, T., & Sedikides, C. (2011). Dropping the weight stigma: Nostalgia improves attitudes toward persons who are overweight. *Journal of Experimental Social Psychology, 48*(1), 130–137.

Williams, B. C. (2015). The Roper-Logan-Tierney model of nursing: A framework to complement the nursing process. *Nursing, 45*(3), 24–26.

Further reading

Hind, M., & Wicker, P. (2000). *Principles of perioperative practice.* Edinburgh: Churchill Livingstone.

Porock, D., & Palmer, D. (2003). *Cancer of the gastrointestinal tract: a handbook for nurse practitioners.* London: Whurr.

Chapter 17

Patients requiring colorectal and anal surgery

Katie Adams and Fiona Hibberts

KEY OBJECTIVES OF THE CHAPTER

At the end of the chapter the reader should be able to:

- describe the anatomy and physiology of the lower gastrointestinal tract
- briefly explain specific investigations for patients with colorectal and anal disorders
- briefly explain causes, conditions and surgical interventions
- give examples of assessment procedures for patients undergoing colorectal and anal surgery
- highlight specific pre- and postoperative management
- assist in the education and discharge planning of patients.

Areas to think about before reading the chapter

- What are names that patients and the public might use for the gastrointestinal tract?
- What strategies can the nurse use to help a patient understand the function of the gastrointestinal tract?
- How might you alleviate embarrassment that may be caused when intimate procedures are being performed?

Introduction

This chapter will provide information for nurses who are caring for patients on a surgical ward that specializes in colorectal and anal surgery. It will focus on surgical interventions that are carried out when all other methods of treatment have been ineffective or are, indeed, inappropriate. The chapter is underpinned by the professional standards of practice and behaviour for nurses and nursing associates that the Nursing and Midwifery Council (NMC) expects every registrant to adhere to as stipulated in *The Code* (NMC, 2018). This chapter will also include endoscopic practice, and both diagnostic and therapeutic procedures will be outlined.

There are many different techniques and practices in the field of gastroenterology; therefore, surgical procedures may have slightly different names, according to their origin. It is important to use this book in conjunction with current evidence-based practice and research.

For the purpose of this chapter, the assessment framework is based on the Roper, Logan and Tierney model of nursing, as described in Williams (2015), as this remains best practice in the ward environment. The generalized pre- and postoperative management remains the same as for any patient undergoing colorectal and anal surgery, and only specific problems will be highlighted following discussion of the disease or organ dysfunction.

Investigations

There are many investigative procedures that a patient may undergo in order to diagnose a disorder and enable

Table 17.1 Investigations of the lower gastrointestinal tract undertaken prior to surgical intervention

Investigation	Surgery
Abdominal X-rays	GI tract
CT scan	GI tract
MRI	Lower GI tract
Colonoscopy	Lower GI tract
Sigmoidoscopy	Lower GI tract
Proctoscopy	Lower GI tract
Ultrasound	Abdomen and GI tract
Proctography	Lower GI tract
Transit study	Lower GI tract

the surgical team to plan the relevant course of action or surgical intervention (Table 17.1). The diagnosis is not always initially clear and differing investigations can help to reach the final diagnosis.

The patient requires a full explanation of the proposed investigation, in order to make an informed decision about whether to consent to and proceed with the test or not. Patients will be required to give verbal and often written consent. Informed consent will involve a discussion with the patient, outlining what the test will look at specifically, the risks involved and the potential outcomes of the test, and, indeed, not having the test at all. Alternatives to the test should also be discussed with the patient. The Department of Health provides guidance for consent in their document *Reference guide to consent for examination or treatment* (Department of Health and Social Care, 2009). The most common investigations are briefly described below.

Certain investigations utilize ionizing radiation (X-rays) to create images, including plain X-rays, computed tomography (CT) scans and fluoroscopy such as Gastrografin enemas or small bowel studies. The patients most at risk from these types of procedure are female patients during their reproductive life who might be knowingly or unknowingly pregnant, as there is an increased possibility of affecting a fetus through pelvic X-rays. Consequently, any abdominal or pelvic radiography should be carefully considered and only carried out if absolutely essential. Female patients of reproductive age (even if sexual activity is not readily admitted) should have a urinary or blood β-HCG test prior to any ionizing radiation investigation. A patient being pregnant is not an absolute contraindication to having an investigation involving radiation, however the risks, benefits and alternatives should be carefully

considered, and usually there are alternatives, such as an MRI or ultrasound. On any request for these investigations, clinicians should include details of menstruation dates, in order for the radiographer to adhere to the 10-day rule guidance (Royal College of Radiologists, 2013).

X-rays

An X-ray involves using radiation (X-rays) to take 2D pictures of the patient, such as an abdominal X-ray. X-rays react differently depending on how dense the tissues are, for example bone is dense and appears white on X-rays, in contrast to bowel gas which has almost no density and appears black. When investigating soft tissue and organs of the abdominal cavity, it is often necessary to use a contrast medium such as barium sulphate or Gastrografin, both of which appear white and dense on X-rays, to highlight the spaces and cavities in the gastrointestinal (GI) tract.

Abdominal X-rays are useful in detecting abdominal fluid levels, bowel gas, constipation and obstruction. Chest X-rays can detect free gas under the diaphragm, which can suggest bowel perforation or be present following surgery. Chest X-rays are also used to check the position of the tip of a nasogastric tube to ensure that it is in the stomach and has not inadvertently been inserted into the lungs.

Nursing issues. As with all tests which use radiation, consideration must be given to check if the patient might be pregnant (see above). The position of the patient also needs to be considered; for example, with a chest X-ray to look for free gas in a bowel perforation, the patient should be sitting up for 15 minutes prior to the test to enable any free gas to float upwards, giving the best chance of seeing free gas. It is important to ensure that the patient understands, has given their consent and taken any preparation required for the test (medications, enemas or a full bladder, for example).

Computed tomography (CT) scan

This scan provides a computerized picture of a part of the body, which is achieved by combining fine X-rays, often with a contrast medium, and is one of the most common abdominal investigations performed for patients with GI symptoms. 'Slices' of the abdomen are produced and are useful for showing the interior anatomy of a patient, including abnormalities such as tumours, bowel or urinary tract obstructions, vascular blockages or infected organs.

Contrast can be given in various ways depending on what the CT has been requested for, including orally, intravenously, via a stoma or rectally. Most of these are administered once the patient is in the radiology, with the exception of oral contrast, which the patient will usually need to take around an hour prior to the scan and so is usually given on the ward. It is worth checking the timing of oral contrast and its concentration as this can vary depending on the scan, and the contrast is usually given in a more dilute form than for other contrast studies (see below). Radiological contrast mediums can affect the kidneys, so care should be taken to assess the patient's renal function prior to administration.

Magnetic resonance imaging (MRI)

MRI is a method of imaging which relies on the magnetic features of water molecules within tissues to create images of the body and does not rely on ionizing radiation as with CT scans or X-rays. It is especially useful when either ionizing radiation is contraindicated (for example when a patient may require multiple scans, or when pregnant) or for certain areas of the body, like the liver or pelvis, where it can provide particularly detailed images. Within colorectal surgery it is most commonly used to image the pelvic structures, such as with rectal and anal tumours or other disorders of the anal canal, namely perianal fistulas.

Nursing issues. Patients having an MRI will often need to be starved prior to their scan, so it is best to check this with the radiology department or treating team before the scan. The scan itself takes longer than a standard MRI, for example up to 20–30 minutes for a pelvic MRI, and is usually within a closed narrow tunnel so patients can sometimes feel claustrophobic whilst the scan is taking place. An MRI can affect some types of metal, like a pacemaker, but not others, like the metallic staples used during a bowel anastomosis, and the treating team will need to take this into account when organizing any MRI. Ensuring this is documented on the patient's notes is important to ensure effective communication between the ward and radiology department.

Colonoscopy, sigmoidoscopy, proctoscopy

The interior of the gastrointestinal tract can be investigated through the use of an endoscope, which is a luminous flexible fibreoptic instrument that can be inserted via the rectum or a stoma to allow inspection of that part of the gut with the images then relayed to a television screen. The fibreoptic endoscope is often used to reach areas previously inaccessible with other instruments, as it has greater flexibility and the end of the endoscope can be moved and adjusted to navigate the intricate twists and turns of the bowel. Instruments can also be passed through a special tube within the endoscope, to obtain biopsies or perform other procedures such as polypectomy.

For this investigation to be successful, the bowel should be clear of its normal faecal contents. For sigmoidoscopy, an enema, aperient (laxative) or suppositories may be

given to allow the patient to effectively evacuate their lower bowel and rectum of faecal contents. For colonoscopy, bowel cleansing solutions are given prior to the investigation, in combination with an altered diet, usually to a low-residue diet or clear fluids, the day prior to the procedure. This procedure is usually performed to detect any abnormalities of the colon, or to investigate rectal bleeding, changes in bowel pattern, anaemia or the cause of an obstruction, e.g. a cancer.

Nursing issues. Cleansing of the lower colon may be contraindicated in patients in whom there are symptoms of a potential blockage in the bowel. Causes of a blockage can include a colonic cancer or a narrowing due to inflammatory bowel disease or diverticular perforation. An assessment of the patient needs to be made prior to requesting the investigations and prescribing appropriate bowel cleaning medications. After the tests, the patient may feel uncomfortable, with a bloated sensation, associated wind pains and, occasionally, nausea.

Contrast studies

Radio-opaque contrast mediums are often used for radiological studies of the gastrointestinal tract. Liquid preparations of either barium sulphate (not water soluble) or Gastrografin (water soluble) can be given via a variety of routes, most commonly orally or rectally, but can also be given via a fistula or stoma.

Gastrografin enema/barium enema

Either barium or Gastrografin is introduced into the rectum and retained by the patient while radiological studies are undertaken to detect disorders of the rectum and large intestine. It is particularly useful in assessing strictures, obstruction, or a volvulus but is contraindicated where there is a potential risk of perforating the bowel.

Nursing considerations. If barium is used for radiological studies in the rectum, special attention should be paid to ensure that the rectum is emptied prior to the procedure, and that constipation following the procedure is avoided by increasing fluid intake and removing the contrast medium by a cleansing enema.

Proctogram

Barium or Gastrografin paste is introduced into the rectum and the patient may also be given contrast to drink. This can highlight the presence of an enterocele, rectocele and any anatomical disorder of the rectum and is often used to assess patients with pelvic floor disorders and evacuation difficulty.

Bowel transit studies

In order to investigate the amount of time food takes to work its way through the gastrointestinal tract, radio-opaque markers in capsules are given to the patient and swallowed. After 5 days, a plain abdominal X-ray is taken to see if any of the markers are still within the gut. Slow gut transit, resulting in constipation, can be diagnosed by assessing the number and distribution of any retained markers, or evacuation disorders diagnosed if markers are retained within the rectum.

Stool specimens

These are usually obtained and cultured to detect infective organisms, occult blood or faecal fats collection. The stool specimen may be a single sample or be part of a series of specimens.

Colorectal and anal disorders

Small intestine

Anatomy and physiology

The small intestine is a long, muscular, tubular organ which runs from the gastric pylorus through to the caecum, by terminating at the ileocaecal valve. It consists of the same layers as throughout the intestinal canal, which have been described in detail in Chapter 16. However, the submucosa and mucosa differ, as their main function is absorption and to assist in the final stages of digestion. The small intestine is divided into three main sections – the duodenum, jejunum and ileum – and is approximately 2.5 cm in diameter, and approximately 3–8 m in length.

The mucosal layer has an increased surface area created by folds and villi that help in the absorption of intestinal contents. In between the villi are small pits lined with glandular epithelium, referred to as glands or crypts (crypts of Lieberkühn), their main function being the secretion of intestinal digestive enzymes.

These digestive enzymes leave the intestinal walls vulnerable to enzymatic action. Therefore, the walls of the small intestine are protected by alkaline secretions from Brunner's glands in the duodenum, and mucus throughout the small intestine, which have the effect of neutralizing the acid and enzymes.

Normal function

Food is propelled along the small intestine by peristalsis. This action involves muscular activity by rhythmic, relaxing and propulsive movement. These actions allow the food to be mixed and broken down for absorption and move the chyme through the small intestine. Intestinal juices are secreted to assist in the digestion of carbohydrates and proteins. Fats are converted into fatty acids and

monoglycerides by the action of pancreatic lipase. Bile salts then assist in converting them into a water-soluble form, for absorption by the villi. The small intestine is responsible for absorbing approximately 90% of the nutrients through the villi by a variety of processes. This is facilitated by the secretion of enzymes, particularly the pancreatic enzymes, amylase and protease, that chemically assist the breakdown of food into smaller molecules.

Abnormal function

Increased peristalsis may cause colic and diarrhoea, which can result in the malabsorption of nutrients. Sometimes, abdominal surgery causes a paralytic ileus, thereby preventing the passage of food and reducing the absorption of nutrients.

Small bowel obstruction

Intestinal obstruction refers to the blockage or slowing down of the normal flow of intestinal contents and may be partial or complete (Table 17.2). The intestine above the blockage becomes dilated, and secretions accumulate, causing stagnation of the contents or even reverse flow. The bowel beyond or distal to the obstruction collapses and loses its function. The intestinal contents build up as the bowel dilates and can cause vomiting, eventually faeculent in nature. Over half of small bowel obstructions are said to be caused by adhesions, either congenital or more commonly caused by previous surgery. Other causes include hernias (both those that can be seen outside the abdomen (external), or within the abdominal cavity itself (internal)), diverticular disease and cancer of the large intestine.

Clinical manifestations

Small bowel obstruction is often referred to as either mechanical or functional and may be diagnosed by observing for clinical manifestations, particularly vomiting faeculent fluid, absence of faeces, colicky pain and abdominal distension. Mechanical bowel obstruction is a physical cause for the bowel to be blocked, either from within the bowel (tumour, foreign body, the bowel structuring down) or from without (such as adhesions or hernia). Functional bowel obstruction is where the lumen of the bowel is intact, but there is a loss of normal function or peristalsis, leading to a similar build up in fluid within the small bowel as with mechanical obstruction. In the small bowel functional obstruction is termed a paralytic ileus and within the large bowel, pseudo-obstruction.

Clinical manifestations depend on the degree of obstruction and portion involved. In acute small bowel obstruction there is a rapid onset, associated with severe symptoms of colicky pain, nausea, vomiting leading to a loss of electrolytes and dehydration. Often the blockage can be complicated by interference with the blood supply

Table 17.2 Small bowel obstruction — causes and surgical interventions

Cause	Intervention
Mechanical — blockage of the lumen	
Foreign body	Laparotomy, excision and removal, repair
Mechanical — lumen wall altered by disease	
Crohn's disease — strictures	Small bowel resection or strictureplasty
Intussusception	Reduction or resection and anastomosis
Meckel's diverticulum	Reduction, repair or resection
Volvulus	Small bowel resection
Neoplasms	Resection, excision of tumour and end-to-end anastomosis
Mechanical — occurring outside the lumen	
Strangulated hernia	Reduction and repair or resection
Adhesions	Division of adhesions
Neoplasm	Resection, excision of tumour and end-to-end anastomosis
Paralytic	
Previous surgery	Decompression by nasogastric intubation
Infection	Withhold all food and fluid; antibiotics
Mesenteric ischaemia	Surgical resection and anastomosis

to a section of small intestine, which may result in ischae-mia, tissue necrosis and the threat of perforation. If the patient progresses to the point of developing bowel ischaemia, this type of obstruction requires immediate surgical intervention. Clinical manifestations of chronic or partial small bowel obstruction present with a slower onset, as the lumen gradually or intermittently obstructs. Symptoms progressively become worse as the condition develops and occasionally will require surgery but is less urgent in nature.

Diagnosis

A detailed history, abdominal examination and abdominal X-rays are often all that is required, particularly in patients with adhesional obstruction where they may have presented with similar symptoms on multiple previous occasions.

Mechanical obstruction

Mechanical obstruction can occur anywhere in the small intestine and may be simple in nature or complicated by strangulation. This type of obstruction arises from either an internal blockage that occludes the lumen, or an exter-nal pressure to the lumen of the bowel. The additional feature of strangulation implies that the not only the lumen of the bowel is occluded, but that the blood supply

to the bowel has also become affected and at this stage the bowel can rapidly progress to the point of perforation. The types of mechanical obstruction are discussed below.

Adhesions. This is the most common cause of patients developing small bowel obstruction. These result from for-mation of scar tissue within the peritoneal cavity. This usu-ally occurs during the inflammatory response of healing, when scar tissue becomes attached to part of the intestine. It is associated with previous surgery, presence of infection, inflammation or injury. Occasionally patients are born with adhesions, termed congenital adhesional bands, but this is less common. Clinical manifestations result when the intes-tine becomes twisted or kinked; they depend on the degree of obstruction but generally include nausea, vomiting, abdominal cramp pain and distension. Diagnosis is by abdominal X-ray or CT scan. Intervention is by operating to divide the adhesions to free the intestine if the obstruction does not settle with conservative management.

Strangulated hernia. Another common cause of small bowel obstruction, this is a weakness in the muscle wall which allows peritoneum and bowel to protrude, which in some patients leads to strangulation. If a hernia becomes irreducible and constricted, this reduces the blood supply (termed strangulation) and causes ischae-mia, necrosis and gangrene of the contained omentum or loop of bowel. Clinical manifestations also include colicky pain and increased swelling of the herniation. Diagnosis can be through abdominal examination alone, but may require X-rays, an ultrasound or CT scan. Intervention is by reduction and repair of the hernia at an operation, possibly with resection of the affected bowel or omentum if they have become unviable.

Foreign body. This type of obstruction is rare and can be due to gallstones or a food bolus that has not been digested and remains lodged in the small intestine, causing a blockage. Intervention is by surgical laparotomy to deal with the underlying cause.

Crohn's disease strictures. The formation of scar tissue as a result of frequent exacerbation of the disease results in narrowing of the lumen of the small intestine. Intervention is by small bowel resection, strictureplasty or, if accessible, by endoscopic dilatation, with the aim of relieving the obstruction whilst preserving as much small bowel as possible.

Intussusception. This is caused by telescoping of the intestine, often very close to the ileocaecal valve, and occurs frequently in young infants. One portion of the bowel prolapses into the lumen of another portion, which may block as a result. Specific clinical manifestations include those already described, but it may also present with blood in the stools and a palpable lump felt through the abdominal wall. Diagnostic investigations include an ultrasound during which a 'target' sign can be seen. Intervention is often non-operative and may include colonic Gastrografin to attempt to reduce the bowel, or by operation if non-resolving or if there are signs that the bowel might be developing ischaemia.

Meckel's diverticulum. This is a congenital condition where there is incomplete closure of the yellow stalk, a duct that links the yellow sac with the midgut of the embryo, leaving a sac which protrudes from the wall of the ileum. Its length can vary from 2 to 50 cm, and it is susceptible to inflammation. It is often asymptomatic, but it may present similarly to appendicitis, or intestinal obstruction. Intervention is by surgical resection of the affected part of the bowel.

Neoplasms. New growth of tissue (tumour) may be benign or malignant and is uncommon in the small bowel and may eventually lead to an obstruction. Diagnosis may require a CT or MRI, with a colonoscopy or push enteroscopy to reach the lesion for biopsy if needed. Intervention is by resection, excision of the tumour and anastomosis of the bowel, with or without a stoma — usually laparoscopically. Further treatment may be necessary with chemotherapy.

Functional obstruction

Paralytic obstruction (paralytic ileus). This condition is an absence or decrease in peristaltic action, which results in bowel contents not flowing efficiently through the small intestine. Although not strictly a specific complication, it is appropriate to mention it at this point, as the condition is associated with abdominal surgery, infection or mesenteric ischaemia. Clinical manifestations include those already discussed but may be complicated by fever, dehydration, electrolyte imbalance and respiratory distress. Diagnosis is by abdominal examination and abdominal X-ray or CT. Intervention includes symptomatic management, bowel decompression, fluid and electrolyte infusions and avoidance of certain medications such as opiates.

Nursing intervention. Many patients admitted with small bowel obstruction are treated as surgical emergencies, therefore time to improve nutritional and fluid levels is restricted. Fluids lost through vomiting or diarrhoea should be replaced and electrolytes corrected by intravenous infusion. The patient should initially be encouraged to abstain from taking food or fluids orally until bowel function returns. A nasogastric tube on continuous drainage and intermittent suction is usually inserted to allow decompression of the bowel. Vital signs are monitored, and pain control management evaluated.

Occasionally, surgical intervention, e.g. laparoscopy or laparotomy with or without resection, and with either anastomosis or stoma, is required if the paralytic ileus results in a complication such as ischaemia or perforation.

Inflammatory bowel disease

Inflammatory bowel disease usually refers to two disorders — Crohn's disease and ulcerative colitis — although there are other forms.

Crohn's disease

Originally identified in 1932 by the American physician Burrill B. Crohn, this disease is often considered together with ulcerative colitis; however, it has a different aetiology and clinically presents differently. It can affect any part of the digestive system, from the mouth to the anus, but is most common in the small intestine, particularly the terminal ileum. The diseased segments are often separated by normal bowel segments and can appear as isolated 'skip' lesions in other parts of the intestine. The inflammation may cause excessive production of fibroblasts and angiogenesis, i.e. new capillary buds, and is histologically distinguishable by the formation of a granuloma. Clinically, there is a thickening of the bowel wall and mucosal lining, giving a cobblestone appearance at the advanced stage. There is also a danger of the affected section of bowel forming abscesses that may rupture or narrowing of the lumen through fibrosis and transmural damage, causing fistulae or sinuses (Chang et al, 2015).

Crohn's disease is particularly common in young adults, although it can occur at any age and in both sexes equally, and in developed countries, with higher frequency in white people and the Jewish population. There is still much speculation as to the cause of the disease, but, like many other disorders, it is multifactorial, with genetic and environmental factors. Many genes have been identified and it can be associated with autoimmune disorders, food additives, allergens and individual response to stress (Chang et al, 2015).

Clinical manifestations. Clinical symptoms of the disease are insidious and often well advanced before the patient is diagnosed. The patient may present to the doctor complaining of tiredness associated with lethargy and sometimes a persistent elevated temperature.

Other specific symptoms include abdominal pain that is often described as similar to cramp, particularly after meals. This is the result of peristalsis following the intake of food, and the inability of the contents to flow through a narrowed section of bowel. Some patients will complain of chronic mild pain which is persistent in nature, occurring between the cramping spasms, and some may have a painful and ineffective desire to empty the rectum (tenesmus). Chronic inflammation of parts of the intestine and oedema may result in diarrhoea. The patient will often admit to having lost weight as a result of withholding food to avoid the cramping pain. This may lead to malnutrition and anaemia, as the patient may already be malnourished due to malabsorption of nutrients through the small intestine. Diagnosis is through patient history, physical examination, radiological studies such as CT and MRI, colonoscopy and ileoscopy, blood tests (leucocytosis, erythrocyte sedimentation rate (ESR), haemoglobin, C-reactive protein (CRP)), and stool specimens for infective organisms, fat content and occult blood.

Complications. Complications may arise due to obstruction, perforation, malabsorption, melaena due to bleeding ulceration, and the formation of abscesses. Other effects of the disease may present as skin ulceration and infection, iritis, arthropathy, and perianal sepsis in the form of anal fistulae.

Intervention. The vast majority of patients are treated medically, long term, with 5-aminosalicylic acid (5-ASA) compounds, steroids, and immunosuppressants such as azathioprine, and monoclonal antibodies such as infliximab. Up to 70% of patients will, however, at some point in their life require surgical intervention. This may include segmental resection of small bowel, subtotal colectomy or total colectomy with formation of an ileostomy, strictureplasty or surgery for perianal disease. Patients may require surgery on many separate occasions (more than 50% in an attempt to ease symptoms of the disease). As medical management of Crohn's disease improves, the overall incidence of surgery is decreasing, especially the requirement of emergency surgery.

Ulcerative colitis

This term is used to describe diffuse inflammation and multiple ulcerations of the superficial mucosa and occasionally the submucosa of the large intestine and rectum. The mucosa becomes oedematous and reddened with bleeding, and eventually becomes ulcerated. This ulceration results in the large intestine developing numerous continuous lesions that eventually cause muscular hypertrophy, which will shorten, narrow and thicken the bowel. The patient will have periods of exacerbation and remission. There is a danger of toxic dilatation, especially in the transverse colon in severe acute disease, which may result in perforation (Overbey et al, 2014). Inflammation from ulcerative colitis starts in the rectum and extends further up the large bowel to a differing degree between patients and to varying amounts during the patient's life. Unlike Crohn's disease, which can have skip lesions, the inflammation in ulcerative colitis (UC) spreads as a single area of inflammation from the rectum extending proximally. Also unlike Crohn's disease, ulcerative colitis affects only the large bowel within the gastrointestinal tract, unless it affects the entirety of the large bowel, in which case it may then also affect just the last part of the small bowel, termed 'backwash ileitis'.

Aetiology and incidence. There still an unclear aetiology in ulcerative colitis but is most likely a combination of patient genetic susceptibility and subsequent environmental factors leading to an immune response to colonic bacteria. As in Crohn's disease, ulcerative colitis has a familial tendency with a ten-fold risk of developing UC if you have a first-degree relative affected, and commonly affects young adults to the middle-aged. Other conditions such as arthritis, ankylosing spondylitis, pyoderma gangrenosum and hepatitis may be associated with ulcerative colitis (Lynch & Hsu, 2018), as well as an increased lifetime risk of developing colorectal cancer.

Clinical manifestations. These are similar to those described in Crohn's disease but, histologically, crypt abscesses are seen, which can become necrotic and ulcerated. There is intermittent tenesmus with urgency and cramping pain. Loose bowel action may occur, often 10−20 times daily. Rectal bleeding may be present, sometimes leading to anaemia. Eventually, the debilitating progression of the disease may extend to such a degree that it affects normal activities of living and social interactions. It can also be so advanced that fistulae and abscesses may be present.

Colonoscopy is the diagnostic tool of choice, where the disease activity can be graded, and biopsies taken. If the inflammation is severe, often a flexible sigmoidoscopy is performed instead, due to reservations on performing the procedure on patients who have active colitis, with a theoretical increased risk of perforating the bowel.

Intervention. Medical intervention has the goal of reducing ongoing inflammation, termed remission, and preventing relapse, termed a 'flare' of ulcerative colitis. 5-

ASA compounds are the main anti-inflammatory drug in the management of ulcerative colitis and can be given either orally or rectally depending on the degree and extent of the inflammation. Corticosteroids, such as prednisolone, hydrocortisone and budesonide, can additionally help reduce inflammation alongside 5-ASAs and help induce remission. Steroids may be required intravenously if the patient does not respond to initial oral medication, and then gradually converted back to oral medication and tapered off eventually if the patient goes into remission. Like Crohn's disease, newer immune modulators, which alter the body's inflammatory response within the bowel, are also available either when steroids have failed to work or as a way of avoiding steroids. Immune suppressive drugs include azathioprine, mercaptopurine and methotrexate, and if a patient is taking these for some time they will require frequent blood tests to ensure that their bone marrow is not suppressed, making them more susceptible to infections. There are now immunologically tailored drugs, in the form of antibodies such as infliximab, adalimumab and ustekinumab, which are used commonly in both Crohn's disease and ulcerative colitis and function through targeting specific pathways involved in inflammation.

If medical therapy does not bring about remission, termed refractory colitis, or the disease has been active for the most part of 20 years, when the patient may then have an increased risk of developing adenocarcinoma of the colon and rectum, surgery may then become advisable. In the urgent setting, the inflammation within the bowel may become so severe that the lining of the bowel becomes a source of significant sepsis or is at risk of acute perforation (fulminant colitis), in which case an emergency operation may be required.

For patients with a long history of ulcerative colitis, where they may have had multiple flare-ups requiring hospital admission, may have abnormal cellular change within the bowel (dysplasia) or not be able to completely come off steroids, they will often be referred to a colorectal surgeon to discuss removal of their large bowel. As ulcerative colitis is a disease of the large bowel, by removing the entirety of the large bowel (colon and rectum), the patient will in effect be cured, an operation termed a proctocolectomy. Once the decision to remove the large bowel has been made, the surgeon and patient must then decide together how best to manage the output of the small bowel. Some patients may wish to have an ileostomy which they then plan on keeping long term and therefore no further surgery is required following the proctocolectomy. A large proportion of patients wish to keep their gut function as normative as possible, and still be able to open their bowels through the anus. For these patients the most common solution is the formation of a J-pouch ileo-anal anastomosis (Fig. 17.1). This technique involves using the last part of the small bowel to create a reservoir which is

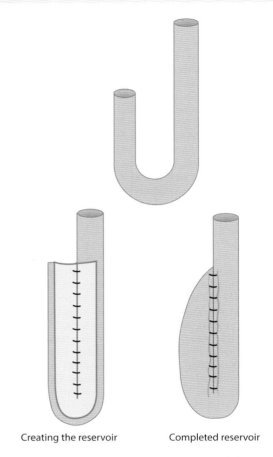

Creating the reservoir   Completed reservoir

Figure 17.1 Ileal pouch—anal anastomosis. J pouch (two sections of small bowel to form the pouch).

then joined on to the anus, and allows small bowel contents to build up within the pouch prior to the patient having the sensation to open their bowels, if the small bowel were attached straight to the anus the patient would likely have near constant diarrhea and/or incontinence.

These patients will most commonly undergo a two-stage procedure. In the first stage, the colon and rectum are removed (proctocolectomy) with formation of the J-pouch, which is then anastomosed to the anal canal (ileal-pouch anal anastomosis), with finally a defunctioning ileostomy created more proximally, so that the pouch can heal in place without having to function as part of the GI tract at the same time. The second stage is then to reverse the ileostomy, once the pouch has healed, typically around two to three months later.

For fulminant colitis, the patient is often unwell in hospital and will likely require antibiotics, possibly blood transfusions, and will have a poor nutritional state. These patients require an operation to remove their large bowel, but without the added operative time and complexity of removing the rectum and creating a pouch, as there would be significant pelvic inflammation associated with their active disease. Therefore they undergo a subtotal colectomy, where the large bowel up to the distal sigmoid/upper rectum are removed, but the rectum remains in place, and the end of the small bowel is brought out onto the surface of the skin as an ileostomy. When the rectum is closed over, the ongoing inflammation will usually resolve, but this may take some time, during which mucous can still build up with the rectal stump and if the pressure builds up sufficiently this can cause the rectum to burst — a stump blowout. For this reason, the surgeon may bring the end of the rectum to the skin or leave a tube through the anus for a few days after the operation.

Once the patient has recovered from this operation, they may then elect to proceed to have the remainder of their rectum removed and either keep the ileostomy or proceed with a pouch, with or without a defunctioning ileostomy whilst the pouch heals.

The whole procedure may be performed in three stages, whilst a more elective operation may be complete in just two stages or, rarely, one stage if no covering loop ileostomy is formed.

- *Stage 1* includes the colectomy, preservation of the rectum and anal sphincter, and formation of ileostomy.
- *Stage 2* includes the formation of the reservoir and loop ileostomy. This may be easily closed when the reservoir or pouch has healed. Stages 1 and 2 can be performed in one operation for elective cases.
- *Stage 3* is closure of the loop ileostomy.

Ileostomy

In this operation, ileum is brought through an opening to the abdomen, onto the surface of the skin. It is usually performed following pan-proctocolectomy or total colectomy, when the diseased or inflamed bowel has been removed, e.g. in ulcerative colitis or Crohn's disease. The opening is higher up the bowel (ileum); therefore, bowel contents are more fluid, as the water has not been absorbed via the large colon.

Pre- and postoperative care of patients with inflammatory bowel disease

Specific preoperative assessment

If the patient has been in a period of exacerbation for some weeks, they may already be dehydrated and malnourished. Therefore, nursing intervention should include replacement of fluids and blood, and a nutritional support programme undertaken prior to surgical intervention;

this may include parenteral nutrition. If the patient is not in a state of exacerbation, then a low-residue diet is encouraged, with small portions several times a day. Antibiotics are often prescribed as a prophylactic measure. In both types of surgery involving the formation of an ileostomy and ileal pouch–anal anastomosis, psychological preparation and support from the stoma therapist should be an integral component of care planning.

The stoma therapist will also be involved in marking the site for the ileostomy, i.e. in siting it appropriately for the patient in terms of clothing, previous surgery and body fat folds and distribution. Assessing the patient's needs and matching these with the types of ileostomy appliances and pouches available is also important. A vital part of preparation for this type of surgery includes providing education and knowledge of the disease and surgical interventions in a language that the patient will understand and respond to by asking appropriate questions. There are many patient information leaflets available from organizations such as the Ileostomy and Internal Pouch Association of Great Britain and Ireland, and Colostomy UK, as well as the manufacturers of stoma products.

One of the problems that may arise with this type of surgery and formation of ileostomy is anxiety in the patient who feels that they may have lost control over faecal elimination, therefore increasing the risk of body image disturbance (Box 17.1).

Specific postoperative interventions

Eating and drinking. Following an urgent operation, in the immediate postoperative period the patient may have a nasogastric tube in position, which will be on continuous drainage and may be aspirated every 4 hours. This will ensure that there is no retention of gastric fluid, which would otherwise cause abdominal distension. Fluid loss will be from stoma drainage, so fluids will need to be replaced by intravenous infusion. This method of replacing fluids will be necessary until there is evidence of bowel activity following surgery. Fluids are often given orally in small amounts and gradually increased if there is no abdominal distension, discomfort or vomiting. If distension and intolerance to fluids does occur, then the patient is restricted from taking oral fluids until the distension subsides. If this is not resolved, the patient may require intravenous nutritional support or occasionally further surgical intervention, as the bowel may be obstructed. Diet is commenced once oral fluids are tolerated and this may initially be a low-residue, high-calorie diet, until the patient has become adjusted to their altered digestive function.

Elimination. The management of an ileostomy involves observation of the stoma for any signs of stoma necrosis, oedema and/or retraction. The stoma colour should remain a healthy pink; if the stoma changes to a bluish/black colour, this may indicate ischaemia and that

---

Box 17.1 **Specific issues related to having a stoma**

- Increased anxiety due to possible presence of odour and flatulence from the ileostomy.
- Increased anxiety associated with possible visibility of the stoma appliance through clothing.
- Anxiety associated with adapting to the ileostomy and ability to apply coping mechanisms.
- Anxiety regarding relationships with partners and expressing sexuality.

Specific objective will be to preserve the patient's body image and empower the patient in retaining sense of control over bowel function.

Nursing intervention and rationale

- The possibility of odour is one problem that causes considerable anxiety, and in order for the patient to control the odour, it is important that they change the bag regularly, and have knowledge of odour-proof bags and deodorants that are available for use when the bag is emptied and changed.
- Advice should be given on which types of food can be eaten that will reduce odour, e.g. orange juice and yogurt. Some foods should be avoided, such as cabbage, onions, beans and garlic, in order to avoid associated embarrassment of flatulence.
- The patient should be educated as to what foods may cause an increase in flatulence, and period of time between ingestion and production of flatus. If flatus is difficult to control, it can lead to increased social embarrassment.
- The patient should also be taught to anticipate the need for correct bag and deodorant filters to be attached, therefore minimizing the effects of flatus by releasing flatus through the deodorized filter.
- The patient should be educated as to how to conceal the bag/pouch underneath a stretchy layer of clothing. This will hold the bag/pouch next to the skin surface, thereby reducing the bulk. This will have the effect of enhancing body image by enabling the patient to dress acceptably in clothes that they already have.
- Discussion should be encouraged with the patient and family regarding the normal emotional response to an ileostomy. This gives the opportunity for negative feelings to be explored and accepted. Coping strategies should be addressed with the patient and their family, as these may need to be altered, adapted or new methods adopted.
- Specialist advice and information on other specialist organizations should be offered, as contact with others in a similar situation will reduce some of the isolation that the patient may be feeling. It will also increase the patient's awareness of the condition being manageable.
- Specialist advice should also be provided on how to manage the ileostomy in normal occupation, social and sexual activities. This will enable the patient to consider coping strategies for these activities, therefore helping to ensure successful outcomes.
- Ensure patients have the contact details of their local stoma therapist for advice and follow-up.

---

the stoma is at risk of developing tissue necrosis. If tissue necrosis does occur, then surgery is required to remove the ischaemic bowel. Sometimes, tissue surrounding the stoma becomes oedematous, and this can cause the skin to stretch the blood vessels resulting in occlusion of the blood supply to the stoma. The bag size should be checked, when the oedema subsides, for a correctly fitting appliance. It is important that all fluid loss is measured and documented in order to calculate the patient's fluid replacement requirements for every 24 hours.

The stoma should also be observed for any signs of retraction. This can be caused by poor healing of the suture line, poor nutrition, or due to technical problems with formation of the stoma. The patient may have been on steroid drugs for some time, and therefore will be more susceptible to wound breakdown (Shanmugam et al, 2015).

Personal cleansing and dressing. Skin integrity is very important for patients with an ileostomy. The skin surrounding the stoma is vulnerable to excoriation if the stoma bag is not positioned correctly and faeces leak onto the skin surface. This is more likely to occur if the diet is not correct and faeces are more fluid, containing enzymes and digestive secretions. It is important that the stoma bag is the correct size and fits to the contours of the skin. Sometimes, problems can be avoided by using a drainable bag, skin sealant and/or barrier paste.

Sexuality. There is a possibility that the patient may experience some sexual dysfunction following surgery, and this can be associated with damage to nerves at the time of surgery or from the psychological impact of an altered body image. It is important, therefore, that opportunities are given to the patient and family for full, open and honest discussion of their ability to adapt to the ileostomy.

Wound. Particular attention should be paid to sutures around the stoma, ensuring that they are not too tight, causing wound breakdown.

Additional specific complications

Other complications include stoma necrosis, oedema and retraction, as previously described. Sometimes, acute obstruction can occur as a result of paralytic ileus or oedema.

Skin excoriation can occur as a result of diarrhoea and poor wound healing, or wound breakdown due to long-term malnutrition. If the patient and their family have a knowledge deficit regarding the condition and aftercare, it is possible that there may be adverse psychological implications with respect to acceptance of both the ileostomy and alteration of body image.

Education and discharge planning

Prior to discharge, documentation should indicate that the patient does not have a fever or any condition that would delay recovery, and that they will be able to progress satisfactorily in their own home. This should reduce the risk of readmission. Also, education and advice should be given on how to manage the stoma. A routine should be established for changing the bag, with all equipment ready prepared. The surrounding skin should be cleaned with warm water. The used bag should be sealed in a plastic bag and disposed of in the dustbin, not flushed down the toilet. Supportive literature highlighting these points and contact numbers may also be given.

There are no restrictions on diet, but the patient should be advised to avoid any food that produces wind or discomfort. There are no problems with travel, but the patient should make certain that they have all the equipment for changing the bag to hand. It is usual to return to work 6–8 weeks after the final operation. Patients who have a pouch formation may return to work in between operations, depending on how they feel.

A full explanation should be provided to patients of how to use community facilities, special organizations and support groups, and how to seek advice or contact appropriate health professionals for support if they are worried about their progress.

Large intestine

Anatomy and physiology

The large bowel begins as the caecum once joined by the last part of the small bowel, the terminal ileum, in the right lower abdomen, and is also where the appendix is attached. There are two main sections to the large bowel, the colon which resides in the main abdominal peritoneal cavity and continues towards the anus as the rectum, residing in the pelvis, below the peritoneum. The large bowel traverses the abdomen around its periphery, travelling up the right side as the ascending colon, across the superior aspect inferior to the stomach as the transverse colon, and then down the left abdominal wall, the descending colon. Once in the left lower abdomen the colon

meanders in a redundant arc or S-shaped segment of bowel, the sigmoid colon before finally reaching the rectum and finally anus.

Its muscular component consists of circular and longitudinal muscle that together help to propel the bowel content. Its mucosa contains no villi but has goblet cells that secret mucus to aid the passage of intestinal residue, which may stay in the colon for several days, depending on gut motility.

Normal function

Absorption of water from the end products of digestion is approximately 1 L in 24 hours. Faeces are propelled along the colon by the action of peristalsis. Whenever food enters the stomach, a reflex action occurs that opens the ileocaecal valve. This action causes the food to be passed along the small intestine and into the colon. Larger peristaltic movements occur four to five times daily.

An additional function of the large intestine is to synthesize vitamin K in the presence of stercobilinogen and bacteria. Vitamin K is absorbed through the gut wall into the bloodstream and has an important function in clotting.

Abnormal function

Peristalsis may slow down, causing the excess water to be absorbed from the colon, resulting in constipation; or quickened, resulting in diarrhoea, altering the bowel elimination pattern.

Constipation

The stool becomes very hard and may become impacted, causing infrequent bowel actions and, depending on the cause, may result in complete absence of defecation. Other terms used to describe constipation include feeling bloated or full, and experiencing difficulty or the inability to pass a hard stool.

Causes of constipation. Constipation may be due to poor dietary fibre intake, poor mobility, some types of medication (particularly, strong analgesic preparations, antidepressants, and iron supplements), or damage or abnormality of the nerve supply (Table 17.3). Other more serious bowel conditions may mimic the features of constipation such as tumours or strictures

Diarrhoea

Diarrhoea is the passage of liquid or soft and often frequent stools, sometimes associated with urgency. This condition should be recognized as potentially harmful, and consideration should be given to the loss of water and electrolytes. Potassium depletion and dehydration, if not replaced adequately, can have very serious consequences, especially for small children and the elderly.

Causes of diarrhoea. Diarrhoea may be due to infection (viral or bacterial), diet (such as spicy foods), irritable bowel

323

syndrome, diverticular disease, ulcerative colitis, Crohn's disease, carcinoma, radiation, overactive thyroid gland, malabsorption, or side-effects from medication, e.g. antibiotics and NSAIDs (see Table 17.3).

Elderly patients are particularly vulnerable to alteration in bowel elimination pattern, especially when in hospital. This is thought to be linked to changes in lifestyle imposed through the hospital environment, e.g. different eating patterns and diet, reduced or limited mobility, increased anxiety and inability to cope with stress.

Pathology

Diverticular disease

Diverticular disease, or diverticulosis, is the presence of pouch-like herniations of mucosa through the muscular layer of the colon, which can become inflamed, termed diverticulitis or haemorrhage from a diverticular bleed. Diverticular disease is very common, particularly in areas with a Western diet, such as the UK, USA and Canada, with approximately half of adults over the age of 60 demonstrating features of diverticular disease. They are thought to be associated with a low-residue diet and constipation causing changes in colonic pressure, although there is still some uncertainty on their exact aetiology.

Whilst it used to be thought to be a disease of more elderly patients, in general diverticulosis is steadily becoming more common in younger patients, even in their 20s and 30s, with the reason for this not fully understood. Diverticulosis can affect any part of the large bowel, but is most common in the sigmoid.

Diverticulitis occurs when the diverticula become inflamed and may even perforate, potentially causing a local abscess, pelvic abscess or pus and/or faecal matter throughout the peritoneal cavity. Patients who are affected often present with a cramp-type pain over the sigmoid colon in the left iliac fossa, where occasionally a mass is palpable. A CT scan will usually demonstrate the pattern of inflammation associated with the diverticulitis, as well as any associated complications such as an abscess or perforation. Treatment is typically initially conservative and usually involves antibiotics, intravenously if the patient cannot tolerate oral diet or is systemically unwell, as well as management of any complications, such as drainage of an abscess performed by the radiologists either with ultrasound or CT scan.

Surgical intervention. If the patient fails to respond to initial management or if when they present there are signs of a significant perforation or undrainable abdominal abscess, then an operation may be required. Traditionally patients would undergo an open laparotomy

Table 17.3 Diarrhoea and constipation — causes and interventions

Cause	Intervention
Diarrhoea	
Infection	Antibiotics
Diet	Avoid hot spicy foods and alcohol
Irritable bowel syndrome	Avoid stress, coffee and alcohol
Ulcerative colitis	Steroids, surgery, ileostomy
Crohn's disease	Steroids, surgery
Carcinoma	Surgery
Metabolic disorders	Medication
Malabsorption	Avoid certain food, e.g. fats
Medications	Identify causative drug
Constipation	
Diet	High-fibre diet, education
Medication	Avoid drugs that affect gut motility
Nerve damage	Surgery
Obstruction/carcinoma	Surgery
Iron supplements	Alternative iron replacement therapy

with removal of the affected segment of colon and the proximal end brought out onto the abdomen, as an end stoma, termed a Hartmann's operation. Many patients will still require this operation, but another option that patients may now have is a laparoscopic operation, where the bowel may be joined at this initial operation as an anterior resection, with or without a defunctioning ileostomy for reversal at a future time (Box 17.2).

Appendicitis

Appendicitis is acute inflammation of the appendix, a tubular projection of bowel approximately 5–10 cm long attached to the caecum. Its function originally was to digest cellulose, in herbivores, but this function diminished when consumption of meat was increased in the diet (Alexander et al, 2006). However, it does fill with faeces and empties on a regular basis. Problems occur when faeces or foreign bodies become lodged in the tubular lumen, or the lymphoid tissue around the base becomes inflamed and causes obstruction; the lumen then becomes inflamed and painful. Left untreated the appendix can become gangrenous and eventually perforate, causing pus and faecal content to spread throughout the abdomen. In a few patients, their own bodies may try to seal off the appendix from the rest of the abdomen by forming acute adhesions to the appendix, with either the omentum or other parts of the bowel, usually the small bowel. In these patients, when they present, this cluster of bowel, omentum and appendix may be palpable as a mass.

Appendicitis can present at any age, although generally is more common in children and in the elderly and is slightly more common in males.

Clinical manifestations. Appendicitis can present in a variety of ways, depending on the age of the patient, position of the appendix, cause of the appendicitis and any concurrent health issues. It may vary from a slow onset with vague abdominal pain, nausea, loss of appetite, or sometimes very acute with more sudden onset of pain. Typically the pain starts in the centre of the abdomen around the umbilicus and then over time becomes more localized to the right iliac fossa. If the appendix has perforated, then infected fluid may

have spread throughout the abdomen and the patient may report that whilst their pain had initially localized to the right iliac fossa, it may have spread throughout the abdomen again as they began to feel more unwell.

Systemic symptoms can include loss of appetite, nausea, vomiting, rigors, with signs including tachycardia, fever, tachypnoea, and with blood tests demonstrating a raised white cell count, especially neutrophilia and raised CRP. Importantly, normal blood tests and physical parameters do not necessarily exclude acute appendicitis.

Investigation and diagnosis. Whilst the diagnosis of acute appendicitis is a clinical diagnosis, given the variety of ways in which it can present there is often some uncertainty; in these cases radiological investigations can help either exclude other causes, such as an ultrasound to look for gynaecological causes (ovarian cysts, ovulation pain) in younger women or CT to exclude bowel tumours or diverticulitis in the more elderly.

Intervention. The main objective is to reduce the associated pain and infection by giving appropriate antibiotics and analgesics, and to replace fluid loss prior to surgery.

Surgical intervention. Appendicectomy is the management of an inflamed or infected appendix, because of the high risk of perforation leading to peritonitis, which can be life-threatening and constitutes a surgical emergency and will usually be performed laparoscopically.

Peritonitis (inflammation of the peritoneum)

The peritoneal cavity is a potentially sterile environment that, once contaminated by infected pus and bacteria, faecal fluid and products of digestion, becomes inflamed and irritated, producing copious amounts of serous fluid. This serous fluid and leakage from rupture or perforation has the potential of spreading throughout the peritoneal cavity, and, if bacteria are present, the resulting toxins will be absorbed through the peritoneum. Peritonitis is the end effect with a variety of causes, however all patients with peritonitis require urgent medical attention and intervention. Common causes include perforation along the course of the gastrointestinal tract, such as perforated duodenal ulcer or perforated sigmoid diverticulitis, or

---

Box 17.2 **Large bowel disorders**

Diverticular disease

- *Indications for surgery*: haemorrhage, perforation, peritonitis, abscess formation, fistula formation, obstruction.
- *Types of surgery*: Hartmann's procedure.

Large bowel obstruction

- *Indications for surgery*: cancer, diverticular disease, inflammatory bowel disease, benign tumours.
- *Types of surgery*: segmental resection of colon, abdominoperineal resection, colostomy formation, Hartmann's procedure, bypass surgery (palliative).

inflammation of the pancreas with leakage of digestive enzymes (pancreatitis).

Clinical manifestations. Pain associated with peritonitis can be very severe and immediate, although somewhat diffused at first. It is quickly followed by symptoms of shock with associated nausea, vomiting and loss of fluids and electrolytes. Body temperature is elevated, and the patient is extremely lethargic and weak. Initial increased motility of the gastrointestinal tract is evident, but this is followed by decreased activity known as paralytic ileus, a temporary loss of smooth muscle tone resulting in the abdomen becoming rigid and tender.

Investigations and diagnosis. Commonly a chest X-ray will be requested, this should be done if possible after the patient has been sitting up for at least 15 minutes so that any free gas within the peritoneal cavity will have had the chance to rise up through the abdomen to sit under the diaphragm and be detected once the chest X-ray is taken, seen as a rim of gas between the diaphragm and the liver on the right or stomach on the patient's left. Free gas on a chest X-ray will be able to demonstrate that there has been a perforation, but not necessarily the cause. Caution: if a chest X-ray is done soon after a patient has had an operation, especially laparoscopically, they will have free gas still within the abdominal cavity, which will be seen on an X-ray. Often a CT scan will be performed, which will be able to detect both free gas and often the underlying cause.

Surgical intervention. Peritonitis constitutes a surgical emergency, along with appropriate antibiotic therapy and fluid and electrolyte replacement. Often the patient will need an operation (with the exception of acute pancreatitis), with either a laparoscopy or laparotomy performed. Patients can often be profoundly unwell with peritonitis, and often more so following an operation, and consideration should be given as to whether the patient will require a period of time in intensive care or the high-dependency unit following their operation.

Colorectal carcinoma

Bowel cancer is the second most common cause of death from cancer in the UK and is responsible for over 10% of all cancer deaths (Cancer Research UK, 2016). Over 42,000 patients are diagnosed in the UK each year and is the fourth most commonly diagnosed cancer. Generally, the incidence of bowel cancer increases with age, peaking at ages 85−89, and is more common in Caucasians than Black or Asian people. Over half (57%) of patients diagnosed with bowel cancer will survive more than 10 years after their diagnosis, and the mortality rate from bowel cancer is predicted to fall by 23% from 2014 to 2023.

Aetiology and incidence. Colorectal carcinoma is commonest in people over the age of 60 years and has a slightly higher incidence in men, with 1 in 15 men and 1 in 18 women being diagnosed in their lifetime, but it is also becoming more common in younger patients. Generally, adenocarcinoma accounts for 90−94% of cases, and the theory is that a substantial number of colorectal cancers arise from adenomatous polyps, i.e. benign tumours that develop from normal colonic mucosa.

Cancer of the large bowel is due to a variety of factors: predisposing genetic factors, and dietary and environmental factors. Other risk factors include processed meat, drinking alcohol and eating too little fibre, as well as being overweight or obese. Smoking, ionizing radiation and too little physical activity are also associated with higher rates of bowel cancer.

Patients in whom there is a family history of bowel cancer may be at higher risk than the general population of developing bowel cancer. Someone with two first-degree relatives with bowel cancer will have a two-fold increase in the risk of being diagnosed with bowel cancer, and in approximately 10% of patients there will be specific mutations found, such as hereditary non-polyposis colorectal cancer patients (HNPCC, or often called Lynch syndrome). In certain families there are extremely high rates of developing bowel cancer with polyposis syndromes, and in whom there have been specific genetic mutations detected, with approximately 3% of patients who are diagnosed with colorectal cancer falling into this group.

HNPCC is due to inherited mutations in the DNA mismatch repair sequences. Slight variations of the mutation between families and patients causes variations in the incidence of bowel cancer and other associated cancers with this syndrome, such as endometrial, ovarian, small bowel, hepatobiliary, urinary and skin cancers. Over two-thirds of patients with HNPCC will eventually be diagnosed with colorectal cancer.

Polyposis syndromes contain a variety of inherited conditions, where genetic mutations lead the patient to develop hundreds, if not thousands, of adenomas within the GI tract and especially in the large bowel. Whilst these adenomas themselves are not malignant, they have a preponderance to eventually undergo malignant transformation, and the sheer number present makes those with the mutation at very high risk of developing colorectal cancer. The most common is familial adenomatous polyposis (FAP), where thousands of polyps line the entire large bowel. FAP is associated with a mutation in the *APC* gene. Patients with the gene mutation have a 7% risk of having developed colorectal cancer by the age of 21 and 93% by the age of 50. These patients and their families are usually counselled and offered a complete large bowel resection in early adulthood. Other polyposis syndromes include Peutz−Jeghers, familial juvenile polyposis, serrated polyposis syndrome and hereditary mixed polyposis syndrome, each with their own pattern of risk of colorectal and other associated cancers.

Despite the increasing awareness of genetic mutations associated with developing colorectal cancers, the majority of patients who are diagnosed will be sporadic, with no significant family history.

The general percentage distribution of the cancers within the large bowel is shown in Fig. 17.2. It can be seen that rectal/rectal—sigmoid cancers account for approximately 30% of cases reported, followed by 25% in the sigmoid colon (Cancer Research UK, 2016).

Colorectal cancers are classified using the TNM staging system, which is one of several classification systems and provides a more accurate description of the tumour itself and its relation to other organs than does the older Dukes' classification system. The tumours are classified into four stages, as shown in Box 17.3.

Clinical manifestations. Symptoms are often vague and often patients will have had symptoms for some time prior to presenting to their GP, with patient often embarrassed or attributing their symptoms to other causes such as haemorrhoids. Patients most commonly present with rectal bleeding, or a change in bowel habit; this may be either constipation, diarrhoea or alternating between the two. Even without overt rectal bleeding, patients may have an iron deficiency anaemia, either symptomatic with fatigue and shortness of breath, or more commonly through routine blood tests.

Some abdominal discomfort may occur, especially if the tumour is large and causing pressure on soft tissue and nerves, although this is less common as patients are often diagnosed prior to this.

Investigations. Investigation into patients with colorectal cancer involves confirming the diagnosis and determining staging. The TNM staging (Tumour Nodes Metastases) system incorporates the tumour's local extent, such as size and involvement in any adjacent organs, any lymph node involvement and the presence of any distant metastases. Confirmation of the diagnosis involves a biopsy of the tumour, usually via colonoscopy. A CT scan of the chest, abdomen and pelvis will allow assessment of the primary tumour as well as any nodal or metastatic disease, most commonly the lungs and liver. In rectal cancer, patients may additionally undergo an MRI of the pelvis as this is more suited to assessment of pelvic organs. Occasionally patients will need additional investigations in certain cases, such as PET CT (which is a sensitive method to detect small metastases throughout the body) or an MRI liver if there are unclear lesions on the CT scan that may be potential metastases.

Treatment options. Following staging, patients will often have their case discussed by a multidisciplinary team (MDT) to determine the best treatment options to put forward to the patient. The MDT will often incorporate the presence of colorectal surgeons, medical and clinical oncologists, specialist nurses, radiologists, pathologists, and other specialists, if required.

There are a variety of potential treatment options for patients with colorectal cancer depending on the disease extent and patient fitness. For patients without metastases, surgery by removing the segment of affected bowel is the mainstay of treatment, termed a resection. The principle of a colorectal resection is to remove the entire segment of bowel with the affected bowel, and supplying blood supply with its lymph nodes. This allows for full staging of

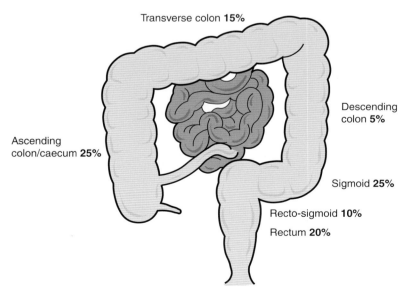

Transverse colon **15%**

Descending colon **5%**

Ascending colon/caecum **25%**

Sigmoid **25%**

Recto-sigmoid **10%**

Rectum **20%**

Figure 17.2 Distribution of cancers of the large bowel. (From Butcher (2003), with permission.)

Box 17.3 **TNM classification of stages of colorectal tumours**

Primary tumour (T)

Pathological staging

TX Primary tumour cannot be assessed
T0 No evidence of primary tumour
Tis Carcinoma *in situ*: intraepithelial or invasion of lamina propria
T1 Tumour invades submucosa
T2 Tumour invades muscularis propria
T3 Tumour invades through the muscularis propria into the subserosa, or into non-peritonealized pericolic or perirectal tissues
T4 Tumour directly invades other organs or structures and/or perforates the peritoneum

Ultrasound staging (u)

uT0 Benign tumour
uT1 Invasion into but not through the submucosa
uT2 Invasion into but not through the muscularis propria
uT3 Invasion into perirectal fat
uT4 Invasion into adjacent organs

Regional lymph nodes (N)

NX Regional lymph nodes cannot be assessed
N0 No regional lymph node metastasis
N1 Metastases in 1—3 regional lymph nodes
N2 Metastases in 4 or more regional lymph nodes
uN0 No metastatic perirectal node
uN1 Metastatic perirectal nodes

Distant metastases (M)

MX Distant metastases cannot be assessed
M0 No distant metastases
M1 Distant metastases

(From Taylor et al (2002).)

the tumour as well as reducing the chance of the tumour recurring. Surgery includes right or left hemicolectomy, transverse colectomy, anterior resection and abdomino-perineal excision of colon, depending on the position of the tumour (Figs. 17.3–17.6).

There are various routes via which a patient may undergo a bowel resection; traditionally this was via an open operation, termed a laparotomy, usually with an incision down the centre of the abdomen. More commonly now patients will be offered laparoscopic surgery, where the operation is typically performed with small incisions only, and usually the largest incision will be purely to accommodate the removal of the segment of bowel being resected. Other options now include single incision laparoscopic surgery, natural orifice surgery and robotic surgery.

Where there is a high-risk tumour or more extensive disease, patients may require additional treatment such as radiotherapy and/or chemotherapy, which may occur before or after surgery. In patients who are too unfit to undergo a bowel resection, other options are available, such as radiotherapy for rectal cancers or colonic stents to stop the bowel lumen from occluding. Patients with early tumours now may also undergo removal of the tumour from inside of the bowel with endoscopic or trans-anal procedures.

Screening. Patients have the best chance of survival, with no disease recurrence, if their bowel cancer is diagnosed at an earlier stage. The symptoms of bowel cancer, especially at an early stage, can be very mild or even absent. Screening is a method to try to detect bowel cancers in patients who may not have any symptoms, with the ability to detect even very early stage cancers and polyps. In England, Wales and Northern Ireland patients over 60, and in Scotland over 50 years old, up until the age of 75 are invited to take part in the national screening

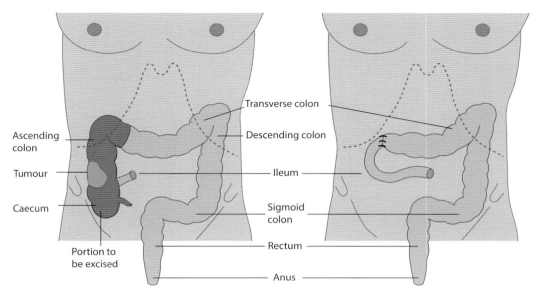

Transverse colon
Descending colon
Ascending colon
Tumour
Ileum
Caecum
Sigmoid colon
Rectum
Portion to be excised
Anus

Figure 17.3 Right hemicolectomy.

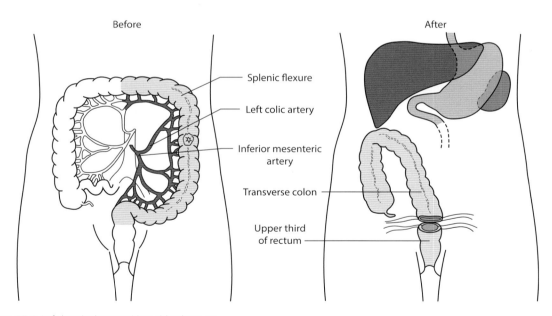

Before

After

Splenic flexure
Left colic artery
Inferior mesenteric artery
Transverse colon
Upper third of rectum

Figure 17.4 Left hemicolectomy/sigmoid colectomy.

programme. This involves a stool test which is designed to pick up even small amounts of blood and invite those patients to undergo a colonoscopy. In addition men and women aged 55 are offered a flexible sigmoidoscopy to detect lesions in the lower part of the large bowel. Both of these tests aim to diagnose patients at an earlier stage and thus improve the outcome for the patient and the general population.

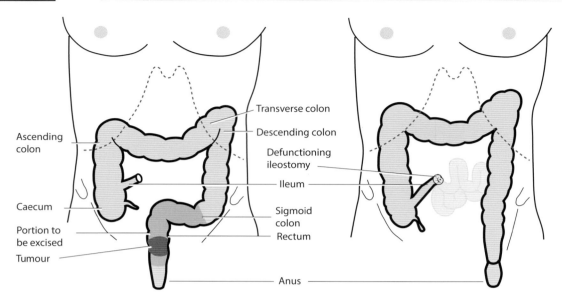

Figure 17.5 Anterior resection with defunctioning ileostomy.

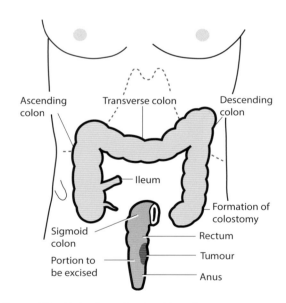

Figure 17.6 Abdominoperineal excision of rectum.

Pre- and postoperative care of patients undergoing colonic surgery

Specific preoperative assessment

Surgery is the most common treatment for colorectal cancer. The tumour is removed along with the surrounding margin of tissue. If early diagnosis and intervention occurs, patients with TNM stages 1 and 2 have a good prognosis, and do not require further treatment. Multidisciplinary teams are involved in providing the best care for patients, and the nurse is central to advocate for the patient, asses their needs and communicate discussions with the patient.

The nurse has an important role in facilitating and documenting the provision of information, teaching activities, physical examination, laboratory tests or diagnostic procedures, informed consent, psychological preparation, physical preparation of the gastrointestinal tract and skin, and administration of medications. These are important areas that enable the patient to proceed safely through surgery.

Bowel preparation may be indicated to prevent infection and remove faecal matter. This is achieved by administering an enema/colonic irrigation, or prescribed bowel preparation (polyethylene glycol, sodium picosulphate or phosphate solutions). During these procedures some patients may need careful monitoring, due to possible unpleasant side-effects and fluid loss (Box 17.4). See section on bowel preparation for colonoscopy.

Stoma formation and management

Stoma is the Greek term used to describe a mouth or opening – in this context an opening in the abdominal wall through which contents of the bowel are evacuated.

Colostomy. A healthy piece of colon is brought through an opening onto the abdomen. It may be referred to as single-barrel, double-barrel or loop colostomy that is supported by a rod, and can be temporary or permanent. A temporary colostomy is performed to give time for the colon to recover and heal prior to resuming its functions. A permanent colostomy is usually performed following removal of part of the bowel, particularly following removal of a malignant tumour. The position of the colostomy can vary according to the area of colon that is affected.

Nursing issues. Optimum management is for all patients who are to undergo bowel surgery and formation of a stoma have the condition and implications discussed with them and their family. However, in some emergency situations, this is not possible. In most hospitals a specialist nurse in stoma therapy is available for assessment, education and counselling both before and after surgery. The stoma therapist may also advise on the most appropriate position for formation of the stoma. Consideration should be given to position of the incision line, bones, scars, skin creases/folds/fat, activities of the patient and type of clothes the patient wears.

All patients who have a stoma formed should receive the appropriate educational material, which will enable them to understand what changes have occurred to their body, what activities they may safely pursue and how to deal with minor complications.

Specific postoperative nursing interventions

Eating and drinking. Oral fluids maybe restricted but should return to normal as soon as possible following surgery. A good indication to commence oral fluids and diet is when the patient has bowel sounds and passes flatus. It is important, therefore, that the patient receives intravenous fluids to replace fluid and electrolyte loss. There is

also a potential risk of paralytic ileus resulting from handling the bowel during surgery. This may be managed by resting the bowel. If the patient has resumed oral fluids, these maybe withheld, and intravenous fluids recommenced until bowel sounds again return.

The advice for patients with a colostomy is similar to that already described for patients with an ileostomy. However, depending on the stage of the disease and extent of surgery, some patients may need further nutritional supplements of protein, calories and carbohydrates.

Elimination. Particular management of the stoma has already been discussed in the section referring to the formation of an ileostomy. However, it is important that the patient is educated and given the option to choose which appliance to use, and how to remove and change the appliance. Supervision and education are usually provided by the stoma therapist together with nurses working in specialized colorectal surgical wards.

Change of body image and sexual activity. A major area of concern relates to the patient's acceptance of the colostomy from an early stage. Some patients may wish to discuss the aspect of sexual rehabilitation. Common fears are those of impotence and appearing mutilated and consequent effect on their sexuality. Examples have previously been given and are highlighted in Box 17.1.

Skin care. The risk to skin integrity around the stoma has already been discussed under management of an ileostomy. However, if the patient has a perineal suture line, there is an increased risk of wound infection or necrosis. This area is also very painful for the patient, due to the presence of sutures and drains; therefore, along with appropriate analgesics, a specialized cushion maybe used, for example, a Valley cushion.

Box 17.4 **Specific issues related to preoperative bowel preparation (if required)**

- Potential risk of infection if bowel is not adequately cleansed/operation cancelled due to inadequate preparation.
- Potential loss of fluid and electrolytes due to physical preparation/dehydration from the cleansing solutions.
- Potential risk of abdominal perforation caused by physical preparation.

Specific objective will be to ensure that the bowel is clean/clear prior to surgery and to minimize the side-effects of vomiting, abdominal pain and contamination.

Nursing intervention and rationale

- Ensure the physical cleansing preparation procedure is correctly carried out and instructions for any laxatives or irrigation carefully followed and monitored. The result of the preparation should be fully documented, and any difficulty in carrying out the procedure should be reported to the surgeon who is performing the surgery.
- All fluid loss associated with diarrhoea and vomiting should be recorded on appropriate documentation, thereby ensuring that fluid and electrolytes can be replaced by intravenous infusion. Antiemetics may be used to relieve excessive nausea and vomiting.
- Identify characteristics of the abdominal pain, e.g. location, duration and intensity, and provide appropriate analgesics, ensuring effectiveness is evaluated. Any associated discomfort through diarrhoea is relieved by ensuring the anal area is clean and dry following any bowel action and by providing anaesthetic creams and protective barrier creams.

Additional specific complications. Other complications include the risk of pulmonary complications, paralytic ileus, wound infection, stoma necrosis, and breakdown of the anastomosis/suture site.

Education and discharge planning

Educational advice is similar to that given for inflammatory bowel disease, especially if a colostomy has been formed. Instruction should be given as to how and when to change the appliance/pouch, irrigate the stoma if necessary, and clean the surrounding skin. Used appliances/pouches are disposed of by placing them in a sealed bag for refuse collection.

Dietary advice is important so that the patient can control the intake of certain foods that may give rise to excessive wind, constipation or loose bowel action.

Supportive literature and contact numbers may also be given for use in case of an emergency, or if the patient is worried about their condition and needs support and advice.

Rectal surgery

Polyps

Polyps occur from the mucous membrane and are small growth projections that are more common in the large intestine, i.e. sigmoid and rectum. They are often benign; however, they can be the precursor in the development of malignant polyps and cancer of the bowel. Fig. 17.7 illustrates the sequence of a benign polyp becoming malignant.

Clinical manifestations. Polyps are often asymptomatic, although they may bleed, and so the patient presents with rectal bleeding. Symptoms are determined by the number of polyps, position and size.

Investigations. These include rectal examination, proctoscopy, sigmoidoscopy, colonoscopy and occasionally CT scans specifically tailored to look at the lining of the large bowel (CT colonography).

Surgical interventions. Most polyps are able to be removed endoscopically, with the use of endoscopic instruments that can be passed down the working channel of a colonoscope. Polyps can be assessed using special light settings during colonoscopy, narrowband imaging, to assess their malignant potential and suitability for endoscopic resection. Endoscopically these suitable polyps can be removed, even if quite large, by specially trained endoscopists. Closer to the anal verge other options for removal of polyps are possible. Patients with large rectal polyps may be offered trans-anal minimally invasive surgery (TAMIS), where an operating port, similar to a large laparoscopy port, is inserted through the anal canal to allow the surgeons to operate on the rectum and remove lesions as needed. Sometimes neither of these approaches will be appropriate and patients may require bowel resections, particularly if a polyp is thought to be malignant.

Perianal abscess

An abscess is formed as a result of an infection forming in the tissues around the anal canal, either in the ischioanal fossa or closely related to the anal sphincters. These usually occur as a result of blocked anal glands, but can be part of underlying disease, such as Crohn's disease or tuberculosis.

Clinical manifestations. These include a very painful site, raised temperature and oedema. There may be an associated malodorous discharge from the rectum. Abscesses may be associated with a perianal fistula.

Intervention. This requires excision and drainage of the abscess. If a fistula has developed, this may require surgery at a later date. Antibiotics are rarely required, except where there is significant cellulitis and induration despite adequate surgical drainage.

Fistula

A fistula is an abnormal opening between two epithelial surfaces, but commonly in this condition it is an opening

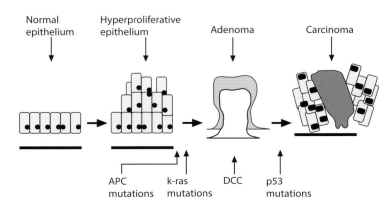

Normal epithelium Hyperproliferative epithelium Adenoma Carcinoma

APC mutations   k-ras mutations   DCC   p53 mutations

Figure 17.7 Polyp cancer sequence. Proposed adenoma to carcinoma sequence in colorectal cancer. Adenomatous polyposis coli (*APC*) gene mutations and hypermethylation occur early, followed by k-ras mutations. Deleted in colon cancer (*DCC*) and *p53* gene mutations occur later in the sequence, although the exact order may vary. (From Jones (1998), with permission.)

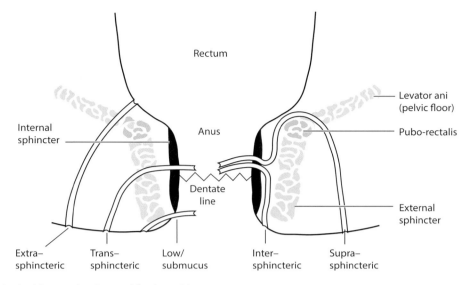

Figure 17.8 Anal sphincters showing anal fistula positions.

at the cutaneous surface near the anus (Fig. 17.8). Fistula is common in Crohn's disease, but most are caused by a local crypt abscess and infection.

Clinical manifestations. These include a rise in temperature and associated pain with a presenting abscess. Sometimes a rectal discharge is present, which often causes excoriation of the surrounding skin and pruritus.

Surgical intervention. This will often take the form of incision and drainage if there is an abscess, and excision or laying open of the fistula tract to allow healing by secondary intention. The insertion of a seton, or suture material threaded through the fistula tract, allows the tract to drain and it can then be laid open surgically (Hibberts & Carapeti, 2003). If the fistula tract contains too much anal sphincter beneath it to allow it to be safely cut open, then there are a multitude of other surgical options, each with their own benefits and drawbacks, with most having a failure rate of between 40% to 60% over time. Other approaches include fistula plugs, fistula glue, video-assisted debridement of the tracts, shortening the tract and either covering or clipping the internal openings. The key to surgical intervention is to eradicate the infection by facilitating drainage, however this must be weighed up with preserving continence. This is why careful examination and assessment of the amount of anal sphincter muscle involved is important. The anal sphincter complex is examined by endoanal ultrasound (structure) and anorectal physiology (function) (Hibberts et al, 2019; Solanki et al, 2019).

Fissure

A fissure is a tear in the lining of the lower anus, exposing the underlying anal sphincter. It is often due to straining on defecation with hard stools. A fissure will typically occur in the midline in most patients, either anteriorly or posteriorly, with the exception of patients with Crohn's disease in whom they may be at any orientation in the anal canal.

Clinical manifestation. There is extremely sharp pain on evacuation of faeces, so much so that patients often describe the sensation of trying to pass glass. It may be managed by local application of a nitrate gel, such as glyceryl trinitrate, or calcium channel blockers, such as diltiazem. These creams work by relaxing the anal sphincter, reducing the spasm and increasing the blood supply to heal it. Mild laxatives may be used initially to soften the stool and increased consumption of water to prevent constipation is advised. The patient should be shown correct toilet positioning: knees up higher than hips, elbows on knees and avoidance of straining.

Surgical intervention. This may sometimes be required, although many fissures resolve themselves. Operations to improve fissure healing include reducing the pressure in the lower anal canal, a sphincterotomy, either through chemical means by paralysing lower internal anal sphincter with an injection of Botox, or physically dividing/cutting the lower internal anal sphincter laterally, in order to relax the muscle at the point of the fissure. The implications of undergoing this type of surgery must be discussed with the patient as temporary or permanent faecal and flatus incontinence may result.

Haemorrhoids (piles)

These are cushions of spongy connective tissue and blood vessels in the anus which, with prolonged straining and hard stools, can descend down the anal canal and cause bleeding. Sometimes they become large enough to protrude from the anus and may become constricted, thrombosed and painful. This condition is associated with constipation and poor toilet positioning and technique, whereby straining to pass a stool increases the intra-abdominal pressure, resulting in their prolapse.

Clinical manifestations. There may be evidence of fresh blood and increased pain when opening the bowel and some patients describe a heaviness or itching of the anal canal during the day.

Investigations. These include digital rectal examination, proctoscopy and colonoscopy or sigmoidoscopy, mostly to exclude other more serious conditions.

Intervention. Many patients manage the condition themselves by local applications of topical medication to lubricate, anaesthetize and shrink the haemorrhoids. If medical advice is sought, this would include health promotion of a high-fibre intake and possibly a bulk laxative before consideration of surgery to remove external, thrombosed and strangulated haemorrhoids.

Surgical interventions. There are many options for surgical intervention in the management of haemorrhoids depending on their size and extent. Smaller internal haemorrhoids can be banded (small elasticated bands to shrink the haemorrhoids), and larger external ones ligated or excised with a haemorrhoidectomy.

Nursing implications. Nurses must be aware that straining to defecate and constipation contribute to the development of haemorrhoids. Pregnant women should be encouraged to remain free from constipation. Following any form of haemorrhoid surgery patients should be aware to monitor for excessive bleeding and avoid constipation and straining when opening their bowels for the first couple of weeks.

Complications. Haemorrhoids may rupture or thrombose, but most of these resolve spontaneously and conservative treatment is all that is required.

Pilonidal sinus

Pilonidal sinus is a blind-ending subcutaneous cavity communicating with the skin and may contain hair. It is most frequently situated over or close to the tip of the coccyx, in between the buttock cheeks in the natal cleft. Abscess formation is common following irritation and subsequent infection.

Clinical manifestations. These include pain and discharge associated with abscess formation, and often affect males during adolescence, and there is a strong familial component. Individuals who have a lot of hair in between their buttocks are also at greater risk of developing this.

Intervention. This includes a course of appropriate antibiotics and analgesics if there is no abscess present and only the presence of cellulitis. Abscesses should be drained surgically and the wound allowed to heal by secondary intention. Aims of elective surgery for pilonidal sinus are excision of the sinus and to reduce the

angulation of the natal cleft. Many techniques have been described, from simple laying open the sinus to primary suturing, and also various reconstructive flap techniques. Recurrence is common after surgery, and the more complex techniques, although more demanding, seem to result in a better outcome long term.

Education and discharge planning

Following rectal surgery, patients should be given advice on how to prevent further complications arising or indeed recurrence. It is important that they recognize that straining and constipation should be avoided; therefore, they must pay particular attention and defecate in response to the initial sensation. The risk of constipation will be lessened by increasing fibre intake in their diet, taking regular exercise and using medications (sparingly) to soften the stool. Patients should observe for any bleeding and seek help if this becomes severe or persistent. It is of particular importance that personal hygiene to the anal area is attended to frequently in order to avoid the risk of infection. Washing the area with warm water is soothing and cleansing and taking warm baths will reduce pain and keep the anal area clean and promote healing.

Enhanced recovery following colorectal surgery

Colorectal surgery led the way in enhancing patient recovery following surgery. In 1997, Professor Kehlet, Chief of Surgery in Denmark, led a multimodal programme that improved the outcomes following major surgery, reduced the complications following surgery and therefore reduced the length of stay in hospital for patients. 'Enhanced recovery', rapid or accelerated recovery, is a blanket term which encompasses a number of principles, with the ultimate aim of returning the patient back to their preoperative state without compromising any discharge criteria, so facilitating a speedier discharge from hospital and reduced complications. Enhanced recovery is a multidisciplinary approach to coordinating the patient's pathway preoperatively and continues post-discharge. The aims are to speed recovery of the patient by effective pre-assessment, early nutrition and early mobilization, and ultimately to shorten the length of hospital stay by lessening complications of decreased mobility, e.g. chest infections, pressure ulcers, deep vein thrombosis, and long periods of pre- and postoperative fasting which compromise nutrition and can slow down healing. Kehlet and Wilmore (2002), Nygren et al (2005, cited in Massen et al, 2007), and Wilmore and Kehlet (2001) were the original research papers, and the approach continues to be supported by the literature and NHS Enhanced Recovery (NHS, 2016).

The principles at each stage of the enhanced recovery programme are as follows:

Preoperatively

- Preoperative optimization, which also includes managing the patient's expectations and planning goals. Any nutritional deficits and issues addressed preoperatively will also assist in the patient's recovery.
- Cardiopulmonary exercise testing (CPET) to establish the patient's anaerobic threshold score, as it is an excellent predictor of mortality from cardiovascular causes (Levett et al, 2018). This then enables a decision to be made about where the patient will spend their first night postoperatively, e.g. back on the ward, overnight in intensive recovery, or in the intensive care unit.
- Pain control and assessment of current drug therapy, polypharmacy and co-morbidity.
- Nutritional assessment and referral to a dietitian preoperatively if necessary. Carbohydrate-loading drinks and supplements are given preoperatively.
- Discharge planning, so that the patient has a plan for going home/discharged back to the community/ returning to their norm.

On the ward: preoperatively

- No routine bowel cleansing. In certain operations the patient may have a rectal enema only. This significantly reduces the risk of electrolyte imbalance, dehydration and fluid balance issues (Birch, 2017; NHS, 2016). Carbohydrate loading drinks given preoperatively.
- Minimize preoperative fasting times.

In surgery

- Nasogastric tubes and pelvic drains are not used routinely (Ljungqvist & Hubner, 2018).
- Urinary catheters are removed the day after surgery (or slightly longer in rectal surgery); this significantly reduces the risk of urinary retention and longer-term urinary problems (Ljungqvist & Hubner, 2018). High thoracic epidural analgesia is more commonly used, to prevent complications of opioids, e.g. delayed gastric emptying and nausea, and paralytic ileus. Using a higher thoracic insertion also reduces the risk of motor block and further delays to returning to the patient's norm (Ljungqvist & Hubner, 2018).
- Laparoscopic/minimal invasive incisions and surgical techniques are the preferred choice. If open procedures are undertaken, then transverse incisions are used as opposed to midline incisions. This change of incision,

alone, reduces postoperative wound pain and reduces the physiological and surgical stress response of the body from the surgery. It also aids improved mobility as there are no large surgical wounds, and reduces the risk of wound infection.

- Intraoperative fluid management is by oesophageal Doppler monitoring, as this enables a more accurate fluid balance, preventing fluid overload and therefore facilitating a quicker recovery.

Postoperatively

- Return to normal nutrition as soon as possible should be encouraged, supplemented with high-energy drinks.
- Goal-orientated exercise is encouraged, e.g. time out of bed and walking.
- A goal-orientated diary should be completed by the patient.
- As there are fewer complications in the postoperative period, the patient will be discharged home sooner without changing traditional discharge criteria.
- After discharge, patients are telephoned and asked a number of standard questions which will highlight any potential complications or issues. This regular communication allows speedy access to the surgical team if any issues are identified, and so prevents re-admission to hospital (Birch, 2017).

All colorectal surgery, regardless of its complexity, and all patients, regardless of their co-morbidities, are suitable to go into an enhanced recovery programme. The programme may require adaptation; however, all patients should be able to reap some benefit. Due to the success of this programme internationally within colorectal surgery, the same principles are now routinely applied to other types of surgery, e.g. urology, upper gastrointestinal and gynaecology.

All specialist nurses should incorporate the principles of enhanced recovery within their practice and care of the patient, from preoperative assessment and preparation to postoperative pain, wound, stoma and nutrition care. Discharge planning is part of the nurse's responsibility and begins as soon as the decision for surgery is made (Birch, 2017).

SUMMARY OF KEY POINTS

- This chapter has described the pathophysiology of the lower gastrointestinal tract. Diagrams have been used to facilitate understanding and dysfunction of the organs and surgical interventions have also been discussed.
- Some guidance has been offered to assist the nurse to use a problem-solving approach in assessing, planning care, setting goals and initiating intervention for those

(Continued)

(cont'd)

patients who undergo surgery for a variety of disorders of the lower gastrointestinal tract.

- Finally, patient education and preparation for discharge has been highlighted, suggesting that it is necessary to focus on the importance of health promotion. Patient education plays an important part in preventing complications from arising and in dealing with the implications of failed surgery that may require further intervention.

REFLECTIVE LEARNING POINTS

Having read this chapter, think about what you need to know and what you still need to find out about. These questions may help:

- How do you make a referral to a clinical nurse specialist for a patient with a newly formed stoma?
- What is your role as coordinator of discharge planning?
- What are the advantages and disadvantages of preoperative bowel cleansing (preoperative bowel preparation)?

References

Alexander, M. F., Fawcett, J. N., & Runciman, P. J. (2006). *Nursing practice: hospital and home: the adult* (3rd edn.). Edinburgh: Churchill Livingstone.

Birch, J. (2017). What is an Enhanced Recovery Nurse? *Gastrointestinal Nursing*, 15(6), 43–50.

Butcher, G. P. (2003). Gastroenterology. *Edinburgh*. Edinburgh: Churchill Livingstone.

Cancer Research UK. (2016). Bowel cancer incidence by anatomical site. Available at: <www.cancerresearchuk.org/health-professional/cancer-statistics/statistics-by-cancer-type/bowel-cancer/incidence#heading-Four>

Chang, C. W., Wong, J. M., Tung, C. C., et al. (2015). Intestinal stricture in Crohn's disease. *Intestinal Research*, 13 (1), 19–26.

Department of Health and Social Care. (2009). Reference guide to consent for examination or treatment (2nd edn.). Available at: <www.gov.uk/government/publications/reference-guide-to-consent-for-examination-or-treatment-second-edition>

Hibberts, F., & Carapeti, E. A. (2003). Caring for the patient with an anal fistula. *Gastrointestinal Nursing*, 1(9), 26–28.

Hibberts, F., Deschamps, N., & Williams, A. (2019). Pelvic floor investigations for bowel dysfunction: part 1 endoanal ultrasound. *Gastrointestinal Nursing*, 16 (10), 19–25.

Jones, D. J. (1998). *ABC of Colorectal Diseases*. London: Wiley Blackwell.

Kehlet, H., & Wilmore, D. W. (2002). Multimodal strategies to improve surgical outcome. *American Journal of Surgery*, 183(6), 630–641.

Levett, D.Z.H., Jack, S., Swart, M., et al; Perioperative Exercise Testing and Training Society (POETTS). (2018). Perioperative cardiopulmonary exercise testing (CPET): consensus clinical guidelines on indications, organization, conduct, and physiological interpretation. *British Journal of Anaesthesa*, 120(3), 484–500.

Ljungqvist, O., & Hubner, M. (2018). Enhanced recovery after surgery: ERAS principles, practice and feasibility in the elderly. *Aging Clinical and Experimental Research*, 30(3), 249–252.

Lynch, W.D. & Hsu, R. (2018). Ulcerative colitis/NCBI online resource. Available at: <www.ncbi.nlm.nih.gov/books/NBK459282/>

Massen, J., Dejong, C. H. C., Hausel, J., et al. (2007). A protocol is not enough to implement an enhanced recovery programme for colorectal resection. *British Journal of Surgery*, 94(2), 224–231.

NHS. (2016). *Enhanced recovery*. Available at: <www.nhs.uk/conditions/enhanced-recovery>

Nursing and Midwifery Council. (2018). *The Code. Professional Standards of Practice and Behaviour for Nurses, Midwives and Nursing Associates*. Available at: <www.nmc.org.uk/globalassets/sitedocuments/nmc-publications/nmc-code.pdf>

Nygren, J., Hausel, J., Kehlet, H., et al. (2005). A comparison in 5 European centres of case mix, clinical management and outcomes following either conventional or fast track perioperative care in colorectal surgery. *Clinical Nutrition*, 24(3), 455–461.

Overbey, D., Govekar, H., & Gajdos, C. (2014). Surgical management of colonic perforation due to ulcerative colitis in pregnancy. *World Journal of Gastrointestinal Surgery*, 6(10), 201–203.

Royal College of Radiologists. (2013). *Radiation and the Early Fetus*. Available at: <www.rcr.ac.uk/system/files/publication/field_publication_files/BFCR%2813%294_radiation.pdf>

Shanmugam, V. K., Fernandez, S. J., Evans, K. K., et al. (2015). Post-operative wound dehiscence, predictors and associations. *Wound Repair and Regeneration*, 23(2), 184–190.

Solanki, D., Hibberts, F., Williams, A. (2019). Pelvic floor investigations for bowel dysfunction: part 2 anorectal physiology, 17(5), 24–31.

Taylor, I., Garcia-Aguilar, J., & Goldberg, S. (2002). *Colorectal Cancer – Fast Facts* (2nd edn.). Oxford: Health Press.

Williams, B. C. (2015). The Roper-Logan-Tierney model of nursing: A framework to complement the nursing process. *Nursing*, 45(3), 24–26.

Wilmore, D. W., & Kehlet, H. (2001). Management of patients in fast track surgery. *British Medical Journal*, 322 (7284), 473–476.

Further reading

Birch, J., & Black, P. (2017). *Essential Stoma Care*. Harrow: St Marks Academic Institute.

Cox, C., Steggall, M., & Coutts, A. (2012). *Fundamental Aspects of Gastrointestinal Nursing*. London: Quay Books.

Gastrointestinal *Nursing* journal. London: Mark Allen Group.

Ong, P., & Skittrall, R. (2017). *Gastrointestinal nursing: a lifespan approach*. London: Routledge.

Wicker, P., & O'Neill, J. (2011). *Caring for the Perioperative Patient* (2nd edn.). Oxford: Wiley.

Relevant websites

Colostomy support & information: www.colostomyuk.org

Ileostomy and Internal pouch support & information: iasupport.org

Crohn's and Colitis UK: www.crohnsand-colitis.org.uk

Guts UK Charity: gutscharity.org.uk

Chapter | **18** |

Patients requiring surgery on the renal and urinary tract

Janice Minter

KEY OBJECTIVES OF THE CHAPTER

After reading the chapter the reader should be able to:

- give an overview of the anatomy and physiology of the kidney and lower urinary tract
- list the functions of the kidney
- discuss renal and urological investigations and the preparation required by the patient
- describe the pre- and postoperative care for individuals undergoing surgery on the kidney and lower urinary tract
- discuss discharge advice that would be given to individuals following surgery on the kidney and urinary tract.

Introduction

During the last 30 years the field of urology has undergone extensive growth as a surgical specialty. As technological advancement has occurred, surgical intervention has moved away from conventional open procedures to minimally invasive and non-invasive surgery for a variety of nephro-urological conditions. The use of improved screening and diagnostic tools has, however, seen surgery for certain conditions become more radical, with an overall improved prognostic outcome. This chapter addresses the management and treatment of individuals with specific renal and urological conditions and explores the nursing interventions and care.

Anatomy and physiology of the urinary tract

The urinary tract consists of:
- two kidneys
- two ureters
- the urinary bladder
- the urethra.

The kidneys

In addition to their primary function of urine production, the kidneys perform a number of other vital functions:
- maintenance of fluid, electrolyte and acid–base balance
- assist the liver to detoxify poisons infiltrating the body
- excretion of drugs and poisons
- maintain adequate blood volume and blood pressure
- produce the hormone erythropoietin
- metabolize vitamin D to its active form (Velho & Velho, 2013).

The kidneys are situated on the posterior abdominal wall on either side of the vertebral column, between the twelfth thoracic and third lumbar vertebrae. The right kidney is normally slightly lower than the left due to displacement by the liver. The kidney is approximately 14 cm long, 6 cm wide and 3 cm thick, and weighs between 135 g and 150 g in adults. The adrenal glands are situated immediately above each kidney.

Each kidney is surrounded by a protective capsule made up of fibrous connective tissue, along with an additional layer of perinephric fat; these layers help to cushion and protect the organ against direct trauma. The renal arteries, renal veins, lymphatic supply and the nerves both enter and leave the kidney at the renal hilum, which is recognized as an indentation on the medial, concave border of the kidney. The funnel-shaped upper end of the ureter also enters at the hilum and expands to become the renal pelvis.

Two distinct areas lie beneath the capsule of the kidney: the outer cortex and the inner medulla body making up the renal parenchyma. Within the medulla there are 8–18 wedge-shaped structures evident, called the medullary pyramids. These drain into minor and then major calyces, which are hollow protrusions of the renal pelvis. The calyces distend as the urine collects within them, leading to peristaltic contraction of the smooth muscle in the walls of the calyces and renal pelvis. The urine is then projected forward from the renal pelvis into the ureter.

The nephron

The nephron is the functional unit of the kidney and each kidney contains approximately 1 million nephrons. The nephron consists of a 'tuft' of capillaries called the glomerulus and the renal tubule. The renal tubule can be subdivided into five distinct regions:

- The *Bowman's capsule* forms the spherical, dilated upper end of the tubule, which surrounds or invaginates the glomerulus. The glomeruli lie in the cortex of the kidney and originate from an afferent arteriole; once filtered, the blood then leaves the glomerulus via the efferent arteriole. The efferent arteriole, in turn, branches into a thick capillary network which surrounds the renal tubule and is involved in the reabsorption process. The entire structure is 150 mm in diameter with a vast glomerular capillary surface area of approximately 5000–15,000 cm^2 per 100 g of tissue. It is suggested that the glomerular capillaries are far more permeable to water and solutes than are the extrarenal capillaries. The capillary endothelium lies on a basement membrane and on the other side of the membrane rests the epithelium which lines the Bowman's capsule. The glomerular epithelium has foot-like structures

projecting from it known as pedicles; they lie on the basement membrane and are separated by filtration slits. Selective filtration is achieved within the first part of the nephron. In total, 170–180 L of plasma in 24 hours is filtered by the glomerulus at a rate of 125 mL/min; thus, the filtrate within the Bowman's capsule is an ultrafiltrate of plasma. The glomerular membrane is permeable to water and other small molecules but is not permeable to blood cells or to proteins, which are only filtered if the kidney is diseased. The glomerular filtrate has approximately the same pH, osmolarity and solute concentrations as plasma.

- The *proximal convoluted tubule* extends from the Bowman's capsule for a length of 12–14 mm and is lined throughout its length by columnar epithelial cells. These cells are adapted on the inner surface to create a border of microvilli (finger-like projections), which increases the surface area inside the proximal tubule, where most of the solute reabsorption takes place. The volume of glomerular filtrate is reduced by 75–80% in the proximal tubule, and active reabsorption of glucose, sodium, phosphate, chloride, potassium and bicarbonate occurs.

- The *loop of Henle* extends from the proximal convoluted tubule, dips down as the descending limb into the medullary region of the renal parenchyma, and forms a U-shape before coursing back up into the cortex via the ascending limb. The columnar cells within the loop of Henle are flatter and have fewer microvilli on the internal surfaces. Passive reabsorption of water, sodium and chloride takes place in the loop of Henle.

- The *distal convoluted tubule* extends from the ascending limb of the loop of Henle and is 4–8 mm in length. Reabsorption of water is controlled here by antidiuretic hormone, a secretion from the posterior lobe of the pituitary gland. The reabsorption of sodium is controlled by the secretion of aldosterone, a hormone secreted by the adrenal cortex.

- The *collecting tubule*—the distal convoluted tubule leads into the collecting ducts which pass through the renal medulla. Antidiuretic hormone secretion regulates reabsorption of water from the collecting tubules and is independent of sodium reabsorption.

The result of this complex process of filtration, selective reabsorption and secretion is the production of urine.

The ureters

The two ureters are hollow muscular tubes which extend from the renal pelvis to the posterior wall of the bladder, entering the bladder at its base. Each ureter is approximately 30 cm long, 6 mm in diameter and lies behind the peritoneum.

The wall of the ureter is composed of three layers:

- inner layer of transitional epithelium
- middle layer of thick muscle
- outer layer of connective tissue.

Peristaltic contractions in the muscle layer of the ureter propel the urine that has drained from the calyces into the renal pelvis and down the ureter into the bladder. The ureters enter the bladder at an oblique angle, thus preventing reflux of urine back along the ureter and into the kidney.

The bladder

The bladder lies low in the pelvis, expanding upwards and forwards in the abdominal cavity during filling, and is held in place by strong ligaments. In males, the bladder lies in front of the rectum and the bladder neck surrounds the prostate gland. In females, the bladder lies in front of the vagina and uterus (Turner, 2009).

At the base of the bladder is a small triangular area known as the trigone, representing the area between the two ureteric orifices and the internal urethral meatus. This area changes little in size during the filling stage but is highly sensitive to stretch and is the area irritated by the presence of foreign bodies, e.g. indwelling urinary catheters (Fillingham & Douglas, 2004).

The bladder is a smooth, distensible, muscular sac lined with mucosa that stores urine temporarily. It is lined with transitional cell epithelium which acts as a protective barrier and allows a stretch facility as it fills with urine. The second submucosal layer is constructed of connective tissue and is known as the lamina propria. The third layer consists of smooth muscle bundles, known as the detrusor muscle. The detrusor muscle contains both longitudinal and circular fibres, which are thought to be distributed throughout the bladder wall (Sam & LaGrange, 2018). The detrusor muscle has a unique function, as it facilitates stretch during the filling phase of the bladder (Turner, 2009). There is also a voluntary component in controlling the storage and emptying ability of this muscle. The superior surface of the bladder is covered by the peritoneum when empty, but during the filling phase the peritoneum lifts upwards and backwards and is therefore not a 'true' layer of the bladder.

The bladder and the urethra function together as a complex unit for the storage and expulsion of urine. The bladder neck differs in males and females and its role in the maintenance of continence is not clearly understood; however, it might have some impact on maintaining closure pressure while the bladder fills with urine.

The urethra – female

The function of the urethra is to convey urine from the bladder to the exterior. The female urethra is approximately 3–5 cm in length and lies anterior to the vagina. The external urethral meatus opens between the clitoris and vaginal orifice. The urethra is lined with transitional epithelium and with squamous epithelium nearer the external meatus. The external sphincter mechanism is made up of musculature within the urethra in conjunction with the levator ani muscle of the pelvic floor; these combined structures are paramount in the mechanical maintenance of urinary continence. The integral urethral muscle maintains urethral closure, and the pelvic floor muscle increases that closure capacity during a raise in intra-abdominal pressure, e.g. on coughing, laughing and jumping. It is important to note that urine is only found in the urethra during micturition, and during the filling phase of the cycle it remains empty and closed.

The male urethra will be discussed in Chapter 19.

Renal and urological investigations

Urinalysis

Simple urinalysis is a non-invasive test using a chemically impregnated strip to measure the urine pH and to detect the presence of blood, glucose, protein, bilirubin, urobilinogen, ketones, leucocytes and nitrites (Yates, 2016). It is important to use a clean container to collect a fresh specimen of urine for testing, so avoiding contamination of the specimen. The colour, consistency and smell of the urine should also be noted during routine analysis, and the findings documented. Some things to observe for are a cloudy appearance, an offensive or 'fishy' smell, blood and possibly mucus-like strands, which may all be indicative of a urinary tract infection.

Urine specimens for culture

If a urinary tract infection is suspected, the collection of urine for culture to identify the offending organisms is indicated. Ideally, a specimen should be obtained before antibiotic therapy is commenced. Urine specimens for culture are usually either a midstream specimen of urine (MSU) or a catheter specimen of urine (CSU) and should be collected in a way that avoids contamination of the specimen with new bacteria.

Midstream specimen of urine

The procedure should be explained to the patient to gain consent and to provide reassurance. The patient is asked to clean the prepuce or vulva (according to local policy), and then to collect the middle part of the void in a sterile container; this is to reduce the number of contaminants in the specimen. It is argued by a number of researchers that cleansing prior to collection is unnecessary, as routine cleansing appears to make little difference in contamination rates (Leaver, 2007). It is also suggested that many patients fail to understand what is required, making the specimen invalid (Fillingham & Douglas, 2004).

The urine should be sent to the laboratory as soon as possible, with the specimen labelled correctly and accompanied by the appropriate investigation request form. Rapid growth of microorganisms will occur at room temperature and lead to an invalid culture; therefore, specimens should be kept refrigerated at 4°C if transport is delayed.

Catheter specimen of urine

A specimen of urine is obtained by withdrawing 3–5 mL of urine via the 'sampling port', found in the catheter drainage system. The equipment used must be sterile and in most instances a needle and syringe is required. The specimen is then transferred to a sterile container for transit to the laboratory. Some local policies recommend that a sterile swab (chlorhexidine based) is used to clean the sample port before and after use (Fillingham & Douglas, 2004).

Early morning urine

The first urine voided in the morning is collected for three consecutive days. Early morning urine (EMU) is more concentrated and therefore provides a better medium to locate specific types of cells, e.g. tuberculosis or malignant cells.

24-hour urine collection

This is the collection of the total volume of urine voided in a 24-hour period and is of value in the diagnosis of a number of renal and urological conditions, e.g. renal calculi/stone disease and impaired renal function. The patient is asked to void, the time is noted and this first specimen is discarded. All urine voided for the next 24 hours is collected in a large specimen container. The patient is asked to void at the end of the 24 hours, and this specimen is included in the collection. Care should be taken not to spill any preservative present in some of the containers, as it may be corrosive.

It is essential that *all* the urine collected in this time frame is kept, as the overall results will be invalid if an incomplete picture is presented. It is important that the nurse and patient have a full understanding of the procedure.

Urinary flow rate

This test measures the rate and volume of urine voided in millilitres per second and is an important investigation to support in the management of the individual with urinary outflow problems (British Association of Urological Surgeons, 2017a). Various types of equipment can be used to measure the flow rate, e.g. rotating disc or dipstick, and all entail the individual voiding into the funnel of a monitoring machine.

Preparation of the patient involves:
- full explanation of what the procedure entails
- ensuring a comfortably full bladder, but avoiding overdistension and consumption of large volumes of fluid prior to the investigation
- instructing the patient to void into the flow rate machine
- maintaining privacy while the patient voids.

Ideally, patients should produce a series of three successive flow rates in order for a more accurate assessment (Fillingham & Douglas, 2004).

Table 18.1 Blood tests	
Blood test	**Rationale**
Haemoglobin	Reduced in anaemia, which may occur as a result of urinary tract bleeding, e.g. in bladder or kidney cancer
White blood cells	Raised in infection, e.g. urinary tract infection
Urea, creatinine and electrolyte estimation	Relates to renal function, e.g. creatinine is raised in renal impairment or failure
Prostate-specific antigen	Raised in prostate cancer
Liver function tests	Performed in suspected liver metastases
Calcium	Raised levels may correlate with stone formation
Blood group	Blood transfusion may be required before, during or after surgery
Clotting screen	Particularly important if patient is taking anticoagulants

Blood tests

Blood analysis is an important part of the investigation of the individual requiring surgery for a renal or urological condition. Blood tests commonly performed are shown in Table 18.1.

Renal function studies

Evaluation of renal function includes measurement of plasma urea and creatinine. Renal damage may occur before plasma urea and creatinine levels rise; therefore, creatinine clearance (normally 125 mL/min), which closely correlates to the glomerular filtration rate (GFR), is a more reliable indicator of renal function. This is calculated from measurement of urine volume, plasma creatinine and urine creatinine. Twenty-four hour urine collection and a blood sample are also required.

Radiological investigations

Plain abdominal X-ray of kidneys, ureters and bladder

A plain abdominal X-ray is taken, to include the kidneys, ureters and bladder (KUB). This is particularly useful for detecting urinary calculi (90% are radio-opaque). It is also useful immediately prior to surgery for stone removal, to check on stone location.

Intravenous urogram

An intravenous urogram (IVU) is a commonly performed urological investigation for the individual with renal stones, haematuria, urinary tract infection or a urinary tract tumour. Following a plain abdominal film, contrast medium containing iodine is injected intravenously and a series of films taken as the contrast medium is excreted by the kidneys and through the urinary tract.

The preparation of the individual varies between departments. It is also dependent on the individual's general health and whether other medical conditions are present, e.g. diabetes, impaired renal function. A full explanation of the procedure must be given and time taken to answer any queries. Patients are normally fasted for 4−6 hours and the bowel should be clear of faecal matter to avoid obscuring the film with air and colon content. If bowel preparation is required, the method employed should follow individual patient assessment and local policy/protocol.

An allergic reaction to iodine in the contrast medium can be severe and may result in cardiac arrest. X-ray departments must be fully equipped for cardiac/respiratory resuscitation. Approximately 20% of patients do experience some reaction, such as nausea or skin irritation, to the contrast medium. It is therefore vital that any history of allergy is highlighted before the procedure is undertaken.

Renal scanning (renogram)

In this procedure, radioisotope-labelled substances that are known to be selectively taken up and excreted by the kidney are injected intravenously. The compound used is then detected and measured by a gamma camera, and information regarding kidney function is obtained, e.g. structure and function of the kidneys and differential kidney function.

The patient should be given adequate information and support prior to undergoing the procedure, and instructions regarding disposal of urine following the scan must be made clear to the patient and ward/departmental staff. Most nuclear medicine departments will provide instructions on the appropriate disposal of urine.

Computerized tomography

In computerized tomography (CT) scanning, specific areas of the body are X-rayed at different angles using high-resolution imaging. Two-dimensional cross-sectional images are reconstructed by computer. In urology it is a particularly useful investigation when planning management/treatment of renal, prostate, testicular and bladder tumours.

Patient information prior to the procedure is of the utmost importance, as the machinery used can be very claustrophobic due to the confined space, and many patients find this distressing.

Ultrasound scan

High-frequency sound waves are transduced through a probe over the area being investigated, e.g. kidney, bladder. The reflected image is analysed by computer and displayed on a monitor.

Ultrasound scanning is a useful and valuable diagnostic investigation as it can differentiate between solid and cystic masses and is used to assess urinary tract obstruction, e.g. hydronephrosis, urinary outflow obstruction.

Patient preparation for ultrasound is minimal. An explanation of the procedure, which is non-invasive in most instances, must be given. When undertaking bladder ultrasonography, it should be noted that the bladder lies low in the pelvis when empty and expands upwards and forwards in the abdomen when it fills; a full bladder is therefore important in order for the sound waves to be transmitted. If the patient has a urinary catheter *in situ*, it should be clamped for approximately 1 hour prior to the investigation and the patient asked to drink moderate volumes of fluid to aid the bladder-filling process.

Retrograde pyelography

This procedure is usually performed under general anaesthetic following cystoscopy. A small-bore catheter is passed up the ureter to the renal pelvis; contrast medium is injected into the upper renal tract and X-rays taken of the renal pelvis and pelviureteric junction (British Association of Urological Surgeons, 2017b).

Retrograde pyelography is a useful investigation in the management of patients with a suspected obstruction within the upper urinary tracts. It may also be used to obtain urine samples from each kidney, e.g. for cytological analysis in patients with suspected renal carcinoma.

Preparation of the patient is as for a general anaesthetic. Following the procedure, the patient should be observed for any signs or symptoms of urinary tract infection, which can occur as a result of instrumentation of the urinary tract, i.e. loin pain, pyrexia and pain on voiding. Allergic reaction to the contrast medium also needs to be observed for.

Antegrade urography

Antegrade urography is performed when an obstructed ureter has been diagnosed or is suspected. Ultrasound is used to locate the renal pelvis. A fine-bore needle is inserted into the renal pelvis and a cannula passed over the needle to allow contrast medium to be injected and X-rays taken. If an obstruction is diagnosed, a nephrostomy tube can be placed to allow drainage of urine from the renal pelvis. If a patient is nervous, a pre-procedure sedative may be given, and analgesics will be required afterwards (Fillingham & Douglas, 2004).

Renal arteriography

Renal arteriography involves injection of contrast medium through a fine catheter, which is inserted into the femoral artery and passed via the abdominal aorta to the renal artery. A series of X-rays can then be taken. The films give an outline of the renal blood supply and are useful in the diagnosis of renal artery stenosis and renal tumours.

Although the procedure is performed under local anaesthesia with sedation, it is highly invasive. If complications arise, further intervention may be necessary; therefore, the patient is fasted for 4−6 hours. A full explanation of what to expect is given to the patient and informed consent obtained. Following the procedure, bedrest is maintained for up to 12 hours, as there is a risk of haemorrhage from the puncture site. If leakage occurs at the femoral artery puncture site, a longer period of bedrest may be necessary. Pedal pulses in the foot are checked to evaluate peripheral blood supply, and blood pressure, pulse, puncture site and capillary return are monitored half-hourly initially until stable (Beynon & Nicholls, 2004).

Renal biopsy

Renal biopsy may be undertaken in the assessment of the individual with renal disease. The procedure can be performed under X-ray control, ultrasound or CT scanning, and a local anaesthetic is used to anaesthetize the area down to the kidney capsule. Preparation of the patient involves obtaining informed consent following a full explanation of the procedure.

Blood specimens pre-procedure are obtained for:
- full blood count
- clotting screen
- blood group and save serum for crossmatch.

In some centres it is advocated that bedrest is maintained for 24 hours following the procedure. Blood pressure and pulse are recorded half-hourly initially and at reduced intervals thereafter if within the patient's normal parameters. A good fluid intake should be encouraged following the procedure (if not medically contraindicated) and observations made of urine output, noting any haematuria.

Cystoscopy

Cystoscopy involves direct visualization of the bladder and urethra and is undertaken in the individual with a urological problem, e.g. haematuria, lower tract obstruction, or follow-up check cystoscopy for bladder cancer. A rigid or flexible cystoscope is used, and the procedure is performed under either a local or general anaesthetic. The bladder is examined and, if abnormal, biopsies are taken for histological examination. Preparation of the patient involves obtaining informed consent following a full explanation of the procedure. The patient is prepared for either a general or local anaesthetic. Following the procedure, patients might experience urethral discomfort and voiding difficulties. The patient is encouraged to drink 2−3 L in 24 hours (unless medically contraindicated), and the urine should be examined for evidence of haematuria. Any pre-existing urinary tract infection is treated with prophylactic antibiotics.

Specific investigations relating to surgical interventions are summarized in Table 18.2.

Nursing assessment of the individual requiring surgery for a urological condition

The initial patient assessment provides an ideal opportunity for the nurse to establish the nurse−patient relationship. The way in which the patient is approached when the patient attends the preadmission clinic or on admission to the ward is extremely important. The patient

Table 18.2 Specific investigations related to surgical interventions on the kidneys or urinary tract

Surgical intervention	Investigation
Pyeloplasty	Intravenous urogram — this will confirm diagnosis by demonstrating hydronephrosis on the affected side Renogram — this will measure overall contribution of the obstructed kidney to renal function Urea and electrolyte estimation — to determine renal function Full blood count — to exclude anaemia and treat infection prior to surgery Group and crossmatch — blood will be available if required
Nephrectomy	Blood • group and crossmatch 2–4 units • urea and electrolyte estimation • full blood count • clotting screen Midstream specimen of urine Intravenous urogram Ultrasound Renogram Computerized tomography (CT) scan
Laparoscopic nephrectomy	Blood • group and crossmatch 2 units • urea and electrolyte estimation • full blood count • clotting screen Intravenous urogram Ultrasound Midstream specimen of urine ECG
Percutaneous nephrolithotomy	Urea and electrolyte estimation — to assess renal function Full blood count — to exclude anaemia Clotting screen — it is important to establish prior to the procedure that the patient does not have a clotting disorder nor is taking aspirin/anticoagulants regularly Group and crossmatch 2 units of blood — blood will be available should the patient require transfusion Midstream specimen of urine — if a urinary tract infection is present, the appropriate antibiotics can be prescribed Intravenous urogram — this will demonstrate the location and size of the stone and whether it is causing an obstruction Plain abdominal X-ray — this is done prior to the procedure, to show location of the stone
Extracorporeal lithotripsy	Blood clotting screen, urea, creatinine and electrolyte estimation Midstream specimen of urine Blood pressure recorded Kidney, ureter and bladder X-ray to locate current position of stone
Cystectomy and ileal conduit urinary diversion	Blood • urea and electrolyte estimation • liver function tests • full blood count • group and crossmatch 6 units • blood glucose • clotting screen

(Continued)

Table 18.2 Specific investigations related to surgical interventions on the kidneys or urinary tract—cont'd

Surgical intervention	Investigation
	Urine • midstream specimen of urine • cytology Chest X-ray ECG Ultrasound of kidneys/bladder or intravenous urogram CT scan

interview and collection of patient information should be done in an environment that provides privacy and maintains confidentiality. The nurse must use good clear communication, as this may be able to allay fears, minimize discomfort and enable individual adjustment (Dougherty & Lister, 2015).

An assessment should explore the patient as a 'whole' being, addressing physical, psychological, emotional, social and cultural needs; the impact of the patient's urological condition on these needs should then be established. Patient assessment is usually performed using a 'model of nursing' and various assessment frameworks that are relevant to the patient experience and/or need.

The assessment undertaken will gather information that includes the following:
- Recording of baseline observations:
  - temperature
  - pulse
  - respirations
  - blood pressure
  - urinalysis
  - weight
- Relevant personal details, including past medical and surgical history.
- Current health status: how well does the patient feel?
- Breathing: does the individual have any respiratory problems? How much exertion causes breathlessness?
- Eating/drinking: is the patient overweight/underweight? What is their usual fluid intake in 24 hours, and what type of fluid do they normally drink? Fluid intake is particularly important for the individual experiencing urinary frequency and urgency, or those with renal stones and/or recurrent urinary tract infections.
- Level of independence/dependence and home circumstances: it is important to establish whether help will be required during the convalescent period after surgery, so that the best possible arrangements can be organized.

- Is the urological condition causing/contributing to mobility problems? The individual with carcinoma of the prostate might have metastatic bone disease causing pain and often restricted mobility.

Elimination

For many patients this is a very sensitive and often embarrassing subject to discuss, but one very much impacted upon by urological disease. A voiding history should be undertaken, which includes information on patients' experiences of urinary frequency, urgency, hesitancy, dysuria, nocturia and haematuria. Patients should be asked to describe their urinary stream when voiding: is the stream strong, do they have to strain to void, do they feel empty on completion? Is urinary leakage or urinary incontinence a problem? Many patients find this a disturbing disease symptom and hide their problem from society, family, friends, and even from themselves (Fillingham & Douglas, 2004). Patients often need support, empathy, clear guidance and good clinical advice when tackling this urinary symptom. Signs and symptoms of urinary tract infection also need to be observed for, e.g. pyrexia, dysuria and offensive-smelling urine. Bowel habits/function should also be assessed, as constipation can be a major contributing cause of urinary symptoms.

Sleeping

Sleep is often affected in some patients experiencing urinary tract disease. In the initial assessment it should be established if sleeping is interrupted by the need to void, and, if so, how many times the patient needs to get up at night.

Body image/expressing sexuality

Urological disease and various types of incontinence can significantly affect patients' quality of life as it can affect both their physical and psychological needs (Stewart, 2018). Sensitivity is required when exploring this issue, although it is paramount that the nurse addresses and guides the patient through this care activity and does not take the easy route of avoidance. It should be established if the patient is sexually active, as some minor and intermediate urological procedures can have a direct impact on sexual function. Retrograde ejaculation is often experienced following transurethral resection of the prostate gland or bladder neck incision, which could render the patient infertile. There is also the risk of impotence/erectile disorder following surgery to combat both bladder and prostatic cancer. Having a urethral catheter *in situ* following surgery impacts on sexual function, but also might have a more profound effect on the patient's personal body image. Sexual function and activity, and the impact of surgical intervention, are topics that the surgical nurse should be able to tackle with all patients in their care (RCN, 2018).

Surgical interventions on the kidney

Pyeloplasty

Pyeloplasty is the operation performed through a loin incision, or via a laparoscopic approach, to relieve an obstruction at the pelviureteric junction, often caused by a ring of fibrous tissue (Fig. 18.1). The defect can be a congenital anomaly or the result of repeated infection or injury; this results in dilatation within the renal pelvis due to a narrowed ureter, inhibiting the free flow of urine.

Signs and symptoms of pelviureteric junction obstruction include:
- loin pain, often associated with a large fluid intake
- infection, due to stasis of urine in the renal pelvis
- nausea and vomiting
- impaired renal function.

Specific preoperative nursing care

Psychological/communication
A full explanation is given of what to expect pre- and postoperatively, and time is taken to answer any questions and allay any fears the patient might have.

Controlling body temperature
Any pre-existing urinary tract infection should be treated with an appropriate antibiotic.

Specific postoperative nursing care

Pain control/communication
The surgical approach is a loin incision, and pain control is particularly important if complications due to reduced mobility are to be avoided. It has been shown that a continuous intravenous or subcutaneous opioid infusion, or patient-controlled analgesia (PCA) provides improved postoperative pain relief for the majority of patients (Wood, 2010). The patient's pain should be assessed and then the patient is assisted into a position in which they feel comfortable. The wound drain, nephrostomy tube (if present) and urethral catheter should be secured to avoid dragging and causing unnecessary pain.

Breathing
It is important that the physiotherapist's teaching of deep breathing exercises is reinforced by nursing staff, because the position of the surgical incision is such that the individual is at risk of developing a chest infection. The patient should be observed for signs of respiratory depression. This is particularly important if an opioid infusion is used to control pain.

Bleeding and shock
The kidney is highly vascular, and therefore carries a risk of haemorrhage. To monitor for signs of shock, blood

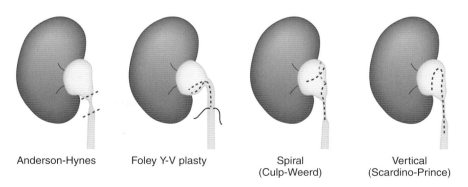

Anderson-Hynes   Foley Y-V plasty   Spiral (Culp-Weerd)   Vertical (Scardino-Prince)

Figure 18.1 Types of pyeloplasty. (Reproduced from Khan et al (2014).)

pressure and pulse should be recorded half-hourly. The frequency of the checks can be reduced as the patient's condition allows.

Eating and drinking

Intravenous fluid replacement is necessary in the initial postoperative period. Fluids and diet can be gradually reintroduced when bowel sounds are present. An appropriate antiemetic should be prescribed and administered if the patient feels nauseous.

Elimination

An accurate fluid balance is maintained to avoid dehydration/overhydration. The colour and consistency of the urinary output should be observed for blood loss, as a blood transfusion may be necessary if haematuria persists. The patient will have either a nephrostomy tube or a double-J stent *in situ*.

Nephrostomy tube. A nephrostomy tube allows external drainage of urine from the renal pelvis. The tube must be kept patent to avoid overdistension of the renal pelvis and the associated potential breakdown of the new surgical anastomosis. Dressings to the site should be performed aseptically with a non-adherent dressing, and then secured to avoid kinking or accidental removal of the nephrostomy tube. Approximately 10–12 days after surgery the tube is clamped for 24 hours, and if the patient does not experience pain or develop pyrexia, the tube is removed. In some centres a nephrostogram is performed prior to clamping, to ensure healing has taken place and the ureter is patent. Any leakage of urine from the nephrostomy tube site should subside within 24 hours. If urinary leakage persists, a drainage bag, e.g. a urostomy bag, can be applied to the site. The patient is reassured that the drainage will decrease and a dressing can then be applied.

Double-J stent. The double-J stent extends from the kidney down the ureter and into the bladder. The stent is normally left *in situ* for up to 3 months. Following stent insertion, the patient may experience urinary frequency, urgency and haematuria. Suprapubic pain or discomfort can also be a problem. An increased fluid intake is encouraged and oral analgesics given for pain/discomfort. These symptoms should resolve within 48 hours. The patient will attend day surgery for stent removal under a local anaesthetic.

Patient education and advice on discharge will be discussed following the section on nephrectomy.

Nephrectomy

Nephrectomy is the surgical removal of the kidney, and is performed through a loin incision, abdominal incision or laparoscopic route.

Indications for nephrectomy include the following:

- Renal cancer – this accounts for around 9% of all urothelial cancers and includes disease of the renal

parenchyma and the urothelium. Within the renal parenchyma, adenocarcinoma accounts for around 80% of disease, with nephroblastoma (Wilms' tumour) making up another 15%. Within the urothelium of the renal pelvis and the ureter, transitional cell carcinoma accounts for the highest percentage of disease. Surgery in all cases may be radical and involve removal of the kidney, adrenal gland, perinephric fat, lymph nodes, ureter and removal of tumour from the inferior vena cava.
- Non-functioning kidney – this may be as a result of a chronic infection that has destroyed renal tissue.
- Renal injury, causing haemorrhage.
- Live donor renal transplant.

Specific preoperative nursing care

Psychological/communication

The prospect of losing a kidney is extremely worrying for most individuals, as they are concerned about what will happen if the other kidney becomes diseased or injured. Time must be taken to address these psychological concerns, and provide the patient with appropriate and accurate information in the process of gaining informed and evidence-based consent.

Specific postoperative nursing care

Maintaining a safe environment

There is a potential risk of haemorrhage due to the highly vascular nature of the kidney. The wound dressing and wound drain(s) should be observed for blood loss. The amount of wound drainage is measured and recorded. The wound drain is removed when 24-hour drainage is less than 50 mL. Blood pressure and pulse are recorded quarter- to half-hourly initially and the frequency reduced as the patient's condition dictates.

Pain control/communication

Pain control after nephrectomy is crucial, as uncontrolled pain can lead to increased anxiety and muscle tension, which further exacerbate pain. The recovery process can be delayed, as the open surgical approach leaves the patient with a large incision/wound that can cause problems associated with reduced mobility, e.g. deep vein thrombosis, and risk of chest infection (Dougherty & Lister, 2015). To avoid the patient experiencing severe pain and discomfort, pain assessment and management must be effective. A continuous intravenous, subcutaneous or epidural opioid infusion can be most useful in controlling pain. Patient-controlled analgesia gives patients independence and involvement in their pain management. However, patients who receive PCA following surgery must be able to understand the concept and be willing to follow instructions for using the device (D'Arcy, 2008).

Breathing

The loin incision, below the level of the twelfth rib, is in close proximity to the diaphragm, pleura and the muscles involved in respiration. This contributes to the potential risk of respiratory problems in the postoperative period. The respiratory rate and effort must be observed and recorded, and any problems acted upon quickly. It is important to reinforce the physiotherapist's teaching of deep breathing exercises and to encourage the patient to cough; good positioning and effective analgesia are important in achieving this. As soon as their general condition allows, patients should be nursed in an upright position to further aid chest expansion. Pneumothorax is a complication associated with this surgery, and therefore regular respiratory monitoring is an essential component of the nurse's observation of the patient.

Elimination

An accurate fluid balance must be maintained to provide an early indication of dehydration or fluid overload. The presence of a urethral catheter allows accurate measurement of urinary output, and is necessary for bladder healing to take place at the area where the ureter has been incised if a radical procedure has been performed. Hourly urine volumes are measured initially, and if output falls below 30 mL/hr, medical staff should be informed. The urethral catheter will normally remain in situ for between 48 and 72 hours.

Eating and drinking

Intravenous fluid replacement is necessary in the initial postoperative period. Fluids and diet can be gradually reintroduced, normally on the day or following postoperative day. An appropriate antiemetic should be prescribed for nausea and vomiting.

Complications

Complications of nephrectomy include the following:

- *Haemorrhage/shock*: this is caused by a reduction in circulating blood volume.
- *Pneumothorax*: the pleura may be damaged during the procedure, resulting in a pneumothorax. This can occur when the procedure has been difficult. On return to the ward the patient will have an underwater seal chest drain in situ.
- *Chest infection*: this is often as a result of poor chest expansion after surgery and may be a consequence of inadequate pain management.
- *Wound infection*: this may result if a pre-existing infection has not been treated appropriately, or if bacteria are introduced during changing of the wound dressing.
- *Urinary tract infection*: the presence of a urethral catheter increases the incidence of urinary tract infection.

- *Deep vein thrombosis*: this may be as a result of reduced mobility. The wearing of thromboembolic deterrent (TED) stockings (Dougherty & Lister, 2015) and prophylactic anticoagulant administration can help to reduce the risk of a thrombosis occurring.

Laparoscopic nephrectomy

Laparoscopic nephrectomy is a well-accepted technique for treating a renal malignancy. The procedure is performed under a general anaesthetic and involves three or four small abdominal incisions being made to provide access for surgical instruments through one of the port sites which is used to detach the kidney and ligate the blood vessels. The intact kidney is enclosed in a bag and removed through an incision, or placed in an impermeable sac and removed through one of the port sites (NICE, 2005).

Open nephrectomy has inherent operative and postoperative complications. The main advantages of laparoscopic nephrectomy are claimed to be shorter operation time, less blood loss, quicker mobilization, less postoperative pain, shorter hospital stay and thus earlier resumption (Anderson, 2008).

Robotic nephrectomy

Robotic surgery is an extension of laparoscopic surgery, with advantages that overcome some of the drawbacks of laparoscopy. It is a recent innovation in urology developed in the USA. During a robotic procedure, the surgeon sits at the console; while watching the monitoring system, the surgeon moves the handles in the directions he/she wants to move the surgical instruments. The surgeon has a range of motion and fine tissue manipulation characteristic of open surgery, but it is performed though small keyhole ports. It gives the surgeon enhanced 3D visualization, improved dexterity, precision and access, and increased range of movement and reproducibility (Ogden, 2016). The patient may experience similar benefits to laparoscopic surgery, including reduced hospital stay, less blood loss, less scarring, reduced postoperative pain, and faster recovery and return to normal activities.

Specific patient education and advice on discharge following nephrectomy/ pyeloplasty

Written information should be available, which is given in addition to individual verbal advice by nursing and medical staff. Understanding should be evaluated and information reinforced as necessary.

Advice is given regarding the following:

- *Rest and activity*: the patient may feel weak and tired after surgery and should be aware that this is expected. As their strength returns, activity should be increased, with the aim of returning to a normal routine within 3–4 weeks.
- *Wound healing*: before discharge the patient will be informed whether the sutures are dissolvable or will need to be removed. If sutures are to be removed, an appointment should be made with the practice nurse at the GP's surgery or with the district nursing service, usually 7–10 days postoperatively. The patient is instructed regarding the need to observe the wound for signs of infection, e.g. redness, discharge. Appropriate dressings are provided if required.
- *Elimination*: the patient is advised to drink 2 L in 24 hours (unless medically contraindicated). If signs of urinary tract infection occur, e.g. pain/burning when voiding, urinary frequency or pyrexia, then the GP should be consulted and an appropriate antibiotic prescribed if indicated.
- *Return to work*: this will depend on the type of work in which the patient is employed. The difference in physical demands requires that a manual worker has a longer period of convalescence than a sedentary worker.
- *Sexual activity*: this can be resumed when the individual feels adequately recovered from surgery.
- *Driving*: driving insurance policies have restrictions following surgery; therefore, individual policies should be referred to. It is advisable not to drive for approximately 3–4 weeks or until one is able to perform an effective emergency stop.
- *Follow-up*: a follow-up appointment is given for 4–6 weeks after surgery. This is to ensure that recovery has taken place and to arrange any further investigations that may be necessary.

Urinary tract calculi

The incidence of urinary tract calculi is estimated at 12% of world population and is more common in men than in women. Around 12,000 of hospital admissions every year are those affected and will require hospitalization due to pain, obstruction or infection (Cunningham et al, 2016). Calculi or stones can occur at any point within the urinary tract (Cunningham et al, 2016).

Factors predisposing to calculi formation include:

- metabolic causes, e.g. an increased excretion of calcium, urate and cystine in the urine
- urinary infection
- hyperparathyroidism.

Signs and symptoms include:

- renal pain/colic – this can be severe pain of sudden onset which radiates from the loin to groin; the pain causes distress and is often accompanied by nausea and sweating
- urinary tract infection – may be recurrent
- haematuria.

Conservative management of renal colic

The patient's pain should be relieved by adequate analgesics, and an antiemetic drug prescribed to control any nausea. A high fluid intake of 2–3 L in 24 hours is recommended, to try to flush out the stone (i.e. a stone small enough to pass through the renal tract). All urine voided is strained, and if the stone is passed, it can be collected and sent for biochemical analysis. Urinary infection should be treated with an appropriate antibiotic.

Indications for surgery include:

- the stone is too large to pass through the urinary tract, therefore constituting a potential risk of obstruction
- recurrent urinary tract infection, which is difficult to treat while the stone acts as a nucleus for microorganisms
- recurrent renal colic.

Surgical management of urinary tract calculi

Surgical management depends on the size and location of the stone within the urinary tract. In recent years, as technology has progressed, methods of stone removal have moved towards minimally invasive surgery, i.e. percutaneous nephrolithotomy (PCNL), and non-invasive management, i.e. lithotripsy. For some patients it may be appropriate to combine methods; for example, for an individual with a large staghorn calculus, the initial treatment is a PCNL followed by lithotripsy at a later date to deal with the remaining stone fragments.

Conventional open surgery, e.g. nephrolithotomy, is now a relatively rare procedure.

Percutaneous nephrolithotomy

This procedure involves removal of the calculus under direct X-ray vision and is usually performed under a general anaesthetic. A percutaneous nephrostomy tract is established and enlarged using graduated dilators. This allows a nephroscope to be passed. Stones are removed using grasping forceps passed down the nephroscope. If the stone is too large, it can be fragmented using ultrasonic lithotripsy or electrohydraulic lithotripsy. Following the procedure, it is usual for a nephrostomy tube to be left *in situ* to allow drainage of blood and urine. The nephrostomy tube is clamped on the first postoperative day and removed on the second postoperative day if the patient is pain-free at the site and there is no leakage around the nephrostomy tube (Champion & Longhorn, 2004).

Table 18.3 Preoperative nursing care plan for an individual undergoing percutaneous nephrolithotomy

Patient problem	Expected outcome	Action/rationale
Communicating		
Potential anxiety due to admission to hospital and impending surgery	Patient is able to express fears and anxieties and will feel safe and informed regarding surgery	Discuss preoperative and anticipated postoperative care Give the patient the opportunity to express any anxieties and fears and provide a relaxed non-threatening environment Provide information — use diagrams if indicated (Hayward, 1975; British Pain Society, 2013) Ensure that consent is informed
Breathing, eating/drinking		
Potential respiratory problems due to inhalation of gastric contents while unconscious, or underlying respiratory disease	Gastric contents will not be inhaled Respiratory problems will not be exacerbated	Reinforce deep breathing exercises taught by the physiotherapist Fast for 6 hours (diet), 2 hours (fluid) prior to general anaesthetic (Association of Anaesthetists of Great Britain and Ireland, 2010)
Controlling body temperature		
Potential postoperative infection, e.g. urine	Temperature will be between 35.5°C and 37.5°C Early detection and treatment should infection occur	Record temperature preoperatively and report if outside normal parameters Perform urinalysis — obtain MSU; if nitrates present (adhere to local policy) administer prophylactic antibiotics as prescribed Bath/shower to be taken prior to theatre
Mobility		
Decreased mobility postoperatively could lead to circulatory problems and potential risk of pressure ulcer occurrence	Patient will remain as mobile as condition permits and risk of pressure ulcer occurrence will be minimized	Assess pressure ulcer risk using an appropriate assessment tool Encourage mobility and foot and leg exercises to aid venous return Measure and fit with TED stockings (Dougherty & Lister, 2015)
Elimination		
Potential risk of incontinence due to loss of voluntary muscle control while unconscious	Patient will remain continent	Give patient the opportunity to void prior to administration of premedication/transfer to theatre Ensure the patient has had a bowel action within 24 hours of theatre

(Continued)

Table 18.3 Preoperative nursing care plan for an individual undergoing percutaneous nephrolithotomy—cont'd

Patient problem	Expected outcome	Action/rationale
Maintaining a safe environment		
Inability to maintain own safety while sedated/unconscious	Safety of the patient will not be compromised	Ensure the following: • Correctly labelled identity bands are worn • Patient's consent form is signed • Wedding ring is covered with tape • Prostheses are removed, e.g. dentures, contact lenses • Baseline observations and weight are recorded • Any allergies are recorded • Patient's medical notes, blood results, X-rays and nursing documentation are available • Patient is positioned correctly on canvas

For pre- and postoperative nursing care, see care plans illustrated in Tables 18.3 and 18.4.

Complications of percutaneous nephrolithotomy

- *Haemorrhage*: bleeding occurs in all cases, but the risks are increased with longer operation time and multiple stone retrieval. A blood transfusion may be necessary depending on the preoperative haemoglobin and estimated blood loss. Regular monitoring of the nephrostomy tube drainage and site should occur in the first 24 hours postoperatively.
- *Infection*: pre-existing infective stones can result in bacteraemia once disturbed. It is important that appropriate antibiotics are commenced prior to the procedure and continued postoperatively.
- *Pneumothorax*: the risk of pneumothorax increases if the puncture to the kidney during the procedure is above the level of the twelfth rib and appears to have higher incidence on the left kidney (Palnizky et al, 2013). An underwater seal chest drain may have to be inserted to draw air from the pleural space.

Patient education and advice on discharge following percutaneous nephrolithotomy. If written information is available, this should be given to the patient on admission (or before) to ensure they are prepared for the postoperative 'journey'; this is provided in addition to any verbal advice given by the nursing and medical staff. Time must be taken to evaluate the individual's understanding and to reinforce the information as required.

Advice is given regarding the following:
- *Wound healing*: the patient is given instruction on observing the nephrostomy tube site for signs of infection,

e.g. redness, discharge and pain. The area should be kept covered with a non-adherent dressing until a scab forms. Appropriate dressings should be provided by the nursing staff for the patient to take home.
- *Elimination*: there may still be blood present in the urine in the initial days following surgery; this is normal, but it should noticeably decrease in the first 3–5 days. The patient should be aware of the signs and symptoms of urinary tract infection, e.g. urgency, frequency, and pain on voiding. If an infection is suspected, the GP should be consulted, as a course of antibiotics may be necessary.
- *Fluids and diet*: a fluid intake of 2–3 L in 24 hours is recommended, to maintain an increased urinary output, which in turn will flush out any blood or stone fragments that might be present. Long-term maintenance of this level of fluid intake might be beneficial in the prevention of future stone formation.
- *Return to work*: this will depend on the occupation of the patient. Manual workers will require longer than the individual with a more sedentary occupation.
- *Sexual activity*: this can be resumed when the individual wishes and feels recovered from surgery.
- *Driving*: individual driving policies should be referred to, as there may be restrictions following a general anaesthetic and surgery.

Extracorporeal lithotripsy

Lithotripsy involves focusing shockwaves, which travel through water, onto the stone, under X-ray or ultrasound control. The shockwaves cause the stone to disintegrate

Table 18.4 Postoperative nursing care plan for an individual following percutaneous nephrolithotomy

Patient problem	Expected outcome	Action/rationale
Breathing		
Potential problems with breathing following anaesthetic and surgical intervention	Patient's airway will remain clear Early detection should problems occur	Patient to be positioned ensuring clear airway is maintained Observe and record respiratory rate {1/4}–{1/2}-hourly initially and decrease frequency as patient's condition dictates Administer oxygen therapy as prescribed Encourage deep breathing exercises to aid lung expansion
Maintaining a safe environment		
Inability to maintain own safety after surgery and potential risk of shock, e.g. due to blood loss	Early detection and treatment if shock occurs	Observe and record patient's pulse and blood pressure {1/4}–{1/2}-hourly initially and decrease frequency as condition dictates Report to nurse in charge/doctor if blood pressure and pulse are outside normal parameters Report changes in patient's peripheral colour and responsiveness Monitor colour/consistency of urine drainage from nephrostomy tube to estimate blood loss Administer blood transfusion if prescribed Follow local protocol regarding blood transfusion
Communicating		
Potential risk of pain/discomfort following surgical intervention and presence of nephrostomy tube	Pain/discomfort will be controlled to level acceptable by the patient	Assess degree of pain/discomfort using verbal and non-verbal communication (McCaffery, 1983; Gregory, 2012) Give analgesics as prescribed and evaluate effectiveness Position patient as feels comfortable, ensuring nephrostomy tube is well secured to avoid traction
Controlling body temperature		
Potential infection following surgical intervention and presence of nephrostomy tube	Temperature will be between 35.5°C and 37.5°C Early detection and treatment should infection occur	Monitor temperature 1–4 hourly Report to nurse in charge if outside normal parameters Observe urine, nephrostomy tube site and IV site for signs of infection Note colour, consistency, smell of urine Note redness, discharge at nephrostomy and IV site Give antibiotics as prescribed

(Continued)

Table 18.4 Postoperative nursing care plan for an individual following percutaneous nephrolithotomy—cont'd

Patient problem	Expected outcome	Action/rationale
Eating/drinking		
Potential nausea/vomiting/ dehydration following anaesthetic and surgery	Patient will not feel nauseated or vomit Patient will feel adequately hydrated	Observe patient for signs of nausea Provide vomit bowl, tissues, mouthwash and ensure privacy Administer antiemetic as prescribed and evaluate effectiveness Maintain intravenous fluids as prescribed, discontinue when normal diet and fluids have been resumed Encourage 2–3 L oral fluids in 24 hours
Elimination		
Potential inability to void following surgery Potential blockage of nephrostomy tube due to clots/debris	Patient will void urine within 12 hours of surgery Nephrostomy tube will remain patent and will be removed 48 hours following surgery	Maintain an accurate fluid balance chart Encourage fluid intake of 2–3 L in 24 hours (intravenous fluids and oral fluids initially) Observe colour and consistency of urine Clamp nephrostomy tube on the first postoperative day, on doctor's instructions, following abdominal X-ray Remove nephrostomy tube on second postoperative day if pain has not been experienced since clamping and there is no leakage of urine around the tube Apply non-adherent dressing to drain site Observe for excessive leakage
Personal cleansing		
Potential problem meeting personal hygiene needs following surgery	Hygiene needs will be met	Assist the patient as necessary, maintaining dignity and promoting independence

into fragments small enough to pass down the ureter (Cunningham et al, 2016).

Since its inception in the early 1980s, there have been great technological advances in the method of delivery of the shockwave system and the efficiency of stone treatment has also improved. The first-generation lithotripter used extracorporeal shockwaves to break up the stones. The patient would be positioned on a chair in a water bath with repeated shockwaves delivered through the water. A general or epidural anaesthetic is required for this procedure, as it can be painful and the treatment might take rather a long period of time.

The second-generation lithotripter, 'extracorporeal piezo-lithotripsy', fragments the stone using shockwaves generated across small ceramic piezoelectric crystals. The patient is positioned so that the affected area is in contact with water, which is integral to the lithotripsy machine. Ultrasound is used to locate the stone. The shockwaves emitted are weaker and the focus area for the treatment to the stone is smaller; this results in a less painful and better tolerated treatment, which does not require a general anaesthetic to be administered in most patients. Many of the newer-generation systems work in a similar way to the piezoelectric lithotripter, using electromagnetic energy to break up the stone.

Large stones require repeated treatments (e.g. up to five treatments) to break up the stone into small fragments, which will then pass through the urinary system. The treatments are usually carried out on an outpatient basis, each treatment lasting approximately 45–60 minutes, unless contraindicated, e.g. in patients with impaired renal function or those who have a solitary kidney.

Preparation for the procedure is minimal. Prior to the procedure, a full explanation of what to expect is essential. Preparation for the procedure involves the patient attending a pre-assessment clinic, where a full clinical history is undertaken.

Many patients who have previously undergone painful procedures or operations for stone removal are understandably very cautious and anxious. For some patients it will be necessary to position a double-J stent prior to lithotripsy, to avoid ureteric obstruction caused by stone fragments at the lower end of the ureter. The stent is inserted under a general anaesthetic and is positioned between the kidney and bladder on the affected side. On completion of lithotripsy treatment, admission is then arranged for the removal of the stent.

Patient education and advice following lithotripsy

- *Pain*: following the procedure, some pain may be experienced as the stone fragments pass down the ureter, causing colic-like discomfort. Analgesics are prescribed for the patient to take home.
- *Risk of infection*: prophylactic antibiotics are given, as most stones have a bacterial component and shattering these can result in urinary tract infection and possibly septicaemia. The importance of completing the course of antibiotics is stressed. The GP should be consulted if pyrexia develops and increased pain is experienced.
- *Elimination*: the patient is advised to drink 2–3 L in 24 hours to help flush out stone fragments and clear any blood in the urine.
- *Activity*: normal activity can be resumed the next day, with a return to work within a few days.

Surgical management of bladder cancer

Bladder cancer is one of the most common urological malignancies and is found in around 3% of the total number of cancer cases, accounting for around 10,187 new cases per year (Anderson, 2018). There is an overall higher incidence of bladder cancers within industrialized societies, with a peak age occurrence at around 65 years of age. The risk is higher in men than in women, but in recent years the incidence in women has increased. The most common form of carcinoma diagnosed is transitional cell carcinoma (TCC), accounting for around 90% of all malignancies, and these tumours are often papillary in nature.

Some of the presenting problems associated with bladder cancer are:

- painless haematuria
- cystitis and urinary infection
- outflow obstruction – causing problems with voiding urine
- ureteric obstruction – causing back pressure within the kidney

- non-specific problems – weight loss, anorexia, anaemia, pyrexia.

Surgical management of bladder cancer can take several routes, depending on the stage and grade of the diagnosed tumour. However, all patients diagnosed with the disease need support and reassurance throughout their 'journey', and the ability to provide effective and honest information is essential.

Transurethral resection of bladder tumours

In superficial disease, tumours are managed by transurethral resection, using diathermy to remove the diseased tissue and cautery to stem the bleeding vessels, under a general or spinal anaesthetic. Patients will normally return to the ward with a urethral catheter *in situ* along with a bladder irrigation, which flushes out any excess bleeding and maintains catheter patency. The irrigation is normally in place for up to 24 hours and the catheter remains *in situ* for the initial 24 hours.

Complications of transurethral resection of bladder tumours

It is extremely important that nurses are aware of the complications of this procedure, as frequently it is the prompt action of the nurse which prevents these occurring.

Complications include the following:

- *Postoperative haemorrhage*: this can be moderate if a diathermized blood vessel in the bladder mucosa is not cauterized during surgery. A blood transfusion might be required if bleeding is prolonged.
- *Clot retention of urine*: the patient will have a distended bladder and severe suprapubic pain caused by clots obstructing the urethral catheter. 'Milking' the drainage bag tubing is often successful in dislodging clots. A bladder washout may be necessary to dislodge and evacuate the clots, and must be performed using an aseptic technique.
- *Urinary tract infection*: it is important that appropriate antibiotics are prescribed preoperatively if the patient is known to have infected urine, therefore reducing the risk of postoperative bacteraemia or septicaemia. Principles of risk reduction should also be enforced when managing the urethral catheter and irrigation systems.

Patient education and discharge planning following transurethral resection of a bladder tumour

Discharge planning begins prior to admission if possible. It is important that the patient's home situation and social circumstances are known so that appropriate arrangements for discharge can be organized.

Information booklets should be available and provided to the patient in the outpatient department, at the pre-assessment clinic prior to admission, or in the ward. It must be stressed that any written information must not be a substitute for verbal advice and discussion, as time must be taken to evaluate understanding and to make sure that the patient is well informed and aware of the operative procedure and the required follow-up care and management of the disease.

Advice is given regarding the following:

- *Activity*: it is important to remember that this surgery is not a minor procedure and this is a fact that many patients and healthcare professionals find difficult to understand because there is no visible operative wound. A gradual return to normal activity over a period of 1−2 weeks is recommended. If the patient still works, and depending on whether it is manual or sedentary work, a further 2−3 weeks' convalescence may be required.
- *Fluids and diet*: a fluid intake of 2−3 L in 24 hours (providing there are no medical contraindications) should be continued for up to 2 weeks after discharge. A diet high in fibre is advised, to avoid becoming constipated and to avoid straining, as this could result in episodes of fresh bleeding in the bladder, for up to 2 weeks after surgery.
- *Sexual activity*: this can be resumed 2 weeks following surgery if the patient feels comfortable.
- *Return to driving*: individual insurance policies should be consulted, as some may require a longer period of abstinence than the 2 weeks advised.

Patients should be advised to consult their GP should there be any unexpected blood loss in the urine or a burning sensation when voiding, as both are symptoms of a urinary tract infection which might require antibiotic therapy.

The patient will be given an outpatient appointment, usually at 2 weeks, for histological results. Check cystoscopy is normally undertaken at 3 months following initial resection, to monitor tumour recurrence, and a course of intravesical chemotherapy might also be administered to reduce tumour recurrence.

Surgical management of advanced bladder cancer

For more advanced bladder cancer, the surgical treatment options are:

- cystectomy and formation of a neobladder
- cystectomy and formation of an ileal conduit urinary diversion.

Both types of surgery are indicated for multiple superficial bladder tumours which are not kept under control by intravesical chemotherapy or transurethral resection and for T2 or T3 staged bladder tumours following radiotherapy (Blandy, 2009). Total cystectomy is a radical procedure and involves removing the bladder, lower ureters, prostate and urethra in men. In women, the bladder, lower ureters, urethra and reproductive organs are removed. Radical pelvic node dissection may also be indicated.

Cystectomy and formation of a neobladder

Formation of a neobladder for treatment of bladder cancer involves removal of the native bladder and replacement with a new bladder constructed from bowel. Bladder substitutions are becoming increasingly common, however this is classified as major surgery (Turner, 2009). The outcome criteria need to be discussed with the patient before proceeding, as there are several postoperative problems associated with this surgery, e.g. high pressures within the neobladder causing ureteric reflux and renal tissue damage, urinary incontinence, and the need to perform intermittent catheterization. Overall outcomes in both men and women have proved to be satisfactory (Mills & Struder, 2000; Nayak et al, 2018), although numbers performed are not large, and most success appears to have been achieved in the larger specialist urological centres. This form of reconstructive surgery is currently used more often in the UK for patients requiring intervention for congenital anomalies and for those with intractable incontinence.

Cystectomy and formation of an ileal conduit urinary diversion

This is the main form of diversional surgery offered to patients requiring cystectomy, and therefore greater focus is given to the nursing care and management of this patient group. There are around 2000 'urostomies' formed annually (Fillingham & Fell, 2004), and following their surgery patients will be required to wear a stoma appliance to collect the urinary output from the ileal conduit.

The native bladder is removed, as discussed above, and the ileal conduit is formed by anastomosing the ureters to an isolated loop of the ileum. The other end of the loop is brought onto the abdominal surface to form the urinary stoma.

Management of the patient undergoing such radical surgery involves the ward nursing team working closely with the multidisciplinary team, particularly the stoma therapist.

It should be clear from the outset to the patient that, due to the nature of this surgery, pelvic nerve damage can result in erectile dysfunction for many men, and both men and women may experience a reduced libido and have difficulty in reaching orgasm following surgery.

Specific preoperative nursing care

Ideally, admission to hospital should be 1 day prior to the procedure, so that the patient can be safely prepared for such extensive surgery.

Psychological/communication

If possible, patients should be admitted to an area where they are familiar with the clinical staff. It is important that the nurses involved in the patient's care are knowledgeable regarding the impending surgery and inherent implications, and are able to communicate honestly and openly with the patient. The patient's significant family/friends should be included in pre-operative discussions, if the patient agrees, so that any fears they may have are allayed, so allowing them to offer support and understanding in the recovery period and beyond.

Stoma formation can have a major impact on an individual's life both physically and psychologically. Difficulty may be experienced in coming to terms with an altered body image and changes relating to sexuality and sexual function. Many healthcare professionals might feel unable to discuss aspects of care relating to altered body image and sexuality, and this may be due to a lack of knowledge, embarrassment and the possible perceived embarrassment of the patient (Salter, 2010). Input from the stoma thera-pist is vital in managing this aspect of the patient's care and management.

Maintaining a safe environment

If the patient has had persistent haematuria prior to sur-gery, this might result in significant blood loss and conse-quent anaemia. A preoperative blood transfusion may therefore be necessary.

Breathing

Because of the nature of the surgery, the operating time may be 3−4 hours or longer. Recovery from the anaes-thetic and surgery is often influenced by the general health of the patient. The anaesthetist and physiotherapist will be made aware of any pre-existing respiratory problems during their preoperative assessments. Elective mechani-cal ventilation may be indicated in the immediate post-operative period. If the patient smokes, this should be actively discouraged prior to surgery.

Elimination

Preoperative bowel preparation may be necessary, as a section of the ileum is resected during the procedure. However, it is argued that bowel preparation is no longer required and can even lengthen hospital stay (Shafii et al, 2002; Large et al, 2012). In many units the method cho-sen is dependent on the 'surgeon's preference'.

Whichever method is chosen, it is vital that the patient is adequately hydrated. Ideally, individual assessment should occur and bowel preparation should be tailored to meet individual needs.

Eating/drinking

A low-residue soft diet is begun 1 day preoperatively until flatus is passed. An intravenous infusion should be commenced 12 hours prior to surgery, to avoid dehydration.

The role of the stoma care nurse

The stomatherapist will be involved with the patient and family as soon as the decision for surgery is made, so early referral is essential. Areas covered within the sto-matherapist's role include giving preoperative information about appropriate appliances, patch testing for these appliances and siting of the stoma. The Royal College of Nursing's *Clinical Nurse Specialists: Stoma care* (RCN, 2009) state that siting should be undertaken by nurses who have taken a relevant academic and clinically assessed stoma course.

Counselling skills are important to enable the nurse to build a rapport with the patient, partner and other family members. Alteration in body image and sexual function can have psychological implications and the stoma thera-pist should use their communication, listening, assess-ment and questioning skills to explore these stoma-related issues (Vujnovich, 2008).

Specific postoperative nursing care

Postoperatively, if their general condition allows, the patient is returned to the ward/high dependency unit, where one-to-one nursing care should be undertaken for the first 24 hours. The patient will have an assortment of tubes and drains *in situ*. These include:

- triple-lumen line for central venous pressure readings/ total parenteral nutrition feeding
- peripheral intravenous infusion
- epidural/intravenous opioid infusion
- ureteric stents
- wound drains
- oxygen therapy.

Breathing

The patient should be observed for signs of respiratory depression. This is particularly important if an opioid infusion is used to control pain. Oxygen therapy is administered as prescribed.

Maintaining a safe environment

Blood pressure, pulse and central venous pressure recordings are monitored as frequently as the patient's condition dictates. The amount of drainage from the wound drains is measured and recorded, and the wound dressings observed for evidence of oozing. Wound drains are removed when drainage is minimal. A blood transfusion may be necessary, and this will depend on blood loss and the patient's preoperative haemoglobin level.

Pain control/communication

A return to independence in activities of daily living is realistic only if pain is controlled to a level acceptable to the patient. Epidural analgesia, an opioid intravenous infusion, or PCA is most effective in the initial postoperative period.

Elimination

Two ureteric stents will be *in situ*, and their function is to splint the ureteric–ileal anastomosis and allow healing to take place. The stents protrude through the end of the stoma and are observed in the stoma bag. The stents are sutured in position (dissolvable sutures) and remain *in situ* for approximately 10 days. An accurate recording of urine output is maintained, with hourly measurements initially. Ureteric stents should not be flushed unless indicated by the stomatherapist or the consultant urologist.

The stoma is checked for viability. This should include:
- *colour*: the stoma may be bruised initially but should look red in colour within the first 48 hours after surgery
- *temperature*: the stoma should be warm, moist and soft to touch.

The patient should be involved in the care of the stoma as soon as this appears to be appropriate, i.e. the patient is emotionally and physically prepared. Further information on stoma care can be found in Chapter 17.

Eating/drinking

The patient is kept on sloppy diet until flatus is passed—normally between 1 and 2 days postoperatively and then gradually increased. If the patient has a prolonged ileus or is in a poor nutritional state, parenteral nutrition may be prescribed.

Controlling body temperature

Prophylactic intravenous antibiotics should be given at induction of the anaesthetic and a course continued postoperatively, to reduce the risk of infection.

Complications

Complications after cystectomy and ileal conduit diversion can be divided into those associated with major abdominal surgery and those associated with ileal conduit surgery.

Complications associated with major abdominal surgery

Complications associated with major abdominal surgery include:
- chest infection
- haemorrhage
- wound infection
- prolonged ileus
- anastomosis leak
- wound dehiscence
- intestinal obstruction
- deep vein thrombosis
- septicaemia
- pulmonary embolism.

Complications associated with ileal conduit surgery

Complications associated with ileal conduit surgery include the following:
- *Stoma necrosis*: postoperatively, a dark purple stoma suggests a poor blood supply, and urgent medical attention should be sought. Surgery may be necessary to remove a pregangrenous section of bowel.
- *Prolapse*: surgical intervention to refashion the stoma may be necessary if it is not possible to manage the prolapse by manual reduction and use of a firm abdominal support.
- *Retraction*: this can result in unmanageable leakage problems, and refashioning of the stoma is often necessary.
- *Stenosis*: constriction of the outlet of the stoma can lead to reabsorption of urine, infection and dilatation of the upper urinary tract. It may be possible to dilate the stoma using a finger or a catheter, but often surgery is necessary.
- *Skin excoriation*: this may be caused by a reaction to the bag adhesive or skin protective agent, or repeated contact with urine, and patients should be aware of the need to seek advice before problems become more difficult to resolve.

Specific patient education and advice on discharge following cystectomy and ileal conduit urinary diversion

Discharge is usually 7 days following surgery. However, for some patients, recovery may take longer, if complications have arisen. It is vital that discharge planning commences on admission or before, if the best possible arrangements are to be made for the individual's convalescence.

Patient education and advice on discharge are given as for major abdominal surgery. Specific information is necessary regarding further management of the urinary stoma. This information is normally given by the stomatherapist, who will continue to care for the patient or arrange continuing care in the community. It is important that nurses in the ward are able to reinforce information and answer any questions the patient may have.

Advice is given regarding the following:

- *Skin care*: maintenance of skin integrity around the stoma is extremely important. If the appliance is ill-fitting, urine will be in constant contact with the skin, resulting in excoriation. To prevent this happening, the size of the appliance opening should be appropriate to the size of the stoma.
- *Stoma equipment*: the patient is given information on how to obtain further supplies of stoma equipment, and prescription details are passed on to the GP.
- *Urinary output*: if blood is seen in the urine, or urinary output decreases or stops, then medical attention must be sought immediately. Mucus is naturally produced from the stoma, and a fluid intake of 2−3 L per day can help to reduce the amount of mucus. Individuals who are diabetic should be aware that urine from the stoma is not suitable for testing, as sugar is absorbed into the conduit (Burch, 2013).
- *Activity*: return to normal activity should be gradual over a period of several weeks. If patients wish to continue a strenuous job or sporting activity, they should be assessed on an individual basis. There are no restrictions on activities such as swimming.
- *Driving*: if seat belts are uncomfortable, aids which can relieve pressure are available from car accessory shops.
- *Altered body image/sexual activity*: erectile disorders/ impotence, loss of libido and problems associated

with body image may cause significant distress. The patient may require ongoing counselling and referral to appropriate agencies if necessary.

- *Follow-up*: the patient will be seen in the outpatient department between 4 and 6 weeks after surgery and at 3-monthly intervals for a year after.

Conclusion

Urology as a specialist area of practice has evolved in the last 30 years, and nurses have played a major role in the development and delivery of appropriate care and management programmes. Patient outcomes have improved with the advent of technological advances in diagnostic screening, minimally invasive techniques and, in some cases, radical treatment options. Ongoing advancement in specialist nursing practice within the field of urology will see the role of the nurse developing in new practice areas in the next decade, giving even more focus on specialist care to those experiencing urological disease.

SUMMARY OF KEY POINTS

- An understanding of the anatomy and physiology of the kidney and lower urinary tract is essential before the most appropriate investigations can be performed, diagnosis is obtained and relevant surgery undertaken.
- This chapter includes both invasive and non-invasive treatments for urological conditions, encompassing new technology and techniques.
- Sensitive nursing care is required, particularly when dealing with the profound change in body image and sexual function experienced with surgery such as cystectomy.

References

Anderson, C. (2008). *Laparoscopic nephrectomy* [Online]. Available at: <www.keyholeurology.co.uk/kidneycancertreatment.html#laproscopic>

Anderson, B. (2018). Bladder cancer: overview and disease management Part1: non-muscle invasive bladder cancer. *British Journal of Nursing, 27*(9), S27−S37.

Association of Anaesthetists of Great Britain and Ireland. (2010). *AAGBI safety guideline preoperative assessment and patient preparation. The role of the anesthetist*. Available at: <anaesthetists.org/Portals/0/PDFs/Guidelines%20PDFs/Guideline_preoperative_assessment_patient_preparation_anaesthetist_2010_final.pdf?ver = 2018-07-11-163756-537&ver = 2018-07-11-163756-537>

Beynon, M. R., & Nicholls, C. (2004). Urological investigations. In: S. Fillingham, & J. Douglas (Eds.), *Urological nursing* (3rd edn). Edinburgh: Baillière Tindall.

Blandy, J. P. (2009). *Lecture notes on urology* (6th ed.). Oxford: Blackwell Scientific.

British Association of Urological Surgeons. (2017a). *Performing a maximum urinary flow rate test (uroflowmetry)*. Available at: <www.baus.org.uk/_userfiles/pages/files/Patients/Leaflets/Flow%20rate%20measurement.pdf>

British Association of Urological Surgeons. (2017b). *Cystoscopy and retrograde X-ray studies (uretero-pyelography)*. Available at: <www.baus.org.uk/_userfiles/

pages/files/Patients/Leaflets/Retrograde
%20ureterography.pdf>

British Pain Society. (2013). *Guidelines for pain management programmes for adults.* Available at: <www.britishpainsociety. org/static/uploads/resources/files/ pmp2013_main_FINAL_v6.pdf>

Burch, J. (2013). *Stoma care* (2nd ed.). Blackwell Publishing.

Champion, J., & Longhorn, S. (2004). Urinary tract stones. In: S. Fillingham, & J. Douglas (Eds.), *Urological nursing* (3rd edn). Edinburgh: Baillière Tindall.

Cunningham, P., Noble, H., Kadhum Al-Modhefer, A., & Walsh, I. (2016). Kidney stones: pathophysiology, diagnosis and management. *British Journal of Nursing, 25*(20), 1112–1116.

D'Arcy, Y. (2008). Keep your patients safe during PCA. *Nursing, 38*(1), 50–55.

Dougherty, L., & Lister, S. (2015). *The royal marsden hospital manual of clinical nursing procedures* (9th edn). Oxford: Blackwell.

Fillingham, S., & Douglas, J. (2004). *Urological Nursing* (3rd ed.). Edinburgh: Baillière Tindall.

Fillingham, S., & Fell, S. (2004). Urological stomas. In: S. Fillingham, & J. Douglas (Eds.), *Urological nursing* (3rd edn). Edinburgh: Baillière Tindall.

Gregory, J. (2012). How can we assess pain in people who have difficulty communicating? A practice development project identifying a pain assessment tool for acute care. *International Practice Development Journal, 2*(2). Available at: <www.fons.org/ Resources/Documents/Journal/ Vol2No2/IDPJ_0202_06.pdf>

Hayward, J. (1975). *Information – a prescription against pain.* RCN Study of Nursing Care Series. London: Royal College of Nursing.

Khan, F., Amed, K., Lee, N., Challacombe, B., Khan, M. S., & Dasgupta, P. (2014). Management of ureteropelvic junction obstruction in adults. *Nature Reviews Urology, 11*, 629–638.

Large, M. C., Kiriluk, K. J., DECastro, G. J., et al. (2012). The impact of mechanical bowel preparation on postoperative complications for patients undergoing cystectomy and urinary diversion. *The Journal of Urology, 188*(5), 1801–1805.

Leaver, R. (2007). The evidence for urethral meatal cleansing. *Nursing Standard, 21*(41), 39–42.

McCaffery, M. (1983). *Nursing the patient in pain.* Adapted for the UK by Beatrice Sofaer. London: Lippincott Nursing Series Harper and Row.

Mills, R. D., & Struder, U. E. (2000). Female orthotopic bladder substitution: a good operation in the right circumstances. *The Journal of Urology, 163* (5), 1501–1504.

Nayak, A. L., Cagiannos, I., Lavellee, L. T., et al. (2018). Urinary function following radical cystectomy and orthotopic neobladder urinary reconstruction. *Canadian Urological Association Journal, 12*(6), 181–186.

National Institute of Health and Care Excellence (NICE). (2005). *Laproscopic Nephrectomy* [Online]. Available at: <www.nice.orguk/Guidance/ipg136>

Ogden, C. (2016). *The evolution of robotic surgery* [Online]. Available at: <https:// urologists.co.uk/surgical-robots-the-evolution-of-robotic-surgery>

Palnizky, G., Halachmi, S., & Barah, M. (2013). Pulmonary complications following Percutaneous Nephrolitotomy: A prospective study. *Current Urology, 7*(3), 113–116.

Royal College of Nursing. (2009). *Clinical nurse specialists: Stoma care.* London: Royal College of Nursing.

Royal College of Nursing. (2018). *Older People in Care Homes: Sex, Sexuality and Intimate Relationships* (2nd ed.). London: Royal College of Nursing.

Salter, M. (2010). Optimizing patient adjustment to stoma formation siting and self management. *Gastrointestinal Nursing, 8*(10), 21–25.

Sam, P., & LaGrange, C. (2018). Anatomy, Abdomen and Pelvis, Bladder Detrusor Muscle [online]. *StatPearls* (Internet). Available at: <https://www.ncbi.nlm. nih.gov/books/NBK482181>

Shafii, M., Murphy, D. M., Donovan, M. G., & Hickey, D. P. (2002). Is mechanical bowel prep necessary in patients undergoing cystectomy and urinary diversion. *BJU International, 89*(9), 879–881.

Stewart, E. (2018). Assessment and management of urinary incontinence in women. *Nursing Standard, 33*(2), 75–81.

Turner, B. (2009). Nursing care and treatment of patients with bladder cancer. *Nursing Standard, 23*(37), 47–56.

Velho, A., & Velho, R. (2013). Anatomy and Physiology series: the kidney and lower urinary tract. *Journal of Renal Nursing, 5*(2).

Vujnovich, A. (2008). Pre and post-operative assessment of patients with a stoma. *Nursing Standard, 22*(19), 50–56.

Wood, S. (2010). Postoperative pain 2: patient education, assessment and management. *Nursing Times, 106*(46), 14–16.

Yates, A. (2016). Urinalysis: How to interpret results. *Nursing Times,* Online issue 2, 1–3.

Relevant websites

Bladder & Bowel UK: www.bbuk.org.uk/ UK

British Association of Urological Nurses: www.baun.co.uk

Cancer Research UK: www.cancerhelp.org. uk

The Continence Foundation: www. continence-foundation.org.uk

Men's Health Forum: www.malehealth.co. uk

Orchid Cancer Appeal: www.orchid-cancer.org.uk

Prostate Cancer UK: www.prostatecancer. org.uk

Sexual Advice Association: www.sexualad-viceassociation.co.uk

Chapter | 19 |

Patients requiring surgery on the male reproductive system

Ashleigh Ward

KEY OBJECTIVES OF THIS CHAPTER

After reading this chapter, the reader should be able to:

- give an overview of the anatomy and physiology of the male reproductive system
- describe the pre- and postoperative nursing care for individuals undergoing surgery on the prostate gland, penis and scrotum
- explain discharge advice that would be given following surgery on the prostate gland, penis and scrotum
- have greater understanding of the psychological impact of surgery.

Areas to think about before reading the chapter

- How might a man's sexuality be impacted after surgery on the male reproductive system?
- What is the role and function of the prostate gland?
- What hormones influence the male reproductive system?

Introduction

This chapter addresses the care, management and treatment of men with specific conditions of the male reproductive system. Nursing care related to these specific conditions will be discussed, including the psychological needs of the man when addressing sexuality and altered body image, and the need for sensitive and empathetic management of this client group. This chapter will cover surgery to the four main structures of the male genitourinary system:

- The accessory glands, specifically the prostate
- The testes and associated ducts
- The penis
- The urethra

Common preoperative investigations for each surgery to each structure are outlined in Table 19.1.

It is also important to note that some women can be born with male anatomy and so male reproductive surgeries can be performed on both men and women. However, limited research exists to advise on the pre- and postoperative needs of the female patient population in these circumstances.

Care of the patient following prostate surgery

Anatomy and physiology of the prostate

The prostate gland surrounds the urethra just inferior to the bladder neck. The size of the prostate varies considerably – it

Table 19.1 Common investigations related to surgical interventions of the male reproductive system

Surgical intervention	Investigation
Transurethral resection of the prostate gland (TURP)	Blood tests • Group and crossmatch 2 units • Urea and electrolyte estimation • Full blood count • Prostate-specific antigen Digital rectal examination Urinary flow rate Midstream specimen of urine ECG Chest X-ray Ultrasound of urinary tract
Radical prostatectomy (open, laparoscopic or robot-assisted laparoscopic)	As above
Urethroplasty	Blood tests • Group and crossmatch 2 units • Urea, creatinine and electrolytes • Full blood count Urinary flow rate Midstream specimen of urine Cystourethroscopy Urethrogram
Penile surgery for incontinence	Blood tests • Blood glucose estimation • Hormone levels: testosterone, follicle-stimulating hormone, luteinizing hormone Doppler ultrasound Cavernosogram
Scrotal surgery including vasectomy, vasovasostomy and exploration for suspected torsion of testes	Semen analysis Scrotal ultrasound if torsion indicated

increases in size at puberty, and in the adult is approximately 15 g in weight. It is described as being donut-shaped and has a diameter of approximately 3 cm. The outer zone of the prostate (the lateral and posterior portions) consists of glandular tissue, and the inner zone (the middle of the prostate) is made up of mucosal glands. The prostate is surrounded and encased by an outer fibrous capsule.

The gland produces milky, slightly acidic secretions which contain enzymes (e.g. acid phosphate, hyaluronidase and fibrinolysin) and many additional components (e.g. citrate, calcium and prostate-specific antigen (PSA)). The fluid makes up approximately 10–20% of the ejaculate and is thought to help neutralize the acidity of the vagina and to stimulate the mobility of the sperm (Abourmarzouk, 2019; Olmsted et al, 2000); it is also thought to be responsible for

the characteristic smell of semen. The prostate gland is reliant on adequate levels of circulating testosterone for it to function effectively.

The prostate gland can often undergo benign hyperplastic change, which can result in urinary outflow obstruction. The precise science to how this occurs is still unknown, but changes in hormone levels in ageing is thought to contribute to this.

Pathophysiology and epidemiology of prostate cancer

The incidence of prostate cancer is increasing across the developed world at a faster rate than most other cancers (Ferlay et al, 2015), though this is thought to be due to developments in diagnostic techniques rather than a genuine increase in the likelihood of having prostate cancer (Moller et al, 2007; Mistry et al, 2011). Due to the influence of PSA testing, incidence trends are unpredictable (Moller et al, 2007; Mistry et al, 2011; Ferlay et al, 2015). However, there is agreement that incidence will continue to increase.

There are many risk factors proposed for increasing the risk of prostate cancer, including ethnicity, age, genetic predisposition and affluence.

Though ethnicity is an acknowledged risk factor for prostate cancer (Leitzmann & Rohrmann, 2012; Mottet et al, 2015), migration studies also show that prostate cancer incidence increases when low-risk populations migrate to higher-risk countries (Brawley et al, 2007; Giovannucci et al, 2007; Whittemore et al, 1995), indicating the role of health culture and behaviour in PSA testing and subsequent diagnosis.

As cancer develops as a result of a cumulation of genetic changes within a cell, age is also considered the greatest risk factor for prostate cancer (Leitzmann & Rohrmann, 2012). However, the introduction of PSA testing has led to a gradual decrease in age and also, stage of prostate cancer at diagnosis (Shafique & Morrison, 2013; EAU guidelines, 2019).

Unlike other cancers, affluence is associated with a higher risk of prostate cancer (Dutta et al, 2005; Shafique et al, 2012). The reason for this is unknown, though it can be speculated that affluence is related to a greater awareness of prostate cancer and PSA testing and so a greater likelihood of diagnosis.

Currently, the UK operates an opportunistic screening protocol, which is defined by Mottet et al (2015) as the individual case finding of prostate cancer initiated by the patient or the physician.

Urological investigations and assessment of the prostate

Though prostate cancer is notoriously asymptomatic (Forbat et al, 2012), benign prostatic hyperplasia is commonly associated with a range of symptoms related to outflow obstruction caused by enlargement of the prostate.

Signs and symptoms of prostate outflow obstruction are:

- *Urinary frequency*: needing to void urine often, usually more than 10 times daily
- *Nocturia*: waking at night to void, usually more than twice
- *Urgency*: sudden and strong desire to void
- *Poor urinary stream*: often worse early morning and may need to strain

- *Hesitancy*: experiences a delay in voiding although desire is present
- *Urinary tract infection*: residual urine caused by bladder obstruction increases risk of infection
- *Dysuria*: pain on voiding, which may be caused by infection
- *Urinary incontinence*: occurs as a result of overdistension, with overflow incontinence as a result
- *Acute retention of urine*

The severity of symptoms can be assessed and evaluated using the International Prostate Symptom Score (IPSS), which consists of seven questions related to the severity of symptoms (Fig. 19.1). A separate question is asked regarding the bothersomeness of symptoms. The maximum possible score is 35 and a score below 20 is regarded as severe. Digital rectal examination of the prostate gland will provide useful information regarding the size, consistency and anatomical limits of the prostate gland. Examination of the abdomen should also be undertaken to detect a palpable bladder that might also indicate chronic retention of urine.

As men age, the prostate naturally increases in size. Generally, levels of PSA in the bloodstream correlate with the size of the prostate (though some events can lead to temporary elevation, such as recent ejaculation, urinary tract infections and cycling). Therefore, PSA testing is also used as a first step in the diagnosis of benign prostatic hyperplasia (BPH) in symptomatic men. BPH is the natural enlargement of the prostate as a result of ageing, leading to symptoms. Therefore, when a person has an abnormal PSA level both BPH and prostate cancer should be considered by clinicians. As BPH is commonly managed in primary care, very little is known about the epidemiology of the disease.

As PSA tests provide an indication of the size of the prostate, PSA testing can provide an appropriate starting point for investigations (Mottet et al, 2015; Gravas et al, 2018). PSA testing is not a cancer-specific test. As men age, the prostate naturally increases in size. Levels of PSA in the bloodstream generally correlate with the size of the prostate. However, PSA testing is controversial as it is widely accepted as the cause of an increased incidence and prevalence of prostate cancer (Mottet et al, 2015; Mistry et al, 2011; Moller et al, 2007; Brewster et al, 2000) and is associated with complications from prostate biopsies (Loeb et al, 2013), a reduction in quality of life (Heijnsdijk et al, 2012), and has shown no survival benefit in some studies (Ilic et al, 2013).

Additionally, some methods of prostate cancer biopsy have shown poor levels of accuracy. Twelve core biopsy techniques have only 43% accuracy (Serefoglu et al, 2013). Although targeted biopsies have potential for increased accuracy (Siddiqui et al, 2015), the introduction of targeted biopsies could still leave one third of prostate cancers underdiagnosed.

	Not at all	Less than 1 time in 5	Less than half the time	About half the time	More than half the time	Almost always	Patient score
1 Incomplete emptying Over the past month, how often have you had a sensation of not emptying your bladder completely after you finished urinating?	0	1	2	3	4	5	
2 Frequency Over the past month, how often have you had to urinate again less than 2 hours after you finished urinating?	0	1	2	3	4	5	
3 Intermittency Over the past month, how often have you found you stopped and started again several times when you urinated?	0	1	2	3	4	5	
4 Urgency Over the past month, how often have you found it difficult to postpone urination?	0	1	2	3	4	5	
5 Weak stream Over the past month, how often have you had a weak urinary stream?	0	1	2	3	4	5	
6 Straining Over the past month, how often have you had to push or strain to begin urination?	0	1	2	3	4	5	
7 Nocturia Over the past month, how many times did you most typically get up to urinate from the time you went to bed at night until the time you got up in the morning?	0	1	2	3	4	5+	
Total IPSS							

	Delighted	Pleased	Mostly satisfied	Mixed	Mostly dissatisfied	Unhappy	Terrible
Quality of life due to urinary symptoms If you were to spend the rest of your life with your urinary condition the way it is now, how would you feel about it?	0	1	2	3	4	5	6

Figure 19.1 Chart for recording the International Prostate Symptom Score.

Treatment of benign prostatic hyperplasia

In most cases, benign prostatic hyperplasia can be managed using medications, namely alpha-1 adrenoceptor blockers or 5-alpha reductase inhibitors. These medications can be used separately or in combination to relieve symptoms. Surgical management is indicated where symptoms continue to be severe, medication ceases to be effective or the patient's quality of life is reduced. Transurethral resection of the prostate (TURP) is the accepted treatment and it would be rare for a man to require radical prostatectomy for this today.

TURP is performed under general or spinal anaesthetic, and a cystoscopy is undertaken prior to transurethral resection, to allow direct visualization of the bladder and to detect any abnormalities. Using traditional methods, the obstructing part of the prostate gland was removed along with the bladder neck using a cutting loop and diathermy to control the bleeding. Removal of the bladder neck then results in retrograde ejaculation. TURP is a challenging procedure, but when undertaken by a skilled and competent urologist it is generally considered safe. Additionally, controversy is still ongoing as to when an open TURP procedure is indicated. In recent years, technological advances such as UroLift have seen TURP procedures change dramatically (Gravas et al, 2018). For example, UroLift involves the stapling or implanting of the prostate gland away from the urethra (Urolift, 2019). As this is classified as a minor procedure, surgical treatment for BPH is now moving towards being a day surgery procedure, and as the technology integrates into practice, nurse consultants may choose to perform this procedure. However, these new procedures are only indicated for patients with prostates measuring less than 100 g — greater than this, traditional methods of TURP are required.

Treatment of prostate cancer

Patients eligible for curative treatment will be given the choice of all treatment options, including active surveillance where appropriate. Active surveillance was introduced to minimize the overtreatment of men caused by PSA screening protocols (Mottet et al, 2015). Where curative treatment is not required, men will eventually enter into the palliative pathway where they may benefit from a range of non-surgical treatments. Though active surveillance was introduced to prevent overtreatment, repeated blood tests and biopsies mean that active surveillance can be considered a form of overtreatment in itself.

Three methods currently exist for treating prostate cancer with curative intent: radical prostatectomy, traditional radiotherapy and brachytherapy. However, brachytherapy is currently recommended as a treatment for low-grade prostate cancers only (Mottet et al, 2015).

Surgery is the traditional method of prostate cancer treatment. Surgical techniques used to perform radical prostatectomy vary across the UK, with some regions still performing open prostatectomy as standard. However, all regions of the UK endeavour to deliver robot-assisted laparoscopic prostatectomy (RALP) using the da Vinci technology, which is considered the gold standard treatment internationally.

External beam radiation therapy (EBRT) and stereotactic ablative radiotherapy (SABR) are variations of traditional radiotherapy where several treatments are delivered over a period of time. EBRT is used throughout Scotland, though some Health Boards are currently trialling SABR. Radiotherapy is currently delivered over eight weeks, though trials are currently underway to assess the delivery of radiotherapy over a two-week period. Although radiotherapy was always an available treatment for prostate cancer, technological advances in the last 10–15 years have placed radiotherapy on an equal footing with surgery.

In previous years, orchidectomy, a procedure for surgical castration, was a routine treatment for men with advanced prostate cancer. Though in recent years this approach is not as popular due to improvements in hormone therapy and the emergence of chemotherapy in the treatment of prostate cancer, this treatment should still be offered to patients.

Postoperative care following prostate surgery

Technological advances have led to substantial changes in postoperative care for patients. For example, surgical intervention for BPH can now be completed as a day case and RALP has led to a substantial reduction in length of hospital stay and complications and side-effects from surgery.

Typical considerations for pre- and postoperative nursing care for individuals undergoing surgery on the prostate gland is outlined in the care plans in Tables 19.2 and 19.3.

Following prostate surgery, clear instructions of the time that the urinary catheter will stay *in situ* should be sought and reflected in local policy, as it is likely to differ within care organizations. The possibility of erectile dysfunction needs to be discussed prior to any surgery taking place and this counselling is usually undertaken by a clinical nurse specialist or a sex therapist. Psychological support is important for all pre- and postoperative patients but is paramount for men on active surveillance.

Complications of transurethral resection of the prostate gland

It is extremely important that nurses are aware of the complications of prostate surgery, as frequently it is the prompt action of the nurse which prevents more serious

Table 19.2 Preoperative nursing care plan for an individual undergoing surgery on the prostate gland

Problem	Expected outcome	Action/rationale
Communication		
Potential anxiety due to hospital and impending surgery	Patient is able to express anxieties and fears and will feel safe and informed about his operation	Discuss preoperative and anticipated postoperative care Provide a non-threatening relaxed environment in which the patient will feel able to express his anxieties and ask questions Provide information, using diagrams if necessary (Hayward, 1975) Ensure that informed consent is obtained before administration of a premedication Provide environment conducive to restful sleep
Breathing, eating/drinking		
Potential respiratory problems due to: • inhalation of gastric contents while unconscious • underlying respiratory disease	Gastric content will not be inhaled Respiratory problems will not be exacerbated	Report any breathing problems the patient may be experiencing Reinforce deep breathing exercises taught by the physiotherapist Fast for 6 hours (diet), 2 hours (fluid) prior to general anaesthetic (Phillips et al, 1993) or in line with local guidelines
Mobility		
Decreased mobility could lead to circulatory problems and increase the risk of pressure ulcer occurrence	The patient will remain as mobile as condition permits, and risk of deep vein thrombosis and pressure ulcer occurrence will be minimized	Perform pressure ulcer risk assessment Perform mobility risk assessment as per local policy Encourage mobility during preoperative period Reinforce physiotherapist's teaching of leg exercises Measure and fit with anti-embolism stockings if appropriate (Doughty & Lister, 2008)
Controlling body temperature		
Potential postoperative infection, e.g. urine	Temperature will be between 35.5°C and 37.5°C Early detection and treatment if infection occurs	Record temperature preoperatively and report if outside normal parameters Perform urinalysis — obtain MSU if nitrates present on dipstick Prophylactic antibiotics to be given as prescribed Bath or shower to be taken prior to theatre Clean theatre gown/bed linen to be provided

(Continued)

Table 19.2 Preoperative nursing care plan for an individual undergoing surgery on the prostate gland—cont'd

Problem	Expected outcome	Action/rationale
Elimination		
Potential risk of incontinence due to loss of voluntary muscle control when unconscious	Patient will remain continent during anaesthesia	Ensure patient has had a bowel action within 24 hours of theatre Give patient the opportunity to void prior to administration of voluntary muscle premedication/transfer to theatre
Maintaining a safe environment		
Inability to maintain own safety while sedated/unconscious	The safety of the patient will not be compromised	Ensure the following: • Correctly labelled identity band is in place • Patient's consent form is signed • Wedding ring is taped • Prostheses are removed, e.g. dentures, contact lenses • Baseline observations and weight are recorded • Any allergies are documented • Patient's medical notes, blood results, X-rays and nursing documentation are available • Patient is positioned correctly on canvas

and even life-threatening situations. Ahyai et al (2010) provides a review of these complications and a brief summary of these are included below.

TURP or TUR syndrome

A potentially fatal syndrome caused by absorption of irrigation fluid (usually 2000 mL or more) leading to symptoms such as confusion, dyspnoea, arrhythmia, hypotension and seizures. Treatment includes elimination of excess water in circulation through use of loop diuretics, or in severe cases, through use of hypertonic saline solutions (Demirel et al, 2012).

Postoperative haemorrhage

This can be severe as the prostate gland is very vascular. It is vital that blood transfusion is readily available.

Clot retention of urine

Patients should be encouraged to increase their fluid intake for at least 3 weeks following surgery (Olapade-Olaopa et al, 1998). If clot retention becomes a problem,

these should be removed with use of irrigation (Scholtes, 2002) or scopes (Lynch et al, 2010) as appropriate, and older methods of clot removal such as 'milking' the catheter should not be used.

Urinary tract infection

Prophylactic antibiotics should be considered postoperatively to reduce the risk of postoperative bacteraemia or septicaemia.

Deep vein thrombosis and pulmonary embolism

These are potential complications following pelvic surgery, but are often overlooked in patients undergoing TURP.

Infertility

Bladder neck resection/prostate resection can cause retrograde ejaculation, where semen travels into the bladder instead of down through the distal urethra. Following surgery, patients may experience dry orgasms. This does not

367

Table 19.3 Postoperative nursing care plan for an individual undergoing surgery on the prostate gland

Problem	Expected outcome	Action/rationale
Breathing		
Potential risk of problems with breathing due to anaesthetic/surgical intervention	Patient's airway will remain clear Early detection of hypoventilation	Position patient ensuring clear airway is maintained Observe and record respiratory rate 1/2 – 1 hourly initially and decrease as patient's condition dictates Administer oxygen therapy as prescribed Follow anaesthetist's instructions regarding position if patient has had a spinal anaesthetic, i.e. length of time patient is to lie flat Encourage deep breathing exercises
Maintaining a safe environment		
Inability to maintain own safety after surgery Potential risk of shock and haemorrhage, e.g. due to blood loss	Patient's safety will be maintained Early detection of signs of shock/haemorrhage	Observe and record pulse and blood pressure 1/2 – 1 hourly and decrease as patient's condition dictates Report to nurse in charge/doctor if blood pressure and pulse are outside normal parameters Monitor colour/consistency of urine for blood loss or blood clots Administer blood transfusion if prescribed and follow local protocol Report changes in patient's peripheral colour and responsiveness
Communication		
Potential risk of pain and discomfort due to surgical intervention and presence of urethral catheter	Pain/discomfort will be controlled to a level acceptable to the patient	Assess degree of discomfort/pain experienced by use of verbal/non-verbal communication Position patient as he feels comfortable Ensure catheter is patent – observe urinary drainage Secure urethral catheter to avoid traction Give analgesics as prescribed and evaluate effectiveness
Controlling body temperature		
Potential difficulty maintaining body temperature in immediate postoperative period Potential infection following surgical intervention and presence of urethral catheter	Temperature will be between 35.5°C and 37.5°C Early detection and treatment should infection occur	Monitor temperature 1 hourly, and decrease as condition dictates Observe urine for signs of infection, i.e. note colour, consistency and odour Inspect IV cannula site for signs of infection; note any discomfort, redness, discharge Instruct patient regarding catheter toilet using soap and water; to be performed twice daily Give antibiotics as prescribed

(Continued)

Table 19.3 Postoperative nursing care plan for an individual undergoing surgery on the prostate gland—cont'd

Problem	Expected outcome	Action/rationale
Eating and drinking		
Potential risk of nausea and vomiting due to anaesthetic Potential risk of dehydration following surgery	Patient will not feel nauseated and will not vomit	Observe patient for signs of nausea Administer antiemetic as prescribed and evaluate effectiveness Monitor IV fluids as prescribed Commence oral fluids when fully awake (if general condition allows) and increase as tolerated Discontinue IV fluids when oral intake is 2 L in 24 hours and diet is tolerated
Elimination		
Potential risk of clot retention following surgery Potential inability to void following removal of urethral catheter Potential inability to eliminate faeces normally	Urethral catheter will remain patent Patient will void urine within 12 hours of catheter removal Patient will eliminate faeces normally before removal of urethral catheter	Maintain an accurate fluid balance chart Maintain bladder irrigation – rate to correspond to colour of urine Discontinue bladder irrigation on the 1st postoperative day if blood loss in the urine is decreasing Observe colour and consistency of urine – if clot retention occurs, perform bladder washout using an aseptic technique, following local protocol Ensure patient does not strain to have his bowels open Administer aperients as prescribed and evaluate effectiveness Remove urethral catheter as directed by clinician and consider procedure Instruct patient to use a urinal when he voids and maintain an accurate record of urinary output
Personal cleansing		
Potential problem performing hygiene needs	Hygiene needs will be met at a level acceptable to the patient	Assist as necessary, maintaining dignity and promoting independence Instruct patient regarding how to perform catheter toilet using disposable wipes, soap and water
Mobility		
Potential complication of reduced mobility following surgery, e.g. pressure ulcer, chest infection and deep vein thrombosis	Independence in mobility will be achieved at a level acceptable to the patient	Assess pressure ulcer risk using recognized assessment tool Use aids as necessary Assist in promoting independence Anti-embolism stockings to be supplied and worn if appropriate Reinforce deep breathing exercises as taught by the physiotherapist

mean that the person is infertile, rather they will need additional support for conception.

Incontinence

This occurs due to damage of the external sphincter and, if severe, may require additional surgical intervention.

Patient education and discharge planning

Discharge planning should begin prior to admission though this is not possible in all cases, for example in those with acute retention. It is important that the patient's home situation and social circumstances are discussed if the best possible discharge planning arrangements are to be made.

In most surgical wards and departments, information booklets are made available to patients requiring surgery. It must be stressed that any written information should be provided in addition to verbal advice and discussion, as time must be taken to evaluate understanding and make sure that informed consent is gained. The Nursing and Midwifery Council (NMC) (2018) require nurses and nursing associates to act in partnership with those people who are receiving care, to help them gain access to relevant health and social care, information and support when they may need it.

Advice should be provided on the following:

- *Activity*: It is important to remember that prostate surgery is a major surgical intervention, a fact that patients, and sometimes healthcare professionals, often find difficult to understand because they will not always see a wound. A gradual return to normal activity over a period of 2–3 weeks is recommended. If the patient still works and depending on whether it is manual or sedentary work, a further 2–3 weeks' recovery may be required.
- *Fluids and diet*: Providing there are no medical contraindications, a slightly higher than normal fluid intake of up to 3 L per day should be encouraged for 2–3 weeks following surgery. This will help the raw area in the prostatic bed to heal and will also clear any blood still present in the urine. It is not unusual to have some blood in the urine for about 10 days; this will clear with fluids and healing time. A diet high in fibre is advised, to avoid constipation and straining when opening the bowels, as this may contribute to fresh bleeding from the prostatic bed.
- *Pelvic floor exercises*: Instruction should be given in the different types of exercise that will help to strengthen the pelvic floor musculature. Relevant advice sheets are often available, and some men may be referred to a continence physiotherapist.

- *Sexual activity*: Activities involving ejaculation can resumed 2 weeks following surgery. It should be stressed that retrograde ejaculation is not a reliable form of contraception and an alternative method should be used if necessary. It should also be noted that this surgery carries a high risk of erectile dysfunction though newer procedures such as robotic surgery and UroLift are reducing this.
- *Return to driving*: Individual insurance policies should be consulted, as some may require a longer period of abstinence than the 2 weeks advised.

Patients should be advised to consult their practice nurse or GP should there be an unexpected episode of haematuria, or dysuria on voiding, as both might indicate a urinary tract infection, though some healthcare organizations prescribe prophylactic antibiotics for prostate surgery as standard. An outpatient appointment for 4–6 weeks is usually provided, and patients will normally be asked to perform a urinary flow rate assessment to evaluate the effectiveness of the surgery on the patient's urinary flow. Due to prostate regrowth in BPH, men having TURP, UroLift, or similar may require a second procedure. For men undergoing UroLift, this equates to approximately 1 in 10 men, and often men will undergo a repeat UroLift procedure.

For patients undergoing open surgery for either radical prostatectomy or retropubic prostatectomy (the open surgical treatment for BPH), additional care will be required to the abdominal wound. Patients will generally need additional analgesics to prevent problems arising from reduced mobility. Fluids and diet are reintroduced on the first postoperative day. The wound is observed for signs of infection and the wound drain is removed only when minimal drainage has occurred over a 24-hour period, and patients are likely to have an extended hospital stay that could be twice as long as patients having laparoscopic radical prostatectomy or TURP.

Care of the patient following scrotal surgery

Anatomy and physiology of the testes and associated ducts

The testes are the sex glands of the male. They have two functions:
- production of androgens, which are the male sex hormone (testosterone)
- production of the male reproductive cell (spermatozoa)

The paired testicles sit within the scrotum and a midline septum divides the two compartments. The scrotum is suspended outside the body below the penis. The testicles are suspended in the scrotum by the spermatic cord; the blood, nerve supply and spermatic drainage run through this structure. Arterial blood supply is via the testicular artery and drainage is via the testicular vein. The testes are surrounded by two layers of connective tissue, the tunica albuginea and the tunica vaginalis: they help protect the testicle against injury and cushion the structures during movement.

There are two distinct cell types within the testicle:
- *Sertoli cells*: responsible for the production of spermatozoa and found within the seminiferous tubules of the testes
- *Leydig cells*: found in the interstitial tissue between the seminiferous tubules responsible for the production of testosterone

The tubules and ducts from each testicle converge at the posterior aspect of the gland and form the epididymis, where the sperm is stored and matures. The epididymis is a coiled tube approximately 6 m in length and is divided into the head, body and tail. The head of the epididymis receives sperm from the testes and storage occurs within the body and tail regions. The epididymis expands near its tail to become the vas deferens.

The vas deferens is a small muscular tube approximately 45 cm long that begins in the scrotum, travels a course through the inguinal canal into the pelvic cavity and ends where it joins within the duct of the seminal vesicle to form the ejaculatory duct. The ejaculatory duct opens into the urethra on either side of the verumontanum, which is a raised structure found on the posterior wall of the prostatic urethra. The two seminal vesicles are located behind the prostate gland beneath the bladder base and are approximately 5−7 cm in length. Seminal fluid, secreted by the seminal vesicles, is viscous, alkaline, and yellowish in colour, and contains nutrients and enzymes. This fluid is thought to aid sperm motility and makes up around 60% of the ejaculatory volume.

Pathophysiology of scrotal and testicular conditions

Scrotal conditions include varicocele, hydrocele, testicular torsion and cancer of the testes.

Varicocele

A varicocele is formed when the veins of the pampiniform plexus, which drain the testes, become varicosed and distended (Masson & Brannigan, 2014). It is most commonly found in the left side and is possibly due to an incompetent or absent valve mechanism at the end of the left testicular vein. A varicocele can also be formed as a result of venous obstruction due to a renal or retroperitoneal tumour.

Hydrocele

Hydrocele is a collection of fluid in the tunica vaginalis, the outer covering of the testes. In many cases the cause is unknown, although it can occur secondary to trauma, infection and tumour. In most cases, the patient is asymptomatic, but for some patients the hydrocele may be so large it causes a dragging pain and discomfort in the scrotum. The size of the swelling can also cause patients some embarrassment.

Torsion of the testes

Though testicular torsion can be diagnosed at any age, it is generally more common in young men (Somani et al, 2010). It is caused by excessive mobility of the testicle, allowing it to twist on its mesentery and interfere with the blood supply. If treatment is delayed, this can lead to infarction of the testicle.

Testicular cancer

This is the most common neoplasm in young, adult men (Park et al, 2018) and the most common presenting symptom is a testicular lump or swelling (Wise, 2018), with incidence continuing to steadily increase. As most testicular tumours are prone to metastatic spread, radiotherapy and chemotherapy are often recommended in addition to surgical intervention.

Urological assessment and investigations for scrotal and testicular conditions

Most scrotal or testicular conditions are visually obvious or obvious following manual manipulation of the scrotum and testes. However, further information is provided below on assessment and investigation of testicular conditions that may not be visible:

Varicocele

This is often described as feeling like a 'bag of worms' in the scrotum and this can be felt on examining the patient whilst they are standing. Men undergoing investigations for infertility will have to have the presence of a varicocele excluded. Infertility caused by varicoceles are due to raised temperatures as a result of this condition, leading to poor spermatogenesis (Masson & Brannigan, 2014). Other signs and symptoms include a sensation of dragging or general scrotal discomfort or ache and scrotal swelling.

Torsion of the testes

Testicular torsion should always be assumed until proven otherwise. Signs and symptoms include sudden acute pain in the scrotum, referred pain in the lower abdomen or groin, testes are tender to the touch and/or the scrotum is red, swollen and oedematous.

Testicular cancer

Men and boys are encouraged to check their testes monthly to identify any unusual masses, and some countries and charities have released campaigns to encourage this during masturbation or sexual encounters. Where an unusual mass is detected, biopsies should be taken to confirm cancer.

Treatment of scrotal and testicular conditions

Treatments for conditions of the scrotum include ligation of the varicocele and excision of a hydrocele:

- *Ligation of the varicocele*: This is recommended only when symptoms are present. Surgical intervention involves ligation of all veins except one in the inguinal canal, and surgery can be performed under local or general anaesthetic.
- *Excision of the hydrocele*: Initially hydroceles are treated through aspiration of the fluid using a trocar and cannula on an outpatient basis. However, the fluid generally reaccumulates and surgery is required to excise and plicate the hydrocele sac.

For conditions involving the testes, orchidopexy and orchidectomy are generally required.

- *Orchidopexy*: Where testicular torsion is suspected, surgical exploration through a surgical incision allows assessment of the viability of the testes and, if viable, an orchidopexy is performed. An orchidopexy is the fixing of the testicle to the scrotal wall using sutures. During the procedure, the other testicle should be examined and an orchidopexy performed on this testicle also if considered at risk of torsion.
- *Orchidectomy*: Where testicular torsion is suspected, surgical exploration through a surgical incision allows assessment of the viability of the testes and if the testes is found to be infarcted, it is removed. Orchidectomy is also the recommended treatment in cases of testicular cancer. Additionally, orchidectomy was once used in the treatment of advanced prostate cancer. Though this is no longer commonly recommended due to the advent of hormone therapies and chemotherapies for treatment of advanced prostate cancer, many healthcare professionals believe that patients should still be presented with this as a surgical treatment option.

Though not strictly a treatment for scrotal or testicular conditions, it is important to take this opportunity to note vasectomy and vasovasostomy surgeries as the most common surgical intervention involving the scrotum and testes:

- *Vasectomy*: Rather than being a treatment for a scrotal condition, vasectomy is used to sterilize men. Vasectomies are commonly performed under local anaesthetic and an incision is made in the scrotum. The vas deferens is located and approximately 1 cm removed from the epididymal end, which is then turned back on itself and ligated to prevent the tube from re-joining.
- *Vasovasostomy*: Vasovasostomy is the procedure to reverse a vasectomy and should be performed under a general anaesthetic. An incision is made in the scrotum or lower abdomen, the ends of the vas deferens are located and re-anastomosed. Vasovasostomies are rare and usually follow a significant life change. Men should be cautioned that vasovasostomy procedures do not guarantee reestablishment of fertility. Dickey et al (2015) provide a comprehensive review of the evolution of vasovasostomy.

Postoperative care, complications, patient education and discharge planning

Postoperative care following scrotal surgery is similar to care following penile surgery. Please see the appropriate section later in this chapter for more information.

In addition to this, specific fertility advice is required for those undergoing vasectomy. Prior to vasectomy it is important that it is fully understood by all relevant parties that a vasectomy is considered a permanent form of contraception and many places require both the patient and their partner to sign a consent form prior to surgery. Following vasectomy, alternative contraception is advised until success of the procedure has been confirmed by a semen analysis.

Also, for those undergoing orchidectomy, it should be made clear to all men how this will affect their fertility.

Care of the patient following penile surgery

Anatomy and physiology of the penis

The penis is an elongated organ consisting of three spongy cylindrical bodies — two dorsal corpora cavernosa and one corpus spongiosum — which surrounds the urethra. The corpora act as storage reservoirs for blood and are surrounded by the Buck's fascia, a tough connective tissue layer. The enlarged head of the penis is known as the glans penis and the urethra opens at its end. The glans penis is covered by the prepuce or foreskin, which is removed during the procedure of circumcision.

Penile erection occurs when there is an increased activity of the sacral parasympathetic nerves, causing vasodilation of the arterioles and constriction of the dorsal veins of the penis. The corpora cavernosa and spongiosum fill with blood, and the penis becomes erect. At ejaculation, detumescence occurs and the penis returns to the flaccid state.

All the above structures are key to the production and transportation of viable sperm. At ejaculation, approximately 3 mL of semen is produced, which contains around 200 million sperm. The whole process of sperm production from inception to completion takes around 74 days.

Pathophysiology and epidemiology of penile conditions

Raising awareness of penile conditions is important so that men do not experience unnecessary poor health, and as a society we become more aware of these conditions that have an enormous effect on men's quality of life.

Erectile dysfunction

Erectile dysfunction, the persistent or recurrent inability to achieve or maintain an erection sufficient for satisfactory sexual activity, is a common disorder, particularly as a person ages (Bella et al, 2015). Other risk factors include diabetes mellitus, vascular disease, Parkinson's disease, multiple sclerosis, pelvic surgery, drugs such as alcohol and antihypertensives, anxiety and stress.

Priapism

Priapism is defined as a persistent painful erection, not associated with sexual desire. The corpora cavernosa becomes engorged as a result of venous congestion and the glans penis and the corpus spongiosum remain flaccid. The condition is often extremely painful and can be frightening for the patient. Priapism is a urological emergency, as a delay in treatment increases the risk of erectile dysfunction and necrosis. Usually the cause is unknown, but risk factors include sickle cell trait, leukemia, tumour within the penis causing blockage, drugs such as marijuana, antihypertensives and anticoagulants, and some treatments of erectile dysfunction.

Phimosis

Phimosis is the term given to the inability to retract the foreskin over the glans penis. The condition is often not detected until the individual is sexually active and complains of painful erections. The individual may also present with balanitis, i.e. inflammation of the foreskin, which is often as a result of inadequate hygiene. Patients who present with phimosis, may require circumcision if the phimosis cannot be reversed.

Paraphimosis

Paraphimosis occurs when the foreskin is retracted over the glans penis and cannot be pulled forward again, resulting in a swollen glans penis and foreskin. The condition usually occurs following sexual intercourse, masturbation, catheterization or medical intervention (e.g. cystoscopy or TURP). Patients should be aware of this potential problem in the postoperative period and ensure that the foreskin is maintained in the forward position. Early diagnosis of paraphimosis can often be treated conservatively with gentle compression to reduce the oedema and manipulation of the foreskin using an anaesthetic gel. If this fails, then surgical intervention will be necessary and usually circumcision is performed.

Peyronie's disease

Plaques of fibrous tissue form in the sheath of the corpora cavernosa of the penis, which adhere to the overlying Buck's fascia (Nehra et al, 2015). This results in penile curvature on erection, and the patient may experience pain and difficulty achieving penetration during sexual intercourse. Aetiology of the condition is unknown, although it can be associated with retroperitoneal fibrosis and Dupuytren's contracture.

Penile cancer

Most penile cancers occur under the foreskin on the glans penis. Therefore, circumcision is thought to be preventative or protective measure, though cancer can occur on any part of the penis. Due to the superficial nature of most tumours, those that are diagnosed early can usually be successfully treated. Fewer than 700 men per year are diagnosed with penile cancer in the UK, though this is steadily increasing. Of these men, approximately 20% are recorded as dying of their cancer each year. Risk factors for penile cancer include human papilloma virus (HPV), presence of a foreskin, age 60 years or over, phimosis, poor personal hygiene, multiple sex partners, and smoking or using tobacco products. As a result, it is thought that most penile cancers are preventable.

Urological assessment and investigations

Most penile conditions are visible to the naked eye and so in most cases limited investigations are required. Where penile cancer is suspected, biopsy should be taken to confirm this.

Due to the range of risk factors for erectile dysfunction, further assessment and investigation is required. If psychogenic causes are suspected, a nocturnal penile tumescence study should be considered. This involves penile strain gauges being attached to the penis and linked to a computer to monitor night-time erections, which occur naturally during periods of rapid eye movement sleep. Generally, this is performed over several nights and patients may be required to undertake this as inpatients. If physiological causes are suspected, blood tests, Doppler ultrasound to measure penile blood flow, and cavernosogram to identify erectile deformity should be considered. Blood tests should measure levels of testosterone, follicle-stimulating hormone and luteinizing hormone levels to exclude hormonal imbalances. Blood glucose estimation is also undertaken to exclude diabetes mellitus.

Treatment

Treatment of penile conditions is largely condition specific, though some conditions may require multiple treatments.

- *PDE-5 inhibitor*: Regardless of suspected cause, a PDE-5 inhibitor, such as Viagra, should be offered to all men with erectile dysfunction providing there are no contraindications.
- *Psychosexual counselling*: This is recommended particularly where psychogenic causes of erectile dysfunction are indicated.
- *Lifestyle advice*: This should also be offered to persons with erectile dysfunction to improve health and, as such, lessen any causal factors such as poor diet and exercise.
- *Other treatment of erectile dysfunction*: Other recommended treatments change rapidly and advice should be sought from the most up-to-date European Association of Urology (EAU) guidelines on male sexual dysfunction (Hatzimouratidis et al, 2019) with consideration given to patient preference.
- *Shunt procedure*: Initial interventions to manage priapism include to wash blood clots out with saline through the insertion of a large bore cannula into the corpus cavernosa under sedation. If unsuccessful, a combination of vasoconstrictors and aspiration is used. If still unsuccessful, a urologist will then surgically perform a 'shunt' procedure to create a venous bypass for the blood to escape through. The long saphenous vein is divided and anastomosed to the corpus cavernosum. This may lead to permanent erectile dysfunction and the patient must be fully informed of this prior to the procedure.
- *Circumcision*: This is the surgical removal of the foreskin and is indicated as a treatment for balanitis, phimosis,

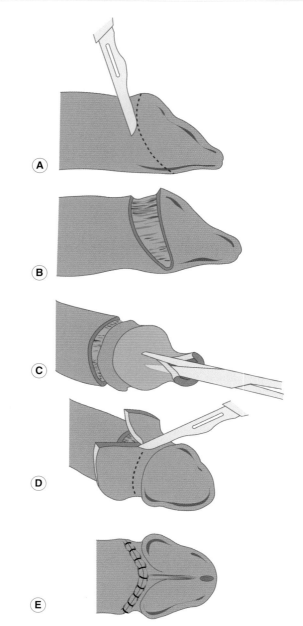

Figure 19.2 Circumcision. (Reproduced from Blandy (1991) by courtesy of Blackwell Science Ltd.)

and paraphimosis (Fig. 19.2). It is also commonly performed in male infants for religious and ritual beliefs. Specific complications include haemorrhage due to the close proximity of the procedure to the dorsal vein and frenular artery, painful erections in the postoperative

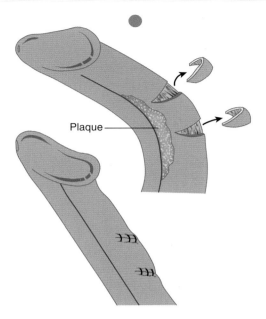

Plaque

Figure 19.3 Nesbit's procedure. (Reproduced from Blandy (1991) by courtesy of Blackwell Science Ltd.)

period (analgesia should be prescribed to treat this) and oedema, which can be relieved or prevented through use of supportive underwear.

- *Nesbit's procedure*: Surgical treatment for Peyronie's disease is usually Nesbit's procedure and is indicated if penile deformity on erection is such that sexual intercourse is impossible or the patient has erectile dysfunction. The operation involves making an incision in the Buck's fascia, on the opposite side to the curvature, leaving the fibrotic plaque intact (Fig. 19.3). Circumcision is often performed at the same time. The procedure results in a shortening in the length of the penis and the patient must be fully informed of this prior to surgery.
- *Lue procedure*: An alternative to Nesbit's procedure, the Lue procedure involves the division of the fibrous plaque with inlaying of saphenous vein in the created space. The advantage of this surgical approach is that there is no shortening of the penis.
- *Penile cancer*: Surgery is the most common treatment for penile cancers. Surgical treatment varies substantially dependent on location, type and grade. Surgical procedures include laser therapy, circumcision, glans resurfacing and wide local excision. In some cases, removal of the glans penis (glansectomy) or removal of the penis itself (penectomy) is required.

Postoperative care following scrotal and penile surgery

As always, good postoperative care begins with good pre-operative care. Preoperatively, patients should receive:

- *Psychological care*: Patients and their partners (where relevant) are often frightened, embarrassed and/or anxious about hospitalization and the impending surgery. It is very important that patients can express any fears and anxieties they may have. Therefore, nurses should provide a relaxed and supportive environment. It can be the role of the nurse to also give emotional and psychological support, but this can also fall to counsellors or psychologists as appropriate. Nurses must be able to recognize their limitations here and be able to refer on.
- *Reducing risk of post-surgical infection*: The perineal and scrotal area should be cleansed prior to surgery, and patients may be prescribed antiseptics for use in a preoperative bath and the area should be shaved (Masterson et al, 2017).

Postoperative care includes, but is not limited to, scrotal support, pain control, wound care, and elimination.

- *Scrotal support*: Following surgery to either the penis or scrotum, patients should be fitted with a correctly fitting scrotal support. It can be useful to record the patient's waist size prior to surgery. Where a scrotal support is not available or recommended, net pants or briefs and a wound dressing pad may suffice.
- *Pain control*: It is unacceptable for patients to experience postoperative pain. Pain should be assessed and controlled with the administration of adequate prescribed analgesics. Nurses should manage analgesia using both verbal and non-verbal communication as appropriate. A correctly fitted scrotal support should relieve pain and enable the patient to mobilize more comfortably. Wound drains should also be secured well to avoid pulling. It should be noted that penile and scrotal pain is often accompanied by nausea. If present, an appropriate antiemetic should be prescribed.
- *Wound care*: Dressings should usually be left intact for 24–48 hours unless otherwise indicated, e.g. signs of infection evident. The wound is then left exposed or redressed with a non-adherent dressing in accordance with patient preference. Usual care should be taken to prevent infection during wound care and indications of infection should be treated promptly. Wound drains should be removed when drainage over a 24-hour period is minimal. It is normal for the area to appear bruised following surgery and patients should be pre-warned of this to avoid undue distress. Additionally, showers rather than baths are recommended where dissolvable sutures are used.

- *Voiding*: It is expected that patients will pass urine within 12 hours following surgery, providing they have adequate fluid intake. Patients are often anxious about voiding postoperatively due to fear of pain. If this occurs, nurses should ensure that patients are pain-free, assist patients into a comfortable position, remove restrictive dressings, and ensure privacy. Voiding postoperatively can cause patients to feel faint so nurses should always remain near the patient in case assistance is needed.
- *Defecating*: It is important that patients are advised not to strain following surgery in case sutures rupture. However, fear of rupture can lead to constipation. Therefore, laxatives can be prescribed to reduce associated anxieties.

Complications of penile and scrotal surgery

Key postoperative complications include haematoma formation, haemorrhage, retention of urine, infection, urethral damage and psychological disturbance.

Haematoma formation

Haematomas can form postoperatively, and these require evacuation in an operating theatre.

Haemorrhage

Due to extensive vasculature of the area, if haemorrhage occurs, pressure should be applied to the area and medical attention sought.

Retention of urine

To prevent retention of urine, privacy, assistance with removing dressings and pain control are required. Where retention continues despite other measures, insertion of an intermittent urinary catheter is indicated.

Infection

Usual treatment of a wound infection is recommended if indicated, and patients should not be discharged home with untreated pyrexia. This is particularly important in men who have had insertion of penile implants or have had skin grafts. When left untreated, the prosthesis can erode through the end of the penis and may cause damage to the urethra, and skin grafts may become necrotic.

Urethral damage

Urethral damage may occur during surgery. Where this occurs, a urethral or suprapubic catheter is inserted for 1 week, though may be required for longer if damage is extensive.

Psychological disturbance

Expectations of surgery are not realized for some patients, and this can lead to considerable psychological trauma. Referral to an appropriate professional should be made.

Patient education and discharge planning following penile and scrotal surgery

If written information is available, this should be given to the patient on admission (or before). Time must be taken to evaluate the patient's understanding of the surgery and to reinforce appropriate information as necessary. Following penile and scrotal surgery, discharge can be on the same day or within 72 hours of surgery. Advice is generally given with regards to wound care, hygiene, pain control, activity, sexual activity, return to work and driving.

- *Wound care*: Instruction is given regarding the need to observe the wound for signs of infection, and if infection is suspected patients should seek guidance from their practice nurse or GP. The patient should be aware that it can take up to 3 weeks for sutures to dissolve. A clean scrotal support or supportive pants should be worn for 2 weeks or longer, and changed as appropriate, as it often takes this time for bruising to subside. Depending on the complexity of the wound, a district nurse may have to visit to monitor the wound.
- *Hygiene*: A shower is recommended for the first 3 days. If patients would prefer to take a bath, soaking of the wound should be discouraged until the suture line has healed.
- *Pain control*: Advice is given on the frequency with which analgesia should be taken and patients should be advised that good pain control should completely absolve the pain, and that poor pain control could lead to further complications. Patients should seek support from their practice nurse or GP for additional support with pain control.
- *Activity*: The patient should be aware of his own limitations, and a gradual return to normal activity is recommended. Contact sports, e.g. football or rugby, should be avoided for at least 2 weeks and up to 4 weeks following vasectomy reversal. Following penile reconstructive surgery, the surgeon will inform each patient of what is expected of them regarding their return to physical activity. Activity following penile reconstruction should not be generalized as each patient's recovery will differ.
- *Sexual activity*: Sexual intercourse can be resumed 1−2 weeks following discharge for most procedures. Following insertion of penile implants, abstinence is advised until the patient is reviewed at the 6-week outpatient appointment. The patient may be advised

to attempt intercourse before the review so that he can report on the outcome.

- *Return to work*: This very much depends on the type of work in which the patient is employed. For example, if he is a manual worker and this involved heavy lifting, then he will require longer than an individual with less strenuous employment.
- *Driving*: Individual driving insurance policies should be referred to. Driving is discouraged until an emergency stop can be performed without straining.

Care of the patient following urethral surgery

Anatomy and physiology of the urethra

The urethra is a long, thin tube that begins at the bladder neck and extends through the penis to the glans penis. The primary role of the urethra is to carry urine and semen from the bladder or testes to outside the body.

Pathophysiology and epidemiology of urethral strictures

A urethral stricture is a narrowing of the lumen of the urethra, usually as a result of scar tissue formation. Causes of urethral strictures include trauma to the urethra (sometimes caused by surgery or by urolithiasis), catheterization (iatrogenic), or by infection.

Urological assessment and investigations

Signs and symptoms of urethral strictures include poor urinary stream, which may be thin, forked and forceful, difficulty in initiating voiding, postmicturition dribbling, urinary retention or feeling of incomplete bladder emptying, and repeated urinary tract infections.

Treatments

Treatment of urethral strictures includes dilation of the urethra, urethrotomy, self-dilation, meatotomy/meatoplasty, and urethroplasty.

Dilation of the urethra

This procedure, which involves regular dilation of the urethra using graduated steel or plastic bougies, is often the treatment of choice for patients who may be unsuitable for alternative management. It is normally performed on an outpatient basis with local anaesthetic gel.

Self-dilation of the urethra

In this procedure, the patient is taught to self-dilate the urethra using a lubricated disposable catheter. The technique is simple to learn and should cause minimal discomfort. However, successful self-dilation as a treatment depends on a skilled teacher and motivated patient. Patients are often encouraged to self-dilate following surgical procedures for urethral strictures. Following surgical procedures, patients usually perform this procedure twice weekly for the first month following healing, then weekly. Flow rate assessment is performed usually 3-monthly to evaluate.

Urethrotomy

Urethrotomy is used in the initial and long-term management of urethral strictures. An endoscopic knife (optical urethrotome) is used under vision to cut the stricture along its length. The procedure is usually performed under general anaesthetic. Postoperatively, the patient will have a urethral catheter *in situ* in line with surgeons' instructions (though usually 48 hours) and patients will usually remain in hospital during this period. Patients should be advised that it is normal to find some blood in the urine initially. Overall, this offers the patient short-term relief from their stricture and is often required to be performed repeatedly.

Meatotomy/Meatoplasty

Meatotomy (incision) or meatoplasty (surgical reconstruction) are used to treat strictures found at the meatus. Postoperatively, patients will have a urinary catheter *in situ* for at least 24 hours.

Urethroplasty

Urethroplasty is an open operation to reconstruct the urethra, and the surgical technique used will depend on the length, severity and location of the stricture (Collins, 2004). If the stricture is short, i.e. 1.5 cm or less, the area can be excised and an end-to-end anastomosis of the urethra can be performed. Where the stricture is longer than 1.5 cm, a substitution urethroplasty is performed. This involves a perineal incision to expose the affected area, which is excised and substituted with grafted skin e.g. buccal mucosa from inside the mouth, skin from behind the ear or skin from the penis or scrotum. The procedure can be performed in one or two stages, depending on the difficulty of the surgery and the type of skin used for the graft.

Postoperative care following urethral surgery

To ensure the best recovery, preoperatively patients should have good psychological care, skin preparation, defecation, and infection advice.

- *Psychological care*: The patient must be given time and the opportunity to express any anxieties they might have regarding the impending surgery and expected outcome.
- *Skin preparation*: The perineal and scrotal area should be cleansed prior to surgery, and patients may be prescribed antiseptics for use in a preoperative bath and the area should be shaved (Masterson et al, 2017).
- *Defecation*: If the patient is constipated prior to surgery then laxatives should be prescribed to avoid straining postoperatively.
- *Infection*: Prophylactic antibiotics should be prescribed preoperatively.

Postoperatively, patients should receive care and advice regarding pain, potential haemorrhage or haematoma, wound care, defecation, voiding, and mobility.

- *Pain*: The combination of an opioid infusion and a non-steroidal anti-inflammatory drug (NSAID) is often the most effective approach to treatment of pain. Patients who have had surgery to the urethra may experience some pain or discomfort on voiding following removal of the catheter due to that contact of urine with the healing tissues.
- *Haematoma formation*: Haematomas can form postoperatively, and these require evacuation in an operating theatre.
- *Haemorrhage*: Due to extensive vasculature of the area, if haemorrhage occurs, pressure should be applied to the area and medical attention sought. A foam compression dressing is often used and is generally most effective in helping to reduce swelling following surgery.
- *Wound care*: The wound dressing is left intact for 3 days if possible. The wound drain is removed when drainage is minimal. The wound is examined each day and healing evaluated. A bath should be taken daily from the fourth day postoperatively and a fresh supportive dressing applied. A corrugated drain is often used and the amount and type of drainage in the wound drain should be recorded.
- *Defecation*: Patients should be advised of the correct hand-washing technique and the importance of perineal cleansing following defecation to avoid wound contamination.
- *Voiding*: A urethral and/or suprapubic catheter will remain *in situ* for up to 3 weeks and the urethral catheter should be secured to avoid damage to the urethra caused by pulling. It is important that the

catheters remain patent so a fluid intake of 3 L of fluids per day is advised. A urethrogram is performed prior to removal of the catheter to ensure that a fistula has not formed. If the urethrogram is satisfactory, the urinary catheter is removed, or the suprapubic catheter is clamped until a voiding pattern has been established. Prior to removal, a urinary flow rate assessment should be performed.

- *Mobility*: To reduce the risk of damaging the urethra, mobility is minimal for the first few days postoperatively. Instruction is given regarding leg and deep breathing exercises, and anti-embolism stockings should be worn and subcutaneous heparin prescribed, to reduce the risk of a deep vein thrombosis occurring.

Patient education and discharge planning following urethral surgery

In addition to the recommended patient education and discharge planning following penile and scrotal surgery, patients should also receive the following information:

- To avoid damaging the new graft, activities involving sexual stimulation of the penis should not resume until at least 6 weeks after surgery.
- Sitting for any length of time should be avoided including when driving long distances.
- If any problems are encountered with voiding, e.g. retention of urine, a suprapubic catheter should be inserted, and the patient seen by the operating urologist as soon as possible.

Conclusion

The field of urological surgical nursing is a progressive and expanding specialty. As nurse involvement in specific surgical urological procedures increases, it is essential that nurses have a sound knowledge base of the reproductive system and the disease processes which may require surgery. This chapter has provided the reader with such information.

SUMMARY OF KEY POINTS

- Benign prostatic hypertrophy and erectile dysfunction are among the most common diseases to affect men beyond middle age.
- The symptoms experienced by these conditions often greatly affect the individual's quality of life.

(Continued)

(cont'd)

- Several treatment options are available for the treatment of benign prostatic hypertrophy and erectile dysfunction.
- Penile and scrotal surgery particularly can be very frightening and embarrassing from the individual patient and it is the nurse's role to help to create a supportive environment for the patient.
- Psychological preparation and support for men undergoing surgery to the male reproductive system is paramount.

REFLECTIVE LEARNING POINTS

Having read this chapter, think about what you now know and what you still need to find out about. These questions may help:

- How might you approach the issue of sex and sexual activity with a man (and, if appropriate, his partner) who is to undergo urological surgery?
- How might a referral to a continence physiotherapist be made in the place where you work?
- What is your local policy and procedure regarding skin preparation prior to urological surgery?

References

Abourmarzouk, O. M. (2019). *Blandy's urology*. Oxford: Wiley-Blackwell.

Ahyai, S. A., Gilling, P., Kaplan, S. A., Kuntz, R. M., Madersbacher, S., Montorsi, F., et al. (2010). Meta-analysis of functional outcomes and complications following transurethral procedures for lower urinary tract symptoms resulting from benign prostatic enlargement. *European Urology, 58* (3), 384−397.

Bella, A. J., Lee, J. C., Carrier, S., Benard, F., & Brock, G. B. (2015). CUA practice guidelines for erectile dysfunction. *Canadian Urological Association Journal, 9*(1−2), 23−29.

Blandy, J. P. (1991). *Lecture notes on urology* (4th edn). London: Blackwell Scientific.

Brawley, O., Jani, A., & Master, V. (2007). Prostate cancer and race. *Current Problems in Cancer, 31*(3), 211−225.

Brewster, D. H., Fraser, L. A., Harris, V., & Black, R. J. (2000). Rising incidence of prostate cancer in Scotland: Increased risk of increased detection? *British Journal of Urology International, 85*(4), 463−473.

Collins, P. (2004). Reconstructive surgery for urinary tract defect. In S. Fillingham, & J. Douglas (Eds.), *Urological nursing* (3rd edn). Edinburgh: Baillière Tindall.

Demirel, I., Ozer, A. B., Bayar, M. K., & Erhan, O. L. (2012). TURP syndrome and severe hyponatremia under general anaesthesia. *British Medical Journal Case Reports*, 2012.

Dickey, R. M., Pastuszak, A. W., Hakky, T. S., Chandrashekar, A., Ramasamy, R., & Lipshultz, L. I. (2015). The evolution of the vasectomy reversal. *Current Urology Reports, 16*(6), 40.

Doughty, L., & Lister, S. (2008). *The Royal Marsden Hospital Manual of Clinical Nursing Procedures* (7th edn). Oxford: Wiley-Blackwell.

Dutta, R., Philip, J., & Javle, P. (2005). Trends in prostate cancer incidence and survival in various socioeconomic classes: a population-based study. *International Journal of Urology, 12*(7), 644−653.

Hatzimouratidis, K., Giuliano, F., Moncada, I., Muneer, A., Salonia, A., & Verze, P. (2019). *Male sexual dysfunction*. Arnhem: European Association of Urology.

Ferlay, J., Soerjomataram, I., Dikshit, R., Eser, S., Mathers, C., Rebelo, M., et al. (2015). Cancer incidence and mortality worldwide: Sources, methods and major patterns in GLOBOCAN 2012. *International Journal of Cancer, 136*(5), E359−E386.

Forbat, L., Place, M., Kelly, D., Hubbard, G., Boyd, K., Howie, K., et al. (2012). A cohort study reporting clinical risk factors and individual risk perceptions of prostate cancer: Implications for PSA testing. *British Journal of Urology International, 111*(3), 389−395.

Giovannucci, E., Liu, Y., Platz, E., Stampfer, M., & Willett, W. (2007). Risk factors for prostate cancer incidence and progression in the health professionals follow-up study. *International Journal of Cancer, 121*(7), 1571−1578.

Gravas, S., Cornu, J. N., Drake, M. J., Gacci, M., Gratzke, C., Herrmann, T. R. W., et al. (2018). *EAU guidelines on management of non-neurogenic male lower urinary tract symptoms (LUTS).*

Arnhem: European Association of Urology.

Hayward, J. (1975). *Information − A Prescription against Pain*. RCN Study of Nursing Care Series. London: Royal College of Nursing.

Heijnsdijk, E., Wever, E., Auvinen, A., Hugosson, J., Ciatto, S., Nelen, V., et al. (2012). Quality of life effects of prostate specific antigen screening. *New England Journal of Medicine, 367*(7), 595−605.

Ilic, D., Neuberger, M., Djulbegovic, M., & Dahm, P. (2013). Screening for prostate cancer. *The Cochrane Database of Systematic Reviews* (1), CD004720.

Leitzmann, M., & Rohrmann, S. (2012). Risk factors for the onset of prostate cancer: age, location, and behavioral correlates. *Clinical Epidemiology, 4*, 1−11.

Loeb, S., Vellekoop, A., Ahmed, H. U., Catto, J., Emberton, M., Nam, R., et al. (2013). Systematic review of complications of prostate biopsy. *European Association of Urology, 64*(6), 876−892.

Lynch, M., Sriprasad, S., Subramonian, K., & Thompson, P. (2010). Postoperative haemorrhage following transurethral resection of the prostate (TURP) and photoselective vaprosiation of the prostate (PVP). *Annals of the Royal College of Surgeons of England, 92*(7), 555−558.

Masson, P., & Brannigan, R. E. (2014). The varicocele. *Urologic Clinics of North America, 41*(1), 129−144.

Masterson, T. A., Palmer, J., Dubin, J., & Ramasamy, R. (2017). Medical pre-operative considerations for patients undergoing penile implantation. *Translational Andrology and Urology, 6* (Suppl 5), S824−S829.

Mistry, M., Parkin, D., Ahmad, A., & Sasieni, P. (2011). Cancer incidence in the United Kingdom: Projections to the year 2030. *British Journal of Cancer, 105* (11), 1795–1803.

Moller, H., Fairley, L., Coupland, V., Okello, C., Green, M., Forman, D., et al. (2007). The future burden of cancer in England: Incidence and numbers of new patients in 2020. *British Journal of Cancer, 96*(9), 1484–1488.

Mottet, N., Bellmunt, J., Briers, E., van den Bergh, R., Bolla, M., van Castern, N. J., et al. (2019). *European Association of Urology guidelines on Prostate Cancer.* Arnhem: European Association of Urology.

Nehra, A., Alterowitz, R., Culkin, D. J., Faraday, M. M., Hakim, L. S., Heidelbaugh, J., et al. (2015). Peyronie's disease: AUA Guidelines. *Journal of Urology, 194*(3), 745–753.

Nursing and Midwifery Council. (2018). *The Code. Professional Standards of Practice and Behaviour for Nurses.* Midwives and Nursing Associates. Available at: <www.nmc.org.uk/globalassets/sitedocuments/nmc-publications/nmc-code.pdf>.

Olapade-Olaopa, E. O., Solomon, L. Z., Carter, C. J., Ahiaki, E. K., & Chiverton, S. G. (1998). Haematuria and clot retention after transurethral resection of the prostate: A pilot study. *British Journal of Urology, 82*(5), 624–627.

Olmsted, S. S., Dubin, N. H., Cone, R. A., & Moench, T. R. (2000). The rate at which human sperm are immobilized and killed by mild acidity. *Fertility and Sterility, 73*(4), 687–693.

Park, J. S., Jongchan, K., Ahmed, E., & Ham, W. S. (2018). Recent global trends in testicular cancer incidence and mortality. *Medicine, 97*(37), e12390.

Phillips, S., Hutchinson, S., & Davidson, T. (1993). Preoperative drinking does not affect gastric contents. *British Journal of Anaesthesia, 70*(1), 6–9.

Scholtes, S. (2002). Management of clot retention following urological surgery. *Nursing Times, 98*(28), 48–50.

Serefoglu, E. C., Altinova, S., Ugras, N. S., Akincioglu, E., Asil, E., & Balbay, M. D. (2013). How reliable is 12-core prostate biopsy procedure in the detection of prostate cancer? *Canadian Urological Association Journal, 7*(5–6), E293–E298.

Shafique, K., & Morrison, D. (2013). Socio-economic inequalities in survival of patients with prostate cancer: role of age and Gleason grade at diagnosis. *PLOS One, 8*(2), e56184.

Shafique, K., Oliphant, R., & Morrison, D. S. (2012). The impact of socio-economic circumstances on overall and grade-specific prostate cancer incidence: a population-based study. *British Journal of Cancer, 107*(3), 575–582.

Siddiqui, M. M., Rais-Bahrami, S., Turkbey, B., George, A. K., Rothwax, J., Shakir, N., et al. (2015). Comparison of MR/ultrasound fusion–guided biopsy with ultrasound-guided biopsy for the diagnosis of prostate cancer. *The Journal of the American Medical Association, 313* (4), 390–397.

Somani, B. K., Watson, G., & Townell, N. (2010). Testicular torsion. *British Medical Journal, 341,* c3213.

Urolift. (2019). *What is the UroLift sytem?* Available at: <www.urolift.com/what-is-urolift>

Whittemore, A. S., Kolonel, L. N., Wu, A. H., John, E. M., Gallagher, R. P., Howe, G. R., et al. (1995). Prostate cancer in relation to diet, physical activity, and body size in blacks, whites, and Asians in the United States and Canada. *Journal of the National Cancer Institute, 87*(9), 652–661.

Wise, J. (2018). Testicular cancer: Symptoms for urgent referral are identified. *British Medical Journal, 362,* k2900.

Further reading and relevant websites

Most good anatomy and physiology textbooks contain good, concise information on the anatomy and physiology of the male reproductive system. However, for a more interactive experience, www.innerbody.com and www.teachmeanatomy.info are recommended.

All nurses caring for persons with conditions of the male reproductive system should be aware of the relevant European Association of Urology guidelines, available from: uroweb.org/guidelines.

Chapter 20

Patients requiring gynaecological surgery

Georgina Lewis

KEY OBJECTIVES OF THE CHAPTER

After reading this chapter the reader will understand:

- the relevant anatomy and physiology of the female
  reproductive system
- specific investigations that may be required by a
  woman undergoing gynaecological surgery
- different types of gynaecological surgery
- what women will experience in hospital and during
  recovery at home
- discharge advice for specific operations
- sexual aspects of gynaecological surgery.

Areas to think about before reading the chapter

- What do you understand by women's health?
- Provide an overview of the menstrual cycle.
- What is the role of the nurse with regards to
  safeguarding?

Introduction

Any surgery is likely to cause anxiety but gynaecological surgery is a particularly sensitive area. Outpatient appointments and admission to hospital often involve vaginal examinations – the most personal of all medical examinations, and a cause of anxiety to many women (Durnell Schuiling & Likis, 2017). It is crucial to gain a woman's confidence and provide a relaxed environment where dignity and privacy are maintained.

Gynaecological surgery may also pose a threat to a woman's concept of her body image, fertility, her role as a woman and as a mother, her sexuality and her relationship with her partner (Fritzer et al, 2013; Cleary et al, 2013). Discussions of sensitive subjects such as sexuality can be forgotten or even avoided by healthcare professionals. Some professionals may fear saying the wrong thing or causing embarrassment. Although every patient will have unique concerns, use of effective and patient-focused communication can be extremely beneficial (Janssen & Lagro-Janssen, 2012). It is vitally important to treat each patient as an individual, to listen to their concerns and, where appropriate, act as their advocate to support holistic care (Box 20.1).

The aim of this chapter is to promote awareness of the wider issues of the psychological effects and related sexuality surrounding gynaecological surgery. Nurses will then be better informed to care sensitively for these women.

Anatomy and physiology of the reproductive system

The female reproductive system consists of the internal genitalia situated in the pelvis – two ovaries, two fallopian tubes, uterus, cervix, vagina – and the external genitalia, comprising the vulva.

The ovaries

The ovaries are the female gonads or sex glands. They are located either side of the uterus, within the pelvic cavity. They measure approximately 3.5 cm in length, 2 cm in depth and 1 cm in thickness. Each ovary is attached to the broad ligament by a thin mesentery, the mesovarian. The blood supply is via the ovarian arteries, which stem from the dorsal aorta on the posterior abdominal wall. The left ovarian vein drains into the left renal vein and the right ovarian vein empties directly into the inferior vena cava.

The ovary is composed of a cortex and medulla. It is surrounded by a layer of germinal epithelium. The ovaries produce ova or eggs and secrete the hormones oestrogen, progesterone and small amounts of androgens.

At birth, each ovary contains at least two to three million primordial follicles. Some of these follicles will develop within the ovarian cortex and become mature cystic follicles. These are known as graafian follicles. The ovum is embedded within the graafian follicle, and, when

mature, one will be released each month, at ovulation, ready for potential fertilization by a sperm.

Ovulation occurs 14 days before the onset of menstruation, midcycle in a 28-day cycle. Some women experience pelvic pain each month when ovulation occurs, known as 'mittelschmerz'. Conception is most likely to occur shortly after ovulation.

The menstrual cycle prepares the uterus for pregnancy. If conception occurs, menstruation does not take place. If the ovaries are removed, menstruation ceases and pregnancy cannot occur.

The menstrual cycle

The menstrual cycle occurs in most women every 28–39 days but may vary from 21 to 42 days. It is controlled by ovarian and pituitary hormones.

Follicle-stimulating hormone (FSH) from the anterior pituitary gland causes the follicle to grow and stimulates the granulosa cells in the graafian follicle to produce oestrogen. As the level of oestrogen rises, it inhibits further production of FSH but stimulates the release of luteinizing hormone (LH), and ovulation occurs.

Accompanying the ovarian and pituitary cycles are a series of changes in the uterine endometrium. When menstruation occurs, the endometrium is shed down to its basal layer and is accompanied by bleeding. Under the influence of oestrogen, regeneration begins, and the endometrium grows thicker. This is the proliferation phase and lasts about 10 days.

Following ovulation and the production of progesterone, the endometrium becomes thicker and the glands more tortuous. This is the secretory phase and lasts about 14 more days, after which the lining is shed again.

After the discharge of the ovum from the graafian follicle, the granulosa cells multiply rapidly and a corpus luteum is formed. The corpus luteum functions as an endocrine gland, secreting oestrogen and progesterone. It persists for about 14 days, after which it degenerates if fertilization has not occurred.

If a pregnancy occurs, the corpus luteum continues to produce both oestrogen and progesterone for about 12 weeks, after which the placenta takes over the production of these hormones.

The corpus luteum is sustained by human chorionic gonadotrophin (hCG), which is produced by the cells of the trophoblast (embryo) from the time of implantation.

Box 20.1 **Questions to open up discussion of sexual anxieties following hysterectomy**

- How will hysterectomy change your life?
- What do you feel is the most important function of your uterus?
- What are your thoughts about losing your uterus?

The fallopian tubes

Two fallopian tubes (also known as uterine tubes) join the uterus just below the fundus of the uterus. Each tube is 10–14 cm long. The end of the fallopian tube distal to the uterus is referred to as the fimbriae and has small finger-like projections. The fimbriae sweep the ovum into the fallopian tube. Fertilization takes place in the tubes, which then carry the fertilized ovum into the uterus, wafted along by the ciliated epithelial cells which line the tubes.

Uterus

The uterus is a hollow, pear-shaped muscular organ lying between the bladder and the rectum. It is made up of the fundus, body and cervix.

The thick muscular wall of the uterus is called the myometrium, while the body of the uterus is lined with a mucous membrane called the endometrium. This is a very vascular layer which differs in thickness throughout the menstrual cycle and is largely shed during menstruation.

The uterus normally lies in an anteverted position, meaning that the long axis of the uterus is directed forwards. It is held in place by muscular and fibrous supports. The muscle is arranged in a spiral form running from the cornu to the cervix, giving a circular effect around the fallopian tubes and cervix, and an oblique effect over the body of the uterus. The important muscular supports are the levator ani muscles. The uterine ligaments include:

- anteriorly – the round ligaments
- laterally – the transverse cervical ligaments
- posteriorly – the uterosacral ligaments.

The broad ligaments, although referred to as a ligament, are folds of peritoneum attaching the uterus to the pelvic side walls, helping to hold the uterine fundus in an anteverted position (Tortora & Grabowski, 2003).

The blood supply to the uterus is derived from two pairs of arteries: the uterine and ovarian arteries.

Cervix

The cervix is the neck of the uterus and extends into the top of the vagina. The cervix is 2–3 cm long and dilates during childbirth to allow the passage of the baby.

The outer surface of the cervix in the vagina is covered with squamous epithelium. Squamous cells begin to grow from beneath the columnar epithelium and gradually replace it. The point at which the squamous cells of the ectocervix (outer cervix) meet the columnar cells of the endocervix (inner cavity) is known as the squamocolumnar junction.

The normal replacement of one type of cell by another is called squamous metaplasia, and where it takes place is called the transformation or transitional zone. During the menstrual cycle the glands in the cervix respond to rising levels of oestrogen by secreting an abundance of mucus. Changes occur in the consistency of the mucus during the cycle This mucus is alkaline and neutralizes the acidic vaginal secretions.

Vagina

The vagina is a muscular canal joining the uterus to the external genitalia. It is about 8 cm long, and normally the anterior and posterior walls are in close contact with one another. They lie in folds called rugae, which expand during sexual intercourse and childbirth.

During the reproductive years, Döderlein's bacilli, a form of lactobacilli, appear in the vagina and produce lactic acid by acting on the glycogen in the epithelial cells. This results in a vaginal environment with a pH of 4, which helps prevent infection.

Vulva

The vulva (meaning 'cover' in Latin) is the collective name given to the external female reproductive organs. The vulva consists of the labia majora, the labia minora, clitoris, vestibule of the vagina, bulb of the vestibule, and the glands of Bartholin. It extends from the mons pubis to the perineum and is bounded by the labia majora.

Specific investigations for patients requiring gynaecological surgery

Pelvic examination

Vaginal examination

The examination is a tool of physical diagnosis and can be performed by either doctors or trained allied health professionals. The examination may be digital (bimanual) or involve the insertion of a speculum.

This is a most intimate procedure and many women have concerns or anxieties regarding this aspect of patient assessment. It is highly advisable to have a chaperone present and essential to gain consent for examination.

It is crucial to provide support and explanation to the woman, always ensure privacy and maintain the woman's dignity. Some women prefer to be told exactly what is happening; others like to be distracted by talking about family or holidays, etc. The more relaxed the patient is, the less uncomfortable the examination. However, it is important to understand that simply advising the patient to 'relax' may be insufficient or even patronizing. It may be better to suggest relaxation techniques or deep breathing exercises as an alternative.

It is advisable that the woman empties her bladder first and is allowed to remove her underclothing in private. A blanket should always be available to maintain her dignity during the examination.

Speculum examination

The clinician will often need to use a speculum to view the cervix, for example in order to take a cervical smear or to obtain a high vaginal swab to test for sexually transmitted infections. The most common type of speculum is a Cusco's or bivalve speculum, which parts the vaginal walls, enabling visualization of the cervix.

Alternatively, a Sims' speculum may be used. This instrument is more commonly used in theatre with the patient in lithotomy but may also be used in clinic with the woman lying in a modified left lateral position. It is used to assess any prolapse of the uterus or vaginal wall. The woman may be asked to cough to demonstrate any signs of stress incontinence.

Bimanual palpation

A bimanual examination is carried out with two hands palpating together, one on the woman's abdomen, pressing down on the fundus (top) of the uterus, and one inside the vagina. The size, position and movement of the uterus are determined via this examination. Other structures such as the ovaries and fallopian tubes are located. Any masses, such as a pregnancy, ovarian cyst or tumor, are noted.

The bimanual examination can be performed with the woman in the dorsal position, in which the woman will be asked to draw her knees up with her ankles together and asked to relax her knees apart.

Cervical screening

This is performed by examining cells from the cervix and identifying early changes, which might lead to squamous cell carcinoma. The aim of the NHS Cervical Screening Programme (NHSCSP) is to reduce the incidence of and mortality from cervical cancer through a systematic, quality-assured population-based screening programme for eligible women (NHS Cervical Screening Programme, 2016).

Cells are taken from the squamocolumnar junction of the cervix, where most precancerous changes originate, and then sent to the laboratory for histological examination. The current standard screening test uses liquid-based cytology. The head of the brush, used to obtain the sample, is put into a small vial containing preservative fluid or is rinsed directly into this fluid. In the laboratory the sample is spun and a random sample of the remaining cells is taken. A thin layer of the cells is then put onto a slide. This is examined under a microscope.

All women during their reproductive years should have a smear test every 3 years from age 25 to 50, then every 5 years until 65 (NHS Cervical Screening Programme, 2016). Routine smears are not usually undertaken during pregnancy, but screening can recommence 3 months postpartum. If a woman has an abnormal result, the frequency of smears is increased.

Sometimes the cervix may appear red. This is a normal physiological state and occurs when there is only a single layer of columnar cells covering the connective tissue and blood vessels. This is an 'ectropion'.

The most common type of abnormal or dyskaryotic cells is cervical intraepithelial neoplasia (CIN). There are three stages of cervical intraepithelial neoplasia.

- *CIN1* refers to cells that have minor changes in cell structure which are the first signs of precancer. In the vast majority of women under 25, low-grade changes will revert to normal without treatment, hence the decision to commence screening above the age of 25 (NHS Cervical Screening Programme, 2016). Where CIN1 is identified, repeat smears may be required more frequently, depending on local policy.
- *CIN2* is the next stage, which usually correlates with moderate dyskaryosis where there are more marked changes. A repeat smear or colposcopy is usually recommended.
- *CIN3* is the most severe preinvasive abnormality and is also known as carcinoma *in situ*. There are definite changes of premalignancy, and one in three lesions will progress to invasive cervical cancer unless the abnormal cells are removed. An urgent colposcopy and biopsy are required to determine whether the malignant cells have become invasive.

Clinical studies have shown that the human papillomavirus (HPV), and in particular strains 16 and 18 of the virus, are responsible for the vast majority of cervical cancers (World Health Organization, 2014). In September 2008 a national immunization programme to protect against HPV was introduced in the United Kingdom for girls aged 12−13 across the UK. In July 2018 it was announced that the immunization programme would be extended to include boys aged 12−13. It is predicted that by vaccinating boys as well as girls, additional cases of HPV-attributable cervical cancer will be prevented in women. There should also be a reduction in the cases of other HPV-attributable cancers for both males and females (Joint Committee on Vaccination and Immunisation, 2018).

It is likely to be many years before the vaccination programme has an effect upon cervical cancer incidence, so women are advised to continue accepting their invitations for cervical screening (NHS Cervical Screening Programme, 2016).

Colposcopy

Colposcopy is the inspection of the cervix and its surrounding tissue with binocular magnification. A microscope is used, which allows magnification of up to 10 times.

Colposcopy is usually undertaken in a gynaecology outpatient department, a specific colposcopy unit or a genitourinary department. The procedure may be undertaken by a doctor or specially trained nurse colposcopist. It is advisable to explain to the woman that the large-looking microscope and its attachments will not go inside her. The procedure is similar to taking a cervical smear, apart from the fact the woman's legs will be in a lithotomy position, i.e. in stirrups. A biopsy may also be taken under local anaesthetic. In many units, the woman may be given the opportunity to view her cervix on a television screen.

Colposcopy is indicated when there have been changes in the cells of the cervix, noted on the woman's smear test. It enables the position and extent of the CIN to be ascertained, so that the correct management is chosen. Increasingly, treatment can be carried out at colposcopy, using local ablative therapy such as cold coagulation or diathermy loop excision, eliminating the need for general anaesthetic.

Discharge advice following colposcopy

• There may be a bloodstained discharge or it may be watery. A panty liner or sanitary towel should be used for sufficient protection. Tampons should not be used for the first period after treatment, to reduce the risk of infection.
• Follow-up is crucial to the ongoing care of women who have had an abnormal smear test. Most women will have a follow-up colposcopy after 6 months and then annual smears for 2 years.
• If the woman has had treatment to the cervix, she should refrain from sexual intercourse for 4–6 weeks to enable the biopsied area of the cervix to heal. Signs of local infection include heavy fresh bleeding or an offensive-smelling discharge.

Pelvic ultrasound scan

Ultrasound is used as a means of examining various organs of the body by means of high-frequency sound waves. These form pictures on a screen and enable any abnormalities to be detected. The uterus and ovaries can be identified and any tumor located and measured. During the menstrual cycle, the growth of a graafian follicle may be observed and the thickness of the endometrium measured, so that the timing of ovulation is confirmed.

A full bladder is necessary as it helps push the uterus and ovaries into a better position for examination. The woman should fill her bladder by drinking 1 L of fluid (not fizzy drinks) during the 2 hours before the appointment. This can be very uncomfortable for the woman.

The procedure takes between 5 and 10 minutes and is not painful but may be uncomfortable. This is because the radiographer has to press firmly, using cold gel, against the abdomen and full bladder, in order to produce a clear picture.

Transvaginal ultrasound scan

This type of scan facilitates a much clearer view of the abdominal organs than an abdominal scan. It is useful in confirming the presence of an early intrauterine or ectopic pregnancy or for identifying a missing intrauterine contraceptive device. An ultrasound scan cannot harm a pregnancy.

The tip of a round-edged probe is covered by a disposable condom, and then inserted into the vagina.

Endometrial biopsy

It is possible to obtain tissue for endometrial biopsy without a general anaesthetic in the outpatient clinic. This may be more suitable for women who do not wish to have a general anaesthetic or for whom a general anaesthetic may be unsuitable, such as elderly women. A narrow plastic pipette is introduced into the endometrial cavity and a biopsy taken. The woman should be advised that this can be uncomfortable but is a relatively quick procedure. The disadvantage of this technique over hysteroscopy is that it is performed blind whereas hysteroscopy facilitates inspection of the whole of the cavity.

Hysteroscopy

A small fiberoptic telescope is passed through the cervix into the uterus. The walls of the uterus are separated with gas or fluid to enable the telescope to view inside the uterus.

Hysteroscopy is increasingly performed as an outpatient procedure, avoiding the need for a general anaesthetic. Additional procedures may be carried out at the same time such as obtaining a biopsy or insertion of an intrauterine device (IUD).

Laparoscopy

This test enables the direct visualization of the pelvic organs using a fiberoptic light and a telescope-like instrument known as a laparoscope. Under general anaesthesia, the woman is catheterized and placed head downwards (in the Trendelenburg position) to allow the upper abdominal contents to fall away from the pelvic organs.

A small incision is made below the umbilicus and carbon dioxide is introduced into the abdominal cavity to obtain a 'pneumoperitoneum'. This helps to displace the intestines and allows the pelvic and abdominal organs to be viewed easily via the laparoscope. Traditionally gynaecologists have chosen to use higher intraoperative pressures (i.e. use more carbon dioxide than other specialties performing laparoscopy), however there is no agreed consensus as to the optimum pressures for the procedure and there have been studies showing that using a lower pressure can reduce some complications including postoperative pain (Kyle et al, 2016).

Additional instruments can be inserted via additional ports – the number and size of which will depend on the procedure being performed. A simple diagnostic procedure may require only one instrument port whereas a more complex procedure (such as hysterectomy) will require additional port(s).

Thorough observation of the pelvic organs can then be undertaken. As an investigation for infertility, methylene blue is injected through the cervix and observed via the laparoscope as it passes through the fallopian tubes and out via the fimbrial ends into the pelvic cavity. The dye illustrates any blockages in the tubes which might prevent the eggs from the ovaries reaching the uterus. If the dye flows through, the tubes are assumed to be patent, although the state of the cilia in the lining cannot be seen. If the test is performed during the follicular phase of the cycle, developing follicles may be viewed.

The woman should be warned that she may feel bloated and have an aching pain around the shoulders. This is quite normal and is caused by the carbon dioxide in the abdomen irritating the phrenic nerve. Paracetamol and hot peppermint water can give relief.

Developments in laparoscopic techniques mean that procedures previously carried out through an open laparotomy including oophorectomy and hysterectomy are now done through laparoscopy, resulting in a quicker recovery time.

Urodynamic investigations

Urinary incontinence (UI) is a common symptom that can affect women of all ages, with a wide range of severity and nature. UI is defined by the International Continence Society as 'the complaint of any involuntary leakage of urine' (NICE, 2015). UI may occur as a result of a number of abnormalities of function of the lower urinary tract or as a result of other illnesses, which tend to cause leakage in different situations. Stress UI is involuntary urine leakage on effort or exertion or on sneezing or coughing. Urgency UI is involuntary urine leakage accompanied or immediately preceded by urgency (a sudden compelling desire to urinate that is difficult to delay). Mixed UI is involuntary urine leakage associated with both urgency and exertion, effort, sneezing or coughing.

Overactive bladder (OAB) is defined as urgency that occurs with or without urgency UI and usually with frequency and nocturia.

Urodynamic investigations measure changes in bladder pressure with changes in bladder volume. This investigation is recommended to demonstrate specific abnormalities before undertaking complex urological procedures (NICE, 2015). A catheter is inserted into the bladder, and a pressure catheter is placed in the rectum to measure abdominal pressure. This eliminates movement artefacts which may be produced if the intravesical pressure alone is measured. The rectal pressure is subtracted from the intravesical pressure to give the detrusor pressure.

The bladder is filled at a fast rate of 100 mL/min. The woman indicates when she first feels the sensation of filling and when her bladder feels full. The water flow is switched off; she then stands up and is asked to cough to demonstrate any urinary leakage. She then sits on the uroflowmeter (a commode-like lavatory) and empties her bladder in private while the peak flow rate and maximum volume pressure are noted.

Video cystourethrography (VCU) can also be carried out, which allows visualization of the urethral sphincter mechanism and demonstrates any associated bladder pathology. This is particularly useful if the patient has previously had continence surgery or there is a medical indication for an X-ray.

Ambulatory urodynamics may be required if the results of normal urodynamics are inconclusive, or the patient still has symptoms and is not responding to treatment. This uses special equipment and lasts for 4 hours. Pressure catheters are placed in the bladder and rectum as for urodynamics but the patient is encouraged to mobilize. Measurements are checked every hour.

Cystoscopy

This procedure involves the thorough examination of the bladder. A cystoscope, a fine telescope-like instrument with a light source, is inserted into the urethra and passed into the bladder. This enables the urogynaecologist to view inside the bladder, and a biopsy may be taken. The procedure may be undertaken under a local anaesthetic in which case a flexible cystoscopy is used or if additional procedures (such as biopsies) are required cystoscopy may be performed under general anaesthetic.

This operation is carried out to investigate the cause of recurrent urinary tract infections or haematuria (blood in the urine). Small polyps in the bladder or a caruncle (a small fleshy lump) at the urethral entrance can be removed during the procedure.

Pregnancy testing

A pregnancy test detects human chorionic gonadotrophin, which is excreted in the urine. The level of this marker hormone in blood and urine reaches its highest point in normal pregnancy between the 8th and 12th weeks. However, modern pregnancy testing kits are now so sensitive that they can detect a level as low as 25–30 IU/L.

Human chorionic gonadotrophin levels in an ectopic pregnancy (i.e. a pregnancy occurring outside the uterus, most commonly in a fallopian tube) are lower than those found at a comparable period of gestation in a normal pregnancy. In instances of suspected ectopic pregnancy, the measurement of serum concentration of the β subunit of human chorionic gonadotrophin (β-hCG) is of great value, especially when used in conjunction with ultrasound scanning.

The level of β-hCG in a viable intrauterine pregnancy doubles approximately every 2 days. At a titre of 1000–1500 IU/L, it should be possible to detect an intrauterine sac on a transvaginal scan. Absence of β-hCG eliminates pregnancy, but levels above 1500 IU/L in the presence of an empty uterus may indicate a pregnancy of unknown location (PUL), often referred to as ectopic, or a very early intrauterine pregnancy. Repeat blood tests may be required after 48 hours to assess both the amount and rate of increase of β-hCG levels.

Rhesus status

The rhesus factor is found in the red blood cells of 85% of the population (rhesus-positive); the other 15% are rhesus-negative (Tortora & Grabowski, 2003). If a mother is rhesus negative and the fetus is rhesus positive and a small amount of fetal blood passes into the mother's blood stream, her body will be stimulated by these foreign cells and she will start to make rhesus antibodies. If the pregnancy continues there will be no harm to the fetus. However, once the antibodies have been produced these could affect future pregnancies. If a subsequent fetus is rhesus negative, there will be no problem as they do not have rhesus antigens. However, a rhesus-positive fetus will have rhesus antigens. The antibodies in the mother's blood will cross the placenta and attack the fetus's red blood cells causing haemolysis (Fig. 20.1).

Rhesus disease may be prevented by the injection of immunoglobulin 'anti-D', which destroys any rhesus-positive cells that have entered a woman's bloodstream. It therefore prevents the woman's body from making the antibodies but must be given within 72 hours of the placenta separating.

Assessment of patient requiring gynaecological surgery

The majority of gynaecological operations are undertaken as planned elective admissions, giving the preadmission team the opportunity to prepare a woman both physically and psychologically for surgery. That being said, gynaecological nursing is a particularly sensitive area, with each patient having unique circumstances and individual concerns or consideration. For certain procedures, including where cancer is a high probability, there may be relatively little time between preadmission and surgery. Finding an empathetic listener can be the first step a woman takes in coming to terms with a difficult diagnosis, be it an unwanted pregnancy or a suspected cancer. Many women find the process of coming for treatment daunting but an effectively run preadmission clinic, which is holistic in nature, can provide invaluable opportunities to inform and prepare the patient whilst including her in the creation of an individual treatment plan (Allison & George, 2014; Gray et al, 2015).

It is important that a full nursing assessment is made as soon as possible after admission and the nurse establishes a rapport quickly so support can be provided for the woman, who may find the situation both distressing and embarrassing (Setchell, 2013).

The woman will visit the clinic, where a practitioner will assess her health status. Ward procedures and the planned surgery will be explained, information leaflets given and any preoperative investigations performed. The National Institute for Health and Care Excellence has produced guidelines for routine preoperative tests based on the American Society of Anesthesiologists' (ASA) grading and grading of surgery booked (NICE, 2016). These may include a full blood count, and group and save for women undergoing major surgery. Here, the laboratory saves some of the patient's blood so that it can be crossmatched with appropriate units of blood in case she should hemorrhage during surgery. Electrophoresis is required for those of Afro-Caribbean and Mediterranean origin to exclude sickle cell disease and β-thalassaemia. Women aged 60 years old or above often require an electrocardiogram to detect any unknown cardiac problems.

In many units, preoperative assessment is performed by the nurse or practitioner. This is to establish a baseline assessment from which change and progress may be compared. It is important to obtain a general medical and social background, as well as a specific obstetric and gynaecological history. An obstetric history listing pregnancies, miscarriages and terminations should be obtained, although some women prefer that any terminations revealed

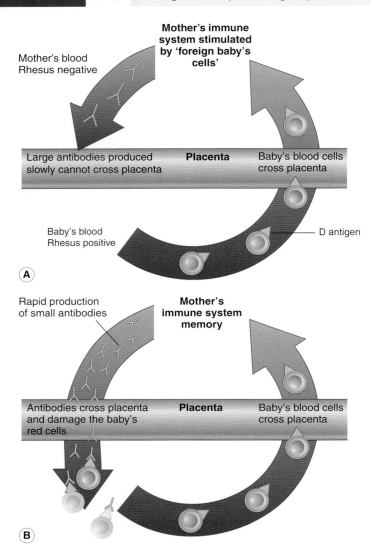

Figure 20.1 Rhesus disease and (A) first and (B) second pregnancies. (Reproduced with permission from Baxter Healthcare).

are not actually recorded. For women undergoing continence surgery, any babies weighing more than 8 lb should be noted and the length of labour and type of delivery are also pertinent. A long labour resulting in a forceps delivery may damage the pelvic floor and urethra. The terms 'gravida', meaning 'pregnancy', and 'para', meaning 'live children', are often used. Thus, a woman described as being G4 P2^{2TOP} means four pregnancies leading to two live children and two terminations.

A menstrual history is also recorded. Every woman has her own idea of what a 'normal' period is like, and therefore it is helpful to ask specific questions such as how many pads/tampons a day she uses during a period. The

length of the period and duration of cycle are important, as is the occurrence of any dysmenorrhoea (moderate–severe period pain) and premenstrual tension.

Any contraception used should be noted. Women using the oral contraceptive pill may be advised to stop taking it before surgery, due to the risk of developing deep vein thrombosis (DVT) following surgery.

An assessment of bowel and urinary function should also be carried out. Many women suffer constipation following surgery. It is helpful to know if a woman suffers from this preoperatively as well, to plan her care accordingly. An overview of a woman's bladder dysfunction is particularly important if she is undergoing continence surgery. Urinary incontinence has been a 'taboo' subject for many years, and women have often been too ashamed or embarrassed to admit that they leak urine. Asking the woman direct questions at an appropriate time will often be a relief to her that the subject has been mentioned. Sometimes, closed questions (questions to which the reply is yes or no) are more useful to elicit information from the woman than are open questions, which may be misinterpreted. For example, the question, 'Do you ever leak urine when you sneeze or during exercise?' is very clear.

Sometimes, assessment may take place while casually talking about another topic or when performing a physical task. Many nurses feel out of their depth discussing sexual matters, but often the patient just wants the opportunity to talk about her experiences and feelings.

Obviously, not all nurses are trained to perform vaginal examinations, but it is a skill with enormous benefits for the woman and the nurse. It may become a basis for a psychosexual nursing assessment without medical staff being present. Many continence and family planning nurses assess pelvic floor function while performing a vaginal examination, and it makes teaching pelvic floor exercises much easier.

The preadmission clinic provides an ideal opportunity for all these assessments to be undertaken by nursing staff. Unfortunately, due to the very busy nature and rapid turnover of most gynaecological wards, a nurse may only have 10–15 minutes to admit each patient, so the assessment must be straightforward and relatively quick.

The model of care based on activities of daily living developed by Roper, Logan and Tierney (2003) is frequently used as an assessment framework for planning care, since it is relatively easy to use. Often 'standard' care plans are used where the care required changes rapidly pre- and postoperatively, to plan care for discharge, and to identify areas where patient teaching is required. However, it is important that the psychological care of the individual woman and her family are also considered.

Integrated care pathways are often used as the basis for planning the care of women admitted for specific procedures. However, nurses must still provide individualized nursing care, based on a holistic assessment that includes the woman's perception of her own anatomy and physiology, with special attention to body image and sexuality.

Increasingly there has been a move towards 'Enhanced Recovery' (ER) in gynaecology. The aim of such programmes is to deliver an optimal surgical pathway designed to minimize the overall physiological and psychological impact of the surgical procedure and therefore to help patients recover sooner. An ER pathway can be divided into three main parts: preoperative patient preparation, perioperative interventions and postoperative

rehabilitation (McDonald, 2015). Preoperatively, the patient will require education and support to facilitate their care. Perioperatively, key elements such as patient warming and fluid therapy can ensure optimal patient care. Postoperatively, key elements of an ER programme include early mobilization, early nutrition, proactive management of pain and nausea and restricted IV fluid administration. Such programmes are deemed to be beneficial to the patient because they promote recovery and beneficial for hospitals/Trusts because they reduce hospital stays and therefore increase bed capacity and reduce costs.

Discharge planning should be commenced at preoperative assessment, to determine, prior to admission, the home environment and what care is available from the family. If the woman has no family or carers — particularly for older women who may live alone — plans should be made at the earliest stage for any support services that may be required on discharge from hospital, by involving a social worker in her care.

However, it is also crucial the patient is not made to feel as though they are 'on a production line', as each patient will have a unique set of needs and requirements.

Minor gynaecological surgery

Hysteroscopy, dilatation and curettage

Hysteroscopy, followed by dilatation of the cervix and curettage of the uterus (D&C), is a common minor gynaecological procedure. It is now commonly performed in outpatient clinics, reducing the need for general anaesthetic.

A telescope is introduced into the endometrial cavity via the cervix, where the size and shape of the uterine cavity and the endometrium can be viewed directly.

This procedure can be used diagnostically where there has been occurrence of postmenopausal bleeding, postcoital bleeding (after sexual intercourse), or any instance of increased bleeding, both during menstruation and between periods (intermenstrual bleeding). It may reveal an endometrial polyp, or the pathology of the endometrial curetting may show an endometrial cancer.

Evacuation of retained products of conception

A modified D&C may also be used as a therapeutic intervention to treat heavy bleeding where the cause is retained products of conception following a miscarriage. This procedure is known as evacuation of retained products of conception (ERPC). It is usually performed under general anaesthetic and uses suction to remove the retained products. An alternative surgical option is a manual vacuum aspiration (MVA) which can be performed under local anaesthetic in an outpatient setting. The National Institute of Health and Care Excellence (2012) advise that, where clinically appropriate, women should be given a choice between these two techniques.

A miscarriage may be described as the expulsion of the fetus from the uterus before it is viable, i.e. before it is capable of independent existence. This is considered to be before 24 weeks' gestation. The correct medical term for a miscarriage is spontaneous abortion, but this can cause additional distress to women, so the term miscarriage is preferred.

The language used when caring for women who have miscarried is always important. It is advisable that the procedure is not referred to as a 'scrape', since this can understandably upset mothers. Women are particularly vulnerable at this time and appreciate health professionals recognizing their loss as significant and as a real baby rather than a fetus.

Women not only need physical and emotional support at this time but also require information to be given clearly, honestly and in a sensitive manner.

Surgical treatment is one of three options the woman should be counselled about, so she can make an informed decision. The other options are conservative or medical treatment.

- *Conservative management*: this should only be offered if the woman is not bleeding heavily. Nature is allowed to take its course and a spontaneous miscarriage occurs. A full explanation must be given of what the woman should expect in terms of pain, bleeding and the expected appearance of the products of conception. She must be given contact phone numbers for the hospital in case the bleeding or pain becomes excessive. A scan is arranged for up to 1 week later, to assess for retained products of conception. This is a natural option and offers women the opportunity of being in control of their bodies with an alternative to medical or surgical treatment. However, some women cannot cope with the psychological effects of carrying a dead baby for possibly several weeks; for these women, one of the other alternatives may be more appropriate.
- *Medical management*: this has developed over recent years and has been shown to be extremely effective. The woman is given combination treatment with the antiprogesterone mifepristone, and prostaglandin E — either orally, such as misoprostol, or vaginally, such as gemeprost (NICE, 2012). The first dose, i.e. mifepristone, is usually given to the woman while in the early pregnancy assessment unit, and she returns to the ward for completion, using misoprostol 36–48 hours later. The woman must be counselled

fully about the effects of the treatment, i.e. that she will have some bleeding and may even miscarry at home. Any products passed must be examined closely for fetal, membranes and placental tissue, to ensure there are no retained products. The woman must be able to return to the hospital at any time should she start to miscarry before the second dose. An advantage of this treatment is that the woman does not require a general anaesthetic, but she will have to experience a process similar to labour during the expulsion of the products.

Loss of a pregnancy, for whatever reason, i.e. miscarriage, stillbirth, ectopic pregnancy or even termination of pregnancy, can cause psychological problems for the woman and her partner for some time after the event. Miscarriage may create problems with a woman's self-concept, inner feelings of failure, loss of faith in her body, and other conflicts in the marriage and family relationships. Guilt is a common feeling and it may take a sympathetic partner and skilled nursing care to help a woman at this time. However, the psychological impact on fathers is often overlooked.

A couple who have had a miscarriage should be advised to wait until the woman has had one normal period before trying for another pregnancy. Different patients will have different feelings. Some may be keen to conceive again as soon as possible, for others it may be too soon. It is crucial that nurses do not assume the attitude, 'Go home and get pregnant again'. The nurse must be aware of all the psychological aspects mentioned above, to ensure they are empathetic and supportive to both parents.

Termination of pregnancy

A similar procedure is also used to perform an early suction termination of pregnancy (STOP) during the first trimester — up to around 12 weeks' gestation. The cervical canal is dilated to take the aspiration cannula, the size used depending on how far the pregnancy has advanced. The vacuum is switched on and the products of conception are dislodged and aspirated. A small curette is then used to check the completeness of the evacuation. The pregnant uterus is obviously enlarged and more vascular, so the risk of uterine perforation and the risk of need for a re-evacuation if not all the products of conception are removed should be explained fully. These procedures are usually performed as day cases under general anaesthesia, but some hospitals do offer the option of a local anaesthetic, which reduces waiting times.

Terminations in the second trimester (13–20 weeks' gestation) can be undertaken by administering mifepristone. This drug causes the embryo to detach, uterine muscles to contract and the cervix to dilate, by blocking the effect of progesterone. The care is similar to that for women undergoing medical management of miscarriage.

Laparoscopic surgery

Laparoscopic adhesiolysis or salpingolysis

This operation is performed via the laparoscope and consists of dividing the peri-tubal adhesions around the upper ends of the fallopian tubes. If the fimbriae are not damaged and the adhesions are not too extensive, the lining epithelium of the fallopian tubes is likely to be intact and its function may be restored. In some cases, a 'lap and dye' (described earlier in this chapter) may be performed at the same time.

Laparoscopic treatment of ovarian cyst

Up to 10% of women will have some form of surgery during their lifetime due to an ovarian mass. In premenopausal women almost all ovarian masses and cysts are benign (RCOG, 2011). The vast majority of patients will benefit from laparoscopic techniques to remove or treat the cyst.

The treatment offered may vary depending on whether or not the cyst is thought to be benign or suspicious, whether or not the woman in postmenopausal, the size of the cyst and the woman's preference. It may be possible to perform an ovarian cystectomy (in which the cyst is removed but the ovary is conserved) which is beneficial for a younger woman who wishes to preserve future fertility. Alternatively, the whole ovary, with or without the tube, may be removed. This is an oophorectomy or, in the case of fallopian tube removal as well the ovary, a salpingo-oophorectomy. The fallopian tube may be removed with the ovary to reduce the potential risk of cancer, as there is some evidence that cancers previously thought to be ovarian start in the fallopian tubes (Erickson et al, 2013).

Some women who have an increased risk of ovarian cancer due to genetic mutations (particularly *BRCA1* or *BRCA2*) may be offered a prophylactic bilateral salpingo-oophorectomy to reduce (although not eradicate) their risk of developing ovarian cancer. For most women, it is appropriate to perform this laparoscopically (RCOG, 2015a; Muto et al, 2017).

Laparoscopic treatment for endometriosis

Endometriosis is a condition which occurs in women of reproductive age where endometrial tissue (that usually lines the uterus) is found outside the uterus. If it is confined to the myometrium, it is called adenomyosis.

Endometriosis may be found on the ovary, broad ligament, bowel and bladder and occasionally has been seen in the lung. In severe endometriosis, the ovaries, fallopian tubes, uterus and bowel are stuck together by dense adhesions. There are several grading systems available which can be used to describe the extent of the endometriosis (Johnson et al, 2017).

The range of symptoms and pain experienced by different women vary considerably. During menstruation, the endometrial tissue is subject to the same hormonal changes as the uterus. The blood released has no way of escape and is reabsorbed into the bloodstream. The inflammation caused gives rise to scarring and adhesions. The deposits may be seen as tiny black spots or as larger cysts, sometimes known as 'chocolate cysts' (endometriomas) from the appearance of altered blood.

There are both pharmacological and surgical management options for endometriosis, which may be used in combination. The treatments offered may vary depending on the patient herself, for example for some women the priority may be to retain fertility, for others pain management may be a priority (NICE, 2017).

If surgical treatment is required, this is usually undertaken under the enhanced vision of the laparoscope. The endometriosis is either destroyed by using diathermy or if the deposits are large enough, by surgically cutting them out and removing them. Risks associated with this surgery include damage to bowel or bladder, often due to adhesions of organs caused as a result of the endometriosis.

Laparoscopic treatment for polycystic ovarian disease

Therapeutic laparoscopy may also be used to treat polycystic ovarian disease. This condition occurs when the ovaries are enlarged and contain numerous cystic follicles. The normal production of oestrogen is affected, resulting in absence of periods (amenorrhoea) or irregular periods (oligomenorrhoea). A woman is considered to have polycystic ovarian syndrome when she has other symptoms in addition to the cysts on the ovaries, such as acne, hirsutism, weight gain, pelvic pain and infertility.

During laparoscopy, multiple holes are made in the ovary ('ovarian drilling'), causing drainage of the subcapsular cysts, which contain high levels of androstenedione. This will lead to a rise in FSH secretion, and, ultimately, spontaneous ovulation should occur. Where ovulation does not occur spontaneously, women often respond to clomifene, even where they were resistant to it before surgery. Although the effect is usually temporary, it allows 'a window of opportunity' for women to attempt conception without having to resort to other, more expensive, infertility options.

391

Laparoscopic sterilization

Female sterilization involves the blocking or excision of the fallopian tubes, thereby preventing the ovum from meeting the sperm and fertilization taking place.

The majority of sterilizations are performed laparoscopically. Occasionally, a mini-laparotomy (8—10-cm scar) may be necessary if access and visualization of the fallopian tubes is difficult. This may be due to the woman being obese, due to previous pelvic surgery or because of previous infections which have resulted in multiple adhesions. In this instance, a stay in hospital of 1 or 2 days will be recommended and heavy lifting should be avoided for about 3 weeks.

Sterilization via a hysteroscopic route (in which flexible metal rods are inserted into the fallopian tubes using a hysteroscope) was an alternative. However, there have been a number of cases of severe side effects including chronic pelvic pain and, as a result, use of this technique has diminished (Dyer, 2018). The Food and Drug Administration (2018) have since imposed a restriction on the use of Essure (the most commonly used product) and the manufacturer discontinued the product in 2018.

Pregnancy following sterilization by laparoscopic tubal occlusion is rare: 2—5 patients per 1000 operations at 10 years (RCOG, 2016). If a pregnancy does occur, there is usually a higher risk of an ectopic pregnancy and the woman should be warned of this possibility. However, sterilization should be treated as a non-reversible procedure and reversal is not available on the NHS. The woman must also be warned of the risk during laparoscopy of damage to adjacent organs or vessels, and advice should be given about pelvic and shoulder tip pain that can develop following laparoscopy.

It is technically possible to carry out sterilization at the same time as a termination of pregnancy or after delivery by caesarean section. However, there are additional risks associated with sterilization at this time, due to increased vascularity of a pregnant uterus. The procedure may be technically more difficult due to the uterus being enlarged and the tubes lying high in the abdomen, increasing the risk of failure. Furthermore, the woman will require additional counselling as the risk of regretting the decision is higher (RCOG, 2016).

Nursing care for minor gynaecological and laparoscopic surgery

Preoperative care

Preoperative care and information is a vital part of the preparation of a woman who is to undergo any gynaecological operation, whether minor or major. This is particularly true of women experiencing a miscarriage or termination. A miscarriage is a problem which occurs suddenly. The woman is admitted to hospital quickly, without time to make plans for the care of any other children. It is important to consider the feelings of both partners and ensure family members have a direct telephone number to the ward. For more detail, see Chapter 4.

Most minor gynaecological procedures are carried out as a day case, although increasingly procedures are being undertaken in the outpatient setting. The nurse must ensure the woman feels relaxed and not part of a conveyor belt, by appearing unhurried and focused on the woman.

Case Study 20.1.

Jane is a 28-year-old woman who is 6 weeks pregnant. This is her first pregnancy (P1 G0). She has been admitted with pelvic pain and it is suspected that the pregnancy is ectopic. She is due to go to theatre for an emergency laparoscopy (+/− laparotomy).

Questions for reflection

What anxieties may Jane have in regard to surgery? And in regard to her future fertility? How can you, as a healthcare professional, support her physically and psychologically?

Postoperative care

Women usually recover very quickly from minor investigations and operations. Providing their observations are stable and vaginal bleeding is not heavy, they may be escorted to the lavatory to pass urine. Once they have tolerated fluids and a light diet, they may go home, usually a minimum of 4 hours after their anaesthetic.

It is important that a partner or friend collects the woman following day surgery, and a written information leaflet containing discharge advice and a contact telephone number should be given to her.

Discharge advice

- It is common to have some bleeding after the procedure, which may be bright red at first and should gradually decrease to a brownish stain.
- If the bleeding becomes heavier than a normal period, offensive smelling or there is a raised temperature, then the ward should be contacted, since these are indications of an infection.
- The woman should be accompanied home and overnight in case of complications developing.

- Sanitary towels rather than tampons should be used, to reduce the risk of infection.
- Mild painkillers such as paracetamol or ibuprofen may be used to relieve any pain.
- It is advisable for the woman to take a few days off work and resume a normal lifestyle and work when she feels ready.

Specific advice following an evacuation of retained products of conception or a suction termination of pregnancy

The advice for women following these two procedures is similar to that for a dilatation and curettage.

- Breast tenderness may be a problem, especially if the miscarriage or termination occurred later in the pregnancy. Women should be warned about this, since it can be a distressing symptom. A well-supporting bra will help reduce discomfort, but it is not usually necessary to take any medication.
- Following a termination, it is crucial that women are offered comprehensive contraceptive advice. They may begin taking the oral contraceptive pill the evening of the operation or the following morning. They should return to their GP 6 weeks after the operation for a general check-up and further contraceptive prescriptions.
- A follow-up hospital appointment is not usually offered unless the woman has had three consecutive miscarriages, or has a miscarriage in the second trimester of pregnancy.
- The Miscarriage Association and SATFA (Support around Termination for Abnormality) have a useful range of booklets.
- Some hospitals have their own miscarriage group run by a bereavement counsellor, and many have an annual remembrance service for all the babies who have died before or at birth in the previous year.

Marsupialization of a Bartholins abscess

The Bartholin's glands lubricate the vulva and lie behind the vestibule, with a duct that opens at the vaginal introitus. They are susceptible to infection by sexually transmitted diseases and also general micro-organisms such as staphylococci and *Escherichia coli*. If the duct becomes blocked, mucous secretions are unable to drain and a cyst is formed. The cyst may resolve or become infected, resulting in a painful Bartholin's abscess, which is often initially noticed during sexual intercourse.

The abscess can be extremely painful and appear hot, red and swollen. The woman may have difficulty in walking, be unable to sit down and is reluctant to pass urine.

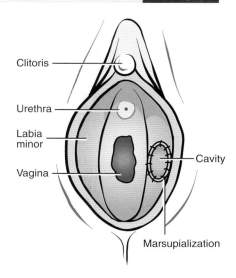

Figure 20.2 Marsupialization of a Bartholin's abscess.

It is preferable not to excise the gland, because it provides lubrication for sexual intercourse. Instead, marsupialization is performed. The abscess is incised, and the walls of the abscess are sutured to the surrounding skin to leave a large orifice to facilitate drainage of the pus (Fig. 20.2).

A new duct forms as healing occurs. During the operation a swab will be taken for microscopy, culture and sensitivity, and antibiotics may be prescribed. The cavity is loosely filled with ribbon gauze impregnated with a solution such as glycerin. This is to keep the skin edges apart so that healing can occur by granulation. If the skin edges heal together before this happens, a sinus can be left under the skin which may harbour recurrent infections.

Postoperative care

This operation is often performed as an emergency, and women usually go home 24 hours later, once they have passed urine. The pack will be removed either by the nurse or by the woman herself. This can be helped by sitting in a warm bath. The area should be kept clean and a hairdryer can be used instead of a towel for drying the area. Antibiotics are not given routinely unless infection is proven. It is probably advisable not to have sexual intercourse for 2 weeks following the operation, so as to avoid reinfection and to allow the area to heal.

Myomectomy

A myomectomy is an operation to remove fibroids from the uterus. A fibroid (also known as a myoma or leiomyoma) begins as a single cell in the endometrium of the uterus, which multiplies to become a mass of muscle and fibrous connective tissue. Most fibroids are no larger than a pea, but they can grow to the size of a grapefruit. Fibroids seem to occur more frequently in West Indian and West African women, although the reason for this is not clear (NICE, 2018a).

It is not entirely clear why fibroids develop, but they are dependent on oestrogen. Before a myomectomy, the woman may be prescribed leuprorelin (Prostap) to suppress the release of oestrogen and cause the fibroids to shrink.

Myomectomy was commonly undertaken as an open procedure via a laparotomy. However, developments in keyhole surgery provide alternatives, including removal of the fibroids via a laparoscope or hysteroscope (depending on the location of the fibroids within the uterus). This has a quicker recovery period when compared to a traditional open technique.

Alternatively, fibroid embolization can be carried out under sedation by a radiologist. Particles are injected into the femoral and uterine arteries which reduces the blood supply to the fibroid causing it to shrink. The rest of the uterus remains unaffected.

Case Study 20.2.

Mrs Smith is a 42-year-old Afro-Caribbean woman with two children from a previous marriage. She has been suffering from painful, heavy periods and been diagnosed with fibroids. Mrs Smith is anaemic due to the bleeding. She is keen to avoid a hysterectomy as she would like to have more children.

Questions for reflection

What types of treatment options may be suitable for Mrs Smith? What can be done preoperatively to optimize her care? What aspects of 'enhanced recovery' may be advantageous to her care?

Reasons for myomectomy

Small fibroids are often asymptomatic and treatment is not required. However, where diagnosis of the pelvic mass is in doubt, where the fibroid is larger than 3 cm or where there are unpleasant symptoms or causing infertility, surgery is recommended (NICE, 2018a).

Menorrhagia (heavy periods) is a common problem caused by the larger area of endometrium that is shed at menstruation. Large fibroids may press on the bowel, causing constipation, or on the bladder, causing urinary frequency or retention.

A myomectomy involves the 'shelling out' of the fibroids and is preferable for women who still want children. If no further pregnancies are desired, then a hysterectomy may be the operation of choice.

During myomectomy, there is a risk of hemorrhage from the incision of the uterine muscle. Women should always be aware of the risk that, if bleeding cannot be controlled, a hysterectomy will be performed. The woman may require a blood transfusion, and therefore this operation is not always advisable for women who do not accept blood products, e.g. Jehovah's Witnesses (although alternatives such as cell salvage can sometimes be used).

If the procedure is performed via a laparotomy the woman will often stay in hospital for 3–5 days, depending on the healing of the wound. However, if the procedure is undertaken as laparoscopic surgery or via hysteroscopic resection of fibroids, the procedure may be carried out as a day case. Since this is minimally invasive surgery, women can return to an active life 7–10 days following surgery and have minimal scars. This kind of procedure is also advantageous because, following laparotomy, any suture lines may weaken the wall of the uterus and may necessitate a caesarean section at subsequent births. There is also a higher risk of further adhesions forming following laparotomy.

If a woman wishes to become pregnant following myomectomy, many gynaecologists recommend that she tries to conceive in the first 3–6 months following surgery, before the fibroids grow again.

Postoperative advice following laparoscopic removal of fibroids

This operation is usually performed as a day case, so the woman should make sure someone is available to take her home. Advice should be given about risks of damage to adjacent organs and how to treat pelvic or shoulder tip pain that can occur following any laparoscopy. It normally takes a woman a few days to recover fully from a laparoscopy, and she should resume normal activities and work when she feels ready.

Hysterectomy

Hysterectomy is the most commonly performed major gynaecological operation. However, with developments in laparoscopic surgery and the use of levonorgestrel intrauterine devices, there are now several alternatives for treatment of menorrhagia and as a result hysterectomy rates for benign causes are dropping (Murkhopadhaya & Manyonda, 2013).

There are various types of hysterectomy (Fig. 20.3), and the type of hysterectomy suggested will depend on the reason for the operation (Box 20.2).

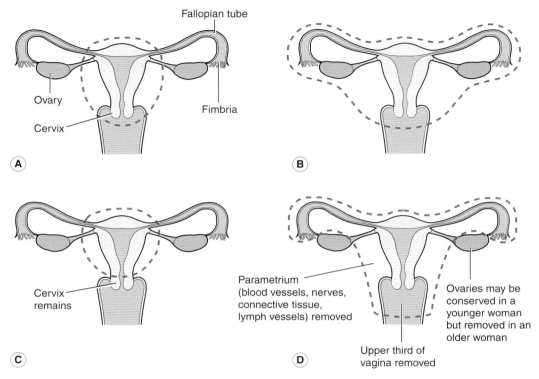

Figure 20.3 Types of hysterectomy: (A) total abdominal hysterectomy; (B) total abdominal hysterectomy and bilateral salpingo-oophorectomy; (C) subtotal hysterectomy; (D) Wertheim's (radical) hysterectomy.

Box 20.2 **Reasons for hysterectomy**

- Painful or irregular periods or episodes of unexplained vaginal bleeding
- Fibroids, which can cause pain, heavy bleeding and occasionally pressure on other pelvic organs, e.g. the bladder
- Uterine prolapse, which may interfere with bladder and bowel function
- Chronic pelvic pain caused by pelvic infection
- Gynaecological cancers of the vagina, cervix, endometrium, fallopian tubes or ovaries
- Occasionally a hysterectomy is performed in an emergency, e.g. in instances of postpartum haemorrhage or following a gynaecological procedure where haemostasis cannot be maintained

---

Total abdominal hysterectomy

This operation involves the removal of the uterus and cervix through a horizontal cut in the abdomen just above the pubic bone, i.e. Pfannenstiel or 'bikini-line' incision. However, some women may require a vertical incision where there is a large abdominal swelling, previous scarring or in cases where cancer is suspected and therefore a complete inspection of the abdomen is required for staging.

Bilateral salpingo-oophorectomy

Bilateral salpingo-oophorectomy refers to the removal of both fallopian tubes and ovaries and is often performed at the same time as a total abdominal hysterectomy, particularly where there is evidence of disease, or if the woman is postmenopausal or approaching the menopause. Oophorectomy prevents ovarian cancer from occurring in the future. For premenopausal women, an attempt is made to conserve the ovaries if they are healthy, so as to avoid a sudden decrease in oestrogen, which could cause severe menopausal symptoms. It has been shown, however, that if the ovaries are conserved, they may have a decreased hormonal function in pre-menopausal women, possibly because their blood supply may be compromised during surgery.

Subtotal hysterectomy

In this procedure, the uterus is removed but the cervix is left *in situ*. Cervical smears are still needed annually to screen for cervical cancer. There have been some claims that, for benign surgery, retaining the cervix may reduce the risk of prolapse in the future, however the evidence behind this is not conclusive (Lethaby et al, 2012).

Radical/Wertheims hysterectomy

This operation is an extended hysterectomy where the uterus, ovaries, fallopian tubes, adjacent pelvic tissue, lymph ducts and the upper third of the vagina are removed. This is necessary in cases of advanced cervical cancer. Further details are described later in the chapter.

Vaginal hysterectomy

This operation involves the removal of the uterus through the vagina, leaving no apparent scar. A vaginal hysterectomy is usually performed where there is prolapse of the uterus. Contraindications to vaginal hysterectomy include a bulky uterus (larger in size than a 14-week uterus) and suspected or known malignancy.

Laparoscopic hysterectomy and laparoscopic assisted vaginal hysterectomy

Laparoscopic hysterectomy was first described by Reich in 1989 and was developed as a minimally invasive alternative to open abdominal or vaginal approach to hysterectomy (Maclaran et al, 2016). Laparoscopic hysterectomy uses 'keyhole surgery' to perform the hysterectomy and then the uterus can be removed vaginally or, after morcellation (cutting it up), through one of the small incisions. This technique may be used for benign or malignant cases, although in cases where malignancy is suspected the specimen should not be morcellated.

There are various types of laparoscopic hysterectomy, depending on the extent of the surgery performed laparoscopically compared to that performed vaginally (Aarts et al, 2015). Depending on the surgical technique the procedure may be conducted entirely through the laparoscopic approach with only the specimen being delivered vaginally or a 'laparoscopic-assisted' technique may be employed where some of the surgery is conducted laparoscopically and some vaginally (for example, where pelvic floor repairs are also required).

There are numerous advantages of the laparoscopic technique including reduced postoperative pain, fewer surgical site infections, reduced blood loss and shorter postoperative hospital stay. This procedure may be undertaken for both benign and malignant disease but has been shown to be of particular benefit for patients with endometrial cancer (NICE, 2010; Asher et al, 2018; Galaal et al, 2018).

Robotic-assisted laparoscopic hysterectomy

An advancement on the laparoscopic technique is the use of robotics. As with laparoscopic techniques, robotic surgery is minimally invasive. However, unlike conventional laparoscopic surgery it is performed by the surgeon sitting at a console (rather than standing at the operating table). The console provides high definition 3D images of the surgical field and the surgery is performed using wristed instruments which are more adaptable and precise than standard laparoscopic instruments.

Advocates of robotic techniques claim that they have many advantages, including more precise instruments, enhanced surgical 3D vision, improved ergonomics and shorter length of hospital stay for patients. Increasingly robotics is being used for a greater range of operations (Sinha et al, 2015). However, it is also expensive and the evidence supporting its use for benign disease is limited (Liu et al, 2014).

Psychological aspects of hysterectomy

All major surgery has implications for an altered body image, but the removal of a uterus can alter a woman's self-image and her perceived femininity and have a profound effect on her feelings of sexuality. The inability to reproduce, even if the woman did not want to, can mark a major life event. To many women, the suggestion of having a hysterectomy provokes fear and horror on account of the misconceptions and old wives' tales surrounding this particular operation. The Ancient Greeks believed the uterus (*hystero*) to be the source of all emotions; hence, the words 'hysteria' and 'hysterectomy'.

The healthcare practitioner is of utmost importance, to uncover anxieties and fears, to correct any myths and misconceptions, and to give clear, accurate advice. Unfortunately, instead of the detailed information women require, they are often only given brief hints about 'not lifting', and important concerns such as when to resume sexual activity are neglected. Some women do not realize that they will no longer have periods following a hysterectomy, and others who have suffered from premenstrual syndrome may mistakenly think that the hysterectomy will cure this problem. However, if the ovaries have been conserved, cyclical symptoms will persist.

Nursing care for major gynaecological surgery

Preoperative care

The importance of preoperative care for minor gynaecological cases has already been discussed earlier in the chapter. Obviously, when a more serious operation is taking place it is even more vital that the woman and her family feel adequately prepared. This is described in more detail in Chapter 4.

A full admission assessment should be undertaken. The patient will require information regarding exactly what will happen. Each patient will respond differently and need different types of support.

It is also necessary to prepare the woman physically for surgery. Bowel preparation may be necessary, depending on the surgery, and local guidelines should be referred to.

There is a risk of DVT following major abdominal and pelvic surgery (NICE, 2018b), so women are measured and fitted for anti-embolism stockings and may be given prophylactic heparin depending on department policy and individual patient assessment. An individual assessment is recommended as for some patients the risk of DVT needs to be balanced against the risk of bleeding.

Patients undergoing major gynaecological surgery are starved prior to surgery to prevent gastric aspiration. ASA (2017) guidelines recommend a minimum of 6 hours for food and 2 hours for clear fluids. All patients should be advised to give up smoking for at least 48 hours before surgery, preferably more.

All women will be required to sign a consent form for the operation after the benefits and serious and frequently occurring risks have been fully explained to her. These should have been explained fully to her during her original outpatient consultation and at preoperative assessment, to ensure that gaining her consent has been a process and not just signing a form (Dimond, 2011; RCOG, 2015b).

In teaching hospitals, medical students are likely to be present at all stages of the patient's care pathway. Some women find it intimidating to discuss their personal symptoms in front of an audience, and the nurse must act as the woman's advocate (Nursing and Midwifery Council, 2018). All women have the right to refuse to participate in the teaching of undergraduates, and if this is the case her wishes should be respected. At some hospitals women may sign a consent form for medical students to perform vaginal examinations while they are in theatre under general anaesthesia. The woman may request a female doctor to examine her and this should be supported where possible. A male doctor should always be chaperoned and it is now recommended that all clinicians, regardless of their gender, should be chaperoned (RCOG, 2015b).

See Table 20.1 for a detailed preoperative care plan for a patient undergoing major gynaecological surgery.

Postoperative care

A detailed postoperative care plan is shown in Table 20.2. Major gynaecological surgery such as hysterectomy, myomectomy or vaginal repair can take from 45 minutes to multiple hours, depending on the specific operation. Oxygen therapy will be required following the general anaesthetic, particularly if patient-controlled analgesia is used, and this will be continued from recovery onto the ward.

The patient will have an intravenous infusion in progress, which will stay *in situ* for 24–48 hours, and occasionally a blood transfusion may be required, depending on the estimated blood loss during the operation. A urinary (Foley's) catheter may be inserted to keep the bladder empty. A Redivac drain may be used. This drain has a vacuum and drains off excess blood from the operation site to prevent formation of a haematoma and is situated close to the wound. However, drains can sometimes increase the risk of infection (due to port site infections) and some surgeons no longer use them as standard but instead use drains dependent on surgical need.

Unless there is particularly heavy oozing from the wound, a light dry dressing will be sufficient covering for the wound for 48 hours. Following a myomectomy, there is an increased risk of the formation of a haematoma. Adhesions may develop later between the intestines and the suture lines on the uterus.

Women who have had a vaginal hysterectomy and/or a vaginal repair may have a 'vaginal pack' (a length of ribbon gauze soaked in glycerin) *in situ*, which is inserted into the vagina rather like a large tampon. This exerts pressure and stops any bleeding from suture points. It may be removed after 24 hours, and this is most comfortably done while the woman sits in a warm bath. The presence of, or removal of, a pack must be documented in the patient's notes.

Strong analgesics will be required for the first 24 hours and morphine sulphate is often administered via an intramuscular injection, or by patient-controlled analgesia (PCA), where the patient can administer the amount required themselves via a pump. In some units, epidurals or other forms of regional anaesthesia such as 'tap blocks' are available. Diclofenac sodium suppositories can be used for their anti-inflammatory and analgesic properties.

Gynaecology patients appear to be more prone to postoperative nausea and vomiting (PONV) (Apfelbaum et al, 2013) and hence antiemetics such as prochlorperazine or metoclopramide may be beneficial. In addition,

Table 20.1 Preoperative care plan for a patient undergoing major gynaecological surgery

Universal self-care	Problem	Aim	Patient activity	Nursing activity requisites
Promote normality	Anxiety related to hospital admission	Alleviate anxiety associated with admission and unfamiliar surroundings and people	Patient to familiarize herself with staff, fellow patients and ward layout	Welcome patient to ward. Introduce to staff and identify named nurse to patient
	Unfamiliar surroundings and disturbance in usual life activities	To give adequate information regarding treatment stay and discharge	Patient is able to ask questions and express anxieties and fears	Explain ward layout and toilets, bathrooms and day room and information about activities, e.g. visiting times, meal times, ward telephone number, etc. Give appropriate explanation of intended treatment and surgery (using information aids if appropriate). Answer questions posed by patient. If unable to, refer to appropriate member of multidisciplinary team Be sensitive to patient's anxieties and fears, which may be expressed in speech or in non-verbal behaviour Discuss any family/social problems arising from admission
Prevention of hazards to life, well-being and functioning	Unprepared for surgery	Safe preparation for theatre	Patient understands rationale for fasting Patient assists in preoperative skin preparation Patient has bath/ shower Patient assists in bowel preparation procedure Patient empties bladder Patient wears operating gown and anti-embolism stockings	Full preoperative nursing assessment: measurement of temperature, pulse, respiration and weight and urinalysis Check consent form is signed and premedication given if required Attach ID band Record results of preoperative investigations: • Full blood count • Sickle cell trait • Urea and electrolytes • ECG if required Ensure any required bowel preparation has been undertaken Patient measured for anti-embolism stockings Fast patient for 6 hours Escort to theatre

Adapted and published with permission from Lisa Stewart.

Table 20.2 Postoperative care plan for a patient following major gynaecological surgery

Universal self-care	Problem	Aim	Patient activity	Nursing activity requisites
Maintain sufficient intake of oxygen	At risk of respiratory insufficiency/infection	Clear airway Independent ventilation	Understands reason for actively performing breathing exercises 4-hourly postoperatively Understands reason for adequate pain relief in order to perform breathing exercises Participates in physiotherapy exercises	Safe administration of oxygen as per anaesthetist's instructions Observe and record respiratory rate, depth and patient colour Reinforce breathing exercises Observe for side-effects such as respiratory depression Offer and assist with mouth care
Prevention of hazards of life, well-being and functioning	At risk of postoperative complications	Maintain patient safety: • haemorrhage • hypovolaemia		Record pulse, blood pressure, patient's colour, level of consciousness according to individual assessment Observe and record Redivac drainage Report any anomalies to senior nursing and medical staff
		• infection		Record temperature Administer antibiotic therapy Remove dressing around 2nd day after operation Remove sutures according to assessment and instructions
		• pain	Understands and uses PCA appropriately	Assess level of pain Monitor and administer prescribed analgesics Assist patient to find comfortable position
		• hygiene		Assist with hygiene needs Maintain patient dignity
Maintain sufficient intake of fluids	Fluid intake affected due to surgery	Adequate hydration and electrolyte balance	Understands reasons for IV hydration until bowel sounds return If able, assists in completion of fluid balance chart	Maintain IV as per prescription Explain rationale for IV hydration to patient Instruct patient to complete fluid chart Check IV patency and cannulation site for signs of infection

(Continued)

Table 20.2 Postoperative care plan for a patient following major gynaecological surgery—cont'd

Universal self-care	Problem	Aim	Patient activity	Nursing activity requisites
			Able to drink fluids independently once IV has been discontinued	Offer and assist with mouth care Monitor patient's record of fluid balance Provide vomit bowls and tissues
Maintain sufficient intake of food	Enforced fasting and temporary anorexia	Balanced diet Adequate calories	Understands reason for being nil by mouth Understands rationale for slow reintroduction of solid foods once bowel sounds have returned Able to participate in menu choice	Keep patient nil by mouth until bowel sounds re-established Observe for signs of paralytic ileus Introduce fluids slowly Offer a light diet, progressing to normal diet
Care associated with elimination	At risk of urinary retention or incomplete voiding	Passes urine normally once catheter is removed	Understands reason for catheter	Close observation of urinary output and catheter patency
			Understands how to care for and empty: • urethral catheter • suprapubic catheter, which is used following a bladder repair operation or occasionally a vaginal repair	Report decrease in urinary output to nursing and medical staff Empty catheter 6 hourly Ensure patient passes urine normally once catheter is removed
	At risk of constipation	Normal bowel action	Is able to assist in completion of fluid chart Understands rationale to prevent constipation: • increased fibre • adequate fluids • to request aperients • increased mobility	Ensure accurate fluid balance chart completed Monitor patient's bowel action Instruct patient on how to complete fluid chart Administer aperients as needed Advise on measures for avoiding constipation
Maintain balance between activity and rest	Enforced rest and limitation on activity due to surgery and associated fatigue following surgery	For patient to appreciate temporary limitations on activity due to surgery	Understands reason for temporary fatigue Understands that usual activities involving abdominal muscles will be altered: • driving • working • cleaning/lifting • sexual intercourse	Explain and reinforce limitations on patient Ensure patient has leaflet and/or advice following major surgery
		To identify discharge facilities and home support	Patient identifies relative or friend to assist in recuperative period at home	Explore with patient family facilities following discharge

(Continued)

Table 20.2 Postoperative care plan for a patient following major gynaecological surgery—cont'd

Universal self-care	Problem	Aim	Patient activity	Nursing activity requisites
			Engages in active exercises Patient understands limitations on independence during convalescence and makes appropriate plans for help after discharge	Encourage balance between adequate mobilization and adequate rest Encourage patient participation in postoperative exercises Confirm home circumstances following discharge
			Inform community/social services to implement discharge plan if required	
Maintain balance between solitude and social interaction	Alteration in usual communication patterns and privacy	To maintain patient social interaction	Patient appreciates alteration in usual patient sociability	Assist in introduction of fellow patients
		To express feelings to nursing staff or friend or relative	Involve relative or friend in communication, if appropriate	Allow time for patient to express her feelings (worries, fears, concerns, etc.)
		To respect patient privacy and solitude	Patient understands rationale for limiting visitors in order to prevent tiring patient	To ensure that patient visiting is promoted yet numbers kept within manageable limits
		To encourage social activities to limit boredom and seclusion		
Promote normality	Potential alteration in body image	Patient feels 'comfortable' with body image, sexual functioning and spirituality	Patient understands temporary limitations on sexual functioning	Provide the opportunity to express feelings/concerns about temporary restriction in sexual functioning
	Loss of body part may lead to grieving			Explore alternative ways of expressing affection if appropriate Involve partner if appropriate
	Temporary physical constraints on sexual functioning related to healing tissues and vaginal discharge Freedom to express spiritual beliefs			Respect patient's spiritual needs

Adapted and published with permission from Lisa Stewart.

acupressure may help and this can be applied to the inner aspect of the wrists using Sea-Bands.

On the day following major surgery the woman will be encouraged to sit out of bed for a short while and encouraged to perform leg exercises, pelvic rocking, i.e. moving hips from side to side, and deep breathing. These will help prevent common postoperative problems such as DVT and chest infections. Early mobilization is also beneficial from an enhanced recovery perspective (McDonald, 2015; Nelson et al, 2016).

When bowel sounds resume, the woman can start sipping water and gradually progress to a light diet. The urinary catheter will be removed, and her intravenous infusion discontinued. A strict fluid balance chart should be maintained until the woman is eating and drinking normally. Some women do contract a urinary tract infection following hysterectomy, and this will be treated with antibiotics. It is important that women empty their bladder fully and squeeze out the last few drops, as this prevents urine being retained in the bladder.

By the second day following surgery, women are usually able to walk to the bathroom and have a shower without too much discomfort. Oral analgesics are now given in conjunction with an anti-inflammatory suppository to control the pain.

Women may worry about 'bursting their stitches' and need reassurance that there are several layers of stitches. They may find it helpful to hold their hand across their abdomen (or hold the sanitary towel in place if they have had a vaginal hysterectomy) when they cough. The sutures used for skin closure are usually dissolvable and therefore do not need to be removed. Similarly, vaginal sutures will dissolve or occasionally fall out. Sometimes a tight one may have to be cut, if the wound feels as if it is pulling. Where staples are used, they can be removed on the 4th–5th day for a horizontal wound, and on the 7th–10th day for a vertical incision.

Many women experience griping 'wind' pain after abdominal or laparoscopic surgery, which can cause considerable discomfort. Hot peppermint water sipped slowly may help, and some doctors prescribe enteric-coated peppermint oil capsules (Colpermin). Walking around and sitting in a warm bath may also help.

Constipation can be a problem and regular lactulose syrup or gentle laxative may be prescribed. Glycerin suppositories can be given if the bowels have not been opened for several days.

It is very common for women to feel 'blue' on the 3rd or 4th day following surgery, and many women find themselves in tears for no apparent reason. They should be reassured that this is a normal reaction, although some women do experience similar feelings again on leaving hospital. For women who have had a hysterectomy and/or bilateral salpingo-oophorectomy and those who are perimenopausal, hormone replacement therapy will help, but there may be deeper reasons for this feeling of depression.

Discharge advice following major surgery

The duration of stay post-surgery will very much depend on the individual patient and the extent of her surgery.

Whatever the situation, it is crucial that the woman, her partner and the rest of her family are aware of what she can and cannot do while she is recovering at home. This should be supported with specific written information, and with an assurance that she can ring the ward for advice at any time. She should also be given the details of any local relevant support networks, e.g. the Hysterectomy Association or the National Endometriosis Society (see Resources section).

The following issues should be discussed with the woman, her partner and family if appropriate.

Bleeding

There may be a vaginal discharge for up to 4 weeks, which will turn from red to a pale brown colour. If it becomes heavier, brighter in colour, or offensive smelling, medical advice should be sought. Occasional red spotting may occur when the sutures fall out. Sanitary towels rather than tampons should be used in order to prevent infection for as long as required. If the woman has not had a hysterectomy, this may be until after the next period.

Resting

It is important that the woman should rest sufficiently during the first 2 weeks, and go to bed for a rest when she feels tired. It is common to feel tired for several weeks after discharge. Some women may need iron tablets following surgery if their haemoglobin level is low.

Exercise

Exercise is important, and any exercises undertaken in hospital should be continued at home, as long as they do not cause undue pain. Some women occasionally feel strange sensations in the abdomen, sometimes described as 'pinging elastic', which is normal. It is advisable to go for short walks, increasing gradually to 45 minutes by 6 weeks after the operation. Swimming may be resumed after about 4 weeks if vaginal bleeding has stopped. Cycling and other light exercises may also be resumed at this stage.

Housework

The woman should not undertake any housework for the first 2 weeks, but, after this, light chores can be safely undertaken. It is very important to avoid lifting anything heavy for the first 4 weeks, and very heavy items, such as shopping, wet laundry, full bin bags or toddlers, should not be lifted for at least 6 weeks. When anything is lifted, it is important to remind the woman to bend her knees, keep her back straight and hold the object close to her, as this avoids straining her abdomen.

Diet

Many women have heard that they will gain weight or develop a 'middle-aged spread' after a hysterectomy. This is a myth, and any weight gain is due to an increased calorie intake combined with a lack of exercise. It is advisable to eat a variety of foods, including fresh fruit and vegetables, to avoid constipation. Some women find prune juice an effective laxative. Other preventative measures, such as drinking at least eight glasses of water per day and taking high-fibre foods, are also recommended.

Work

Some women feel able to return to work 6−8 weeks following surgery, whereas others may need to take further time off. Obviously, some jobs are more strenuous than others and women should judge for themselves when they feel ready. Some employees may allow women to return on a part-time basis initially, which is an ideal way to readjust to the demands of their job.

Driving

A woman should avoid driving until she feels capable of performing an emergency stop. Slamming the foot down on the brake pedal will pull on the abdominal muscles and the woman should be fully in control of this manoeuvre. It is also advisable for the woman to check with her insurance company as they may have their own guidelines.

Sexual activity

All nurses working in specialties where sexuality is a central issue need to realize that patients do have sexual concerns and that nurses can contribute to this crucial aspect of recovery. Some nurses are concerned about violating their patients' privacy regarding sexuality and are anxious that they will be unable to help with questions raised. However, nurses working on gynaecology wards do not have to be sexual therapists. They can help their patients by providing information and understanding about self and body, and its relation to sexuality before and after diagnosis and surgery.

It is vital that each woman is treated as an individual and that assumptions about her sexuality are not made. It is important that an older woman's sexuality is not ignored. Older women may be less likely to initiate discussions about sexual concerns, and therefore the gynaecology nurse must act as a sensitive facilitator. Sexuality in the elderly can be difficult to discuss.

The issue of confidentiality is important for all gynaecology patients, since gynaecology is so intimately related to sexuality. A patient's sexuality should not be recorded on medical or nursing notes, since its inclusion may leave the patients open to negative attitudes from other staff in the future.

It is also important for nurses to take into account any cultural differences between women they care for. Certain ethnic groups find hysterectomy particularly hard to accept, and nurses should be aware of the impact this operation may have on different cultures and communities. Women of West Indian descent view menstruation as a cleansing act, ridding the body of impurities, and so are reluctant to have a hysterectomy. Some also fear they will be 'less of a woman' in the eyes of their men, who may be tempted to look for another 'whole woman'. For this reason, they may not wish their partner or family to know exactly what operation they are having, and all staff should respect their right to confidentiality.

Generally speaking, it takes about 6 weeks to feel both physically and emotionally ready to resume sexual intercourse after major gynaecological surgery, and most gynaecologists recommend this time interval before attempting intercourse. It is important to wait until any vaginal bleeding has stopped, to prevent the risk of infection. The woman's partner should understand the importance of being gentle initially, to avoid undue trauma to the area. Tissue strength is adequate by this time, and the risk of infection is virtually non-existent in the presence of complete healing.

The hormonal effects of oophorectomy, i.e. reduced oestrogen and testosterone, may cause loss of libido, vaginal atrophy and reduction of vaginal lubrication. This may be overcome by hormone replacement therapy or locally applied oestrogen cream. Vaginal dryness may also be helped by using a lubricant such as KY Jelly or Senselle, which will reduce chafing and discomfort, and also increase sensitivity.

Hysterectomy usually includes removal of the cervix, which can slightly decrease the length of the vagina. A change in position may be more comfortable initially, such as the female astride or legs together. Some women do report a decreased sexual response after hysterectomy. This may be because the scar tissue at the surgical site within the vagina is not as tactile and will not engorge and stretch as well as other genital tissues during the excitement and plateau phases of sexual arousal. Sensory nerve pathways to the vagina and perineum may also have been interrupted. While the inner vagina does not contain tactile nerve endings, it has pressure-sensitive nerves that can prompt sexual engorgement. Preoperatively, deep penile thrusting may have been enjoyable because of the pressure it placed on the inner vagina and cervix. Penile thrusting can also produce pleasurable

403

feelings through the movement of internal abdominal organs caused by the motion of the cervix and uterus during intercourse. If this has been part of a woman's enjoyment and arousal pattern, she should be encouraged to focus on other sensations that will assist in building her sexual response.

The character of orgasm for women who have had a hysterectomy may change. This is due to the lack of any uterine contractions but does not usually affect overall satisfaction.

Endometrial ablation

Endometrial ablation is one of several hysteroscopic procedures developed over recent years and increasingly is done in the outpatient setting (Clark & Gupta, 2005; NICE, 2018a). It involves destroying the endometrium and prevents the cyclical regeneration of the endometrium, instead of undertaking a hysterectomy, which is a much more extensive surgical procedure, with an increase in associated risks and recovery period. The endometrial lining of the uterus is removed while the procedure is observed on a video screen via a hysteroscope. In practice, not all the endometrium is removed, so some bleeding will still occur, but this is usually no longer such a problem for the woman as preoperatively. Women will have a hysteroscopy prior to the operation, to ensure their suitability for such surgery.

There are different types of ablation techniques and the method chosen will depend on the surgeon's preference and patient-specific factors. For example, a patient who has intrauterine fibroids may benefit from resection of fibroids in addition to an ablation, whereas for other women without fibroids this may not be required.

Prior to the development of endometrial ablation, the traditional treatments for heavy menstrual bleeding were drug therapy, a dilatation and curettage, or the option of major surgery in the form of a hysterectomy. Endometrial ablation is usually undertaken as a day case and increasingly in outpatient clinics. Consequently, for many women the associated physical, social and psychological implications make it preferable to a hysterectomy. Different techniques have been developed but they are based on the same principle, which involves destroying the endometrium using heat. A list of the different techniques can be found in Box 20.3.

The advantages and disadvantages of having endometrial ablation compared with a hysterectomy are outlined in Table 20.3 and contraindications to endometrial ablation are outlined in Box 20.4.

Balloon endometrial ablation

Following hysteroscopy, a special catheter is introduced via the cervix to the endometrial cavity. Water distends the balloon of the catheter so that it comes into direct contact with the endometrial lining. The water is then super-heated. The heat produced effectively destroys the endometrium.

A newer technique (NovaSure) involves a similar procedure but uses a triangular mesh device which is introduced to the uterine cavity and expands to conform to the endometrial lining. Electrical energy is then delivered to destroy the endometrium as above. The exact duration of the procedure will depend on the size of the uterine cavity, but usually the procedure lasts less than 90 seconds, which is why this method is often used in the outpatient setting.

Levonorgestrel intrauterine system

The levonorgestrel intrauterine system, Mirena, is a T-shaped intrauterine contraceptive device which contains the progesterone levonorgestrel in a sleeve around its stem. Progesterone is released slowly from the core and can be used for both contraceptive purposes and treatment of menorrhagia. It is ideal for older perimenopausal women who require hormone replacement therapy but still need contraception, and has a potential role for some patients with hyperplasia.

If used for women with menorrhagia who do not wish to have surgery, it must be explained thoroughly that the woman may experience erratic, irregular bleeding for the first 3−4 months following insertion. Bleeding then decreases considerably if the woman is able to tolerate this period of uncertainty. The device can be retained for 5 years before replacement is required.

Box 20.3 **Second-generation devices for endometrial ablation**

- Thermal balloons
- Hot saline
- Electrodes (first generation but still in use)
- Microwave devices (infrequently used)

Table 20.3 Comparison between endometrial ablation and hysterectomy

Procedure	Advantages	Disadvantages
Ablation	Can be carried out under sedation and local anaesthetic Greatly reduced need for analgesics Rapid recovery and convalescence No visible scar For many women can be done as outpatient Retains womb, symbol of femininity and fertility Quickly resume sexual function	Potential risk of uterine perforation Cannot guarantee total cessation of periods or sterility May still require hysterectomy for fibroids, menorrhagia and ovarian problems Several contraindications (see Box 20.4)

Hysterectomy	No further periods
	Sterility guaranteed
	No need for further surgery for fibroids, etc.
		Risk of haemorrhage
		Potential wound infection
		Increased anaesthetic time
		Postoperative complications:
		  • chest infection
		  • DVT
		  • constipation
		  • need for strong analgesics
		Altered body image with change in sexual function
		Abdominal scar
		Long convalescence required

Box 20.4 **Contraindications to endometrial ablation**

- Pregnancy or planned future pregnancies
- Any woman with a vaginal prolapse
- Endometriosis or fibroids
- If there is a suspected malignancy, a total abdominal hysterectomy, where biopsies may be taken from other sites in the pelvis, is required
- Active genital tract infection
- Previous uterine surgery causing weakness to myometrium
- Some methods of treatment require no fluid to leak from the uterine cavity during the procedure. Therefore a very dilated cervical os may prevent the ablation device from working.

Vaginal repair surgery/colporrhaphy

Vaginal repair surgery (or colporrhaphy) is a surgical procedure used to treat uterine or vaginal wall prolapse. Prolapses develop due to lack of support for pelvic organs by either the pelvic floor muscles or ligaments. This can be caused by increased abdominal pressure due to pregnancy and labour, persistent coughing or, more frequently, postmenopausally. The uterus may descend into the vagina and even reach the introitus. In severe cases the uterus extends right outside the vagina and is known as a procidentia. A prolapse is often first discovered when a woman complains of 'something coming down'; she may also have pelvic pain, backache, dyspareunia and urinary symptoms such as stress incontinence. There are several types of uterine prolapse:

- *Cystocele*: prolapse of the bladder and anterior vaginal wall.
- *Cystourethrocele*: the urethra descends as well as the bladder, resulting in urinary problems such as difficulty emptying the bladder, recurrent urinary tract infections and stress incontinence. Stress incontinence may be demonstrated while asking the woman to cough when the bladder is full. A small jet of urine is seen to escape from the urethra while a Sims' speculum parts the vaginal walls.

- *Rectocele*: the rectum prolapses through the adjacent posterior vaginal wall. The woman may have backache or a dragging feeling in the pelvic floor and may have difficulty emptying the bowel.
- *Enterocele*: hernia of the rectovaginal pouch into the upper third of the vagina. It may occur without uterine prolapse and occasionally following hysterectomy, where there may be a vault prolapse.

There are also several grading systems used to differentiate between the location and extent of a prolapse (Persu et al, 2011).

Non-surgical treatment

Many women with a slight prolapse have no discomfort and do not require surgical treatment, but do benefit from pelvic floor exercises. A prolapse which is causing discomfort should be treated by surgery unless the woman plans to have another baby, or if she is too old or frail to undergo an operation. In these instances, a polyethylene ring pessary may be inserted into the vagina to support the pelvic organs. The ring pessary needs to be changed every 6–12 months unless there is any bleeding or unusual discharge.

Types of surgery

Traditionally vaginal hysterectomy and pelvic floor repair has been the standard procedure for prolapse repair.

Anterior colporrhaphy

This operation is a repair of the anterior vaginal wall and is designed to cure a cystocele or cystourethrocele, due to urethral sphincter incompetence. The anterior vaginal wall is incised, and a triangular portion of vaginal skin from below the external urethral opening to the front of the cervix is excised. One or two sutures are placed deep around the bladder neck. The edges of the wound are sutured together to provide extra support for the bladder and urethra.

Posterior colporrhaphy

This procedure is used to repair a rectocele, or a rectocele and enterocele. A triangular portion of posterior vaginal wall with its apex at the mid-vaginal level and its base at the introitus is removed by an inverted T-incision to expose the levator ani muscles. These muscles are brought together with one or two interrupted sutures and closed in a Y-shape to avoid narrowing the entrance to the vagina. The operation also involves the excision of any enterocele and repair of the perineal body (perineorrhaphy).

Use of mesh for colporrhaphy

There are several types of mesh, which are manufactured biological or synthetic devices used to reinforce or support tissue during colporrhaphy. However, in July 2018 a period of 'high vigilance restriction' was implemented by NHS Improvement and NHS England meaning that for the vast majority of patients mesh surgery should not be performed. The only exception to this is for those patients where mesh procedures are assessed as being the only viable option. This was due to reports of complications including chronic pain (RCOG, 2018). Further research is currently ongoing.

Continence surgery

Urinary incontinence is highly prevalent worldwide, particularly with advancing age. It can be associated with a stigmatism and be associated with significant reduced quality of life (Irwin et al, 2011). There are several different operations that aim to improve continence, and these may be done vaginally, laparoscopically or via an abdominal or suprapubic approach.

The aims of continence surgery are to elevate the bladder neck and urethra from the pelvis into the abdomen where intra-abdominal pressure can act as an additional closing cone. Surgery should also provide support to the bladder neck.

It is crucial that prior to surgery a thorough assessment has been made of the woman and her complaint to ensure that the treatment offered is the most appropriate for the individual woman.

Women who suffer from urge incontinence (especially those with frequency issues) may benefit from injection of botulinum toxin or 'botox'. This has the effect of relaxing the muscles of the bladder. Injections are administered while observing the bladder via a cystoscopy. The procedure can be undertaken under general anaesthetic or, in some cases, under local anaesthetic. However, the effects are not permanent, and the procedure needs to be repeated depending on the patient's response.

Sling operations are performed to elevate the bladder neck and partly to provide support underneath it. Sling material may be organic (rectus sheath fascia) or inorganic (Silastic or Mersilene). The sling may be attached to the rectus sheath or ileoperitoneal ligaments. The amount of tension in the sling will depend upon whether it is being used to obstruct the outflow or to just support the bladder neck.

Insertion of a 'tension-free vaginal tape' (TVT) has developed as a minimally invasive alternative procedure which promotes a quicker recovery than open suprapubic surgery. Until recently it was being recommended as the first-line treatment option for stress incontinence where conservative management had failed (NICE, 2015). Two small incisions are made suprapubically and a needle is passed from the vagina upwards to take a length of the tape either side of the bladder and provide a sling to the bladder and urethra. This operation is often undertaken under local or regional anaesthesia, to enable the surgeon to adjust the tape in response to increases in abdominal pressure by asking the woman to cough at certain points of the procedure. Recovery time is considerably faster than open suprapubic sling surgery. However, it should be noted that the patient safety alert related to the use of vaginal mesh also applies to TVT (RCOG, 2018). As such, at time of writing there is an ongoing period of high vigilance in the use of TVT, meaning that it can only be used for patients where this procedure is the only viable treatment option.

Burch colposuspension

This operation is usually performed if an abdominal hysterectomy is required and is performed through a suprapubic incision. Sutures are inserted on either side of the bladder neck and urethra, which elevates the paravaginal fascia, and it is sutured to the iliopectineal ligaments. As well as raising the urethra and bladder neck, this procedure elevates the vaginal vault, so any existing anterior vaginal wall prolapse is simultaneously repaired.

The results of this suprapubic operation are better than those for traditional anterior colporrhaphy with bladder neck buttresses, but it requires a longer hospital stay and the use of a suprapubic catheter postoperatively. Women can experience difficulties in voiding urine and so the patient may be discharged home with a suprapubic catheter *in situ* until urinary function is resumed.

Laparoscopic treatment of prolapse

As with other laparoscopic procedures, laparoscopy for treatment of prolapse provides the surgeon with excellent exposure and an ability to see surgical detail. Laparoscopic techniques for prolapse have been shown to reduce blood loss and the need for excessive bowel manipulation making it an excellent method to perform pelvic floor surgery (Manodoro et al, 2011). The types of procedure that can be performed laparoscopically include hysteropexy (in which the uterus remains *in situ* and a mesh is inserted around the uterus to provide support) or sacrocolpopexy (in which the cervix is used to provide support using a mesh). Unlike the mesh used for vaginal repairs or TVT,

this mesh is not subject to the current restrictions imposed by NHS England. These techniques have been shown to provide significant long-term improvement for patients (Rahmanou et al, 2014).

Nursing care for patients requiring vaginal repair and continence surgery

Preoperative care

Preoperative care is very similar to that of women undergoing any major gynaecological surgery. All women will require a full explanation of the proposed surgery, and the chances of success and risks should be honestly discussed so that the woman can make an informed choice before deciding on surgery. Discharge planning should commence at preoperative assessment, since these patients are often elderly.

A midstream urine sample should be sent on admission and antibiotics commenced if necessary. Even if a woman appears 'elderly' to nurses, it should be ascertained whether she is still sexually active. If so, the gynaecologist should be aware of this when they are suturing near the introitus, to prevent future dyspareunia.

Postoperative care

These operations usually take about 45 minutes to 1 hour and the care is very similar to that following an abdominal hysterectomy. A vaginal pack will be *in situ* following a vaginal repair, and if the woman has had bladder surgery, a suprapubic catheter may be *in situ*. This is a fine plastic tube which is inserted just above the mons pubis and has a plastic disc with four sutures attached to the skin to prevent it from falling out.

Pain can be a particular problem for women who have had a posterior repair. Opioids will be prescribed either via a PCA pump, by continuous infusion or by intramuscular injections initially, and diclofenac suppositories are very effective in reducing inflammation and pain. Advising the woman to change her position in bed regularly or maybe lie prone can help, in conjunction with advice from the physiotherapist. Women need reassurance following repair surgery, since the pain and discomfort initially may appear to be worsening due to the bruising and the fact that they are probably moving around more than on the day after the operation.

Following a vaginal repair without bladder involvement, the urethral urinary catheter will be removed in the first couple of days. If a suprapubic catheter has been used, it will be left to drain freely for 3–5 days, depending on the urogynaecologist's preference. After this time, a 'suprapubic clamping regimen' will commence, to test whether normal bladder function has returned. On the first day, the catheter is clamped for an agreed time, e.g. 3 or 4 hours, to observe whether the woman can pass urine urethrally. After this time, the clamp is released and the residual that drains into the bag is measured. Initially, the residual may be larger than the amount of urine voided urethrally, but after a few days the residual usually decreases, and when it is less than approximately 100 mL the catheter may be removed. This is a painless procedure, and the small abdominal wound heals quickly without the leakage of urine that women might expect.

The regimen used in different hospitals may vary, and initially can appear complicated. Time and patience are required while explaining to the woman about clamping and measuring residuals. Women are usually taught how to clamp their own catheter, empty the drainage bag and record their own fluid balance measurements.

Women often need considerable encouragement, especially when they compare themselves with other patients who may be progressing more rapidly. Occasionally, women are unable to pass urine urethrally and these women may go home with their suprapubic catheter *in situ*. They can either leave the catheter on free drainage, or they may continue with the suprapubic clamping regimen, where the familiar home environment often produces better results. They are taught how to strap their catheter correctly, how to use a leg bag during the day and how to change to an overnight bag when necessary. Some district nurses will supervise the clamping regimen.

Where a urethral catheter has been used, residual amounts of urine can be measured, without further catheterization and its inherent risks of introducing infection, by the use of a bladder scanner. Nurses can be trained in the use of a small portable scanner, which is far more comfortable for the woman than being catheterized.

In rare instances of women being unable to pass urine urethrally after at least a month following surgery, intermittent self-catheterization will be taught.

Intermittent self-catheterization

This procedure involves introducing a catheter into the bladder to remove any residual urine. The catheter is then removed until required again. In hospital, this must be done aseptically to prevent cross-infection, but the woman can use a clean technique at home.

Factors such as being well motivated, good cognitive skills, manual dexterity, physical ability and good eyesight are needed for the woman to master the technique

(Newman & Wilson, 2011). Undertaking this procedure is not acceptable to all women, and nurses must take this into account.

Gradually, the woman may find that she is able to empty her bladder fully, and the residual amount of urine may become less and less when she self-catheterizes. She may well only then need to use the catheter when she wakes in the morning.

Many women find that drinking cranberry juice helps prevent cystitis or urinary tract infections developing and there is some evidence that it helps reduce the incidence of UTIs. However, cranberry juice cannot currently be recommended for the prevention of UTIs as the evidence is insufficient (Jepson et al, 2012).

Discharge advice

Women undergoing repair procedures need to be told about their internal sutures since no external wound is visible. They may not understand why precautions about lifting, etc, as discussed on page 392, are necessary.

Bowel habits

Following any vaginal surgery, care needs to be taken to avoid constipation or straining at stool. Some women may like to hold a sanitary towel to support the perineum and they should be encouraged to eat plenty of fresh fruit and vegetables and drink plenty of fluids, particularly water. Some analgesics can also result in changes to bowel habits and some consultants will routinely prescribe gentle laxatives to counteract this.

Pelvic floor exercises

All women having vaginal repair surgery and continence surgery must learn how to perform pelvic floor exercises. This increases muscle volume in the pelvic floor. These can be taught by nurses or physiotherapists. The woman should be instructed to tighten the muscles around the anus as if trying to prevent flatus escaping, and then do the same around the vagina. Asking the woman to imagine she is on the toilet and trying to stop the flow of urine may help her to visualize just what she should be feeling. Once she can manage this, she should be encouraged to hold these contractions for at least 5 seconds, then repeating 5–10 times at least five times a day. Women should be encouraged to do these exercises regularly and visual reminders such as stickers on cupboard doors can act as cues. Women of all ages should develop a habit of performing daily pelvic floor exercises on a long-term basis in order to be effective. They are also especially important after childbirth and can improve sexual enjoyment.

Laparoscopic treatment of ectopic pregnancy

This condition is included under major gynaecological surgery because an ectopic pregnancy is potentially life-threatening for the woman.

What is an ectopic pregnancy?

The word 'ectopic' originates from the Greek *'ektopos'*, meaning 'misplaced', and an ectopic pregnancy occurs when the fertilized ovum implants and develops outside the uterus. For this reason an alternative name for an ectopic pregnancy is 'pregnancy of unknown location'.

In the UK several studies indicate that the incidence is rising. Elson et al (2016) reported 11 ectopic pregnancies per 1000 pregnancies. It is often the result of fibrosis or damage to the cilia in the tube following salpingitis (infection or inflammation of the fallopian tubes). Other contributing factors are shown in Box 20.5.

A woman with a suspected ectopic pregnancy should always be treated as a gynaecological emergency. This is because there is a high risk of sudden rupture of the fallopian tubes, which can lead to a massive intraperitoneal haemorrhage. The woman's symptoms vary according to the site of implantation, although most ectopic pregnancies occur in the fallopian tube. If implantation has occurred within 4–6 weeks of her last period, the woman may not realize that she is pregnant. The first symptoms may include irregular vaginal bleeding and pelvic pain caused by the distension of the tube. Some women arrive at hospital in a state of collapse due to tubal rupture, requiring resuscitation, blood transfusion and immediate surgery by laparoscopy or laparotomy. Symptoms of tubal rupture are listed in Box 20.6.

A diagnosis of ectopic pregnancy can be confirmed using a serum β-hCG pregnancy test, which is accurate 2 weeks after conception, and a pelvic or a transvaginal scan, which will fail to show an intrauterine pregnancy. If the diagnosis remains doubtful, a laparoscopy will be performed. Either an incision is made into the tube and the pregnancy removed — the tube then heals spontaneously — or the damaged tube is removed (salpingectomy). A woman should understand there is a risk that a laparotomy may be required if the tube has ruptured.

Specific preoperative care

Frequently there is no time to fully admit and prepare a woman for surgery, since she may be rushed to theatre as an emergency. Frequent monitoring of vital signs is essential to ensure the woman's condition is assessed accurately. If a woman does come to the ward initially, she needs to be prepared as if for major surgery, since this is always a possibility. Most importantly, her psychological care is paramount.

Women can be very distressed when an ectopic pregnancy is diagnosed, since they are experiencing a multiple loss, i.e. that of a baby and possibly a fallopian tube, leading to concerns about their future fertility. They may be very shocked if they were using contraception and had not even realized they were pregnant. On the other hand, a couple may have been trying to conceive for many years, have had a previous ectopic pregnancy or have been on an IVF (*in vitro* fertilization) programme.

Box 20.5 **Factors contributing to ectopic pregnancy**

- Tubal surgery, including sterilization
- Post-delivery or post-abortion infection
- Pelvic inflammatory disease
- Endometriosis (where endometrial tissue is deposited outside the uterus)
- Previous ectopic pregnancy

Box 20.6 **Symptoms of tubal rupture**

- Sudden severe pain
- Vaginal bleeding
- Shoulder tip pain, caused by irritation of the diaphragm by blood in the peritoneal cavity
- Pallor and signs of shock and blood loss
- Distended abdomen due to bleeding

Postoperative care

Postoperative care will depend on whether the woman has had a laparoscopy or laparotomy. Women usually remain in hospital for 24 hours following laparoscopy and for 2−3 days following laparotomy. It is important that the woman's rhesus status is ascertained before she goes home. Nurses must ensure the woman and her partner are given the appropriate psychological care. This may involve talking about the pregnancy and its outcome or providing the opportunity to meet with a counsellor at a later date. However, the nurse must be aware that women will react differently to this distressing experience and must respect the woman if she does not wish to discuss her feelings at this time.

Specific discharge advice

Sexual intercourse may be resumed once any bleeding has stopped. It is probably advisable for the couple to wait until one or two normal periods have occurred before they try for another pregnancy. The couple may also find it useful to contact the Miscarriage Association (see Resources section).

Treatment for gynaecological cancers

The care of patients with cancer has been an increasing priority for the British government over recent years. The rapid referral system was instigated as part of the NHS Cancer Plan (NHS, 2000), whereby any patient suspected of having cancer must be seen within 14 days. Women with rare cancers, for example cancer of the ovary, fallopian tube and vulva, are referred to cancer centres, which may be a distance from the patient's home, where multidisciplinary teams have developed and maintained the necessary skills and expertise.

Total hysterectomy and bilateral salpingo-oophorectomy are the treatment of choice for women with endometrial cancer. Increasingly this is achieved via the laparoscopic or robotic-assisted approach. The pelvic lymph nodes may also be removed at the same time. A preoperative MRI scan of the abdomen and pelvis is carried out to ensure that the tumour is confined to the endometrium. For stage IC disease and more advanced disease, the surgery is followed by a course of adjuvant radiotherapy treatment, which may be given externally or internally. Table 20.4 illustrates the stages of endometrial cancer. If the woman has an aggressive form of endometrial cancer, for example a serous papillary or clear cell tumour, she may also be given chemotherapy in conjunction with postoperative radiotherapy. If the disease is inoperable, palliative radiotherapy is given to control the bleeding.

A radical or Wertheim's hysterectomy is an extended hysterectomy where the uterus, fallopian tubes, adjacent parametrial tissue, pelvic lymph nodes and the upper third of the vagina are removed. It is usually carried out for early cervical cancer, up to stage IB2. The ovaries may also be removed, depending on the age of the woman. If the woman is younger and wishes to preserve her fertility, an operation to remove the cervix, but retain the uterus, is undertaken. This procedure is called a trachelectomy. A cervical cerclage is inserted at the same time to allow for menstruation but in the event of future conception a caesarean will be required.

Table 20.5 illustrates the International Federation of Gynaecology and Obstetrics (FIGO) classification for staging of cancer of the cervix. For more advanced cervical cancer stage IIA−IV, the treatment may be chemotherapy in conjunction with external radiotherapy and internal radiotherapy, depending on the woman's renal function and general fitness.

Ovarian cancer is the leading cause of death from gynaecological cancer in the UK. This is suspected to be because patients often present at an advanced stage, as unlike cervical cancer there is no screening system and the onset of symptoms is often insidious. The incidence of ovarian cancer is rising, with a lifetime risk of about 2% in England and Wales (NICE, 2011). There is a strong genetic link, with approximately 20% of epithelial ovarian cancers (the most common type) being hereditary (RCOG, 2015a).

Surgical treatment for women who are diagnosed with ovarian cancer will depend on the extent of the disease. A CT scan of the abdomen and pelvis will ascertain this. If surgery is indicated, a laparotomy is performed with a total abdominal hysterectomy, bilateral salpingo-oophorectomy, peritoneal washings, excision of pelvic lymph nodes and omentectomy, as the aim is to achieve complete macroscopic clearance.

Chemotherapy is used alongside surgical treatment options. A course of chemotherapy is usually given postoperatively for advanced disease. Chemotherapy may be given as neoadjuvant therapy if the disease is too far advanced for surgical treatment. A CT scan of the abdomen and pelvis is then undertaken part way through chemotherapy to ascertain if the disease has reduced sufficiently for intervention debulking surgery to be performed. Further chemotherapy is given subsequently.

For younger women with early stage disease, the aim is to provide a diagnosis and, if possible, the remaining ovary, fallopian tube, uterus and cervix are conserved for future fertility. Unfortunately, this may not always be possible and the woman may require additional support and

Table 20.4 FIGO (International Federation of Gynaecology and Obstetrics) staging of endometrial cancer and uterine sarcomas

Stage	Description
Carcinoma of the endometrium	
Ia	Tumour confined to the uterus, no or <{1/2} myometrial invasion
Ib	Tumour confined to the uterus, >{1/2} myometrial invasion
II	Cervical stromal invasion, but not beyond uterus
IIIa	Tumour invades serosa or adnexa
IIIb	Vaginal and/or parametrial involvement
IIIc1	Pelvic node involvement
IIIc2	Para-aortic involvement
IVa	Tumour invasion of bladder and/or bowel mucosa
IVb	Distant metastases including abdominal metastases and/or inguinal lymph nodes
Uterine sarcomas (leiomyosarcoma, endometrial stromal sarcoma, and adenosarcoma)	
Ia	Tumour limited to uterus <5 cm
Ib	Tumour limited to uterus >5 cm
IIa	Tumour extends to the pelvis, adnexal involvement
IIb	Tumour extends to other uterine pelvic tissue
IIIa	Tumour invades abdominal tissues, one site
IIIb	More than one site
IIIc	Metastasis to pelvic and/or para-aortic lymph nodes
Iva	Tumour invades bladder and/or rectum
IVb	Distant metastasis
Adenosarcoma stage I differs from other uterine sarcomas	
Ia	Tumour limited to endometrium/endocervix
Ib	Invasion to <{1/2} myometrium
Ic	Invasion to >{1/2} myometrium

Source: BGCS Uterine Cancer Guidelines: Recommendations for Practice (2017). Based on FIGO Classification by Pecorelli (2009).

counselling to adjust to both the diagnosis and the implications of treatment.

Ovarian cancer is perceived as a chronic illness as it tends to recur. The longer someone goes between one course and the next, the better it is. If the disease does recur, there may be further surgery to remove the recurrence, or further chemotherapy using different chemotherapy drugs. Occasionally, if a woman has a recurrence within the pelvis, she may also receive radiotherapy. Due to the relatively high morbidity of this disease, oncology nurse specialists are paramount in providing both patients and family with support.

Vulvectomy

Vulval cancer accounts for approximately 3% of all gynaecological cancers (Lai et al, 2014). It is usually seen in elderly women over 70 years old, although increasing numbers of younger women are being seen with cancer of the vulva, due to the effects of the human papillomavirus (HPV). The predisposing factors that may contribute to cancer of the vulva are vulval intraepithelial neoplasia (VIN 3 — a precancerous condition), lichen sclerosis, genital warts, smoking and multiple sexual partners. The most common histological type is squamous cell carcinoma, which accounts for 90% of all vulval cancers. Early signs are pruritus or irritation, pain, burning, soreness, bleeding, an ulcer or a lump. There may also be colour changes of the affected area. Elderly women are often reluctant to seek medical help due to embarrassment; consequently, the cancer may be at an advanced state at presentation.

Wide local excision

Precancerous vulval abnormalities such as lichen sclerosis and VIN 3, together with early stages of cancer of the vulva, i.e. tumours with a depth of less than 1 mm, may be treated by surgery which involves a wide local excision. The aim is to remove the abnormal tissue together with a

Table 20.5 FIGO (International Federation of Gynaecology and Obstetrics) classification of cancer of the cervix

Stage	Description
I	The carcinoma is strictly confined to the cervix (extension to the uterine corpus should be disregarded)
IA	Invasive carcinoma that can be diagnosed only by microscopy, with maximum depth of invasion <5 mm[a]
IA1	Measured stromal invasion <3 mm in depth
IA2	Measured stromal invasion ≥3 mm and <5 mm in depth
IB	Invasive carcinoma with measured deepest invasion ≥5 mm (greater than Stage IA), lesion limited to the cervix uteri[b]
IB1	Invasive carcinoma ≥5 mm depth of stromal invasion, and <2 cm in greatest dimension
IB2	Invasive carcinoma ≥2 cm and <4 cm in greatest dimension
IB3	Invasive carcinoma ≥4 cm in greatest dimension
II	The carcinoma invades beyond the uterus, but has not extended onto the lower third of the vagina or to the pelvic wall
IIA	Involvement limited to the upper two-thirds of the vagina without parametrial involvement
IIA1	Invasive carcinoma <4 cm in greatest dimension
IIA2	Invasive carcinoma ≥4 cm in greatest dimension
IIB	With parametrial involvement but not up to the pelvic wall
III	The carcinoma involves the lower third of the vagina and/or extends to the pelvic wall and/or causes hydronephrosis or non-functioning kidney and/or involves pelvic and/or para-aortic lymph nodes[c]
IIIA	The carcinoma involves the lower third of the vagina, with no extension to the pelvic wall
IIIB	Extension to the pelvic wall and/or hydronephrosis or non-functioning kidney (unless known to be due to another cause)
IIIC	Involvement of pelvic and/or para-aortic lymph nodes, irrespective of tumor size and extent (with r and p notations)[c]
IIIC1	Pelvic lymph node metastasis only
IIIC2	Para-aortic lymph node metastasis
IV	The carcinoma has extended beyond the true pelvis or has involved (biopsy proven) the mucosa of the bladder or rectum. (A bullous oedema, as such, does not permit a case to be allotted to Stage IV)
IVA	Spread to adjacent pelvic organs
IVB	Spread to distant organs

When in doubt, the lower staging should be assigned.
[a]Imaging and pathology can be used, where available, to supplement clinical findings with respect to tumor size and extent, in all stages.
[b]The involvement of vascular/lymphatic spaces does not change the staging. The lateral extent of the lesion is no longer considered.
[c]Adding notation of r (imaging) and p (pathology) to indicate the findings that are used to allocate the case to Stage IIIC. Example: If imaging indicates pelvic lymph node metastasis, the stage allocation would be Stage IIIC1r, and if confirmed by pathologic findings, it would be Stage IIIC1p. The type of imaging modality or pathology technique used should always be documented.
Source: Bhatla et al (2018).

minimum 1-cm margin of healthy tissue. Further surgery depends on the size and depth of the tumour and may also necessitate the removal of the inguinal lymph nodes on one (unilateral) or both (bilateral) sides. Many women with VIN 3 have multifocal disease, which means repeated episodes of surgery to try to control the disease.

Radical vulvectomy

A radical vulvectomy is performed for invasive cancer of the vulva. In the past, the vulval tissue was removed *en bloc* in one piece. However, this procedure was associated with significant morbidity and can have a significant impact on patient quality of life (Lai et al, 2014). To reduce this, a triple-incision technique was introduced in the 1980s. This involves the excision of the vulval lesion, together with the left and right inguinal and femoral nodes. In some cases, the terminal end of the urethra and the clitoris are also removed. The degree of surgery depends on the location and extent of the primary lesion, and the surgeon will plan to effect treatment but reduce morbidity and postoperative complications. However, if it is necessary to remove a large area of skin, a skin graft may be required from the thigh or abdomen. Vulvectomy wounds are under a tremendous amount of stress and at high risk of wound breakdown. The statistics on this vary greatly between studies but the consensus is that vulvectomy wounds are at a very high risk of wound breakdown or infection (BGCS & RCOG, 2014; Iavazzo & Gkegkes, 2017).

Preoperative care

Preoperative care will be the same as that for any major gynaecological surgery, but it is obviously vital that women and their partners have a full explanation of the operation and its implications. On admission, both ward and specialist nurses must be involved with the woman's care. A full sexual history and assessment should be undertaken. Women may find it difficult to come to terms with the mutilating effects surgery will have, and considerable time will need to be spent preoperatively in discussion with the whole family. Drawing diagrams of the area to be removed may also help.

If possible, there are advantages to nursing a woman undergoing vulvectomy in a side-room initially, due to the privacy and intensive nursing care required. However, if a woman would rather be with other patients, this should be arranged.

Anti-embolism stockings should be measured for and fitted, since mobility will be impaired by pain and bulky bandages. These patients are often elderly and should be taught deep breathing and leg exercises prior to surgery, to reduce the risks of DVT. Subcutaneous heparin will also be prescribed, as for all patients undergoing major surgery.

Shaving prior to surgery may be required. However, most evidence suggests that this is most beneficial if completed immediately prior to surgery.

Postoperative care

Opioid analgesics will be required postoperatively, either by PCA, infusion pumps or injections, or an epidural may be sited. Intravenous fluid replacement will be required,

since fluid loss may be considerable during this complicated operation. After the initial drowsiness and nausea, drinking and eating may be gradually resumed. A low-fibre diet is necessary to avoid bulky stools and straining.

A urethral (Foley) catheter will be in place and it will remain *in situ* while healing occurs. If the terminal end of the urethra is removed, women may find that urine no longer flows out in a steady stream, so they need to be taught how to squat and sit back slightly to avoid wetting their legs or the floor.

Two drains (one in each groin) are inserted to prevent lymphocyst formation if the inguinal lymph nodes have been removed. The amount of lymph drainage must be measured daily, and the drains are removed once the drainage is less than 50 mL daily. Wound care varies between different units and there appears to be very little published research to recommend the best approach. Nursing staff often take the lead in determining the most appropriate wound care, based on the rationale of promoting healing and reducing wound breakdown, which has been associated with this surgery in the past. Following bathing or showering, the area can be dried thoroughly using a hairdryer. However, if there is any infection present, this practice is not appropriate as the hairdryer can blow microorganisms into the atmosphere. In some hospitals, women return to theatre for a light anaesthetic before removal of sutures, or inhalational analgesia such as Entonox is used. Surgery involving removal of lymph tissue can result in lower limb lymphoedema, whereby lymph is unable to drain properly and collects in interstitial tissue. Advice must be given concerning skin care, as it is imperative to keep the skin supple and moisturized. Special care must be taken to look after the legs, for example attention must be made when cutting the toenails, to prevent any infection and shaving of legs should be avoided. Referral to a lymphoedema specialist nurse may also be made for further treatment and fitting compression hosiery.

Altered body image

All women undergoing vulval surgery may experience an altered body image and require psychologically sensitive care (Lai et al, 2014). Women may find it difficult to look at their new altered appearance, and it is advisable that they try to do so before going home. Many women in this age group are not used to looking 'down below', so sensitive communication is required. If possible, the woman should look with the help of a mirror, in her own time, but with her nurse present if she prefers. It may be better to wait until the staples or sutures are removed, since they can make the scarring look worse. Many women find it hard to visualize what the scar will look like. Due to the fatty, stretchy nature of vulval skin, the remaining skin can be stretched to leave a very neat scar. Women need to be warned that, because the labia have been removed, the opening of the vagina will be more visible. If the clitoris has been removed, the area will now be flat skin, without the usual folds of the vulva. Also, the groin may feel tight at first if lymph nodes have been removed. Many women feel unable to discuss their diagnosis and treatment with family and friends and may benefit from counselling to reduce the impact of postoperative consequences on her lifestyle, body image and self-esteem.

Discharge advice

Discharge planning from the time of preoperative assessment is essential. A specific support group for vulvectomy patients, VACO (Vulva Awareness Campaign Organisation), may assist women to feel that they are not the only ones with this disease. Contact details of VACO are in the Resources section. In general, similar discharge advice should be given as for patients who have undergone major gynaecological surgery.

Sexual advice

It is crucial that, before discharge, there should be discussion about any sexual concerns the couple may have. The psychosexual implications of vulvectomy are of utmost importance, since genitals are intimately associated with a woman's sexuality, body image, gender identity and general quality of life.

Excision of the clitoris is likely to greatly reduce sensation, and the loss of orgasm was note by some studies. The scarred tissue at the remaining vaginal opening can be insensitive to penetration, and a loss of sensitivity in the genital area with persistent numbness and loss of libido may also occur (Aerts et al, 2014).

A woman who has undergone a vulvectomy should be advised that she may resume intercourse when she feels ready, probably 4–12 weeks following surgery. Couples should be advised to compensate for loss of perineal sensation by exploring other erotic areas, i.e. breasts, buttocks, thighs. It has to be remembered that couples may need explicit advice and information rather than vague generalizations about intercourse, since people's sexual experiences vary enormously. Although a detailed discussion such as alternative recommended positions for lovemaking may or may not be accomplished by nurses, depending on their personal expertise and degree of comfort, it is important not to neglect the issue of the patient's altered sexuality. In such circumstances, specialist oncology nurses should be involved.

Case Study 20.3.

Mrs Jones is a married 70-year-old woman, who has undergone a vulvectomy after being diagnosed with a squamous cell carcinoma of the vulva. She is currently on postoperative day 1 but is concerned about how the wound looks and is worried about infection.

Questions for reflection

How can patient education on the part of the healthcare professional promote effective wound healing? How might the surgery and postoperative care influence Mrs Jones's view of herself and her sexuality?

Total pelvic exenteration

Total pelvic exenteration is a major operation which may be considered following a recurrence of a cancer of the cervix or, more rarely, the endometrium. It is carried out if an MRI scan of the abdomen and pelvis and CT scan of the chest have excluded the presence of any metastatic disease elsewhere in the body. A PET scan may also be utilized. The surgery involves the removal of the rectum and distal sigmoid colon, the urinary bladder, all reproductive organs and the entire pelvic floor, and necessitates the formation of both a urostomy and a sigmoid colostomy. Vaginal reconstruction may be performed at the time of operation or at a later date.

The chance of a cure entails great sacrifice on the part of the patient. There are multiple potential complications of surgery (Petruzziello et al, 2014). Potential survival involves the formation of two stomas, with the loss of the vagina, and thus causes drastic alteration to body image, self-respect and sexuality. A multidisciplinary approach to the care of these women is vital from the time that the surgery is planned, including an assessment by a consultant psychiatrist or clinical psychologist. Consultants in gynaecology, oncology, urology and colorectal surgery are involved in the surgery, together with a consultant anaesthetist. Following the surgery, the woman is cared for in an intensive care/high-dependency bed. Specialist nurses are involved with teaching the woman to care for her stomas, together with support from dietitians, physiotherapists and occupational therapists.

The teaching objectives of the nurse include education of the patient regarding anatomy and the changes that will occur as a result of surgery. By discussing the outcomes of surgery, the nurse also encourages the patient to voice her feelings about the impending alterations to body image, eliminatory and sexual functions.

Conclusion

Due to constant developments in women's health, it has been impossible to discuss every gynaecological operation. However, it is hoped that this chapter has provided a straightforward overview of gynaecological surgery and insight into the psychological aspects of care. Conflicts can occur on gynaecology wards where some of the women are longing for a pregnancy, while others are terminating them.

Although many of these operations are considered routine by healthcare staff, it should always be remembered that for each individual woman, surgery on an intimate part of the body can be a major life event. The sexual anxieties of women are often forgotten but should be a crucial focus of care. This will enable the woman to make a full recovery. It is the responsibility of the healthcare professional to ask a woman about her specific anxieties rather than waiting for her to offer them as topics of discussion, and dignity and respect must always be maintained.

SUMMARY OF KEY POINTS

- Gynaecological surgery is an extremely sensitive area, and this should be taken into consideration when caring for patients, and their partners, who are undergoing any form of gynaecological investigations and/or surgery.
- Healthcare practitioners need to be aware of the psychological effects and related sexuality surrounding gynaecological surgery.
- A woman's concept of her body image, her role as a woman and mother, her sexuality and her relationship with her partner can be threatened following gynaecological surgery.
- A general medical, social, obstetric and gynaecological history should be obtained during the assessment process.
- The practitioner should provide an environment in which the woman and her partner are able to discuss any sexual matters.
- The primary goal of gynaecological nursing is to help the woman become independent and self-supporting following her surgery.
- The healthcare professional must maintain a sensitive, non-judgmental attitude at all times.

REFLECTIVE LEARNING POINTS

Having read this chapter, think about what you now know and what you still need to find out about. These questions may help:

(Continued)

(cont'd)

- What key areas does the nurse need to address preoperatively with the woman (and if appropriate her family) to help alleviate preoperative anxiety?
- How might you ensure that the care you offer to women is non-judgemental.
- Outline the biophysical, psychosocial and cultural aspects of care that need to be provided to women with gynaecological or related conditions.

Dedication

This chapter is dedicated to the memory of Sarah Moore (nee McAllister), patient and friend who lost her battle with cervical cancer on Boxing Day 2018, aged 37. Never was there a more poignant example of the importance of recognizing the individual behind every illness. Never forget that behind every patient is an individual person.

Resources

Antenatal Results and Choices
Tel: 0845 077 2290 or 0207 713 7486 via mobile
https://www.arc-uk.org/
Association for Continence Advice
Tel: +44 (0) 1506 811077
Email: aca@fitwise.co.uk
www.aca.uk.com
British Society of Urogynaecology
Tel: 020 7772 6211
Email: bsug@rcog.org.uk
bsug.org.uk
Bladder and Bowel Community
Tel: 01926 357220
Email: help@bladderandbowel.org
www.bladderandbowel.org
British Gynaecological Cancer Society
Email: administrator@bgcs.org
bgcs.org.uk
British Menopause Society
Tel: 01628 890199
thebms.org.uk
Cancer Research UK
Tel (general enquires): 0300 123 1022
Tel (cancer related): 0808 800 4040
www.cancerresearchuk.org/about-cancer/womens-cancer

Fertility Network UK
info@fertilitynetworkuk.org
Tel: 01424 732361
fertilitynetworkuk.org/about
Hysterectomy Association
healthyhappywoman.co.uk/hysterectomy-information
Miscarriage Association
Tel: 01924 200799
Email: info@miscarriageassociation.org.uk
www.miscarriageassociation.org.uk
National Association for Premenstrual Syndrome (NAPS)
Tel: 0844 8157311
Email: contact@pms.org.uk
www.pms.org.uk
National Endometriosis Society
Tel: 020 7222 2781
endometriosis-uk.org

National Osteoporosis Society
Tel (general enquires): 01761 471 771
Tel (helpline): 0808 800 0035
www.nos.org.uk
Royal College of Obstetricians and Gynaecologists
Tel: 020 7772 6200
www.rcog.org.uk
Sands (Stillbirth and Neonatal Death Charity)
Tel: 020 7436 7940
Helpline: 0808 164 3332
Email: helpline@sands.org.uk
www.sands.org.uk
VACO (Vulva Awareness Campaign Organisation)
www.vaco.co.uk

References

Aarts, J. W. M., Nieboer, T. E., Johnson, N., Tavender, E., Garry, R., Mol, B. J., et al. (2015). Surgical approach to hysterectomy for benign gynaecological diseases. *Cochrane Database, 8,* CD003677.

Aerts, L., Enzlin, P., Verhaeghe, J., Vergote, I., & Amant, F. (2014). Psychologic, relational, and sexual functioning in women after surgical treatment of vulvar malignancy: a prospective controlled study. *International Journal of Gynecological Cancer, 24*(2), 372–380.

Apfelbaum, J.L. Silverstein, J.H., Chung, F.F., Connis, R.T., Fillmore, R.B., et al; American Society of Anesthesiologists Task Force on Postanesthetic Care. (2013). Practice guidelines for postanesthetic care: an updated report by the American Society of Anesthesiologists Task Force on Postanesthetic Care. *Anesthesiology, 118*(2), 291–307.

Asher, R., Obermair, A., Franzcog, C. G. O., Monika, J., & Gebski, V. (2018). Disease-free and survival outcomes for total laparoscopic hysterectomy compared with total abdominal hysterectomy in early-stage endometrial carcinoma: a meta-analysis. *International Journal of Gynecological Cancer, 28*(3), 529–538.

Allison, J., & George, M. (2014). Using preoperative assessment and patient instruction to improve patient safety. *Association of Operating Room Nurses, 99* (3), 364–375.

American Society of Anesthesiologists (ASA). (2017). Practice guidelines for preoperative fasting and the use of pharmacologic agents to reduce the risk of pulmonary aspiration: application to healthy patients undergoing elective procedures: an updated report by the American Society of Anesthesiologists Task Force on Preoperative Fasting and the Use of Pharmacologic Agents to Reduce the Risk of Pulmonary Aspiration. *Anesthesiology, 126*(3), 376–393.

Bhatla, N., Aoki, D., Sharma, D. N., & Sankaranarayanan, R. (2018). FIGO Cancer Report 2018. Cancer of the Cervix Uteri. *International Journal of Gynecology and Obstetrics, 143*(S2), 22–36.

British Gynaecological Cancer Society (BGCS) & Royal College of Obstetricians and Gynaecologists (RCOG). (2014). *Guidelines for the diagnosis and management of vulval carcinoma.* London: BGCS/RCOG.

Clark, T. J., & Gupta, J. K. (2005). *Handbook of outpatient hysteroscopy.* London: Hodder.

Cleary, V., Hegarty, J., & McCarthy, G. (2013). How a diagnosis of gynaecological cancer affects women's sexuality. *Cancer Nursing Practice, 12*(1), 32–37.

Dimond, B. (2011). *Legal Aspects of Nursing* (6th ed.). Harlow: Pearson Education Ltd.

Durnell Schuiling, K., & Likis, F. (2017). *Women's Gynecologic Health* (3rd ed.). Burlington, MA: Jones and Bartlett Learning.

Dyer, C. (2018). UK women launch legal action against Bayer over Essure sterilisation device. *British Medical Journal, 360,* k271.

Elson, C.J., Salim, R., Potdar, N., Chetty, M., Ross, J.A., Kirk, E.J. on behalf of the Royal College of Obstetricians and Gynaecologists. (2016). Diagnosis and management of ectopic pregnancy. *BJOG, 123,* e15–e55.

Erickson, B. K., Conner, M. G., & Landen, C. N., Jr (2013). The role of the fallopian tube in the origin of ovarian cancer. *American Journal of Obstetrics and Gynecology, 209*(5), 409–414.

Food and Drug Administration. (2018). *Essure permanent birth control.* Available at: <www.fda.gov/medical-devices/implants-and-prosthetics/essure-permanent-birth-control>

Fritzer, N., Haas, D., Oppelt, P., Renner, S., Hornung, D., Wölfler, M., et al. (2013). More than just bad sex: sexual dysfunction and distress in patients with endometriosis. *European Journal of Obstetrics & Gynecology and Reproductive Biology, 169*(2), 392–396.

Galaal, K., Donkers, H., Bryant, A., & Lopes, A. D. (2018). Laparoscopy versus laparotomy for the management of early stage endometrial cancer. *Cochrane Database of Systematic Reviews, 10.*

Gray, C. E., Baruah-Young, J., & Payne, C. J. (2015). Preoperative assessment in patients presenting for elective surgery. *Anaesthesia and Intensive Care Medicine, 16*(9), 425−430.

Iavazzo, C., & Gkegkes, I. D. (2017). Vulvar cancer and post-vulvectomy complications. In M. A. Farage, & H. I. Maibach (Eds.), *The vulva: Physiology and clinical management* (2nd ed.). Boca Raton: CRC Press.

Irwin, D. E., Kopp, Z. S., Agatep, B., Milsom, I., & Abrams, P. (2011). Worldwide prevalence estimates of lower urinary tract symptoms, overactive bladder, urinary incontinence and bladder outlet obstruction. *BJU International, 108*(7), 1132−1138.

Kyle, E. B., Maheux-Lacroix, S., Boutin, A., Laberge, P. Y., & Lemyre, M. (2016). Low vs standard pressures in gynecologic laparoscopy: a systematic review. *Journal of the Society of Laparoendoscopic Surgeons, 20*(1).

Lai, J., Elleray, R., Nordin, A., Hirschowitz, L., Rous, B., Gildea, C., et al. (2014). Vulval cancer incidence, mortality and survival in England: age-related trends. *BJOG: An International Journal of Obstetrics and Gynaecology, 121*(6), 729−739..

Lethaby, A., Mukhopadhyay, A., & Naik, R. (2012). Total versus subtotal hysterectomy for benign gynaecological conditions. *Cochrane Database of Systematic Reviews, 4*, CD004993.

Liu, H., Lawrie, T. A., Lu, D., Song, H., Wang, L., & Shi, G. (2014). Robot-assisted surgery in gynaecology. *Cochrane Database of Systematic Reviews, 12*, CD011422.

Janssen, S. M., & Lagro-Janssen, A. L. M. (2012). Physician's gender, communication style, patient preferences and patient satisfaction in gynecology and obstetrics: A systematic review. *Patient Education and Counseling, 89*(2012), 221−226.

Jepson, R. G., Williams, G., & Craig, J. C. (2012). Cranberries for preventing urinary tract infections. *Cochrane Database of Systematic Reviews, 10*, CD001321.

Johnson, N. P., Hummelshoj, L., Adamson, G. D., Keckstein, J., Taylor, H. S., Abrao, M. S., et al. (2017). World Endometriosis Society consensus on the classification of endometriosis. *Human Reproduction, 32*(2), 314−322..

Joint Committee on Vaccination and Immunization. (2018). *Statement on HPV vaccination*. Available at: <assets. publishing.service.gov.uk/government/ uploads/system/uploads/attachment_ data/file/726319/JCVI_Statement_ on_HPV_vaccination_2018.pdf>

Maclaran, K., Agarwal, N., & Odejimi, F. (2016). Perioperative outcomes in laparoscopic hysterectomy: identifying surgical risk factors. *Gynecology Surgery, 13*, 75−82.

Manodoro, S., Werbrouck, E., Veldman, J., Haest, K., Corona, R., Claerhout, F., et al. (2011). Laparoscopic sacrocolpopexy. *Facts, Views and Vision in Obstetrics, Gynaecology and Reproductive Health, 3*(3), 151−158.

McDonald, R. (2015). Enhanced recovery clinical education programme improves quality of post-operative care. *BMJ Quality Improvement Reports.* Available at: <bmjopenquality.bmj. com/content/4/1/u208370.w3387>.

Murkhopadhaya, N., & Manyonda, I. T. (2013). The hysterectomy story in the United Kingdom. *Journal of Midlife Health, 4*(1), 40−41.

Muto, M. G., Goff, B., & Falk, S. J. (2017). Risk-reducing bilateral salpingo-oophorectomy in women at high risk of epithelial ovarian and fallopian tubal cancer. *UpToDate.* Available at: <www.uptodate.com/contents/risk- reducing-bilateral-salpingo-oophorec- tomy-in-women-at-high-risk-of-epithe- lial-ovarian-and-fallopian-tubal- cancer>.

National Institute of Health and Care Excellence (NICE). (2010). *Laparoscopic hysterectomy (including laparoscopic total hysterectomy and laparoscopically assisted vaginal hysterectomy) for endometrial cancer: Interventional procedures guidance.* London: NICE.

National Institute of Health and Care Excellence (NICE). (2011). *Ovarian cancer: recognition and initial management.* Clinical guideline [CG122]. London: NICE.

National Institute of Health and Care Excellence (NICE). (2012). *Ectopic pregnancy and miscarriage: diagnosis and initial management.* Clinical guideline [CG154]. London: NICE.

National Institute for Health and Care Excellence (NICE). (2015). *Urinary incontinence in women: Management.* [CG17]. London: NICE.

National Institute for Health and Care Excellence (NICE). (2016). *Routine preoperative tests for elective surgery.* [NG45]. London: NICE.

National Institute for Health and Care Excellence (NICE). (2017). *Endometrosis diagnosis and management.* [NG73]. London: NICE.

National Institute for Health and Care Excellence (NICE). (2018a). *Heavy menstrual bleeding: assessment and management.* NICE guideline [NG88]. London: NICE.

National Institute for Health and Care Excellence (NICE). (2018b). *Venous thromboembolism in over 16s: reducing the risk of hospital-acquired deep vein thrombosis or pulmonary embolism.* NICE guideline [NG89]. London: NICE.

Nelson, G., Altman, D., Nick, A., Meyer, L. A., Ramirez, P. T., Acheson, N., et al. (2016). Guidelines for Postoperative Care in Gynecologic/Oncology Surgery: Enhanced Recovery after Surgery (ERAS). Society Recommendations − Part 2. *Gynecologic Oncology, 140*(2), 323−332.

Newman, D. K., & Wilson, M. M. (2011). Review of intermittent catheterization and current best practices. *Urologic Nursing, 31*(1), 12−29.

NHS. (2000). *The NHS Cancer Plan: a plan for investment, a plan for reform.* London: Department of Health.

NHS Cervical Screening Programme. (2016). *Cancer screening programmes: Colposcopy and programme management* [Online]. Available at: <www.bsccp. org.uk/assets/file/uploads/resources/ NHSCSP_20_Colposcopy_and_Program- me_Management_(3rd_Edition)_(2).pdf>

Nursing and Midwifery Council. (2018). *The Code. Professional standards of practice and behaviour for nurses, midwives and nursing associates.* Available at: <www.nmc.org.uk/standards/code>

Pecorelli, S. (2009). FIGO committee on gynecologic oncology: revised FIGO staging for carcinoma of the vulva, cervix and endometrium. *Internal Journal Gynecology Oncology, 105*(2), 103−104.

Persu, C., Chapple, C. R., Cauni, V., Gutue, S., & Geavlete, P. (2011). Pelvic Organ Prolapse Quantification System (POP-Q) − a new era in pelvic prolapse staging. *Journal of Medicine and Life, 4*(1), 75−81.

Petruzziello, A., Kondo, W., Hatschback, S. B., Guerrerio, J. A., Fiho, F. P., Vendrame, C., et al. (2014). Surgical results of pelvic exenteration in the treatment of gynecologic cancer. *World Journal of Surgical Oncology, 12*(1), 279−287.

Rahmanou, P., White, B., Price, N., & Jackson, S. (2014). Laparoscopic hysteropexy: 1- to 4-year follow-up of women postoperatively. *International Urogynaecology Journal, 25*(1), 131−138.

Roper, N., Logan, W. W., & Tierney, A. J. (2003). *The roper—logan—tierney model of nursing*. Edinburgh: Churchill Livingstone.

Royal College of Obstetricians and Gynaecologists (RCOG). (2011). *Management of suspected ovarian masses in premenopausal women*. London: RCOG.

Royal College of Obstetricians and Gynaecologists (RCOG). (2015a). *Management of women with a genetic predisposition to gynaecological cancers scientific impact paper No. 48*. London: RCOG.

Royal College of Obstetricians and Gynaecologists (RCOG). (2015b).

Obtaining valid consent clinical governance advice No. 6. London: RCOG.

Royal College of Obstetricians and Gynaecologists (RCOG). (2016). *Female sterilisation: Consent advice No 3*. London: RCOG.

Royal College of Obstetricians and Gynaecologists (RCOG). (2018). *Mesh Safety Alert*. London: RCOG. Available at: <www.rcog.org.uk/en/guidelines-research-services/guidelines/mesh-safety-alert/>.

Setchell, M. E. (2013). Pre-operative assessment and diagnostic procedures. In M. E. Setchell, & J. H. Shepherd (Eds.),

Shaw's textbook of operative gynaecology (7th ed., pp. 29—37). Oxford: Elsevier.

Sinha, R., Sanja, M., Rupa, B., & Kumari, S. (2015). Robotic surgery in gynaecology. *Journal of Minimal Access Surgery*, *11*(1), 50—59.

Tortora, G. J., & Grabowski, S. R. (2003). Principles of anatomy and physiology (10th ed.). New York: John Wiley.

World Health Organization. (2014). *Comprehensive cervical cancer control a guide to essential practice* (2nd ed.). Geneva: WHO.

Further reading

Durnell-Schuiling, K., & Likis, F. (2017). *Womens gynecologic health* (3rd ed.). Burlington MA: Jones and Bartlett Learning.

Gupta, S., Holloway, D., & Kubba, A. (2010). *Oxford handbook of women's health nursing*. Oxford: Oxford University Press.

Iavazzo, C., & Gkegkes, I. D. (2017). Vulvar cancer and post-vulvectomy complications. In M. A. Farage, & H. I. Maibach (Eds.), *The vulva: Physiology and clinical management* (2nd ed.). Boca Raton: CRC Press.

Kaschak, E., & Tiefer, L. (2014). *A view of women's sexual problems*. New York: Routledge.

Magowan, B. A., Owen, P., & Thomson, A. (2018). *Clinical obstetrics and gynaecology* (4th edn). Elsevier.

Murray, S., McKinney, E., Holub, K., & Jones, R. *Foundations of maternal-newborn and women's health nursing* (7th ed). Elsevier.

Norwitz, E. R., & Schorge, J. O. (2013). *Obstetrics and gynecology at a glance* (4th ed.). Oxford: Wiley Blackwell.

Oats, J. J. N., & Abraham, S. (2015). *Llewellyn-Jones fundamentals of obstetrics and gynaecology* (10th ed.). Edinburgh: Elsevier.

Olshansky, E. F. (2015). *Women's health and wellness across the lifespan*. Philadelphia: Wolters Kluwer Health.

Royal College of Obstetricians and Gynaecologists. (2016). *Providing quality care for women: Standards for gynaecology care*. London: RCOG.

Spiers, M. V., Geller, P. A., & Kloss, J. D. (2013). *Women's health psychology*. New Jersey: John Wiley and Sons.

Sundar, S., Balega, J., Crosbie, E., Drake, A., Edmondson, R., Fotopoulou, C., et al., (2017). *BGCS uterine cancer guidelines: Recommendations for practice*. BGCS. Available at: <https://www.bgcs.org.uk/wp-content/uploads/2019/05/BGCS-Endometrial-Guidelines-2017.pdf>

Chapter | 21 |

Patients requiring breast surgery

Barry T. Hill

KEY OBJECTIVES OF THE CHAPTER

At the end of the chapter the reader should be able to:

- describe the basic anatomy and physiology of the breast
- demonstrate a basic knowledge and understanding of the investigations used in breast disease
- understand the conditions requiring breast surgery and the reasons for it
- assess the needs of patients undergoing breast surgery, using a model of nursing care
- plan and implement pre- and postoperative nursing care, considering current research and the available evidence
- plan a discharge from hospital
- give appropriate advice, information and education to the patient.

Areas to think about before reading the chapter

- What fear and anxieties might a person have if they have been diagnosed with breast disease?

(Continued)

(cont'd)

- At what age are women invited to take part in breast screening programmes?
- What are the key functions of Breast Care Nurse Specialist?

Introduction

Breast disease is a common occurrence in women and, although less common, it can also impact on men and those who identify as trans and non-binary; accordingly it is likely that most nurses will find themselves caring for patients with breast disease at some point in their career. It is therefore important to have a good knowledge base and understanding from which to work.

The first symptom of breast cancer for many women is a lump in their breast. But it is important to note that 9 out of 10 breast lumps (90%) are benign, which means that they are not cancers (Cancer Research UK, 2017a,b). For the patient, finding a breast lump instils a fear of cancer. It is essential that the patient is cared for in a kind and sensitive manner and a diagnosis is made quickly.

This chapter looks at both benign and malignant breast disease, the different types of surgery and the nursing care of a patient undergoing breast surgery.

Anatomy and physiology

The breasts, also known as mammary glands, exist in both males and females, and are the accessory organ of reproduction. The breasts are situated on either side of the

419

sternum, between the second and sixth rib and overlying the pectoralis major muscle. They are stabilized by a suspensory ligament known as Cooper's ligament, named after Sir Astley Cooper.

The shape of the breast is hemispherical, with a tail of tissue extending towards the axilla. The size varies with the stage of development as well as with age. Size also varies between individuals, and often one breast is larger than the other.

Gross structure

The axillary tail, also known as the tail of Spence, extends towards the axilla.

The areola is the pigmented circular area, approximately 2.5 cm in diameter, situated at the centre of each breast. The colour varies from a pale pink in fair-skinned women to a dark brown in dark-skinned women. The colour darkens during pregnancy. There are approximately 20 sebaceous glands, called Montgomery's tubercles, on the areola which lubricate the nipple.

The nipple lies in the centre of the areola and is approximately 6 mm in length. It is composed of erectile tissue and is highly sensitive. The surface is perforated by the openings of the lactiferous ducts.

Microscopic structure

The breast is made up of three types of tissue — fibrous, glandular and fatty — and is covered by skin.

Fibrous bands divide the glandular tissue into approximately 16–20 lobes. Within each lobe is the milk-producing system. The alveoli are the milk-secreting cells (also known as acini). The alveoli are connected by lactiferous tubules, which then connect to the main lactiferous ducts. The lactiferous ducts are lined with epithelial cells. The lactiferous duct then widens to form the ampulla, which acts as a reservoir for the milk to be stored. The lactiferous duct then continues on from the ampulla and opens onto the nipple.

The glandular tissue of the breast is surrounded by fat. If weight is gained or lost, the shape and size of the breast will vary.

Blood supply

The blood supply to the breast comes from the axillary artery and the internal mammary artery. The venous drainage is through the corresponding vessels into the internal mammary and axillary veins.

Nerve supply

The nerve supply to the breast is mainly by the somatic sensory nerves and autonomic nerves accompanying the blood vessels. The nipple, being the most sensitive part of the breast, is supplied by somatic sensory nerves, whereas the rest of the breast tissue is mainly supplied by the autonomic nerves.

The medial aspect of the breast is served by the thoracic intercostal nerve, which penetrates the pectoralis major to reach the skin. The upper outer quadrant is served by the intercostal brachial nerve, which comes via the axilla.

Lymphatic system

The lymph fluid from the outer quadrants of the breast flows into the axillary lymph nodes and eventually into the nodes in the neck. Lymph fluid in the inner quadrant drains towards the sternum via the inframammary nodes.

The major lymphatic drainage of the breast is to the axilla, and the axillary nodes are divided into three levels:
- Level I — the nodes lie lateral to the lateral border of the pectoralis minor muscle
- Level II — the nodes lie behind the pectoralis minor muscle
- Level III — the nodes are located medial to the medial border of the pectoralis minor muscle.

Physiology of the breast

The breast is influenced by two main hormones: oestrogen and progesterone. Oestrogen stimulates the growth of the breast once a girl has reached puberty. Progesterone has a secondary function in the maturation of the glandular tissue.

The breasts undergo cyclical changes with the menstrual cycle, due to the changing levels of the hormone prolactin, which controls the secretion of the ovarian hormones oestrogen and progesterone. These hormones cause the breast tissue and ducts to enlarge. The breast may change in size and consistency and become tender, swollen and nodular, usually 10–14 days prior to menstruation.

When ovarian activity ceases at the menopause, causing a fall in the level of circulating oestrogen and progesterone, the glandular tissue in the breasts starts to involute and atrophy. The glandular tissue then becomes replaced by fat.

Assessment and investigations

A woman will initially present to her practice nurse or general practitioner with a breast symptom. The GP will assess her and decide whether referral to a breast specialist is appropriate.

According to the National Institute for Health and Care Excellence (NICE) (2019) in their March 2019 'Early and locally advanced breast cancer overview' pathway, a person with early or locally advanced breast cancer should be referred to secondary care even if breast cancer is merely suspected. They will be offered information, advice and support as required. NICE (2018c) suggest in their 'Suspected cancer recognition and referral' pathway that health professionals must discuss with people with suspected cancer (and their carers, as appropriate, taking account of the need for confidentiality) their preferences for being involved in decision-making about referral options and further investigations including their potential risks and benefits. Patients will receive three key pieces of guidance, which include recommendations on cryopreservation to preserve fertility in people diagnosed with cancer; the need to stop systemic HRT in women who are diagnosed with breast cancer if they are taking this medication; and to offer women information and counselling about the possibility of early menopause and menopausal symptoms associated with breast cancer treatments. Following on from here the patient will receive assessment and staging, and then neoadjuvant therapy, which can be either neoadjuvant chemotherapy or neoadjuvant endocrine therapy. The patient may then be offered surgery to the breast and breast reconstruction, or surgery to the axilla, before being discussed at a multidisciplinary team meeting to explore the best course of treatment for receiving adjuvant therapy, which may include chemotherapy, radiotherapy, or biological therapy.

Regarding referral times, some of the UK nations have targets around how quickly patients with breast lumps will be seen. In England, an urgent referral means that patients should see a specialist within 2 weeks. In Northern Ireland, the 2-week wait only applies if the patient is referred for suspected breast cancer. This 2-week time limit does not exist in Scotland or in Wales (Cancer Research UK, 2019c).

Methods of assessment

History taking

Prior to a clinical assessment, a detailed history should be obtained from the patient (Bickley, 2016). This not only gives the clinician the information required to help make a diagnosis and assess the risk factors for developing breast cancer, but also helps to relax the patient.

The details obtained should include:

- patient's age
- past medical history
- family history of breast cancer
- age at menarche
- age at menopause
- date of last menstrual period (LMP)
- use of hormone replacement therapy
- use of the combined contraceptive pill

- number of pregnancies
- age at first pregnancy
- whether she breastfed her babies.

It is also very important to note the woman's presenting symptom, noting the duration of the symptom and whether it is cyclical in nature.

Clinical examination

The environment in which the patient is examined is very important. A gown should be provided to ensure the patient's dignity and the door should be locked to ensure privacy. Regardless of gender, a chaperone must be considered to be present to protect the patient's privacy and dignity (NMC, 2018).

The clinical examination is divided into two parts:

- palpation
- inspection.

The nurse may be required to assist the patient before, during and after examination takes place. The aim is to ensure comfort and offer physical and psychological support.

Palpation

The woman is first examined lying supine on the couch, with her arms above her head. This flattens out the breast tissue, so it is easier to palpate (feel). The examiner, having washed and warmed their hands, uses the flats of the fingers to palpate the whole of the breast tissue with a steady, medium-to-light pressure. This can be done in a variety of different ways: for example, using one hand or both hands; the examiner must find the most suitable method for them. Any lesion found is then examined with the fingertips to assess mobility and fixation. It is important to examine both breasts for comparison. The breast is also palpated when the patient is in the sitting position.

The axillary nodes are then examined either lying down or sitting up, depending on the examiner's preference. The patient's arm is supported to relax the muscles. Nodes are easily missed in a fatty axilla (Bickley, 2016).

According to Görkem and O'Connell (2012), normal and abnormal axillary lymph nodes are commonly seen on mediolateral oblique (MLO) mammograms. Normal axillary lymph nodes are frequently identified and are typically small and oval with a lucent centre due to hilar fat. Abnormal lymph nodes are characterized by high density, absence of hilar fat, and a round, irregular, ill-defined shape with or without intranodal calcifications on the MLO view.

When the patient is sitting up, the supraclavicular area is examined for any enlarged supraclavicular nodes. The hands are then swept down both sides of the chest towards the breasts to assess for any enlarged inframammary nodes.

The Nursing and Midwifery Council (NMC) (2018) advise that registered nurses and nurse associates must work within their scope of practice, identifying their limitations and referring to the wider multidisciplinary team, and work interprofessionally for best patient outcomes. With the advances in continuous professional development, advanced practice, and nurse specialist roles, breast palpation may belong within the nurse's remit, however if it does not the nurse must refer to an appropriate clinical expert.

Inspection

The breasts are inspected with the patient in three positions:

- hands relaxed by the side
- hands in the air
- hands on the hips.

The different positions are important, as changes are sometimes noticed in only one of the positions. Putting the hands on the hips contracts the pectoralis major muscle behind the breast. When this is done, a dimple in the breast may be noted, which has previously not been seen in the relaxed position with the hands by the side.

The size and contour of the breasts are noted, and the breasts are inspected for any skin changes, such as skin dimpling, increased vascularity and skin lesions. The nipple is inspected for any eczematous changes, discharge, crusting and recent inversion. However, some patients will have always had inverted nipples, and this is normal for them. Also, in older people, nipple inversion can be due to hypertrophy of the ducts, but this should be investigated to exclude malignancy.

Breast awareness and breast screening

The nurse plays a role in advising patients about breast awareness. There is a breast awareness five-point code:

- Know what is normal for you.
- Know what to look and feel for.
- Look and feel.
- Report any changes to your GP without delay.
- Attend for routine breast screening if you are aged 50 or over.

Breast cancer screening is currently offered to women from age 50 to their 71st birthday in England. But currently there is a trial to examine the effectiveness of offering some women one extra screen between the ages of 47 and 49 and one between the ages of 71 and 73. Patients will initially be invited for screening within 3 years of their 50th birthday, although in some areas they'll be invited from the age of 47 as part of the age extension trial. Patients may be eligible for breast screening before the age of 50 if they have a very high risk of developing breast cancer (NHS, 2019b).

Investigations

A woman may undergo one or several of the following investigations, depending on her age.

Mammography

A mammogram is a low-dose X-ray of the breast tissue. With modern techniques a dose of less than 1 mGy is used.

A full explanation should be given to the woman prior to the procedure. To obtain the mammogram, the breast must be compressed between two plates while the exposure is made, which may be uncomfortable. Two views are normally obtained. The oblique view is taken across the breast lengthways, and the craniocaudal is looking at the breast from head to toe.

In women under 35 years old, the breast is relatively radiodense, so a mammogram is rarely indicated in women in this age group. If a woman over 35 years old has a palpable lump, a mammogram may be performed.

Ultrasound

Ultrasound is a painless technique which uses high-frequency sound waves. The reflections are detected and turned into an image. A conductive jelly is placed on the breast, and a probe is used to scan the breast. Ultrasound is used if there is a palpable lump in a woman under the age of 35 years. It is also used as an aid to mammography, as it can differentiate between a cystic and a solid lesion.

Other radiological imaging

Magnetic resonance imaging (MRI) scans and scintimammography are other radiological imaging procedures that can be used in addition to mammography. These are not routine investigations and are usually advised by the consultant radiologist.

Fine-needle aspiration

This test is performed in the outpatient department. If there is a palpable lump, the clinician can perform a fine-needle aspiration (FNA). A full explanation is given to the patient prior to the test. The skin is cleaned and a fine needle (21 G or 23 G) attached to a 10-mL syringe is introduced into the skin. Suction is applied by withdrawing the plunger of the syringe. Several passes are made into the lump in different directions, to ensure a good sample is obtained from the lump. The plunger is then released, and the needle is withdrawn. The material is then spread thinly onto slides and left to air dry or is fixed with an alcohol fixative (depending on the cytologist's preference). The cytologist then examines the slides under the microscope and a cytological diagnosis can be made (ACS, 2014).

Results are usually given a numerical scoring (Table 21.1). The advantage of FNA is that, if a cancer is diagnosed, the patient and their family know prior to surgery what they are dealing with and can make an informed choice.

Core biopsy

If the cytology from the fine-needle aspiration is not conclusive, or if a histological diagnosis is required, a core biopsy can be taken.

This procedure can be performed in the outpatient department. A full explanation should be given to the patient prior to the procedure. If a biopsy gun is used, the patient should hear the sound made, as it can cause her to jump if she is not prepared. Local anaesthetic is injected into the breast, and once this has taken effect a small puncture is made by a scalpel blade over the site of the lump. The trocar is inserted through the puncture until the tip touches the tumour, and the central trocar is advanced into the mass. A core of tissue is obtained, inserted into a pot of formalin and sent to the histology department.

Pressure should be applied to the breast to help to prevent bruising, and a pressure dressing should be applied. Extra caution should be taken with patients taking warfarin – their INR (international normalized ratio) needs to be checked prior to the procedure and extra pressure exerted afterwards.

Staging investigations

If a breast cancer is diagnosed, the woman will need to have further investigations to assess if there has been any metastatic spread. These tests are usually performed as an outpatient at the time of diagnosis, and the appropriate treatment can then be planned. The following blood tests are usually performed:

- full blood count (FBC)
- erythrocyte sedimentation rate (ESR)/C-reactive protein/plasma viscosity
- urea and electrolytes (U&Es)
- albumin
- bilirubin
- alanine aminotransferase
- alkaline phosphatase
- gamma-glutamyl transferase
- calcium
- phosphate.

Although ESR is still used in some countries around the world as it is inexpensive and simple to perform, the disadvantage is that it is affected by a variety of factors, including anaemia and red blood cell size, not sensitive to screen. Most Western countries tend to use C-reactive protein as it is the most rapid response to inflammation (complementary to ESR in this regard). There are some disadvantages – the wide reference range may necessitate sequential recording of values, expensive batch processing may delay individual results. Finally, plasma viscosity may be used, the advantage being that it is unaffected by anaemia or red blood cell size; however, this test is expensive, not widely available, and technically cumbersome to perform.

If any of the above tests are abnormal, the following investigations can be arranged, if appropriate:

- *Bone scan*: the procedure involves an intravenous injection of a harmless radioactive isotope, and then, approximately 3 hours later, an X-ray of the whole body is taken. The films are examined by a consultant radiologist to assess for any metastatic spread to the bones.

Table 21.1 Cytology grading

Cytology grade	Meaning
C1	Sample inadequate for testing
C2	Normal breast cells
C3	Cells abnormal but more likely to be benign
C4	Highly suspicious of cancer
C5	Cancer cells present

In 1996, the National Cancer Institute (NCI) proposed five categories for the diagnosis of breast cytology in order to bring a degree of uniformity to the diagnostic reporting (Arul et al., 2016).
The accuracy of fine-needle biopsy depends upon the breast specialist obtaining a sample from the lump, and upon the cytologist accurately grading the cells under the microscope. If the test is positive (i.e. grade C5), then it is almost certain (99.5%) that the lump is a cancer. However, a negative test (i.e. grade C2) does not exclude the possibility of cancer but merely makes the diagnosis of cancer less likely. If the needle biopsy result is graded C1, it usually implies the sample was inadequate for analysis and the test should be repeated (Arul et al., 2016).
Source: National Cancer Institute (2013).

- *Liver ultrasound*: this uses the same technique as with the breast ultrasound, but is used to assess if there has been any metastatic spread to the liver.
- *Chest X-ray*: this is performed to assess for any lung disease.
- If there are any neurological symptoms suggestive of metastatic brain disease, a computerized tomography (CT) scan can also be arranged.

Breast surgery

Breast surgery is performed for both benign and malignant breast disease. The two areas will be looked at separately.

Breast surgery for benign breast disease

Not all benign breast conditions will require surgery: e.g. cysts can be aspirated in the outpatient department. Each breast unit will have its own local policy, so variations may be found.

Ambulatory surgery

Ambulatory (outpatient) care has come on leaps and bounds over the past 25 years. NHS Improvement (2011) recognized that the vast majority of operations for breast cancer (excluding operations for breast construction) can be safely undertaken as a day case procedure or with a single overnight stay. NHS Improvement has been working with clinical teams across England to transform the way in which breast surgery is delivered. This work has been supported by the British Association of Day Surgery, the Association of Breast Surgery and by patients. All the partners have recognized that the transformation is good for patients and good for the NHS. Patients do not need to be admitted to hospital the night before surgery. Equally they want to return to normal life as quickly as possible. The original hypothesis underlying this work was that streamlining could reduce length of stay by 50% and release 25% of unnecessary bed days for 80% of major breast surgery (excluding reconstruction). This goal has been exceeded. Mean length of stay has reduced from 2.35 days to 1.35 days overall. The number of patients with length of stay greater than 1 day has been reduced markedly. Overall bed days have been reduced by more than 40%.

An example of global changes to ambulatory breast care can be seen in Pek et al's 2016 work conducted in Singapore. The study by Pek et al (2016) recognized that ambulatory breast cancer surgery is well accepted and is the standard of care at many tertiary centers. Rather than being hospitalized after surgery, patients are discharged on the day of surgery or within 23 hours. Such early discharge does not adversely affect patient outcomes and has the added benefits of better psychological adjustment for the patient, economic savings, and a more efficient utilization of healthcare resources. The minimal care needed post-discharge also means that the caregiver is not unduly burdened. Unplanned conversions to inpatient admission and readmission rates are low. Wound complications are infrequent and no issues with drain care have been reported. Because the period of postoperative observation is short and monitoring is not as intensive, ambulatory surgery is only suitable for low-risk procedures such as breast cancer surgery and in patients without serious comorbidities, where the likelihood of major perioperative events is low. Optimal management of pain, nausea, and vomiting is essential to ensure a quick recovery and return to normal function. Regional anesthesia such as the thoracic paravertebral block has been employed to improve pain control during the surgery and in the immediate postoperative period. The block provides excellent pain relief and reduces the need for opiates, which also consequently reduces the incidence of nausea and vomiting. The increasing popularity of total intravenous anesthesia with propofol has also helped reduce the incidence of nausea and vomiting in the postoperative period. Ambulatory surgery can be safely carried out in centers where there is a well-designed workflow to ensure proper patient selection, counselling, and education, and where patients and caregivers have easy access to medical services should problems arise after discharge.

The informational needs for women with benign breast disease can be met by information leaflets produced by Breast Cancer Now (see Resources section and Breast Cancer Care (2019)).

The following surgical procedures may be performed for benign breast conditions.

Removal of a benign breast lump

The most common breast lump to be surgically removed is a fibroadenoma, which is a benign fibrous lump. These are solid growths of tissue. They are the most common type of benign breast lump and patients are most likely to get one between the ages of 16 and 24. They do not usually hurt and can sometimes move slightly underneath patients' fingers when they check their breast (BUPA, 2019).

Presentation

Fibroadenomas usually present as a palpable lump, although some may be impalpable and are only detected on mammographic screening. They tend to be smooth, well-circumscribed, firm and mobile lumps. According to Breast Cancer Care (2019a), it's not unusual to have more than one fibroadenoma. They often develop during puberty so are mostly found in young women, but they can occur in women of any age. Men can also get fibroadenomas, but this is very rare. Fibroadenomas are usually painless, but sometimes they may feel tender or even painful, particularly just before a period. Most fibroadenomas are about 1–3 cm in size and are called simple fibroadenomas. When looked at under a microscope, simple fibroadenomas will look the same all over. They do not increase the risk of developing breast cancer in the future. Some fibroadenomas are called complex fibroadenomas. When these are looked at under a microscope, some of the cells have different features. Having a complex fibroadenoma can very slightly increase the risk of developing breast cancer in the future. Occasionally, a fibroadenoma can grow to more than 5 cm and may be called a giant fibroadenoma. Those found in teenage girls may be called juvenile fibroadenomas.

Management

Policies for removal of a fibroadenoma may vary between units. In general, the following policy applies:

- *Observation*: if the clinical examination, ultrasound and fine-needle aspiration (known as the triple assessment) confirm this lump to be a benign fibroadenoma and the woman is under the age of 35 years old, the lump can be left *in situ* and reassessed with clinical examination and repeat FNA in 6–8 weeks' time. Most women, if given the choice, will opt to leave the lump *in situ* as opposed to having surgery resulting in a scar.
- *Excision*: if the fibroadenoma measures over 4 cm, if there is any clinical suspicion, if the woman is over 35 years of age or if the woman wishes to have the lump removed, then excision is advised.

The reason why women over the age of 35 years old are advised to have the fibroadenoma removed is that the risk of breast cancer increases with age.

Surgical treatment

Most fibroadenomas are removed as a day case, if the woman meets the criteria set out for day surgery. A small incision is made over the site of the palpable lump, and the fibroadenoma is shelled out. The wound is then sutured, usually with a subcutaneous dissolvable suture to give the best cosmetic appearance possible. If the lump is near the areola, a subareolar incision is made, which gives a very good cosmetic result.

Specific nursing care

The general nursing care is the same as that for any patient undergoing surgery. Advice should be given regarding wound care, pain control, bathing and so forth. The patient should be advised to wear a supportive non-wired bra, to give support to the breast, so preventing pulling on the scar.

She should be provided with information that meets her specific needs and given a contact number to all should she experience any problems.

An outpatient appointment should be made for 7–10 days postoperatively, for the wound to be checked and for the histology result and local policy must be adhered to. If the histology is benign, it should be clearly explained to the woman that it is not a cancer and that it does not increase the risk of breast cancer.

The same management and nursing care as described above applies to patients having the following:
- lipoma (fatty lump)
- discrete nodularity (thickening of the breast tissue).

Excision of fat necrosis

Fat necrosis is usually caused by trauma to the breast, which causes fat cells to burst open. The body does not recognize these altered fat cells, and so reacts to them as if they were a foreign body. Intense scarring occurs, which feels like a firm irregular lump. The scar tissue then contracts, pulling on the Cooper's ligament, causing skin dimpling. Thus, it mimics a cancer (Akkas & Vural, 2013).

Management

A careful history needs to be taken with special regards to trauma. A mammogram and fine-needle aspiration should have been performed in the outpatient department. If there is still bruising present on the breast, it may be appropriate to reassess the woman in a few months' time. If there is any suspicion, excision is advisable.

Surgical treatment

Surgical treatment is as for removal of a benign breast lump.

Specific nursing care

Specific nursing care is as for removal of a benign breast lump.

Microdochectomy

A microdochectomy (excision of a duct) is performed to excise an intraduct papilloma. Duct papillomas are 'warty'-like growths within a duct. They can either be single or multiple. Currently there is no supporting evidence to suggest that there is any malignancy potential. Microdochectomies are also performed to investigate a bloodstained discharge and to cure a chronic serous discharge.

Presentation

The most common symptom is a spontaneous serous or bloodstained nipple discharge, usually from a single duct.

Management

A mammogram will have been performed in the outpatient department if the woman is over 35 years old, and slides from the discharge will have been taken to send for cytology assessment.

Surgical treatment

A microdochectomy is performed using a small subareolar incision. The duct containing the papilloma is isolated and removed. The wound is then sutured with either a subcutaneous dissolvable suture or an interrupted Prolene suture. This can be performed as a day case, providing the woman meets the day surgery criteria.

Specific nursing care

Specific nursing care is as for removal of a benign lump.

Incision and drainage of a breast abscess

Breast abscesses can occur in the non-lactational or lactational breast.

Non-lactational abscess

These abscesses can occur either in the periareolar region or peripherally. There are several causative factors:

- duct ectasia (a benign condition within the duct, commonly linked with smoking)
- diabetes mellitus
- steroid treatment
- trauma
- infected sebaceous cyst (Dixon & Khan, 2011; Dixon, 2013).

Lactational abscess

The incidence of puerperal mastitis and lactational breast abscesses has reduced in recent years due to improvement in maternal and infant hygiene, a change in feeding patterns and the introduction of early treatment with antibiotics (Dixon & Khan, 2011; Dixon, 2013). The organism most commonly responsible is *Staphylococcus aureus* or *Staphylococcus epidermidis*. Infection starts usually via a break in the skin, e.g. cracked nipple, and then enters via the nipple.

Presentation

The most common time for presentation is within the first month after giving birth. The woman presents with a red, swollen, hot and painful breast. In the later stages there may be a fluctuant mass. The woman may feel unwell, with a pyrexia and tachycardia.

Management

Most breast abscesses can be managed conservatively, but some will still require incision and drainage.

Conservative management. Antibiotics, if given in time, can prevent abscess formation. If there is a fluctuant mass, a fine-needle aspiration can be performed to aspirate some pus, which can be sent for microscopy, culture and sensitivity (M, C and S), and antibiotic treatment is continued. The woman is encouraged to continue breastfeeding from both breasts, as this helps to promote drainage.

Surgical treatment. Occasionally, incision and drainage are necessary if the breast abscess is not resolving with the use of antibiotics. This is usually done under a light general anaesthetic. It is now more common practice for women to be allowed to continue breastfeeding provided that the incision is away from the baby's mouth. Feeding can continue as normal from the unaffected side (NICE, 2018b). Because milk stasis is often the initiating factor in lactational mastitis, the most important management step is frequent and effective milk removal. Sudden cessation of breastfeeding in women with lactational mastitis increases the risk of abscess formation. Additionally, it is also advised by NICE that the infant may continue to feed from the affected breast as several studies have shown that this is generally safe, even in the presence of *Staphylococcus aureus* infection (NICE, 2018b).

Specific nursing care

Postoperatively, the wound will be left open and a daily dressing will be required to lightly fill the cavity to promote healing; local policy and procedure will prevail. The patient should be offered advice and support and appropriate information should be provided (NMC, 2018), and analgesia prescribed to manage pain as well as the provision and utilization of a support bra. Antibiotic therapy should be prescribed only if necessary and advice should be provided to the patient on how to take them properly (NHS, 2019a; NMC, 2018). Adequate pain control should be given, and a supportive bra should be worn.

The woman will require the use of a single room, as the baby will usually accompany her. This reduces the risk of hospital-acquired infection for the baby, gives the mother privacy and causes less disturbance to the other patients.

Psychological support may be necessary, as this can be a difficult and emotional time. Practical support with baby care may be necessary if there is no family support, and referral to a health visitor or social worker may be appropriate.

Breast cancer

Breast cancer is the most common form of cancer among women (Box 21.1).

The latest statistics provided by Cancer Research in 2015 identify that there are 55,122 new cases of invasive breast

Box 21.1 **Breast carcinoma incidence**

- There are around 7700 new breast carcinoma *in situ* cases in the UK every year, that's 21 every day (2013–2015).
- In males in the UK, there were around 30 new cases of breast carcinoma *in situ* in 2015.
- In females in the UK, there were around 7900 new cases of breast carcinoma *in situ* in 2015.
- Incidence rates for breast carcinoma *in situ* in the UK are highest in people aged 65 to 69 (2013–2015).
- Since the early 1990s, breast carcinoma *in situ* incidence rates have almost tripled (186%) in the UK. Rates in males have increased by four-fifths (80%), and rates in females have increased by almost three times (187%).
- Over the last decade, breast carcinoma *in situ* incidence rates have increased by almost half (46%) in the UK. Rates in males have remained stable, and rates in females have increased by almost half (47%).
- Most *in situ* breast carcinomas are intraductal.
- *In situ* breast carcinoma is more common in White females than in Asian or Black females.
- An estimated 63,800 women who had previously been diagnosed with *in situ* breast carcinoma were alive in the UK at the end of 2010.

Source: Cancer Research UK (2019a).

cancer within the UK (Cancer Research UK, 2019a). In 2016 in the UK, breast cancer was responsible for 11,563 deaths (Cancer Research UK, 2019a). However, according to the latest statistics available, 78% of patients survive breast cancer for 10 or more years (females only), between 2010 and 2011, in England and Wales (Cancer Research UK, 2019a). According to Cancer Research UK (2019a), 23% of breast cancer cases are preventable.

Breast cancer affects women and men and can also affect those who have undergone a gender reassignment or who are non-binary. NICE guidelines (NICE, 2018a) have used the term 'women' for recommendations that usually only relate to women (such as breast-conserving surgery) and 'people' in all other cases. However, no discrimination is intended, and recommendations relate to all those who have early or locally advanced breast cancer (NICE, 2018a).

Types of breast cancer

There are several types of breast cancer:
- invasive ductal
- invasive lobular
- ductal carcinoma *in situ* (DCIS)
- lobular carcinoma *in situ* (LCIS)
- Paget's disease of the nipple
- Other rare forms (Macmillan Cancer Support, 2019).

Invasive ductal carcinoma

This is the most common type of breast cancer, usually presenting as a palpable lump. It originates from the epithelial cells lining the ducts within the breast. It breaks out of the duct and into the surrounding breast tissue. As the cancer grows, it can invert the nipple, cause skin dimpling and, in the advanced stage, cause peau d'orange,

where the skin looks like the skin of an orange, eventually leading to ulceration and possible fungation. It has the potential to metastasize. If detected early, the prognosis is improved.

Invasive lobular carcinoma

Invasive lobular carcinoma cancer originates from the lobules of the breast, and behaves the same way as ductal carcinomas, but has the tendency to be bilateral and multifocal.

Ductal carcinoma *in situ* and lobular carcinoma *in situ*

These cancers are pre-invasive conditions. The cancer cells are contained within the ducts or the lobules and have not broken out into the surrounding breast tissue. They do not have the ability to metastasize. They usually do not present as lumps but are picked up on mammographic screening, by the appearance of a cluster of microcalcifications.

Paget's disease of the nipple

This condition presents as an eczema-type rash on the nipple and areolar complex, which progresses to ulceration. Itching, tingling, burning and bleeding are common accompanying symptoms. If there is any doubt, a biopsy should be performed. On histology, malignant Paget cells are found in the epidermis.

Other rare forms

Cancers arising from connective tissue can also be found in the breast. These are known as sarcomas. The breast can also be a site for secondary carcinomas, e.g. malignant melanomas, although this is rare.

Staging

It is known that the smaller and the less advanced the tumour is at the time of diagnosis, the better the prognosis. There are many different systems of staging breast cancer, and each breast unit will adopt the most appropriate system for their practice. One simple system involves dividing breast cancer into four stages (Table 21.2).

Metastatic spread

Cells from the breast cancer can spread via the blood-stream and lymphatic system to other organs in the body. The most common sites for breast cancer metastases are in the axillary, supraclavicular and inframammary nodes, the liver, bones, lungs and brain.

Surgery for breast cancer

There are several types of surgery used in the treatment of breast cancer, which will be discussed below. This is often accompanied by axillary surgery, which will be discussed as a separate issue.

The type of surgery performed depends on:
- patient choice
- size of the tumour in comparison to the size of the breast
- location of the tumour
- age of the patient.

There is no high-quality evidence available at this time to support the timing of breast cancer surgery in relation to the menstrual period.

The different types of surgery will now be discussed.

Breast-conserving surgery (BCS) (wide local excision), also referred to as lumpectomy

Breast-conserving surgery (BCS) is an operation to remove the cancer while leaving as much normal breast as possible (ACS, 2019). Some surrounding healthy tissue and lymph nodes are usually also removed. How much of the breast is removed depends on the size and location of the tumor and other factors. Breast-conserving surgery is sometimes called lumpectomy, quadrantectomy, partial mastectomy, or segmental mastectomy. It is often an option for a woman with early-stage cancer and allows her to keep most of her breast. If the tumour is large, a quadrantectomy may have to be performed, which involves removal of a whole quadrant of the breast. This may involve a significant loss of breast tissue, causing an alteration in breast shape. A Redivac drain is inserted into the cavity to prevent a fluid collection.

Needle-localization biopsy

This surgery is performed when there is an abnormality on the mammogram, such as a cluster of microcalcifications, which cannot be felt. To ensure the surgeon removes the correct area, a fine wire must be inserted into the abnormal area in the breast. On admission, the woman goes to the X-oray department, where she is given a local anaesthetic. Under mammographic control, a fine wire is inserted into the abnormal area. There is a small hook on the end of the wire to prevent it moving. The wire is then taped securely to the breast. At the time of surgery, the surgeon makes an incision and follows the wire down to the tip and excises an area of tissue around it. The specimen is then X-rayed while the woman is still asleep, to ensure the mammographic abnormality has been completely removed (Cancer Research UK, 2019b).

Table 21.2 Staging of breast cancers

Stage	Explanation
0	Indicates that the cancer is where it started (*in situ*) and has not spread
I	The cancer is small and has not spread anywhere else
II	The cancer has grown, but has not spread
III	The cancer is larger and may have spread to the surrounding tissues and/or the lymph nodes (part of the lymphatic system)
IV	The cancer has spread from where it started to at least one other body organ; also known as 'secondary' or 'metastatic' cancer

Different types of staging systems are used for different types of cancer. This is an example of one common method of staging.
Source: NHS (2018).

Mastectomy

Mastectomy is usually performed if the lump is too big to be able to conserve the breast, if the disease is multifocal, or if this is a recurrent breast cancer in the same breast. Some patients will also choose mastectomy, as opposed to breast-conserving surgery, for a variety of reasons, e.g. fear of local recurrence.

There are several types of mastectomy (Table 21.3). The decision regarding the type of mastectomy is usually dependent on the extent of the disease and the position of the cancer. Fig. 21.1 shows a mastectomy scar.

Breast reconstruction

Following a mastectomy, breast reconstruction can be performed either at the time of surgery or at a later date. There are several types of breast reconstruction:

- silicone implants
- tissue expander
- myocutaneous flaps
- nipple reconstruction.

The type of reconstruction depends on the patient's choice, patient's general health, breast size, type of mastectomy performed, condition of the skin on the chest wall, condition of the muscle and the perceived need for radiotherapy.

Silicone implant

This procedure involves insertion of a silicone implant under the pectoralis muscle at the time of mastectomy. This method is only suitable for small-breasted women and is not suitable if a radical mastectomy has been performed or if radiotherapy has been given to the breast in the past.

In the 1990s there was much debate regarding the safety of silicone and the possible harmful effects it may have on the body in the long term. In 1992, the US Food and Drug Administration (FDA) suspended the sale of silicone implants pending investigation. The Department of Health set up an Independent Review Group (IRG, 1998) to review the safety of silicone, and it has found them to be safe. Over the past 10 years more than 30,000 women in France, and thousands of others in countries including Spain and the UK, had breast augmentation with what have turned out to be potentially defective implants in what is now described as a cosmetic surgery horror story. The scandal has sent panic through France's vast plastic surgery industry (Chrisafis, 2011). The company Poly Implant Prosthesis (PIP), based in the south of France, was one of the world's leaders in silicone implant production until last year when it was found to have been cutting corners and saving an estimated £840 m a year by using industrial silicone instead of medical-grade fillers in their breast implants. The casing around the filling was also faulty and prone to rupture or leakage. The company has closed and more than 2000 women have filed legal complaints. A judicial investigation has begun for involuntary homicide over a woman who died from cancer.

Tissue expander

This procedure involves the insertion of a silicone sac under the pectoralis muscle. A commonly used tissue expander is the Becker tissue expander. The sac has a port and valve attached. Saline is injected into the sac via the valve at the time of surgery. Postoperatively, the woman attends the outpatient department to have more saline inserted on a weekly or fortnightly basis to achieve the required size.

The expander has a port (a metal or plastic plug, valve, or coil) that allows the surgeon to add increasing amounts of liquid (a salt-water solution) over time (between 2 and 6 months) until the skin gradually is stretched enough to accommodate the implant (Breastcancer.org, 2019a). Once the required size is achieved, more fluid is inserted. This overexpansion is done for two purposes. First, when the port and valve are removed, some saline is removed at the same time, to match the breast size and to obtain the natural droop of the breast. Secondly, the stretching of the tissues is thought to decrease the incidence of capsule formation.

Table 21.3 Types of mastectomy

Type of mastectomy	Explanation
Total mastectomy	Removal of the breast tissue with some of the overlying skin, including the nipple
Subcutaneous mastectomy	Removal of the breast tissue, keeping the nipple
Radical mastectomy	Removal of the breast tissue, including the pectoralis muscle and axillary contents
Modified radical mastectomy	Removal of the breast tissue, leaving the pectoralis major muscle intact but dividing the pectoralis muscle, so allowing the axilla to be cleared
Salvage mastectomy	Removal of the breast tissue for an ulcerating or fungating lesion in advanced breast cancer, with the aim of improving the quality of life and the relief of distressing symptoms

429

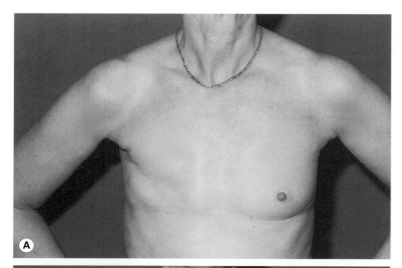

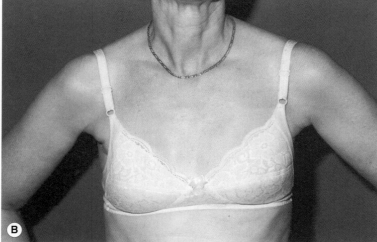

Figure 21.1 (A) A mastectomy scar. (B) Same woman wearing bra with prosthesis.

There are now novel techniques of breast reconstruction using inflation of breast expanders with air (Green et al, 2018). The port and valve can be removed as a day case.

This method of breast reconstruction is used when the skin is of good quality. It is not suitable following a radical mastectomy unless a myocutaneous flap is used. It is not usually advisable following radiotherapy, as the skin and muscle can be fibrosed.

Myocutaneous flaps

This procedure is used to reconstruct the breast when the skin is damaged by radiotherapy or the breast is large. This technique involves taking a flap of skin and muscle, still attached to its blood supply, from another part of the body to reconstruct the breast. An implant can be inserted underneath this flap, if required, but if the breast is small the flap alone may be sufficient to form a breast mound.

There are two types of myocutaneous flaps used in breast reconstruction: the latissimus dorsi flap (LD flap) and the transverse rectus abdominis myocutaneous flap (TRAM flap).

Latissimus dorsi flap. This procedure involves dissecting the latissimus dorsi muscle from the back, keeping it attached to its own blood supply, rotating it on a pedicle and tunnelling it under the skin of the axilla to cover the deficit from the mastectomy site. The donor site can be taken horizontally so the scar can be hidden by a bra strap, or vertically (BreastCancer.org, 2019c), this is the most commonly used myocutaneous flap.

Transverse rectus abdominis myocutaneous flap. This procedure involves dissecting the rectus abdominis muscle, which runs from the pubis to the costal cartilages of the fifth, sixth and seventh ribs. Again, it is kept attached to its own blood supply and tunnelled under the skin to cover the deficit. The abdominal scar is transverse and so is well hidden, and a mesh is inserted to prevent herniation. It has the added benefit of giving a 'tummy tuck' at the same time.

Despite the advantages of this flap in being able to take a large area of tissue and the reduced need of an additional implant, it is not as popular as the latissimus dorsi flap. This is because a longer stay in hospital is required and it has a lower success rate.

While it is the most popular flap reconstruction procedure, according to Breastcancer.org (2019b) the TRAM flap is not for everyone. It is not a good choice for:
- thin patients who do not have enough extra abdominal tissue
- patients who already have had multiple abdominal surgeries
- patients who plan on getting pregnant
- patients who are concerned about losing strength in their lower abdomen
- patients with cardiac failure or vascular disease that has impact on microcirculation and wound perfusion and recovery.

It must also be remembered that if the woman has stretch marks on her abdomen, these will then be visible on her reconstructed breast.

Nipple reconstruction

There are several techniques that can be used to reconstruct the nipple. This is usually performed several months following the initial reconstruction.

The most common method is to use the skin and fat from the reconstructed breast to form the nipple, and a skin graft is taken from the inner thigh to form the areola. The graft can be tattooed to obtain the correct colour if necessary.

There is the potential risk of the graft failing and becoming necrotic. This risk should be explained to the woman prior to surgery. Other techniques have been developed where the areolar complex is tattooed onto the reconstruction and a nipple bud is created from this skin. Further tattooing may be necessary to reshape the areola.

Many women will not opt for nipple reconstruction, preferring to use an adhesive silicone nipple instead when wearing tight-fitting clothes.

See Chapter 24 for specific nursing care regarding reconstructive surgery.

Management of the axilla

Axillary surgery is undertaken for two main reasons:

- for staging and prognostic information, so that adjuvant therapy can be planned — if any of the glands are positive, then adjuvant chemotherapy may be required
- for local control.

If axillary surgery is not performed, radiotherapy may be given to the axilla.

Several complications can arise from axillary surgery or radiotherapy. The possible complications include seromas (fluid collection), reduced arm movement, nerve damage and lymphoedema, the most significant being the development of lymphoedema (Breast Cancer Care, 2019b).

For many years, axillary node clearance was conventional management for early-stage breast cancer. However, during the last few years there has been the development of the sentinel lymph node biopsy (SLNB), which is less invasive and so potentially reduces the morbidity associated with axillary dissection.

Sentinel lymph node biopsy

The sentinel lymph node is defined as the first lymph node into which the primary tumour drains. It is the most likely node to contain metastatic tumour. If the sentinel node is not involved with metastatic disease, the remainder of the lymph nodes should also be negative.

An injection of a blue dye and/or a radioisotope is given several hours before surgery. The theory is that, once injected, the dye and radioactive material will be drawn through the breast to the lymph nodes. The first node it reaches — i.e. the sentinel node — has a blue appearance. The surgeon excises this node and sends it to pathology for a frozen section (microscopical analysis of the node). If this node is positive, the surgeon will proceed with an axillary dissection; if it is negative, no further surgery to the axilla will be required.

Axillary node dissection

A separate incision is made in the axilla to remove the nodes (LII–III) and a single suction drain is inserted to prevent a fluid collection. The drain will need to stay in place until the drainage is less than 50 mL over 24 hours (this takes approximately 5–6 days).

Adjuvant treatments

Adjuvant treatment is decided upon once the histology report is available and will depend on:
- patient choice
- the size and grade of the tumour
- the nodal status
- age and menopausal status
- excision margins
- previous treatment
- oestrogen receptor (ER) status

- HER2 status.

The adjuvant treatments to prevent local and distal disease may include all or a combination of the following.

Radiotherapy

This is a high-dose X-ray treatment which destroys any residual cancer cells that might be remaining in the breast tissue or chest wall. It is a localized treatment which is given to help prevent local recurrence. It is most commonly given following breast-conserving surgery, but is occasionally given to the chest wall following mastectomy. It is commenced once the wound has healed and full arm movement has been achieved; this is usually 4–6 weeks postoperatively.

Chemotherapy

This simply means 'treatment with drugs'. It is a systemic treatment, so, unlike radiotherapy, it treats the whole of the body. A combination of different cytotoxic drugs is used, which kills cells that are dividing rapidly.

Endocrine therapy

Tamoxifen

This is a common and very successful endocrine therapy which has been used for many years. It is anti-oestrogenic as it competes with oestrogen to lock on to the oestrogen receptor site, preventing growth stimulation. Benefits are greatest in women with tumours that are sensitive to oestrogen. It is used in pre- and postmenopausal women. NICE (2018a) advise tamoxifen as the initial adjuvant endocrine therapy for men and premenopausal women with ER-positive invasive breast cancer. They recommend that an aromatase inhibitor is offered as the initial adjuvant endocrine therapy for postmenopausal women with ER-positive invasive breast cancer who are at medium or high risk of disease recurrence. Offer tamoxifen to women who are at low risk of disease recurrence, or if aromatase inhibitors are not tolerated or are contraindicated.

Aromatase inhibitors

Once the menopause has passed, the majority of naturally circulating oestrogen has gone. However, oestrogen is still produced, mainly from fat, under the control of the adrenal gland. The enzyme aromatase converts the androgen androstenedione in the fat into oestrogen. There are three commonly used aromatase inhibitors (AIs) which are licensed for different use, and are only suitable for postmenopausal women:

- anastrazole (Arimidex) – used as a sole therapy or following 2–3 years of tamoxifen

- exemestane (Aromasin) – following 2–3 years of tamoxifen
- letrozole (Femara) – as extended treatment for 3 years following 5 years of tamoxifen.

Monoclonal antibodies

Trastuzumab (Herceptin)

Trastuzumab is a monoclonal antibody which utilizes the natural immune system to kill tumour cells. Some breast cancer cells grow and divide when a protein known as human epidermal growth factor attaches itself to another protein known as HER2. Approximately 20% of breast cancers overexpress HER2. Trastuzumab works by attaching itself to the HER2 protein, preventing the human epidermal growth factor from doing so. This stops the cells from dividing and growing.

It is given to patients who are HER2-positive following adjuvant chemotherapy. It is a 3-weekly infusion and is currently given for 1 year (NICE, 2018a).

Nursing care of a patient undergoing surgery for breast cancer

The general nursing care for patients undergoing breast surgery is the same as for any surgery, e.g. wound care, but there are specific issues that the nurse needs to be aware of in planning the nursing care. See Table 21.4 for a case study of a woman undergoing a mastectomy.

Preoperative information

Ideally, the woman should have been seen by a Breast Care Nurse at diagnosis, who will have explained what to expect, but if not, the nurse carin g for the women should be able to provide this information. Written information should also be provided.

The woman should be given an idea about the possible cosmetic outcome of the surgery. The use of a photo album to illustrate the outcomes of different operations may be of help, but it should be stressed that every person is an individual, so outcomes may differ.

If axillary surgery is planned, the woman should be warned that she may lose the sensation under her arm and along the underside of the upper arm. This can be quite an uncomfortable feeling. Sensation may return in a few months postoperatively, but it may never be fully regained. The woman should also be informed about the use of surgical drains postoperatively. Often, two Redivacs are inserted, one in the breast and one in the axilla, to prevent a haematoma or a seroma (fluid collection). These

Table 21.4 A nursing care plan for a patient undergoing surgery for breast cancer, using the Roper, Logan and Tierney model

Assessment/usual routine	Patients problem	Goal	Nursing action	Evaluation
Maintaining a safe environment				
Ann's skin is healthy and intact	Potential wound infection following surgery	To prevent infection	Use an aseptic technique when dealing with the dressing and caring for the Redivac drains Record temperature 4 hourly Take the dressing down after 24 hours Observe the wound for signs of infection and swelling	Ann remained apyrexial, and the wound healed well with no sign of infection
	Potential development of both seroma and haematoma formation	To minimize the risk of seroma and haematoma	Check drains for patency and measure the amount of drainage every (1/4) hour for the first hour and then, if satisfactory, hourly for 24 hours and thereafter twice daily Change bottle daily and record the output accurately every 24 hours Remove the drain on surgeon's instruction, usually when drainage is <50 mL in 24 hoursOffer oral analgesics prior to removal	The drain remained patent and the loss was within normal limits The bottle was changed daily and the amount recorded The drain was removed 6 days postoperatively
Communication				
Ann settled into the ward well and chatted to the other women She became tearful when talking about losing her breast	Anxiety and fear about losing her breast	For Ann to be able to talk about her breast loss without being tearful	Refer to the Breast Care Nurse Allow Ann to express her feelings Offer Ann the opportunity to see photographs of mastectomy scars Provide written information Explain what to expect postoperatively	Postoperatively, Ann was much less tearful and talked to other patients about her operation
Ann expressed concern about her two daughters developing breast cancer	Fear of her daughters developing breast cancer	To be able to put her fears into perspective and to feel something is being done for her daughters	Give advice on how her daughters can be referred to a family history clinic Provide information on breast awareness	Ann's daughters had both visited their GPs, who had referred them both to family history clinics. Ann felt more positive that something was being done
Mobilization				
Ann is a very active woman who usually does all the		To prevent a frozen shoulder	Refer to a physiotherapist for arm exercises	At discharge, Ann had a good range of movement in her arm *(Continued)*

Table 21.4 A nursing care plan for a patient undergoing surgery for breast cancer, using the Roper, Logan and Tierney model—cont'd

Assessment/usual routine	Patients problem	Goal	Nursing action	Evaluation
housework with little help from the family	Potential risk of a stiff shoulder due to axillary surgery		Encourage the use of the affected arm Encourage the family to help with the housework	and was encouraged to continue the exercises at home
	Potential risk of developing lymphoedema due to axillary surgery	To reduce the risk of developing lymphoedema	Give written information regarding arm care (see Box 21.2)	The written information reassured Ann and made her less anxious
	Pain due to surgery	To be pain-free, or reduce pain, to allow Ann to mobilize and be comfortable and to be able to perform her exercises	Administer regular analgesics orally once tolerating fluids Rest affected arm on a pillow when in bed or sitting in a chair	Ann mobilized well postoperatively and was able to perform her exercises twice a day Her pain was well controlled with regular co-dydramol
Work and play				
Ann works full time as a secretary for an accountancy firm. The firm is having some financial problems and there have been some redundancies	Ann is worried she may lose her job due to her sick leave and is considering early retirement	To return to work as soon as she is able	Encourage Ann to express her fears Refer to a social worker	The surgeon wrote a supportive letter to her boss, who in fact was very supportive and reassured Ann her job was safe
Ann attends a weekly water aerobics class	Ann is concerned the other women will stare at her	To encourage Ann to return to the class	Refer Ann to the Breast Care Nurse for advice regarding swimwear and prosthetics	As yet, Ann has not returned to the class but has bought a new swimming costume
Expressing sexuality				
Ann and her husband have been married for 24 years. They still enjoy a sexual relationship	Ann fears Paul will not want to touch her	To resume normal sexual relations	Encourage Paul to be involved with Ann's care Inform them of the availability of counselling	At her 6-week follow-up, Ann informed the Breast Care Nurse that Paul had been supportive and they had kissed and cuddled but had not had sexual intercourse Ann felt that this would come in time
	Fear of appearing different and people noticing her breast loss	To feel confident about her body image	Encourage Ann to look at and touch the scar and for Paul to be present Refer to the Breast Care Nurse for fitting of a temporary prosthesis Encourage Ann to wear her own clothes	Ann left the ward wearing the same clothes she wore on admission and felt confident An appointment had been made for fitting a permanent prosthesis

(Continued)

Table 21.4 A nursing care plan for a patient undergoing surgery for breast cancer, using the Roper, Logan and Tierney model—cont'd

Assessment/usual routine	Patients problem	Goal	Nursing action	Evaluation
			Advise Ann about voluntary organizations, e.g. Breast Cancer Now	
			Discuss the possibility of breast reconstruction	
Dying				
Devastated by the diagnosis of breast cancer, as she feels so well	Fear of dying	For Ann to have a realistic outlook	Allow Ann to express her fears and to correct any overly pessimistic views	Ann still has a fear of dying and leaving her family behind
			Explain more will be known once the histology result is available	Ann was referred to a counsellor, who is exploring this fear with her further
			Explain the follow-up procedure	
			Encourage Ann to plan for the future	
			Refer to a counsellor if appropriate	

are normally left *in situ* until the drainage is less than 50 mL in a 24-hour period.

A seroma may occur after the axillary drain is removed. The fluid that was previously drained away in the Redivac bottle may collect in the cavity, causing a swelling in the axilla. This causes some discomfort and the feeling of having an orange under the arm. It can be drained by inserting a needle into the area and drawing off the fluid. This should be performed by a doctor or the Breast Care Nurse, who has been trained to drain seromas. The woman should be warned that this may reoccur, so that she is not alarmed.

Potential risk of lymphoedema

Lymphoedema is a chronic and progressive disorder resulting from impaired lymphatic system function. In developed countries, upper extremity lymphoedema is mainly the consequence of breast cancer surgery in which axillary lymph node dissection and radiation alter upper extremity lymphatic flow. According to Cancer Research UK (2017a,b) approximately 1 in 5 people (20%) will have lymphoedema of the arm after breast cancer treatment that includes surgery to remove lymph nodes, and radiotherapy to the lymph nodes.

Lymphoedema is the accumulation of protein-rich fluid in tissues. The impaired function of lymph vessels interrupts the drainage of the lymphatic system that is a part of the circulatory system just like the arterial and venous structures. Lymph vessels remove excess fluid from tissues and transport it back to the circulation. In addition, the maturation of immune cells takes place in the lymphatic system; thus, it constitutes one of the most critical defence mechanisms throughout the body.

Lymph capillaries are in the dermis, woven like a cobweb, then drain to lymphatic vessels in the subcutaneous plane and ultimately to the deeper system and the thoracic duct.

Lymphoedema can either be primary or secondary. Regardless of the aetiology, it is clinically characterized with chronic swelling, localized pain, atrophic skin changes and secondary infections.

Following axillary surgery, the patient should be given information regarding skin care to prevent the occurrence of lymphoedema. The skin care advice for the affected arm is of great importance (Box 21.2).

Potential immobility of the affected arm

The woman should be referred to a physiotherapist, to be shown arm exercises to prevent a frozen shoulder and also to help prevent lymphoedema. These should be encouraged twice daily (Fig. 21.2).

Box 21.2 Skin care advice for the affected arm following surgery

Infection in the patient's 'at risk' arm, hand or breast/chest area can cause swelling, and may damage their lymphatic system, leading to lymphoedema.

The following tips can help with skin care, and reduce the risk of developing an infection:

- Moisturize the skin daily to prevent dry and cracked skin (use a moisturizing cream that suits your skin type)
- Use a high factor sunscreen to avoid sunburn
- Use oven gloves when cooking
- Apply insect repellent to avoid bites and stings
- Wear protective gloves in the garden (particularly when near rose bushes or brambles)
- Take care when cutting nails
- Take care if using wax or a razor to remove hair from under arm as it can damage the skin. Electric razors are gentler on the skin.
- Depilatory (hair removal) cream can be used, but check first that the patient is not sensitive or allergic to the cream
- Keep any cuts or grazes clean and use antiseptic cream; contact GP or breast care nurse if it is thought to be infected
- There is no strong evidence that having injections, taking blood, taking a blood pressure reading or having intravenous fluids in the 'at risk' arm will cause lymphoedema (Breast Cancer Care, 2019b). However, anecdotally, health professionals tend to do these procedures on the non-affected arm, using clinical decision-making skills to decide benefit over risk.
- It is important to exercise the arm and shoulder to prevent lymphoedema gradually, building strength, and guided by health professionals.
- Eat a plant-based diet that emphasizes whole grains and legumes (beans, lentils and dried peas), vegetables and fruit. These foods provide fibre, vitamins and minerals as well as cancer-fighting phytochemicals. Most plant foods are also naturally low in calories and fat which can be helpful for managing weight.
- Eat mostly plant foods. Choose foods that are minimally processed. Aim to make at least half of your grain choices whole grains each day. Choose beans, lentils and dried peas often instead of meat.
- Patients can continue with manicures and bathing as usual. There is no evidence that these increase the risk of lymphoedema.

Source: Breast Cancer Care (2019).

Anxiety

When a woman is given a diagnosis of breast cancer, it completely changes her life. It raises many fears and anxieties which she must learn to cope with.

The high prevalence of psychological morbidity after surgery of breast cancer is well documented (Del Piccolo et al, 2019; Kang et al, 2017; Fallowfield et al, 1986; Maguire et al, 1978). Most breast units have a specifically designated Breast Care Nurse who is specially educated in breast cancer to provide practical advice and support. The effectiveness of the role of the Breast Care Nurse has been well researched and evaluated and has been shown to reduce the incidence of psychological morbidity (NICE, 2018a).

If there is no Breast Care Nurse in post, support may be provided by voluntary organizations such as Breast Cancer Now. The NICE (2018a) advanced breast cancer diagnosis and treatment guideline describes the tests, treatment, care and support that patients with advanced breast cancer should be offered. Specific reference to nursing suggests community-based treatment and supportive care, including recommendations on psychosocial assessment and access to a key worker. In agreement, the *UK Guidance Document: Treatment of Metastatic Breast Cancer* (Coleman et al, 2012) supports the need for all metastatic breast cancer patients to have access to a clinical nurse specialist. From a European nursing practice perspective, the 1st International Consensus Guidelines for Advanced Breast Cancer (ABC1) (Cardosa, et al, 2012) supportive care recommend that every patient with metastatic breast cancer should have access to a clinical nurse specialist with the appropriate skill set.

Altered body image

The breast throughout history has been a symbol of womanhood. It is seen as a symbol of sexuality as well as a symbol of motherhood.

The woman should not be forced into looking at the wound before she is ready. When she feels able to look, she may or may not want her partner with her. Looking at the wound should be handled with sensitivity and understanding. A nurse should be present when this is done. A hand mirror should be available, so the woman can gradually look at the scar before seeing herself in a full-length mirror.

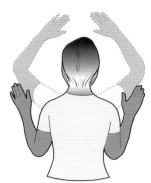

Wall reaching
With your feet apart for good balance, standing very close to, and facing a wall. Slowly 'walk' both hands up the wall, slide hands back down again and repeat

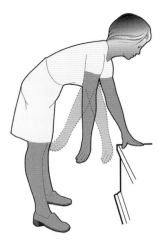

Support yourself with your unaffected arm. Let your other arm hang loosely and swing from the shoulder. Swing forwards, backwards, side to side and in circles

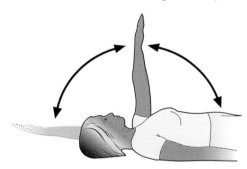

Reaching back
Lying on a firm surface, lift your affected arm to the vertical position then gently back so that it brushes past your ear

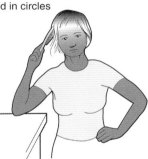

Hair-brushing
Rest your elbow on a table and sit up straight. Start by brushing your hair on one side and progress to brushing the whole head

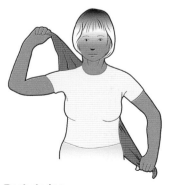

Back drying
Using a towel, practise a back drying movement

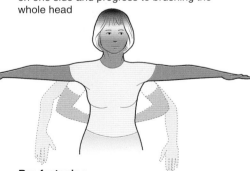

Bra-fastening
Hold your arms out level with your shoulders. Bend at the elbows and slowly reach behind your back to bra level

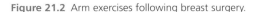

Figure 21.2 Arm exercises following breast surgery.

If a mastectomy has been performed, the woman should be fitted with a soft temporary prosthesis, sometimes called a 'comfie' (Fig. 21.3), as soon as she wishes prior to discharge. Arrangements for fitting a permanent silicone prosthesis should be made for 4–6 weeks postoperatively, when the scar has healed. The woman should be encouraged to wear her own clothes on the ward.

The person and partner may need reassurance that they can resume a sexual relationship as soon as they wish.

Support for the family

This is also a very traumatic time for a partner and family. It is difficult to see someone you care for distressed. The partner and family should be encouraged to take part in the care and be present at consultations (if appropriate). Breast Cancer Now provides a helpline for partners, so this information should be made available (see Resources section and Breast Cancer Care (2019)).

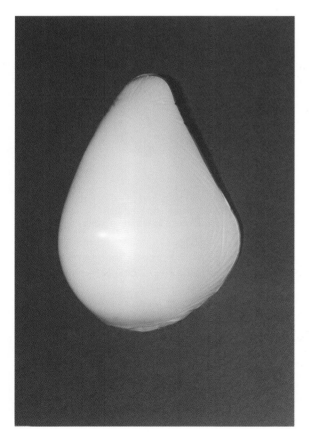

Figure 21.3 External silicone breast prosthesis.

Example of a nursing care plan

Ann is a 58-year-old married woman who was referred to the breast unit by her GP after she had found a lump in her left breast. She was naturally very anxious, as her mother had died from breast cancer at the age of 60. Unfortunately, the mammogram and the fine-needle aspiration confirmed this lump to be a breast cancer.

Ann and her husband were seen by the consultant surgeon and the Breast Care Nurse, who discussed the possible treatment options. They were given time to go away and consider these options. They returned to see the Breast Care Nurse 3 days later for the results of the staging tests, which were normal. Ann and her husband had decided that a mastectomy would be the best option for them, as Ann felt she would constantly worry about the cancer returning in that breast.

The care plan (see Table 21.4) uses the Roper, Logan and Tierney model (Roper et al, 1996). It looks only at the specific nursing care for a patient undergoing a mastectomy.

Discharge planning and advice

Going home is going to be greeted with some pleasure, but it also instils some fear into the woman, as she may feel alone and vulnerable. Her home situation should be assessed to see if any other services are required, e.g. home help.

Advice should be given on resuming normal activities. If the woman usually undertakes housework, this should be avoided or at least undertaken lightly for the first 4–6 weeks until full arm movement has returned. If she is working, she should return to work when able and advised by the medical professional. This is dependent on her duty and responsibilities and the type of job she does. It is advisable not to lift heavy objects with the affected arm, indefinitely. Driving can be resumed normally after 4–6 weeks, once the woman has regained full arm movement and feels she can safely stop the car in an emergency. The woman should seek advice from her surgeon regarding resumption of sporting activities.

Information regarding voluntary organizations, e.g. Breast Cancer Now (see Resources section), should be given to the woman so she has someone she can contact if she needs to talk or wants to receive added written information. If a Breast Care Nurse is in post, the woman should have her contact number so she can call the nurse if she has a problem. It is, however, important to return some control to the woman, so she can develop her own coping mechanisms and not become too reliant on the Breast Care Nurse or voluntary organizations.

A follow-up appointment should be made for the following week after discharge home, so the wound can be checked and the pathology result can be given to the woman. Further treatment can then be discussed. The woman should be reassured that she will have regular follow-up appointments. The follow-up policy will vary between breast units, but on average it is usually 3-monthly for 1 year and then 6-monthly until 5 years, when the patient is discharged.

Conclusion

Caring for women undergoing breast surgery is a very rewarding and challenging experience. It not only gives the nurse the skills to look after a person undergoing surgery but it also has many psychosocial issues involved, which adds another dimension. Any surgery to the breast may cause worry, anxiety and a fear of an altered body image. If the nurse can treat the woman with sensitivity and understanding, it can help to make the whole experience less traumatic.

SUMMARY OF KEY POINTS

- Breast cancer is a common problem, affecting 1 in 9 women in the UK.
- Patients who find a lump will fear breast cancer.
- Treatment should be provided in a specialist breast unit.
- It is important to consider physical, social and psychological needs of patients undergoing breast surgery.
- All patients who have breast cancer should have access to a Breast Care Nurse.
- All patients, especially women, should be encouraged to be breast aware.

REFLECTIVE LEARNING POINTS

Having read this chapter, think about what you now know and what else you still need to find out about. These questions may help:

- How do I make a referral to a Breast Care Nurse Specialist?
- What might be the key concerns that a person with lymphoedema may have as they carry out their activities of living?
- What advice might I give to a woman who wishes to breastfeed after a diagnosis of breast disease?

Useful addresses

Breast Cancer Now (formed by the merger of Breast Cancer Care and Breast Cancer Now)
Fifth Floor, Ibex House
42−47 Minories
London EC3N 1DY
Tel: 0345 092 0800
Helpline: 0808 800 6000
breastcancernow.org
Macmillan Cancer Support
89 Albert Embankment
London SE1 7UQ
Tel: 020 7840 7840
<https://www.macmillan.org.uk/>

References

American Cancer Society (ACS). (2014). *What happens to biopsy and cytology specimens?* Available at: <www.cancer.org/treatment/understanding-your-diagnosis/tests/testing-biopsy-and-cytology-specimens-for-cancer/what-happens-to-specimens.html>

American Cancer Society (ACS). (2019). *Breast-conserving surgery (lumpectomy).* Available at: <www.cancer.org/cancer/breast-cancer/treatment/surgery-for-breast-cancer/breast-conserving-surgery-lumpectomy.html>

Akkas, B. E., & Vural, G. U. (2013). Fat necrosis may mimic local recurrence of breast cancer in FDG PET/CT. *Revista Española de Medicina Nuclear e Imagen Molecular, 32*(2), 105−106. Available at: <https://www.sciencedirect.com/science/article/pii/S2253654X12001655>.

Arul, P., Masilamani, S., & Akshatha, C. (2016). Fine needle aspiration cytology of atypical (C3) and suspicious (C4) categories in the breast and its histo-pathologic correlation. *Journal of Cytology, 33*(2), 76−79.

Bickley, L. (2016). *Bates' Guide to Physical Examination and History Taking* (12th edn). Baltimore: Wolters Kluwer.

Breast Cancer Care. (2019a). *Fibroadenoma.* Available at: breastcancernow.org/information-support/publication/fibroadenoma-bcc72

Breast Cancer Care. (2019b). *Reducing the risk of lymphoedema.* Available at: <www.breastcancercare.org.uk/sites/default/files/publications/pdf/bcc15_reducing_the_risk_2019_web.pdf>

Breast Cancer Now. (2019). *After surgery*. Available at: breastcancernow.org/information-support/facing-breast-cancer/living-beyond-breast-cancer/after-surgery

BreastCancer.org. (2019a). *Implant reconstruction: what to expect*. Available at: <www.breastcancer.org/treatment/surgery/reconstruction/types/implants/what-to-expect>

BreastCancer.org. (2019b). *TRAM flap*. Available at: <www.breastcancer.org/treatment/surgery/reconstruction/types/autologous/tram>

BreastCancer.org. (2019c). *Latissimus dorsi flap*. Available at: <www.breastcancer.org/treatment/surgery/reconstruction/types/autologous/lat-dorsi>

BUPA. (2019). *Benign breast lumps*. Available at: <www.bupa.co.uk/health-information/womens-health/breast-lumps>

Cancer Research UK. (2017a). *Breast cancer symptoms*. Available at: <www.cancerresearchuk.org/about-cancer/breast-cancer/symptoms>

Cancer Research UK. (2017b). *Lymphoedema after breast cancer treatment*. Available at: <www.cancerresearchuk.org/about-cancer/breast-cancer/living-with/lymphoedema-after-treatment>

Cancer Research UK. (2019a). *Breast cancer statistics*. Available at: <www.cancerresearchuk.org/health-professional/cancer-statistics/statistics-by-cancer-type/breast-cancer#heading-One>

Cancer Research UK. (2019b). *Wire-guided excision biopsy*. Available at: <www.cancerresearchuk.org/about-cancer/breast-cancer/getting-diagnosed/tests-diagnose/wire-guided-excision-biopsy>

Cancer Research UK. (2019c). *Your urgent referral explained*. Available at: <www.cancerresearchuk.org/cancer-symptoms/what-is-an-urgent-referral>

Coleman, R. E., Bertelli, G., Beaumont, T., et al. (2012). UK guidance document: treatment of metastatic breast cancer. *Clinical Oncology, 24*(3), 169–176.

Cardosa, F., Costa, S., Norton, L., Cameron, D., Cufer, T., & Fallowfield, L. (2012). 1st international consensus guidelines for advanced breast cancer (ABC1). *Breast, 21*(3), 242–252.

Chrisafis, A. (2011). France's faulty breast implants scandal. *The Guardian*. 14 December 2011. Available at: <www.theguardian.com/lifeandstyle/2011/dec/14/france-faulty-breast-implant-scandal>.

Del Piccolo, L., Mazzi, M., Mascanzoni, A., Lonardi, M., De Felice, M., Danzi, O., et al. (2019). Factors related to the expression of emotions by early-stage breast cancer patients. *Patient Education and Counseling, 102*(10), 1767–1773.

Dixon, J., & Khan, L. (2011). Treatment of breast infection. *BMJ, 342*, d396.

Dixon, J. M. (2013). Breast infection. *BMJ, 347*, f3291.

Fallowfield, L. J., Baum, M., & Maguire, G. P. (1986). Effects of breast conservation on psychological morbidity associated with diagnosis and treatment of early breast cancer. *BMJ, 293*(6558), 1331–1334.

Görkem, S. B., & O'Connell, A. M. (2012). Abnormal axillary lymph nodes on negative mammograms: causes other than breast cancer. *Diagnostic and Interventional Radiology, 18*(5), 473–479.

Green, M., Habib, T., & Raghaven, V. (2018). A novel technique of breast reconstruction: inflation of breast tissue expander with air. *Plastic and Reconstructive Surgery. Global Open, 6* (12), e2036.

Independent Review Group (IRG) Report. (1998). *Silicone gel breast implants*. London: Crown Copyright.

Kang, K. D., Bae, S., Kim, H. J., Hwang, I. G., Kim, S. M., & Han, D. H. (2017). The relationship between physical activity intensity and mental health status in patients with breast cancer. *Journal of Korean Medical Science, 32*(8), 1345–1350.

Macmillan Cancer Support. (2019). *Types of breast cancer*. Available at: <www.macmillan.org.uk/information-and-support/breast-cancer/understanding-cancer/types-of-breast-cancer.html>

Maguire, G. P., Lee, E. G., Bevington, D. J., et al. (1978). Psychiatric problems in the first year after mastectomy. *BMJ, 1* (6118), 963–965.

National Institute of Health & Care Excellence (NICE). (2018a). *Early and locally advanced breast cancer: diagnosis and management*. NICE guideline [NG101]. Available at: <www.nice.org.uk/guidance/ng101>

National Institute of Health & Care Excellence (NICE). (2018b). *Mastitis and breast abscess*. Available at: cks.nice.org.uk/mastitis-and-breast-abscess#!scenario

National Institute of Health & Care Excellence (NICE). (2018c). *Suspected cancer recognition and referral overview*. Available at: pathways.nice.org.uk/pathways/suspected-cancer-recognition-and-referral

National Institute of Health & Care Excellence (NICE). (2019) *Pathway: Early and locally advanced breast cancer*. Available at: <https://pathways.nice.org.uk/pathways/early-and-locally-advanced-breast-cancer>

NHS. (2018). *What do cancer stages and grades mean?* Available at: <www.nhs.uk/common-health-questions/operations-tests-and-procedures/what-do-cancer-stages-and-grades-mean>

NHS. (2019a). *Antibiotics*. Available at: <www.nhs.uk/conditions/antibiotics>

NHS. (2019b). *Breast cancer screening*. Available at: <www.nhs.uk/conditions/breast-cancer-screening>

NHS Improvement. (2011). *Delivering major breast surgery safely as a day case or one night stay (excluding reconstruction)*. London: NHS Improvement.

Nursing & Midwifery Council (NMC). (2018). The Code. Professional standards of practice and behaviour for nurses, midwives and nursing associates. Available at: <www.nmc.org.uk/standards/code>

Pek, C. H., Tey, J., & Tan, E. Y. (2016). Ambulatory surgery for the patient with breast cancer: current perspectives. *Open Access Surgery, 9*, 65–70. available at: <www.dovepress.com/ambulatory-surgery-for-the-patient-with-breast-cancer-current-perspect-peer-reviewed-fulltext-article-OAS>.

Roper, N., Logan, W. W., & Tierney, A. J. (1996). *The elements of nursing* (4th edn). Edinburgh: Churchill Livingstone.

Further reading

BBC. (2018). *How to do a breast examination*. Available at: <www.bbc.co.uk/news/av/health-44384499/how-to-do-a-breast-examination>

British Lymphology Society (BLS): <www.thebls.com>

Cancer Research. (2019). *Breast cancer*. Available at: <www.cancerresearchuk. org/about-cancer/breast-cancer>

healthtalk.org. (2019). *Breast cancer in women*. Available at: <www.healthtalk. org/peoples-experiences/cancer/breast-cancer-women/topics>

healthtalk.org. (2019). *Breast cancer in men*. Available at: <www.healthtalk. org/peoples-experiences/cancer/breast-cancer-men/topics>

Link, J. (2017). *The breast cancer survival manual* (6th edn). New York: St Martins Griffin.

Lymphoedema Support Network: <www. lymphoedema.org>

National Institute of Health & Care Excellence (NICE). (2019). *Breast cancer*. Available at: <www.nice.org. uk/guidance/conditions-and-diseases/-cancer/breast-cancer>

World Health Organization (WHO). (2019). *Breast cancer*. Geneva: WHO. Available at: <www.who.int/cancer/ detection/breastcancer/en/index3. html>.

Chapter | 22 |

Care of patients requiring vascular surgery

Bhuvaneswari Krishnamoorthy

KEY OBJECTIVES OF THE CHAPTER

At the end of the chapter the reader should be able to:

- discuss the physiology of circulation
- provide an overview of the various investigations associated with vascular disease
- describe a number of vascular conditions and their surgery
- discuss the effects of vascular surgery on a person
- outline care provision required for those who are to undergo or have undergone vascular surgery.

Areas to think about before reading the chapter

- What do you understand by peripheral vascular disease?
- How can vascular disease and surgery impact on a person's ability to perform the activities of living?
- Discuss the role and function of the nurse when caring for those undergoing vascular surgery?

Introduction

This chapter aims to address the patterns of peripheral vascular disease, investigations, assessment and treatment. In addition, national and international guidelines for diagnostic, pre- and postoperative nursing care will be discussed. This will include management of patients undergoing radiological intervention, arterial reconstruction and venous surgery (open and endovascular surgical procedures).

Vascular disease is caused by the gradual deposit of fatty tissues inside the blood vessel. This deposit occurs gradually and sometimes without any symptoms until the blood vessels become inflamed and weakened. It is one of the leading causes of death and at the time of writing is projected to become the main cause of death worldwide by 2020 (Valentijn & Stolker, 2012). One of the major causes of death is unhealed venous leg ulcers. According to NHS benchmarking (SIGN, 2010), 39% of district nursing clinical time is spent on wound care, of which 20% relates to venous leg ulcers. Approximately 8% of the whole district nursing workforce time is spent on venous leg ulcers with 2.1 million visits annually (Ousey et al, 2013; NHS England, 2018). The Tissue Viability Nurses' review done at Nottinghamshire Healthcare NHS Foundation Trust concluded that providing staff with e-learning tools, redesigning the leg ulcer assessment and management templates, and implementing a leg ulcer care policy could bring better outcomes with anticipated savings of £19,000 annually per trust (NHS England, 2018).

Most arterial vascular disease is a consequence of the atherosclerotic process. The most common vascular disease is peripheral arterial disease (PAD) and it is reported with a prevalence of 15% in Western countries and up to 30% when studied in elderly population (Conte & Vale, 2018).

The presence of PAD is a strong warning sign for the risk of myocardial infarction, stroke and death and it can significantly affect health-related quality of life (Muir, 2009). The Reduction of Atherothrombosis for Continued Health (REACH) Registry demonstrated that polyvascular disease is common in PAD patients and risk factors are less intensively controlled and undertreated (Valentijn & Stolker, 2012).

Care of patients with end-stage PAD is both challenging and complex. It involves early detection, ongoing monitoring, and knowledge of new developments in diagnostic, radiological, invasive and non-invasive surgical procedures. A major component of care must include measures to reduce the progression of atherosclerosis, which requires a multidisciplinary team approach to achieve successful outcomes.

Physiology of circulation

Blood flow is essential to human life, and blood is circulated to all areas of the body by the pumping action of the heart. Blood flows through arteries, veins and capillaries which compose the vascular bed. Arteries and veins are composed of three layers:

- Tunica adventitia – outer layer of fibrous tissue which gives the vessel support to maintain its shape.
- Tunica media – middle layer consisting of muscle and elastic tissue which regulates the diameter of the vessel by dilatation and constriction.
- Tunica intima – inner layer of endothelium which provides a smooth passage for blood to flow.

The arterial system

The arterial system is responsible for carrying oxygenated blood and nutrients to the body tissues. Arteries help to regulate the blood pressure by expanding with each surge of blood ejected from the heart and then resuming their original diameter.

The arteries branch off into smaller arterioles, which subdivide into the capillary network. The arterioles differ from the larger arteries in that the tunica media layer consists almost entirely of smooth muscle. Blood has to pass through precapillary sphincters before entering the capillary network. These sphincters work in conjunction with the autonomic nervous system to regulate the perfused capillary bed. The capillaries form a network to link the smallest arterioles to the smallest venules.

Capillaries are the simplest of the blood vessels; their walls consist of a single layer of endothelial cells, which have a semipermeable membrane. The capillaries make up the microcirculation, which allows the exchange of nutrients and waste products from the surrounding tissues. When the smaller arteries constrict, there is an increase in peripheral vascular resistance. This is a measure of the friction between the molecules of the blood and the radius and length of the blood vessel. The smaller the radius of the vessel, the greater the resistance to the flow of blood, so altering blood flow.

During vasodilatation of the artery, there is a decrease in diastolic blood pressure and in peripheral vascular resistance, so increasing blood flow.

There is increasing evidence of the important function of the inner layer of the endothelial cells and its role in the development of vascular disease. The endothelium provides a cellular lining to all the blood vessels in the circulatory system and acts as an interface between the blood and the vascular wall. There is evidence that the vascular endothelium helps preserve cardiovascular homeostasis. The healthy endothelial cells express antiplatelet and anticoagulant agents that prevent platelet aggregation and fibrin formation (Yau et al, 2015).

The venous system

The venous system originates in the capillary beds to form venules, which are responsible for removal of waste products from the capillaries. The venules merge to form veins, which carry deoxygenated blood back to the heart.

Veins

Veins have thinner walls, less muscle and elastic tissue, and lie closer to the skin surface than do arteries. Veins also differ in that some, mostly in the limbs and especially the lower limbs, have endothelial valves. These permit blood flow only towards the heart, preventing reflux. The return of blood to the heart is therefore reliant on three factors: patency of the veins, valve competence and contracting surrounding muscles (muscle pump). During exercise, the veins in the leg are compressed by the contracted leg muscles, which act as a 'muscle pump', so allowing blood to be returned towards the heart. Blood is returned from the lower limbs to the right side of the heart via the inferior vena cava by the pumping action of the muscles. This pumping action from the calf and foot muscles compresses the deep veins of the legs, which contain one-way valves, and pushes the blood back to the heart, with backflow being prevented by the valves. These muscular contractions allow emptying of the blood from the superficial veins into the deep veins, via the communicating vessels. The venous system of the leg comprises a superficial system in the skin and subcutaneous fat, and a deep system beneath the fascia. The main superficial leg veins are the long and short saphenous, which form a venous network with other perforating veins, which pass through the fascia to join the deep veins. These deep veins run alongside the arteries and have the same names.

Lymphatic vessels

Lymphatic vessels are thin-walled vessels which arise at the capillaries and also branch into their own circulation. Lymph capillaries, like veins, increase in size and, with the assistance of valves and muscular contractions, transport excess interstitial fluid (lymph) to the venous system via large ducts in the thoracic cavity. Through these ducts, the lymph flows into the inferior vena cava and subclavian vein and finally into the right atrium, where it is recycled into the central circulation. Lymphatic vessels are highly permeable, with large pores which allow the removal of proteins, cellular debris and fat absorption from the intestines. Lymph nodes are situated along the lymphatic system and filter debris from bacteria, viruses and other refuse from lymphatic fluid.

Arterial occlusive disease

Arterial occlusive disease may occur suddenly, following an embolus or thrombus, or insidiously, as in atherosclerosis.

Atherosclerosis

The Global Burden of Disease (GBD) Study, carried out in 2013, demonstrated that peripheral arterial disease was the main reason for more than 40,000 deaths, which is an increase of 155% from 1990 (GBD, 2015). Atherosclerosis is a systemic process which occurs gradually within the arterial wall and has a strong correlation with coronary artery disease and cerebrovascular disease. It mainly affects the aorta, arteries to the lower limbs, and coronary, carotid and renal arteries. Common sites include the aorto-iliac, femoral, popliteal and tibial arteries.

The changes within the arterial wall are identified in three stages:
1. Stage of fatty, lipid streak formation within the intima.
2. Stage of fibrous plaque formation in the subintimal layer, which extends along the artery walls and then protrudes and narrows the lumen.
3. Stage of complication – characterized by endothelial ulceration, calcification, and activation of platelets and leucocytes, leading to thrombus formation.

The process of atherosclerosis results in the arterial walls becoming thickened and hardened, with loss of elasticity and decreased blood flow. However, at the early stage of atherosclerotic development, the fatty streak does not protrude into the artery wall nor impede blood flow and this process is already visible in most people by the age of 20 (Delewi et al, 2013). Additional risk factors, such as endothelial dysfunction, stress, diabetes, hypertension, hypercholesterolemia and smoking, can aggravate these processes and may lead to thrombosis or emboli formation with ischaemia.

Atherosclerosis may play a role in contributing to aneurysm formation, although the true aetiology is thought to be multifactorial. The artery wall becomes weakened, causing a local dilatation of the artery, which can contain thrombus. The aneurysm may rupture as it grows larger and the blood vessel wall becomes thinner, resulting in severe haemorrhage or death. Aneurysms can occur throughout the arterial tree; the most commonly affected vessels are the aorta and iliac arteries, followed by the popliteal arteries.

Aneurysms are classified as *true* or *false*. A true aneurysm occurs when the artery wall becomes dilated and thin but remains intact (Fig. 22.1A−C). Thrombi can collect between the layers of artery, causing a local dilatation. A false aneurysm occurs due to trauma of the three layers of artery wall, which allows blood to leak extravascularly (Fig. 22.1D). Clot formation occurs, and the clot becomes surrounded by periarterial connective tissue; blood then passes into the sac as it flows along the lumen of the artery (Greenhalgh, 1990).

Risk factors

The major risk factors for PAD are age, gender, smoking, hypertension, hyperlipidaemia, diabetes mellitus, obesity, family history of vascular disease and strong chronic smoking history. The National Health and Nutrition Examination Survey of 2000 patients with PAD suggested that more than 95% had at least one of the above-mentioned major risk factors and over 70% of patients had more than two risk factors (Selvin & Erlinger, 2004).

Age and gender

PAD is recognized as a global pandemic which affects over 202 million people worldwide (Fowkes et al, 2013). The

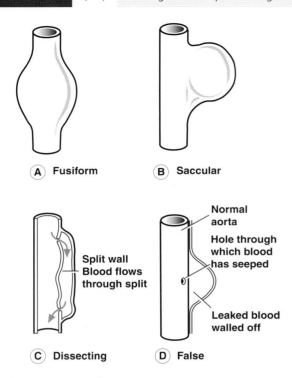

(A) Fusiform   (B) Saccular

Split wall
Blood flows
through split

Normal
aorta

Hole through
which blood
has seeped

Leaked blood
walled off

(C) Dissecting   (D) False

Figure 22.1 Types of aneurysm.

prevalence of PAD is the same in women and men in high-income countries, however it is more prevalent in women than men in low-income countries (Hiramoto et al, 2014). Women with PAD experience faster functional decline with poorer outcomes after lower extremity revascularization surgical procedures than men (McDermott et al, 2011).

Smoking

The relationship between smoking and PAD was first reported in 1911 (Erb, 1911).

Around 50% of PAD may be related to smoking (Willigendael et al., 2004) and the disease develops in smokers 10 years earlier than non-smokers (Lassila & Lepantalo, 1988). Most of the PAD cases result in total or partial amputation (Dormandy, 2000). However, the NICE 2012 guideline concluded that there is extremely limited evidence available to support the use of amputation. It is therefore vital to consider the overall poor results of amputation and it would be useful to discuss the treatment options with the multidisciplinary team before proceeding to surgery (NICE, 2012). Smoking is considered as one of the most modifiable risk factors for PAD and it is vital to motivate for cessation of smoking and an increase in physical exercise, both of which are clearly attainable objectives to prevent PAD (Berger et al,

2013). Nicotine and carbon monoxide have been shown to produce endothelial injury, insulin resistance and lipid abnormalities, leading to the development of atherosclerotic plaque in the arteries (Sebelius, 2010). Smoking should be stopped, and patients informed of the harmful effects of nicotine on their condition. The majority of smokers with PAD are nicotine addicts and require counselling and behavioural support therapy. In addition, nicotine replacement therapy, bupropion or varenicline tartrate and e-cigarettes can help relieve cravings and withdrawal symptoms in order to successfully quit.

Hyperlipidaemia

One of the most important independent risk factors for developing PAD is hyperlipidaemia. The Framingham Heart Study reported that an elevated cholesterol level was associated with a two-fold increase in the incidence of intermittent claudication (Kannel et al, 1970; Cote et al, 2003). The initial step for reducing serum cholesterol should be diet, along with statin drug therapy and active physical exercise. Treatment with statins has shown to improve endothelial dysfunction and reduce levels of nitric oxide, which is related to dyslipidaemia and which, in turn, leads to an improvement in blood flow in the microcirculation (Crismaru & Diaconu, 2015). The Heart Protection Study demonstrated that anti-lipid drug therapy in patients with PAD reduced the rate of major vascular events by about a quarter, independent of the baseline lipid level, and also reduced peripheral vascular events by 16% (Heart Protection Study Collaborative Group, 2007). The American College of Cardiology (ACC) has a class 2a recommendation for the use of fibric acid derivatives for patients with PAD and high triglycerides/low high-density lipoprotein-cholesterol, but normal low-density lipoprotein-cholesterol (Rooke et al, 2011).

Diabetes

Diabetes mellitus (DM) patients with PAD have a 2.5 times higher risk of mortality and morbidity than other patients (Lu et al, 2014). DM patients with poorly controlled blood glucose have been linked with accelerated atherosclerosis and higher rates of cardiac events, which can lead to diabetic foot ulcers with a result of amputation (Weledji & Fokam, 2014). Diabetes patients are more susceptible to atherosclerosis due to drivers such as oxidative stress, endothelial dysfunction, alterations in mineral metabolism, increased inflammatory cytokine production and release of osteoprogenitor cells from the marrow into the circulation (Yahagi et al, 2017). Neuropathy is also common, which causes a lack of sensation, making the patient with diabetes prone to trauma, resulting in foot injuries, infections and non-healing ulcers. Diabetic leg ulcers are usually situated on the bony prominences of the feet, resulting in necrotic wounds. Good blood glucose control reduces the risk of small vessel limb disease.

The National Institute for Health and Care Excellence (NICE) guideline CG147 recommends that diabetes patients with PAD can be a challenge because diagnostic tests are conducted in a variety of healthcare settings. It is therefore vital that assessment tools with inter- and intra-rater reliability, such as ankle–brachial pressure index, post-exercise ankle–brachial index, toe–brachial index and Doppler wave form analysis, are used as diagnostic tools in clinical practice (NICE, 2018a,b).

Foot care advice should be given to all patients with arterial occlusive disease, not only people with diabetes, to help reduce the incidence of injury, and followed up with an information leaflet. The information leaflet can be oral or written and should include the following information: a clear explanation of the person's foot problem, care of the foot and leg, details of whom to contact in case of emergencies, footwear advice, wound care and, importantly, information about diabetes and blood glucose control (NICE, 2015). The nurse can help educate the patient by teaching them how to perform self-assessment and foot care (Fig. 22.2). Patients should be instructed to check their feet daily or, if they are unable to do this for themselves, a relative or carer will need to be taught how to do this. The importance of contacting their nurse, doctor, or foot clinic/podiatrist immediately if problems occur should be stressed.

Hypertension

An increased mechanical stress on the arterial wall due to higher blood pressure in hypertensive patients results in endothelial damage. Those people with PAD and hypertension have an increased risk of developing myocardial infarction and stroke. The main focus for these patients needs to be on decreasing the global cardiovascular risk, rather than only controlling blood pressure and reducing the PAD symptoms. Therefore, it is vital to treat these patients with antiplatelet drugs, ACE inhibitors, statins and, importantly, patients with intermittent claudication should be prescribed pentoxifylline to improve the blood flow in the legs (Topfer & Spry, 2018).

The NICE guidelines recommend that the target clinical blood pressure should be below 140/90 mmHg in patients aged 79 or under with treated hypertension, and a clinical blood pressure below 150/90 mmHg in patients aged 80 or over with treated hypertension (NICE, 2014a,b). If a higher value is noted of between 10 and 15 mmHg, this may indicate an arterial stenosis on the side of the lower reading.

Hyperhomocysteinaemia

Homocysteine is a sulfhydryl-containing amino acid which is an intermediate product in the normal

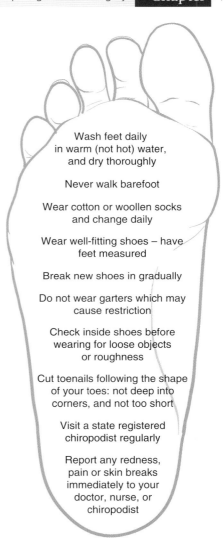

Wash feet daily
in warm (not hot) water,
and dry thoroughly

Never walk barefoot

Wear cotton or woollen socks
and change daily

Wear well-fitting shoes – have
feet measured

Break new shoes in gradually

Do not wear garters which may
cause restriction

Check inside shoes before
wearing for loose objects
or roughness

Cut toenails following the shape
of your toes: not deep into
corners, and not too short

Visit a state registered
chiropodist regularly

Report any redness,
pain or skin breaks
immediately to your
doctor, nurse, or
chiropodist

Figure 22.2 Foot care advice.

biosynthesis of the amino acids methionine and cysteine. Hyperhomocysteinaemia can augment the adverse effects of risk factors such as hypertension, smoking, lipid and lipoprotein metabolism, as well as promotion of the development of inflammation (Baszczuk & Kopczynski, 2014).

The elevated level (above 15 μmol/L) can cause adverse effects on the cardiovascular endothelium and smooth muscle cells with resultant alternations in subclinical arterial structure and function (Ganguly & Alam, 2015). Elevated homocysteine levels should be checked, particularly in patients under 60 years old. A meta-analysis conducted by Li et al concluded a 10% lower risk of stroke and a 4% lower risk of overall cardiovascular disease with folic acid supplementation (Li et al, 2016).

Alcohol

Binge drinking should be avoided, and unit guidelines are now the same for men and women. Both genders are advised not to regularly drink more than 14 units a week. A high-quality study conducted in 19 countries and published in *The Lancet* provides further evidence to support the current UK guidelines advising people to drink no more than 14 units a week (Wood et al, 2018).

Sedentary lifestyle

Physical inactivity is a major risk factor for cardiovascular disease. Regular exercise combined with weight reduction is associated with lowering cholesterol and blood pressure.

Metabolic syndrome

Abdominal obesity in combination with hypertension, dyslipidaemia and glucose intolerance will result in metabolic syndrome. This increases the risk of type 2 diabetes and vascular disease (Alshehri, 2010).

Socioeconomic factors

Social deprivation also increases risk factors for developing peripheral arterial disease, as patients from lower social classes are more likely to eat an unhealthy diet, exercise less and smoke. Low socioeconomic status and high anxiety levels have been found to contribute to development of the disease (Pande & Creager, 2014).

The patient with chronic ischaemia

Clinical features

A patient with chronic ischaemia may have minimal symptoms in the early stages or may develop limb pain, ulceration or gangrene. Clinical features of arterial occlusive disease occur when there is partial or complete occlusion of the artery. The primary symptom of PAD is intermittent claudication. The term 'claudication' derives from the Latin *claudus*, meaning 'lame', which is attributed to the Emperor Claudius, who walked with a limp.

Intermittent claudication

Intermittent claudication (IC) is pain only induced by exercise and experienced in the foot, calf, thigh or buttock, depending on the level of arterial occlusion, when a certain distance is walked. The pain is caused by inadequate blood supply to the muscles and can vary in severity and walking distance. Walking at a brisk pace or on an incline will produce symptoms earlier. Patients frequently refer to their symptoms as an ache, heaviness or dullness of the leg muscles. Intermittent claudication may affect one or both legs, is more common in the calf and is always relieved by rest.

Patients with intermittent claudication may not experience a major handicap to their lifestyle, or their symptoms may even resolve with regular walking exercise. In 5–10% of patients with asymptomatic PAD, IC develops over 5 years and 75% of them will experience stabilization in their symptoms or improvement without any intervention (O'Donnell et al, 2011).

Although some claudicants may initially fear limb loss, only 7 of 100 patients (6 of whom had diabetes) underwent major amputation. If the condition becomes more severe, it may lead to signs of critical ischaemia such as rest pain, ulcers and possible gangrene. In the 1950s, Fontaine classified the signs and symptoms of chronic leg ischaemia into four stages (Box 22.1). It is therefore important that patients with intermittent claudication modify their risk factors at an early stage to help prevent disease progression and also to reduce their chance of suffering a heart attack or stroke.

Rest pain

The true rest pain usually affects the foot or toes of the affected limb as opposed to benign nighttime calf cramps (Peach et al, 2012). Temporary relief may be gained by hanging the limb out of bed or by sleeping in an armchair with the foot down.

As the disease progresses, the blood flow to the leg is reduced such that pain occurs while resting rather than induced by exercise. Patients with ischaemic rest pain initially awake at night with pain in the foot and toes. Pain is continually present when the patient is immobile and prevents sleep occurring, causing rapid deterioration in the patient's morale.

Ulceration and/or gangrene

Arterial disease may ultimately result in tissue loss of the toes, foot or leg. Critical leg ischaemia is a condition which endangers the distal part of the limb, and there is a high risk

---

Box 22.1 Fontaine's classification of ischaemia

Stage 1: asymptomatic
Stage 2: intermittent claudication
Stage 3: severe, persistent rest pain of the foot
Stage 4: ulceration and/or gangrene

that the patient will require toe or limb amputation. The definition of critical leg ischaemia has evolved over time from the first definition written by the European Working Group (1991) to the current definition, written by the Peripheral Academic Research Consortium (Patel et al., 2015):

- Classical signs of ischaemic rest pain requiring analgesia for longer than two weeks.
- Ulceration or gangrene of the lower extremity with ankle systolic blood pressure <50 mmHg and/or toe systolic pressure <30 mmHg.
- Patients with tissue loss as ankle systolic blood pressure <70 mmHg and/or toe systolic pressure <50 mmHg.
- Transcutaneous oxygen (TcPO2) (<20 mmHg of patients with ischaemic rest pain and <40 mmHg for patients with tissue loss).
- Skin perfusion pressure (<40 mmHg or <30 mmHg, respectively).

Investigations

A full medical history is taken, and a clinical examination performed, which will include an electrocardiogram (ECG) to determine cardiac function. An echocardiogram may be undertaken if surgical treatment is necessary. Full blood count, clotting screen, urea and electrolytes, blood glucose, HbA1c in people with diabetes and lipid screening will also be required, as well as routine urinalysis. Thrombophilia screen and homocysteine levels should also be undertaken in younger (<60 years old) patients. Chest X-ray and lung function tests are performed to identify potential respiratory problems prior to surgical intervention.

The limbs are observed for warmth, colour, sensation, movement, and any ulceration or gangrenous changes (Fig. 22.3A–D). Pallor, dusky erythema or cyanosis may be present, with absent or reduced peripheral pulses. Thin, shiny atrophic skin, thick brittle nails and hair loss on the limb may indicate poor tissue nutrition due to reduced blood supply. Capillary refill in the nails indicates perfusion time in the capillary beds; normal refill should occur within 3 seconds. The skin is prone to breakdown, especially from trauma. Tissue loss or gangrene may also be present over areas of high pressure such as metatarsal heads, dorsum of the foot and particularly the heels.

The use of contrast angiography, echo-enhanced colour flow Doppler and duplex sonography is widely regarded as the gold standard investigation in PAD. These investigations are non-invasive techniques which give clear information about both structural and dynamic anomalies in the peripheral arteries (Peach et al, 2012).

Peripheral pulses

Limb pulses are palpated to assess the adequacy and volume of the blood supply at femoral, popliteal, posterior tibial and pedal pulse sites (Fig. 22.4). The absence of pulses or a weak pulse may determine the presence of arterial disease and require confirmation by Doppler ultrasound and ankle–brachial pressure index (Bailey et al, 2014).

The presence of central bruits (abnormal 'whooshing' sounds or murmurs) may be heard with a stethoscope. This turbulent flow, heard over major arteries, may be significant in carotid vessels which are narrowed due to atherosclerosis.

Doppler ultrasound

Doppler ultrasound is a practical non-invasive test using ultrasonic high-frequency sounds emitted from a hand-held transducer probe. It is used to assess the arterial blood supply to the lower limb by listening to the arterial sounds, and for measuring the ankle–brachial systolic pressure ratio, to aid diagnosis and detect the degree of arterial insufficiency. Doppler ultrasound can also be used to ascertain the presence of pedal pulses following intervention such as angioplasty, thrombolysis or reconstructive bypass surgery.

The highest systolic pressure in the arm at the brachial artery is compared with the highest systolic pressure in the ankle at the dorsalis pedis and the posterior tibial artery, to give an ankle–brachial pressure index (ABPI):

$$ABPI = \frac{\text{highest systolic ankle pressure (mmHg)}}{\text{highest systolic brachial pressure (mmHg)}}$$

- normal ABPI >1.00
- ABPI for patients with claudication = 0.5–0.9
- ABPI for patients with rest pain and critical leg ischaemia ≤0.5.

According to the American Diabetes Association consensus statement, the normal range of ABPI falls between 0.91 and 1.3. If the patient has mild disease, it will be in the range of 0.7–0.9, whilst moderate disease will be 0.41–0.69 (American Diabetes Association, 2003).

However, false high readings may be obtained in patients with diabetes, atherosclerosis, and chronic renal disease, as a result of calcification of the arteries, which means the sphygmomanometer cuff cannot fully compress the hardened arteries. ABPI is also known to be a predictor of survival in vascular patients and adding the ABPI into risk calculations based on Framingham score improves the accuracy of cardiovascular risk prediction (Bailey et al, 2014).

Toe pressures

Measurement of toe pressures can be performed to assess arterial blood flow in people with diabetes by using photoplethysmography (PPG). A special small occlusion cuff is usually attached to the first toe, and the PPG sensor uses changes in infrared light to detect blood flow. This

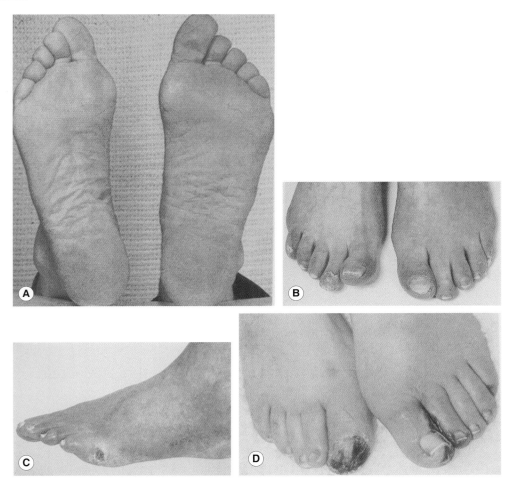

Figure 22.3 Features of critical leg ischaemia. (A) Ischaemic pallor of the sole of the foot. (B) Both feet show changes of ischaemic disease, such as hair loss, skin coarsening and ulceration. (C) Thinning and shininess of the skin around the toes, with ulceration at a pressure point. (D) Patient presenting with rest pain in both feet and gangrenous toes. (Reproduced with kind permission from Bettie Walker, on behalf of William F. Walker, from Walker (1988).)

technique is feasible because distal pedal vessels in people with diabetes are less calcified and incompressible than ankle vessels.

Treadmill assessment

A treadmill is useful in assessing exercise tolerance in patients with intermittent claudication. The patient is asked to walk on the treadmill until they experience claudication pain, and the distance and time are noted. This test can also be combined with a pre- and post-exercise Doppler assessment of the ABPI to confirm diagnosis in patients with a normal resting ABPI. A significant drop

in the ABPI after a treadmill test may indicate an arterial occlusion.

Colour duplex scan

Duplex ultrasonic scanning (US) of the arterial tree with colour flow imaging is a non-invasive technique used to provide more accurate diagnosis of stenosis or occlusion from the aorta to the tibial vessels. The scan demonstrates the direction of arterial or venous blood flow using an ultrasonic probe and displays it as a colour. An increase in velocity of the flow and colour change occur where there is a stenosis. It is usually possible to detect whether a

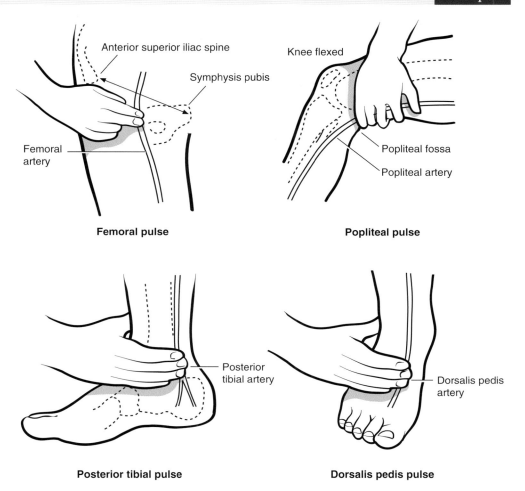

Figure 22.4 Palpation of arterial pulses in lower limb.

lesion is suitable for balloon angioplasty, and, in most centres, duplex scanning has replaced the need for more invasive diagnostic angiography.

The recent three-dimensional US is used for measuring plaque volume, with good intraobserver and interobserver reproducibility. The US has been found to distinguish between the stenosis with a diameter reduction greater than or less than 50% with a sensitivity of 77–82% and a specificity of 92–98% (Hwang, 2017).

Computerized tomography

Three-dimensional computerized tomography (CT) gives detailed information about atherosclerotic calcifications and the extent of arterial stenosis or occlusion. It has some advantages, such as shorter time during examination, and also has

the ability to evaluate the iliac arteries with less operator bias (Hwang, 2017). CT scanning uses a rotating X-ray source, which allows individual slices to be obtained. Spiral CT can also be used and allows continuous rotation while the patient moves through the X-ray beam. A CT scan is useful in the diagnosis of aortic aneurysms, but the contrast medium used can cause problems in patients with impaired renal function.

Magnetic resonance angiography

Magnetic resonance angiography (MRA) is a non-invasive scan. This technique is particularly useful to more accurately detect the size and extent of atheromatous lesions and where patients may be at risk from invasive angiography. MRA is also useful to screen patients for an aortic aneurysm.

451

Angiography

A radio-opaque contrast medium is injected into an appropriate artery, and a series of X-rays is taken of the arteries, demonstrating filling of the vessels and any narrowing or stenosis. A femoral artery approach is normally used to investigate lower limb arteries.

Angiography is usually performed under a local anaesthetic and can be undertaken on a day case basis, depending on the age, social circumstances and clinical condition of the patient. Sedation or general anaesthesia may occasionally be required for very anxious patients. Digital subtraction angiography (DSA) allows greater clarity of the arteries but it has several limitations due to need for an invasive arterial access and associated complications, ionizing radiation and contrast media (Garg et al, 2018). This is a computerized method of angiography without background information, e.g. bones and bowel.

Specific preparation of the patient prior to angiography

- The patient should be fully informed of the length of the procedure and that the injection of dye causes a sensation of heat and some discomfort.
- Fasting is not required prior to angiography. The bladder should be emptied beforehand, as the patient needs to lie very still during angiography.
- Intravenous prophylactic antibiotics will need to be given immediately prior to the procedure in patients with previous synthetic bypass grafts or stents, to prevent infection.
- The nurse may be required to assist the patient prior to the procedure, during the procedure or after the procedure.

Aftercare

- Patients are at risk from haemorrhage, haematoma formation and development of arterial occlusion. Following the procedure, pressure is applied to the puncture site to prevent haemorrhage when the catheter has been removed.
- The patient should be nursed relatively flat in bed and instructed to keep the affected limb straight for 4–6 hours post-procedure, depending on the catheter size used.
- Observations of respiration rate, oxygen saturation, level of consciousness, temperature, pulse rate and blood pressure are undertaken using a National Early Warning Score (NEWS2) system for vital signs:
  - 1/4-hourly for 1 hour
  - 1/2-hourly for 2 hours
  - hourly for 1 hour
  - 4-hourly overnight (non-day care patients).
- Observation of foot pulse, colour, temperature, limb movement and sensation should also be made at these

times and the puncture site carefully monitored for haemorrhage or signs of haematoma formation. The patient should be instructed to call the nurse immediately if any bleeding occurs at the puncture site.
- The patient should be encouraged to drink at least 2 L of fluid in order to flush out the contrast medium from the kidneys.
- At all times the nurse must adhere to local policy and procedure.

Nursing assessment of patients with peripheral vascular disease

Nursing assessments are generally undertaken in a vascular pre-admission clinic for those being admitted for a planned procedure. Patients being admitted to hospital will be experiencing either moderate or severe problems, which may interfere with their activities of living. The impact of the varying stages of the disease is demonstrated within the framework of the Activities of Living model of nursing of Roper, Logan and Tierney (Roper et al, 1981). A functional assessment to identify the patient's self-care ability and lifestyle should be undertaken. Guidelines for these stages of the nursing process, together with planning and implementing care, have been included under each activity. The nurse must adhere to the tenets of the Nursing and Midwifery Council (NMC) (2018) *Code* when planning and providing care, ensuring that the patient is at the centre of all that is done.

Maintaining a safe environment

There is a potential risk of further deterioration in the blood flow to the limbs following admission. Patients with advanced arterial insufficiency are also at risk of developing breaks/ulceration to the skin's integrity, especially the sacrum and heels (Fig. 22.5). This risk is significantly increased in patients with severe ischaemic rest pain who have been immobile and may also have been sleeping in an armchair at night to try to relieve their pain.

Initial limb assessment should be documented (NMC, 2018), and regular observations recorded for patients with severe ischaemia:
- the colour, warmth, sensation and movement of both limbs should be compared
- the dorsalis pedis and posterior tibial pulses should be checked with a Doppler and compared with those in the other limb.

A risk assessment of the patient's skin should be undertaken within 6 hours of admission (NICE, 2014a,b), paying attention to the lower limbs, which will aid in

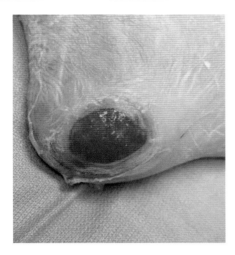

Figure 22.5 Pressure ulceration and gangrene of heel. (From Bhatia, A.C. & Rohrer, T.E. (2005). *Surgery of the skin: procedural dermatology.* Elsevier Inc.)

identifying the high-risk ulcers without delay. The skin should be observed for dryness, infection, oedema, ulceration and gangrenous changes. Detection of any breaks or abnormalities should be reported and documented on a wound assessment chart. Skin ulceration is more commonly found on the toes, malleoli and heels in patients with advanced disease.

An assessment of pressure ulcer risk should be based on clinical judgement and/or the use of validated scales such as the Braden scale, the Waterlow scale or the Norton risk assessment scale (NICE, 2014b). The staff can use an appropriate pressure-relieving mattress, seating and heel protection pad. Patients with rest pain may well present with a high-risk score on admission. Chair nursing should be kept to a minimum and pain relief regularly reassessed to allow the patient to sleep in bed.

All patients presenting with leg ulcers must undergo a full holistic assessment and Doppler assessment to help determine the underlying aetiology of the ulcers.

Communication

Nursing assessment should consider patients' psychosocial needs and also take account of their spiritual, cultural and ethnic requirements. Any social service requirements for home support on discharge, or advice regarding benefit/ mobility allowances, should be assessed and communicated to the appropriate members of the multidisciplinary team, ideally prior to admission to hospital.

Patients may have fears and anxieties about forthcoming procedures. They may also experience varying degrees of pain, which may not be adequately communicated to

the nurse. Patients with severe ischaemia may also fear limb loss as a possible outcome. Social isolation can be a common problem in patients with severe disease affecting their quality of life. The nurse should be aware of factors such as poor mobility, pain, and smoking and drinking habits, which can contribute to a patient's isolation.

Allowing time and privacy for open discussion and providing sufficient information/explanation of proposed procedures will help to allay anxieties. It will also assist patients to make choices about their care and consider any alternatives of treatment. Evaluation of the patient's understanding of their condition is vital to ensuring informed consent and to facilitate active involvement in care and recovery (NMC, 2018). Verbal information should be reinforced where possible with leaflets on various aspects of vascular conditions and treatments; alternative formats should also be made available.

Breathing

Breathing may not be compromised. However, some patients are often lifelong heavy smokers, and this factor, together with restricted mobility in some, will increase the risk of developing chest infections. An increase in respiratory rate and/or production of sputum, as well as any shortness of breath on exertion, should be monitored. Baseline respiratory rate and oxygen saturation levels should be documented.

Eating and drinking

Nutritional and hydration status is a high priority. A baseline admission weight and Body Mass Index (BMI) should be documented. The debilitating effects of severe rest pain and consequent reduced mobility may have resulted in the patient relying on convenience snacks at home. Heavy smokers may also have had appetite suppression, and alcohol intake should be assessed.

Patients with diabetes may require review of their dietary intake, as poorly controlled diabetes will escalate the onset of foot complications and delay postoperative wound healing. Patients who have raised blood cholesterol may also require review of their diet.

A full nutritional assessment by the dietitian will be needed if malnutrition is suspected, as problems such as electrolyte imbalance, delayed wound healing and sepsis can influence the morbidity and mortality of vascular patients.

Eliminating

Poor mobility due to severe ischaemia may prevent the patient from reaching the toilet. Routine urinalysis should be performed to check for glucose, ketones and protein. Urine output should be monitored, as people with vascular conditions frequently have renal impairment.

Constipation may arise in patients with ischaemic pain having regular analgesics, particularly morphine; therefore, the patient should be assessed and an aperient may be prescribed.

Dressing and cleansing

Again, limited mobility and pain may have affected the patient's ability to wash and dress independently.

Controlling body temperature

Temperature on admission should be checked, as elderly patients living alone who have a critically ischaemic limb may have hypothermia. Pyrexia may be an indication of chest, wound or graft infection, or due to limb ulceration or cellulitis.

Mobilizing

Pain is the main factor in reducing the patient's mobility; this is affected to a lesser or greater degree by the extent of the arterial occlusion.

Patients experiencing claudication pain on walking may have only minimal inconvenience to their normal mobility and lifestyle, whereas those affected by rest pain due to severe arterial occlusion and/or ulceration may be totally unable to bear weight on the affected leg.

The following information needs to be obtained during assessment:
- Is the pain related to exercise and is it relieved by resting?
- Does the pain occur in the foot, calf, thigh or buttock on walking, and how far can the patient walk before experiencing pain?
- Does the pain occur at rest and prevent the patient from sleeping at night?
- How has the pain been managed and what analgesics are taken?
- Has the patient had any problems with walking, and have walking aids been required?

Visual pain analogue assessment tools are essential to help establish the severity and type of pain, its effect on the patient and the effectiveness of prescribed analgesics.

Ensure that footwear is appropriate and does not cause undue pressure. This is especially important for diabetes patients, where there is an increased risk due to neuropathy. Special surgical shoes are available to help accommodate wound dressings to the foot.

Working and playing

Depending on severity of symptoms, occupation or hobbies will inevitably be affected in patients with intermittent claudication, whereas reading or watching television may become a strain for those with rest pain.

Sexuality

A male patient with claudication may suffer erectile dysfunction due to internal iliac artery occlusion, and this may also be a complication following surgical repair of an abdominal aortic aneurysm.

Sleeping

Sleep patterns are often disturbed by severe limb pain, either by waking the patient suddenly or by preventing sleep occurring. Hanging the affected limb out of bed or sleeping in an armchair with feet down may provide temporary pain relief but will increase leg oedema.

Dying

Caring for dying patients with advanced vascular disease is challenging due to the complexity of the disease and surgical procedures performed; these patients are potentially associated with substantial morbidity and mortality (Wilson et al, 2017). Some patients may express anxieties regarding proposed major surgery, which may be necessary to save a critically ischaemic limb or prevent stroke or rupture of an aortic aneurysm. A study conducted by Wilson et al (2017) concluded that advanced-stage vascular patients who receive palliative care consultation earlier during the process were less likely to receive mechanical ventilation. This is possibly due to the surgical team and family opting to limit the care and give comfort to the patient who is in the end stage of life.

Management of the patient with intermittent claudication

Patients with intermittent claudication need to adapt their lifestyles to comply with the risk factor modifications previously discussed. Management requires an individualized and holistic approach, focusing on health education and physical and psychosocial needs.

Exercise

Exercise is the mainstay of treatment for patients with claudication and it aids in the development of collateral circulation, which may help prevent ischaemia in the affected leg.

A Cochrane review with 1200 patients from 22 studies demonstrated that an exercise programme with at least two sessions a week can improve the walking distance of vascular patients with claudication by 50–200% (Watson et al, 2008). A Cochrane meta-analysis concluded that a structured exercise programme can have huge benefit on these patients, especially with supervised programmes showing 30–35% greater improvement in walking distance after three months. Therefore, NICE has recommended that all patients with vascular disease with intermittent claudication should be offered a supervised exercise programme during the rehabilitation period (NICE, 2012). Despite the evidence and recommendations, supervised programmes are not readily available in primary or secondary health settings. Some patients may not be willing to wait for symptom improvement with exercise or are more likely to not have access to suitable programmes.

Lifestyle and risk factor management of intermittent claudication

Low socioeconomic status, race, environmental and lifestyle factors are known to be significant risk factors, independent of others, for development of the intermittent claudication which can lead to amputation (Arya et al, 2018). Concordance and control may depend upon a patient's social and cultural situation, which will influence their health behaviour (Ewles & Simnett, 2017).

The role of the nurse in providing holistic care is important, as promoting a healthy lifestyle will enable patients to make lifestyle choices to try to improve their own health and quality of life. Influencing lifelong health beliefs and smoking, eating and exercise habits in this patient group provides a challenge to the nurse. The nurse, whether a novice nurse, nursing associate or an experienced nurse specialist running nurse-led services, will need to gain the patient's active participation in decision-making and actions in order to bring about change to slow disease progression. Factors affecting adherence and understanding of a patient's self-motivation are essential in effecting changed behaviour. Control of this chronic condition and prevention of complications will depend on the careful assessment of the patient's risk factors as discussed earlier, and strategies to manage them, especially smoking.

Medications

Medication concordance is vital, and patients should be advised of the importance of taking medications regularly, such as antihypertensives, diabetes drugs, statins and antiplatelet therapy. The latter medication, such as aspirin combined with clopidogrel, low-molecular-weight heparin, reduces the frequency of thrombotic events in peripheral arteries and reduces overall cardiovascular mortality in claudicants by reducing blood viscosity (Robertson et al, 2012). However, these antiplatelet agents and vasodilators are good in reducing the cardiovascular risk but there is little evidence that these drugs can benefit in treating the symptoms of intermittent claudication (Peach et al, 2012).

NICE 2012 guidelines strongly recommend the use of naftidrofuryl in patients with PAD who have failed to improve with the structured exercise programmes and in patients who do not wish to be referred for angioplasty or surgery. These medications can be prescribed in the primary care, but they should be reviewed after three to six months and discontinued if the patient's symptoms have not improved with this treatment (NICE, 2012).

Stress management

Stress management is also important, as the body's response to life pressures and anxieties is to release adrenaline (epinephrine), which increases the heart rate, blood glucose and cholesterol levels. Consequently, the body becomes stressed, resulting in hypertension, which eventually contributes to the development of atherosclerosis. Offering the patient stress management strategies, such as relaxation techniques, taking regular exercise and avoiding excessive alcohol or food consumption, is equally important.

Pain management

PAD is diagnosed with the persistence of pain; worsening pain is associated with disease progression. It is vital to understand the pathophysiological processes of complex mechanisms which drive the pain in people with vascular conditions. Due to atherosclerotic stenosis to the blood flow in the vessels this leads to muscle ischaemia, increased inflammatory process and subsequently the muscles die off and remodeling of the local nerve endings leads to acute or chronic pain (Seretny & Colvin, 2016). The pain mechanisms – nociceptive, inflammatory and neuropathic – can contribute to the pain but a careful approach needs to be made while choosing the most appropriate analgesic for the patient (Smith et al, 2007).

Nociceptive pain occurs after thermal, chemical or mechanical stimulation of peripheral nociceptors. In people with vascular disease, nociceptive pain is an important element of intermittent claudication, which happens after repeated muscle action or active exercise (Seretny & Colvin, 2016). Inflammatory pain occurs due to the response of the somatosensory nervous system to tissue damage and inflammation. Neuropathic pain results from a lesion or disease of the somatosensory nervous system. Those with vascular conditions with critical limb ischaemia have persistent chronic neuropathic pain (Grone et al, 2014).

Patients with vascular disease with chronic pain are always complex to treat and it is vital to have a multidisciplinary pain management approach. The patient should be treated with maximum pain relief, and regular exercise programmes and activities to improve their quality of life need to be considered as part of the treatment programme (Seretny & Colvin, 2016).

Patient safety checklist before any vascular interventions

Most of the medical errors happen within hospital settings which can be preventable with strict patient safety check measures in place. In 2007, the World Health Organization developed and evaluated a three-stage surgical checklist, demonstrating that surgical infection rates, medical errors and mortality were reduced by using the checklist (Livingston, 2010).

One of the main aims of this checklist is to stop the wrong patient, wrong site or surgical procedures/interventions being carried out due to lack of communications between the multidisciplinary team in the hospital settings (Nagpal et al, 2010). These errors are more frequent in high turnover settings such as day case surgeries, outpatient clinic interventions, etc. The surgical checklist includes five items: team brief (before the patient is brought into theatre), sign in (before induction of anaesthesia), time out (before skin incision), sign out (before the patient leaves the operating room) and the final team brief to avoid any miscommunication. Wrong site surgery is an uncommon event compared to poor communication between the team, and evidence in the literature suggests that communication failures occur every 7–8 minutes and affect up to 30% of interactions in the operating theatres (Hu et al, 2012; Lingard et al, 2004).

It is therefore vital for the team to adhere to hospital policy in carrying out the surgical checklist, which reduces possible errors, promotes teamwork and allows team members to raise concern when there is any problem.

Endovascular intervention

Minimally invasive endovascular intervention treatments are used to open the blocked arteries. The current methods are percutaneous transluminal angioplasty with stenting, endarterectomy, lithoplasty (Shockwave Medical) and Pantheris lumivascular atherectomy.

Percutaneous transluminal angioplasty

Percutaneous transluminal angioplasty (PTA) has become an established treatment for moderate to severe claudication, limb-threatening disease with ischaemic rest pain and to help facilitate healing of ischaemic ulcers. Angioplasty is performed under local anaesthesia and therefore carries a lower overall risk than surgery.

Short stenosis or occlusion of iliac, femoral and popliteal arteries can be effectively treated by angioplasty. The procedure involves the insertion of a balloon catheter, which is passed into the lumen of the vessel, usually via the femoral artery, under local anaesthesia. The catheter is advanced to the site of the atheromatous plaque, and the balloon inflated, dilating the stricture, and hence improving the patency of the lumen of the vessel (Fig. 22.6A).

Other techniques such as atherectomy and insertion of stents can be combined with angioplasty. Atherectomy (Fig. 22.6B) uses high-speed revolving cutters to cut and remove an obstructing thrombus, whereas expandable metal stents with/without drug coating can be inserted to prevent restenosis at the angioplasty site (Fig. 22.6C).

Preparation of the patient prior to percutaneous transluminal angioplasty

- Nursing care and preparation are similar to that provided prior to angiography, except that the patient should be fasted for 2–3 hours prior to the procedure in case complications arise, such as thrombosis/embolus or rupture of the vessel wall, which will require surgical intervention.
- During angioplasty, patients will be required to lie still for a long period of time and therefore will require pressure-relieving aids to prevent skin breakdown of their sacrum and heels if they have severe limb-threatening disease. Pressure on the heel, even for a short time while lying on the X-ray table, can lead to pressure ulceration and necrosis.

Aftercare

- Aftercare is also similar to that following angiography. However, the nurse must be aware of the increased risk of haemorrhage, haematoma or thrombosis, and must report any such occurrences immediately to the surgical team. Pedal pulses should ideally be located using the Doppler ultrasound probe.
- Neurovascular observations are important, such as assessment of the limb for colour, temperature, sensation, movement and pain.
- Assess for abdominal pain, groin pain and back pain including cardiac vital signs (tachycardia, hypotension, etc) to rule out any retroperitoneal bleeding.
- Continued pressure relief for sacrum and heels will be required throughout the period of bedrest in high-risk patients.
- Make sure all the documentation, such as routine observation and continuous monitoring chart, post-anaesthetic observation chart and nursing assessment sheets, is recorded before moving or discharging the patient from the recovery.
- Health education advice should be reinforced before the patient is discharged, and, if necessary, advice given for self-referral to a smoking cessation clinic. Walking exercise should be encouraged to develop collateral circulation.

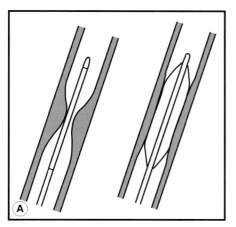

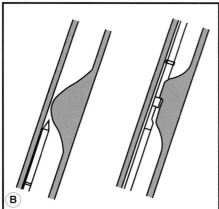

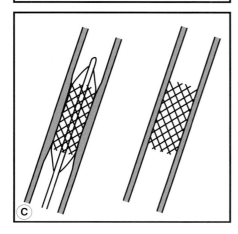

Figure 22.6 (A) Percutaneous transluminal angioplasty. (B) Atherectomy. (C) Stent insertion.

Reconstructive bypass surgery

Patients with ischaemic rest pain, ulceration or gangrenous lesions will require surgical intervention if less invasive treatment is not possible, since, if left untreated, most patients with critical ischaemia will eventually require amputation. The most common cause of claudication is aorto-iliac lesions, which can be treated with endovascular therapy if occlusion is <5 cm of iliac arteries; this gives long-term patency (≥90% over 5 years) with low-risk complications (Indes et al, 2013). For longer occlusion (>5 cm), most hospitals carry out a hybrid procedure which involves endarterectomy and bypass at the femoral level combined with endovascular therapy of iliac arteries. Aorto-bifemoral bypass surgery is indicated if the occlusion extends from the aorta up to the renal arteries, but it is suitable only for fit patients with severe life-limiting claudication (Anderson et al, 2014). If there are no other alternatives, extra anatomic bypass such as axillary to femoral bypass may be considered for extensive lesions, but it is not free of perioperative risk and long-term occlusion (Aboyans et al, 2018).

The other most common occlusion is femoro-popliteal lesions. If there is normal circulation found on the profunda femoral artery, there is no need for any intervention, just exercise therapy is enough. If the occlusion is <25 cm, endovascular therapy should be the first choice, but for better long-term patency surgical bypass with the great saphenous vein should be considered as an option. No direct trials comparing endovascular therapy and surgery are yet available (Aboyans et al, 2018).

Revascularization methods depend on the location and extent of the stenosis/occlusion (Fig. 22.7). Restoring blood flow entails bypassing the stenosed or occluded artery using synthetic graft material or the patient's own long saphenous vein. Patency rates for prosthetic grafts used in narrower more distal arteries in the legs are poor. The operative procedure involves anastomosis of the graft from an area above to an area below the diseased vessel. A vein harvested from the arm can also be used if the leg veins are unsuitable. Due to the presence of valves, the vein is either reversed before insertion, to enable correct direction of blood flow, or the valves are destroyed, and the vein left *in situ*. Synthetic grafts made from polytetrafluoroethylene (PTFE) are now commonly used (Fig. 22.8).

The Zilver PTX trial demonstrated that the 5-year primary patency with conventional and drug-eluting stents was 43% and 66%, respectively (Dake et al, 2016). The 5-year patency after above-the-knee femoro-popliteal bypass is >80% with great saphenous vein and 67% with prosthetic conduits (Klinkert et al, 2004).

Endarterectomy

This is the coring out of the atheromatous plug using a ring stripper inserted into the artery lumen; it is now

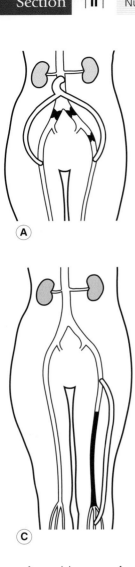

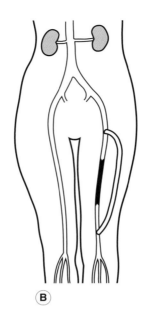

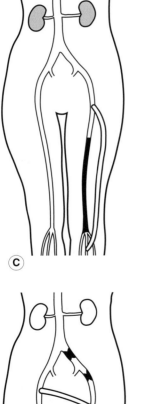

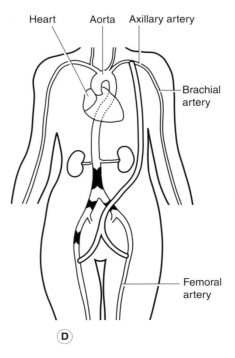

Heart   Aorta   Axillary artery

Brachial artery

Femoral artery

Figure 22.7 Examples of types of reconstructive surgery and types of occlusions: (A) aorto-bifemoral graft; (B) femoro-popliteal bypass; (C) femoro-distal bypass; (D) axillo-bifemoral graft; (E) femoro-femoral crossover graft.

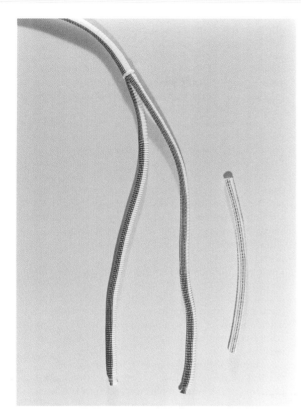

Figure 22.8 Examples of straight and bifurcated axillo-bifemoral PTFE grafts.

more commonly used for common femoral or carotid artery stenosis.

Aorto-bifemoral bypass

This bypass extends from the distal aorta to the common femoral arteries and is performed for stenosis or occlusion of the aorta or iliac vessels, using synthetic graft material. Patients with aorto-iliac disease will often present with bilateral buttock/hip claudication and impotence.

Femoro-popliteal bypass

This bypass is performed for occlusion in the superficial femoral artery.

Femoro-distal artery bypass graft

This bypass is performed for occlusion in distal vessels in patients with severe critical ischaemia who may have accompanying gangrenous lesions in the foot. The graft extends from the femoral artery to either the peroneal or tibial artery in the leg or foot. Distal bypass surgery can be a lengthy and clinically demanding procedure that may also require surgical debridement of gangrenous foot lesions at the end of the arterial reconstruction.

Extra-anatomical bypass graft

Extra-anatomical grafts may be considered for patients who are too unfit for major abdominal surgery and are at risk of limb amputation for critical ischaemia. These synthetic grafts are routed extra-peritoneally through subcutaneous tissue to bypass the diseased vessel. The axillary and femoral arteries lie close to the skin surface, making the procedure more rapid and straightforward than more invasive bypassing. Although this type of bypass is less traumatic for patients, the patency rates are much lower than for aorto-iliac reconstructions for patients with certain co-morbidities, such as advanced age, diabetes, hypertension and ischaemic heart disease (Appleton et al, 2010).

Axillo-bifemoral graft

This graft is performed for aorto-iliac occlusion.

Femoro-femoral crossover graft

This graft is performed for iliac artery occlusion.

Preparation of the patient for bypass surgery

Patients with critical limb ischaemia are at high risk of irreversible ischaemic damage to the leg or foot. It is therefore vital for these patients to be assessed by a vascular multidisciplinary team before making the treatment decision (NICE, 2012); the patient's wishes and aspirations must also be considered. The aim of surgery with critical leg ischaemia should be a pain-free patient with a functioning limb. Primary amputation may need considering as an option if there is severe tissue necrosis which prevents weight-bearing of the foot, fixed flexion deformity of the limb, or in very frail patients with severe medical problems who could not withstand a lengthy anaesthetic. Acquiring informed consent will require lengthy discussion with the patient and relatives (if appropriate), taking into consideration all these factors.

The patient should be fully informed of the bypass technique and the nurse will need to explain all pre- and postoperative care requirements. Due to the complexity of bypass surgery, the use of diagrams as a teaching aid may be useful for explaining the position of the intended grafts.

- Venous mapping using ultrasound technique is undertaken to determine suitability of the patient's saphenous vein as bypass material.

- Psychological support for the patient and their relatives is essential (see Chapter 4). Patients with critical limb ischaemia often experience severe pain at rest, impaired mobility, and loss of independence and control. Patients may have concerns about the progression of the disease and may fear the risk of amputation. It is vital to discuss the management plan, such as recovery with rehabilitation and prosthesis (Aboyans et al, 2018).

- Relief of ischaemic rest pain by adequate analgesics will be necessary. Pain control and rehabilitation should be a priority of care for patients awaiting revascularization to restore blood flow (Aboyans et al, 2018). The impact of pain can vary between patients as pain can be very subjective to the individual. Ischaemic pain is often described as an unbearable, deep burning pain and it affects quality of life. Appropriate pain management needs to adapt, for example the use of either weak or strong opioids depending on the severity of the pain. The nurses need to be observing the bowel pattern of the patients and drugs such as laxatives and anti-emetics can be used to manage the adverse effects of strong opioids (NICE, 2012).

- Nutritional status should be reviewed preoperatively, as a patient with severe ischaemia may be in a malnourished state due to lack of mobility, excessive smoking, severe pain and poor diabetes control. High protein sip feeds should be regularly offered, and a dietician referral made if necessary. Blood glucose levels should be optimized preoperatively in people with diabetes.

- Reassessment of skin, particularly the heels and sacrum, should be undertaken regularly, and appropriate pressure-relieving mattresses provided (NICE, 2014a,b). The size, location and condition of any ulcerated lesions should be clearly documented.

- The weight of bed linen should be kept off limbs by the use of a bed-cradle, and extreme care taken to avoid accidental trauma to the ischaemic limbs. Unlike venous leg ulcers, patients with arterial leg ulceration should not have compression bandaging applied, as this will cause further impairment to the blood supply (Langer, 2014).

- Infection control measures are essential preoperatively. A culture swab should be obtained from any ulcerated lesions, and appropriate antibiotic therapy given if required to minimize the risk of graft infection postoperatively, as this can pose a catastrophic risk to the patient. Many vascular patients have prolonged hospital stays prior to surgery, which will increase their risk of surgical site infections (SSIs).

- Hospital-acquired infection continues to be a major challenge in the NHS, with 300,000 patients a year affected. The human cost is enormous but the financial cost to the NHS is approximately £1−2 billion a year. Many of these infections are preventable; patients should therefore be routinely screened for organisms such as methicillin-resistant *Staphylococcus aureus* (MRSA) and methicillin-sensitive *Staphylococcus aureus* (MSSA) (Thomas, 2018).

- The clinical team should adhere to the local antibiotic guidelines in line with the microbiology and pharmacy protocols for the correct three prophylactic doses. Prophylactic intravenous antibiotics are administered immediately prior to surgery, to prevent graft infection. Antiseptic showers/baths are recommended to help reduce skin microbes preoperatively. Preoperative shaving of nearby areas is no longer recommended. To sterilize the patient's skin, single-use alcoholic chlorhexidine or povidone-iodine need to be used to prevent SSIs (NICE, 2016).

- Deep vein thrombosis (DVT) prophylaxis is usually given in the form of low-molecular-weight heparin and administered in the evening, to avoid the risk of dural haematoma formation if epidural anaesthesia is used. The use of anti-embolism stockings is contraindicated in patients with peripheral arterial occlusive disease.

- Care bundles should be used to improve patient surgical outcomes by putting together evidence-based elements in the surgical pathway, such as antibiotics prophylaxis (in agreement with the local hospital guidelines), no hair removal, normothermia, and good hygiene discipline in the theatre environment (restricted staff numbers, minimal door movements, good theatre ventilation) (Thomas, 2018).

Anaesthetic assessment

In 2014−2015, the NHS carried out 9.9 million operations (Thomas, 2018) and patients undergoing vascular surgery had an increased risk of postoperative cardiovascular adverse complications due to diabetes and smoking risk factors (Smeili & Lotufo, 2015). A full preoperative assessment of the patient's cardiorespiratory and renal function will be required and reviewed by the anaesthetist. Closer monitoring for high-risk patients may necessitate an overnight stay post-operatively on a high-dependency unit.

Immediate aftercare

- The nurse's prime responsibility for the patient after a bypass graft is the early recognition of complications. The patient should be monitored using an NEWS2 system of vital signs.

- Blood pressure and pulse must be monitored half-hourly for 6 hours, then hourly for 12 hours, as hypertension may cause rupture of the anastomosis, and hypotension may reduce patency of the bypass graft.

- Urinary output should be carefully monitored. A urinary catheter will be *in situ* and hourly measurements recorded, as renal impairment is likely in people with vascular conditions, particularly following aortic/iliac bypass where the renal arteries have been clamped in theatre. Depending on the patient, an output of less than 30 mL over 2 consecutive hours should be reported following the EWS protocol. The NEWS2 did not consider that the urine output should be part of the new scoring system because it needs to be tailored to the specific clinical areas (Royal College of Physicians, 2017). The urinary catheter is usually removed by the second or third postoperative day after careful clinical review and once the patient is passing adequate urine with no problems.
- Intravenous fluids are usually given via a central venous line to maintain hydration until the patient is able to drink adequately. Patients who have undergone aortic bypass surgery will require central venous pressure measurement hourly on a high-dependency ward.
- The capillary blood glucose needs to be checked hourly except when it is <5 mmol/L and the sliding scale is stopped. In this case, the glucose level should be checked every 30 minute. 2 hourly blood glucose checks will be required for those with diabetes who normally take insulin or oral hypoglycaemics, until blood glucose levels are stable, and they are able to return to their normal diabetes regimen. A longer sliding scale regimen may be required to optimize wound healing.
- Oxygen is administered as prescribed and pulse oximetry undertaken to measure oxygen saturation levels.
- The limbs should be inspected frequently to detect early signs of ischaemia. Colour, temperature and limb movement should be observed and documented. The foot should be warm and well perfused. Sudden changes in colour, warmth, movement or sensation should be reported immediately. The patient's feet should initially be exposed with the use of a bed-cradle to aid observation, and the heels protected from skin breakdown using pressure-relieving aids. Care should be taken to ensure that the patient's limbs do not knock against the bed-cradle. Peripheral pulses should be located hourly at the dorsalis pedis or posterior tibial using a Doppler probe. The nurse should mark the location of the pulse once identified. Any loss of pulses, or a sudden increase of pain, should be reported immediately to facilitate early intervention. Graft occlusion may have occurred, and graft thrombectomy/embolectomy or further reconstruction may be required. The calf muscle

should be regularly inspected, as reperfusion can occasionally lead to *compartment syndrome*, which would require a fasciotomy to relieve pressure on the microcirculation. Increased calf pain, tenderness, tenseness of the calf muscle and shiny skin accompanied by paraesthesia, or reduced sensation/foot movement should be immediately reported to the surgeons. Two skin incisions are usually made over the calf muscle to split the fascia covering the anterior, lateral and posterior compartments.

- The wound dressing should be checked regularly for any bleeding and if the dressing is wet, and the wound should be inspected for bleeding or haematoma formation. Sudden increase in blood loss through the drainage tubes must also be noted and action taken, as this would indicate rupture of the graft anastomosis.
- Any indication of graft occlusion or rupture of the graft anastomosis constitutes a surgical emergency. The haste of returning the patient to theatre and increase in pain and discomfort will be alarming for the patient. The nurse should ensure that explanations of the need for returning to theatre are calmly and carefully explained to the patient and relatives to allay anxiety.
- Once haemodynamically stable, the patient can be sat upright and encouraged to deep breathe to aid lung expansion and perform gentle foot exercises to help prevent DVT.
- Pain should be assessed, and prescribed analgesics administered regularly, to enable the patient to cooperate with physiotherapy. Epidural or patient-controlled analgesia (PCA) is recommended for effective pain relief for 24−48 hours or until the patient is able to take regular oral analgesics.
- Prophylactic intravenous antibiotics will be prescribed to prevent infection of the graft.
- Paralytic ileus may be present in patients who have had aortic grafts, and therefore the stomach should be kept empty by nasogastric tube aspiration. The patient will be allowed sips of water only. Fluids and diet will be gradually reintroduced as bowel sounds return.
- A nutritious diet should be encouraged to aid wound healing, as soon as the patient is able to eat and drink. High-protein sip feeds will be required for most patients, particularly those who have undergone aortic bypass surgery, who may experience temporary appetite loss.
- Mobility is encouraged 24−48 hours postoperatively, gradually increasing walking distances, although this will depend on the patient's general condition. Regular evaluation of pain relief is essential to allow early mobilization. Patients can sit out of bed after 24 hours postoperatively and should elevate their legs on a footstool following limb bypass surgery, to prevent occlusion of grafts behind the knee. Elevation of feet

when sitting will also help to relieve swelling, as minor reperfusion oedema following reconstructive surgery is common. Lengthy periods of chair sitting should be avoided to prevent pressure ulcer development. DVT prophylaxis with low-molecular-weight heparin is continued. Anti-embolism stockings should not be applied to patients following limb reconstructive surgery unless instructed by the surgeon under strict supervision: they are not recommended for patients with an ABPI of less than 0.7.

- Wound vacuum drains are normally removed 24−48 hours postoperatively.
- A non-adherent clear wound dressing applied in theatre can be left *in situ* for up to 48 hours. If the dressing becomes heavily bloodstained or soiled, it should be replaced, and the wounds should then be inspected for signs of inflammation, avoiding unnecessary handling or contamination of the wound. Otherwise, the clear wound dressing needs to be left *in situ*. The groin wounds are particularly susceptible to infection, especially in those patients who have a high BMI and there is an increased risk of graft infection in these patients. Attention to hygiene in the skin folds of the groin will help to reduce this risk. Sutures should be removed after 12−14 days. Restrictive dressings and compression bandages should not be used on wounds or ulcers on the patient's legs.
- Delayed wound healing despite successful bypass surgery can pose challenges for patients and increases the workload of vascular nurses. Surgical debridement of ulcerated lesions or minor amputation of necrotic toes or tissue lesions may also be required. Frequent assessment of the wound/ulcers and the use of appropriate wound care products, as discussed in Chapter 5, will help to optimize wound healing.
- The use of negative pressure wound therapy has been shown to be successful in reducing wound oedema, improving tissue perfusion and stimulating cell growth at the amputated wound surface; it also encourages the patients to do their physical exercises without fear of injuring the wound (Wise et al, 2017).
- Suitable footwear to accommodate dressings of foot wounds as well as ongoing chiropody and foot care advice, particularly for people with diabetes, should be arranged. Ongoing nutritional support and blood glucose control in those with diabetes is essential to aid healing of challenging wounds postoperatively.
- A case study of a patient undergoing a femoral to distal popliteal bypass is demonstrated in Box 22.2.

Discharge planning

Pre-admission assessment may have identified problems, especially in elderly patients whose mobility may temporarily be more limited after having undergone major bypass surgery.

The main reasons for delay in discharge from hospital to home have remained constant over 20 years regardless of having national guidelines (Shepperd et al, 2013). The majority of delayed discharges from hospital are preventable by having good planning and involvement of effective multidisciplinary team input (Wariyapola et al, 2016).

The multidisciplinary team, in liaison with the patient and patient's relatives or carers, should agree a provisional discharge date and inform community services. A home assessment may be required by the occupational therapist and social worker before discharge.

Health promotion and discharge advice

- Risk factor modification and lifestyle changes have previously been discussed. However, these factors, especially in relation to smoking cessation and foot care, must be re-emphasized to the patient and relatives before discharge. Explanations must be given as to why each risk factor is dangerous and that stopping smoking will increase graft patency (Aboyans et al, 2018). Walking exercise should be encouraged following discharge, as this will also help to maintain graft patency and improve collateral circulation.
- Aspirin or other antiplatelet therapy is usually prescribed to prevent platelet aggregation, improve graft patency and reduce the risk of having a heart attack or stroke. The importance of continuing to take this, along with other medications, e.g. antihypertensive and statin therapy, should be explained.
- Patients should be advised to inform any dentist or doctor they may consult that they have had an artificial graft bypass, as prophylactic antibiotic cover may be required prior to any invasive procedure.
- Information leaflets are recommended to help reinforce patient education and concordance following discharge; other formats should also be made available, such as Braille or large print. Healthcare professional emergency on-call team contact telephone numbers should be included and the patient instructed to make contact in the event of any sudden coolness, numbness or increased pain to the limb, which may indicate graft occlusion.
- Graft surveillance using duplex scanning is recommended following discharge, every 3−4 months for the first two years and then twice a year with ABI/toe pressures for early detection of graft failure in patients who have had vein grafts (McCallum et al, 2017). The importance of this procedure needs to be explained to the patient during the preoperative preparation.

Box 22.2 **Case study of a patient undergoing femoral-distal popliteal bypass graft**

Margaret is 86 years old and lives alone in a ground-floor flat. She was referred by her GP to the vascular outpatient clinic with an ischaemic right leg. For 2 months Margaret had been experiencing pain at night in her right foot, requiring her to hang her leg out of bed in the dependent position. She was also having pain while resting during the day and had developed small ulcerated lesions on her right second and third toes during the last 2 weeks. For 2 years previously, Margaret had been having intermittent claudication in her right calf and her walking distance had reduced to 50 m in the last 3 months.

Until her admission to hospital, Margaret had been able to cook for herself with the aid of her daughter, who undertook shopping for her and lived only 1 mile away. Margaret was finding this increasingly difficult immediately prior to admission owing to pain in her foot which made mobilizing more difficult. Apart from a 20-year history of hypertension treated with nifedipine, and a right total hip replacement 12 years previously, her past medical history was otherwise unremarkable. She had a 30-year history of smoking but had quit in her mid 50s.

On admission, Margaret was noted to be experiencing considerable pain, which initially required dihydrocodeine 30 mg 4-hourly, and paracetamol 1 g 6-hourly. Margaret was still unable to sleep at night due to increasing pain, and was having to get out of bed to sleep in a chair. On her second night in hospital, oral morphine 10 mg was also prescribed 2–3-hourly for breakthrough pain. Margaret was then requiring two to three doses a day and now needed assistance to walk to the bathroom due to increasing drowsiness and unsteadiness in her gait. She had no palpable pulses below her right femoral pulse and her ABPI was 0.25 for her right leg, and 0.70 for her left leg.

A duplex scan revealed a right 50–75% stenosis of the superficial femoral artery and an occlusion of the popliteal artery, which appeared amenable to angioplasty. An angioplasty of the popliteal artery was attempted via a femoral artery approach, but an attempt to re-enter the artery beyond the popliteal occlusion was unsuccessful and the procedure was abandoned. Margaret's pain became considerably worse following the attempted angioplasty, requiring an increase in morphine to four doses daily in addition to regular dihydrocodeine and paracetamol. Her foot became increasingly cyanosed with onset of gangrene to the second toe, indicating that urgent intervention was now required.

Margaret's case was discussed at the multidisciplinary team meeting, where it was felt that reconstructive bypass surgery was the only option left to prevent limb loss. This proposed operation was discussed at length with Margaret and her daughter with the aid of diagrams. Both Margaret and her daughter agreed that surgery was urgently required the following day to restore blood flow in an attempt to reduce her pain and prevent limb amputation. They were warned that despite bypass surgery it would not be possible to save her second toe. Duplex vein mapping was undertaken to assess the suitability of Margaret's long saphenous vein, which would be required for the bypass graft material.

The following day, Margaret underwent a 5-hour operation for a right femoral to distal popliteal bypass using *in situ* long saphenous vein for the graft material. Two vacuum drains were inserted to both the femoral and popliteal wounds. Due to the length of anaesthetic, Margaret was monitored overnight on the high dependency unit. Margaret's pain control was changed to PCA and her vital signs remained stable overnight. She had no palpable pedal pulses but monophasic signals could be heard with the Doppler probe at the dorsalis pedis. Margaret was transferred back to the ward the following morning and her pain was controlled satisfactorily enough to allow her to be recommenced on regular non-opioid analgesics and the PCA stopped after 48 hours.

Margaret made excellent progress postoperatively. The drains were removed the next day and her foot became warm and well perfused. Her pain was now well controlled and she was sleeping well at night. By the fourth day following surgery, Margaret was able to mobilize independently with a walking stick and an occupational therapy assessment was undertaken and a discharge date set for 10 days postoperatively. A duplex ultrasound scan was arranged prior to discharge, which confirmed the bypass graft had remained patent. The ulcerated lesion on her third toe had shown signs of healing and the gangrenous second toe was dry and mummified. Her wound staples were removed prior to discharge. Margaret and her daughter were warned that the gangrenous toe was expected to auto-amputate after discharge. A community nurse was arranged to dress her toes on alternate days following discharge and a follow-up outpatient appointment was made for 6 weeks. Immediately prior to her outpatient appointment, the gangrenous toe had auto-amputated, leaving healthy granulating tissue at the base, and complete healing had occurred of the third toe. A repeat duplex ultrasound was arranged for 3 months following surgery.

Lithoplasty (Shockwave Medical)

This technique combines a balloon angioplasty catheter with the use of sound waves, as used for removal of kidney stones. Studies have demonstrated that calcified stones are more difficult to break, and drug-coated balloons and stents are less effective (Brodmann et al, 2017). The sound waves are produced by the emitters, which are embedded inside the lithoplasty catheter and help to break the superficial and deeper calcifications before inflating the angioplasty balloon. Fracturing the calcification using sound waves allows less pressure on the expansion of the balloon with minimal damage to the arterial wall (Topfer & Spry, 2018).

Pantheris lumivascular endarterectomy system (Avinger, Inc)

This system uses optical coherence tomography (OCT), which is an imaging technology that uses light to provide 3D visual guidance during the endarterectomy procedure (Schwindt et al, 2017). Using this system allows the operator to remove the calcification with less damage to the arterial wall. This system uses less contrast and reduces exposure to the radiation compared with the traditional fluoroscopic imaging guidance. The manufacturer recommends that this procedure is safe for patients with kidney disease compared to the fluoroscopic technique. This Pantheris catheter is 135 cm long with an optical fibre component for the OCT, and the nose cone of the catheter collects all the excised calcification and the tissue from the artery (Topfer & Spry, 2018).

Acute leg ischaemia

Acute leg ischaemia is common in elderly people and requires urgent diagnosis and treatment to restore blood flow to the affected leg in order to prevent limb loss. It can result from thrombotic or embolic event or due to traumatic arterial occlusion. Misdiagnosis of acute leg ischaemia is very common – the Medical Defence Union (MDU) and the Medical Protection Society (MPS) have identified almost 224 cases that resulted in limb loss over a 10-year period (Shearman & Shearman, 2012). Most of the time, misdiagnoses occur due to inconsistent clinical diagnosis and assessment and it is not considered a surgical emergency (Brearley, 2013). Thrombosis of a pre-existing atheromatous plaque is a more common cause of acute lower limb ischaemia than is an embolus.

Signs and symptoms

Classic features frequently associated with the sudden onset of acute ischaemia are the 'six Ps': Pain (always present, persistent), Pallor (cyanosis or mottling), Pulselessness (always present; can you count it?), Paraesthesia (reduced sensation or numbness), Paralysis (reduced power) and Perishing cold (poikilothermia). However, these symptoms may be subtle, so it is vital to compare left and right legs (Brearley, 2013). The limb-threatening symptoms for acute leg ischaemia are reduced muscular power and reduced sensation in the limb (Brearley, 2013).

Diagnosis

The diagnosis of acute leg ischaemia can be done very quickly, simply and reliably by measuring the ankle blood pressure with a pocket Doppler machine and a blood pressure cuff (NICE, 2012). The absence of Doppler signals indicates a threatened limb and requires urgent vascular referral which is mandatory (Brearley, 2013).

A medical history and careful assessment may help elicit an obvious cause of acute ischaemia, although it is not always easy to determine whether acute ischaemia is embolic or thrombotic. If an embolus is suspected, an ECG and urgent abdominal ultrasound may be required. An urgent angiogram or duplex ultrasound, magnetic resonance angiography, computed tomographic angiography or intra-arterial angiography can be ordered to form a basis for treatment planning (NICE, 2012).

Thrombosis

Thrombosis is the commonest cause of acute ischaemia. *In situ* thrombosis can occur on an atherosclerotic stenosis in a patient with a history of claudication, or in a pre-existing bypass graft. Other causes of thrombosis/thromboembolism include clotting disorders (e.g. malignancy), drug-induced thrombosis (e.g. contraceptive pill) (Ramot et al, 2013) or following radiation therapy (Guy et al, 2017). The resulting symptoms are often less severe than from an embolic source, as collateral blood vessels may have developed.

Embolism

An embolism is a thrombus which becomes detached from the left atrium, left ventricle or from an atheromatous abdominal aorta. The embolus travels in the bloodstream and eventually lodges at a major arterial bifurcation such as the common femoral or popliteal arteries. Emboli can become lodged in any vessel, but the lower limbs are more commonly affected.

Management of the patient with acute leg ischaemia

Those with acute leg ischaemia must be discussed and action taken by a vascular surgeon as soon as possible. Even a few hours' delay can make the difference between death or amputation and complete recovery of limb function, and can affect postoperative outcomes (Norlyk et al, 2013; Adams & Lakra, 2018).

Patients are generally categorized into two groups based on the severity of the ischaemia (Earnshaw et al, 2001; Callum & Bradbury, 2000).

- *Acute critical ischaemia* (ischaemia <14 days)
  - No audible ankle Doppler signal *with neurosensory deficit.* These patients require very urgent treatment on the day of admission, e.g. surgical embolectomy or urgent vascular opinion and angiography.

- *Acute subcritical ischaemia* (worsening signs and symptoms <14 days)
  - Patients have ischaemic rest pain, with audible ankle Doppler signal and *no neurosensory deficit*. These patients require prompt intervention, but more time is available to investigate, allowing intravenous heparinization overnight and vascular opinion/angiography the following day.
- *Chronic critical ischaemia* (ischaemia stable for >14 days).

Embolectomy

Embolectomy is undertaken to remove limb-threatening occlusions and may be performed under local anaesthesia to reduce cardiac morbidity. The procedure requires insertion of a balloon-tipped Fogarty catheter after exposure of the artery at the level of obstruction. The uninflated balloon is gently passed proximally and distally within the artery and inflated. The balloon is then partially deflated and pulled through the artery to extract the embolus and any propagated thrombus via the arteriotomy. An arteriogram should be performed to confirm that there is no remaining embolus in the vessel. Fasciotomy is frequently performed with embolectomy to prevent compartment syndrome.

Preparation of the patient

- The patient will need to be prepared for an emergency surgical procedure. This should be calmly and carefully explained to the patient and relatives to allay anxiety.
- Intravenous heparin will be commenced to reduce the risk of further thromboembolic episodes and may be temporarily discontinued immediately prior to surgery to prevent haemorrhage.
- Regular analgesics will be required to help alleviate pain preoperatively.

Aftercare

Postoperative observations and care are similar to those for patients having bypass grafting.

- Minor leg swelling is not uncommon postoperatively. However, severe swelling, paraesthesia, reduced/absent pedal pulses and red, glossy skin in patients without fasciotomy would indicate compartment syndrome. If this increased pressure is not relieved, necrosis and gangrene can occur. The nurse must carefully observe for this and report any occurrence immediately. Other signs and symptoms of compartment syndrome include increased pain when stretching the leg muscles, muscle herniation, muscle weakness, passive dorsiflexion of the foot and foot drop (Kiel & Kaiser, 2019).
- Calf fasciotomy wounds may be dressed with an alginate and secondary dressing until healed. However, larger wounds benefit from topical negative pressure dressings or possibly skin grafting to hasten healing.
- A Roylan foot support splint can be used immediately postoperatively to help prevent or correct foot drop, and regular flexion and extension exercises encouraged.
- Intravenous heparin will be recommenced, and the patient will then be converted on to oral anticoagulants (warfarin). Activated partial thromboplastin time (APTT) levels are monitored regularly, to prevent bleeding from over-administration, or further embolism from under-administration of anticoagulants. The APTT is maintained between 1.5 and 3.5. Heparin administration should be stopped if the APTT result is >7 and the medical staff informed immediately.
- The source of the emboli will need investigation by an echocardiogram and a cardiology opinion may be sought. Long-term warfarin therapy will be reviewed after 3 months.
- A vacuum wound drain may be *in situ* and can be removed 24–48 hours postoperatively. Sutures will be removed 10–12 days postoperatively.

Management of the patient requiring lower limb amputation

Amputation of a limb is one of the oldest surgical procedures recorded in the world. The traumatic amputation and the use of prothesis is found written in Sanskrit texts dating from 1800 to 3500 BC. There are almost 5500 lower limb amputations carried out in England alone every year (National Confidential Enquiry into Patient Outcomes and Death, 2014).

Amputation of a leg is a destructive but sometimes necessary outcome for patients with critical limb ischaemia. It is essential that amputation is viewed as a positive way of improving a patient's quality of life and is often the most effective means of relieving the pain and suffering they may have been experiencing for many months. It is estimated that there were around 25,312 major limb amputations and 136,215 revascularizations across England between 2003 to 2009. Approximately 90% of these were as a result of peripheral vascular disease with risk factors of diabetes (44%), hypertension (39%) and coronary heart disease (23%) (Ahmad et al, 2014).

Each patient needs to be assessed individually, when a decision is made as to whether a bypass operation or amputation is the more appropriate action. The decision to amputate is based on a number of factors and would only be taken if the patient's quality of life cannot be improved by saving their leg, i.e. severe uncontrollable pain, a non-healing, infected, gangrenous ulcer and immobility. The patient with peripheral vascular disease may already be in hospital following failed bypass surgery or may have been coping at home with conservative management until amputation became necessary. Either way, the patient and relatives will probably be familiar with the health professionals involved in their care, and a rapport established. However, some patients will present as an emergency with acute leg ischaemia requiring immediate amputation and will have been denied the time to consider the reality of their situation before amputation is performed.

Amputation cases should be discussed with and involve multiple healthcare providers, ultimately including the surgeon and the patient. Giving consent to amputation requires courage, and helping the patient make an informed choice is vital at this stage. Some patients who are experiencing severe pain will readily accept the need for surgery without delay, whereas others will need more time to reach a decision. In some patients, a decision for surgery will often follow discussion with family members because the patient may be unable to make a rational decision, as a result of confusion from associated sepsis due to gangrene, or because of the effects of strong analgesics to maintain the patient's comfort. In such cases, a final decision will be the surgeon's responsibility, made in collaboration with the patient's family and other members of the multidisciplinary team involved in the patient's care. Occasionally, a patient may refuse or postpone a decision to undergo amputation. The practitioner supporting a person's decision-making should respect these wishes if the patient is fully informed of the possible risks involved in delaying surgery or seek advice to ensure the patient has the capacity to make this decision (NICE, 2018a).

Level selection for amputation

The level of amputation will be discussed with the patient and is determined by the extent of ischaemia, the level at which healing is likely to take place and the patient's mobility and general health (Fig. 22.9). The primary aim of amputation is to remove sufficient diseased, infected and gangrenous tissue to allow stump healing, while at the same time retaining adequate limb length for a prosthesis. The two major amputations performed for critical ischaemia are above-knee (transfemoral) and below-knee (transtibial). Diabetes is a major cause of all amputations in England; there are 5000 major amputations (over 90%) undertaken in England every year (Ahmad et al, 2016) in contrast with 3500 lower limb amputations carried out every year in the USA (Adams & Lakra, 2018). The physiotherapist should be actively involved in this decision, following assessment of functional ability, and in the rehabilitation programme. The introduction of a multidisciplinary prosthetic programme

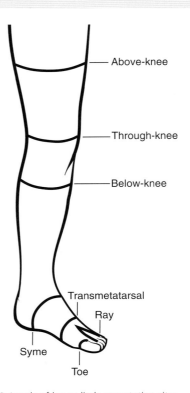

Figure 22.9 Levels of lower limb amputation sites.

for the elderly dysvascular men with transtibial amputation can reduce the time to all primary rehabilitation outcomes, including time to wound healing, initial prosthetic casting, and independent walking (Hordacre et al, 2012)

It is paramount to have close communications across all healthcare disciplines before commencing below-knee amputation. The initial work-up needs to begin in the emergency department or local clinic to recognize whether it is an emergency or elective surgical procedure. The complete assessment of the full clinical picture – vital signs, thorough examinations, assessment of full blood tests, lactic acid, base deficit, blood cultures and radiographic imaging – should be carried out. The surgical services should include orthopedics, general surgery or vascular surgeon with the anaesthetic surgical team. There should be a clear discussion carried out regarding prosthetic devices and postoperative pain, starting with devices such as stump shrinker, limb protector and knee immobilizer (Adams & Lakra, 2018).

Toe, transmetatarsal and metatarsal

Toe, transmetatarsal or metatarsal (Ray) amputations can be performed for localized toe or foot gangrene. Patients requiring this surgery may also require an arterial bypass to increase blood flow and aid wound healing. Suturing of these wounds is usually avoided due to poor skin flap healing or infection. The wound is left to granulate and epithelialize using either an alginate cavity-filling dressing and secondary dressing, or topical negative pressure to hasten healing.

Syme's

This amputation is not commonly performed in patients with ischaemic disease. It involves a disarticulation through the ankle joint at the lower end of the tibia.

Below-knee

This amputation has the advantage of preserving the knee joint, which helps with mobilization and limb fitting.

Through-knee

This amputation is a less traumatic procedure than above-knee amputation, when a below-knee procedure is not possible, as no bony structures need to be divided during surgery. However, this type of amputation is rarely performed, as difficulties can arise with limb fitting.

Above-knee

This amputation can be performed in patients who are likely to have stump healing problems with below-knee wounds.

Hindquarter (hip disarticulation)

Hindquarter amputation may be indicated for severe aorto-iliac ischaemia and involves disarticulation at the hip. This procedure is generally only performed as a life-saving operation.

Preparation of the patient for amputation

Pre- and postoperative care of the patient and their family or carers requires setting short- and long-term goals using a team approach. This will include input from nurses, surgeons, physiotherapist, occupational therapist, social worker, dietitian, prosthetist and counsellor.

Psychosocial preparation

Amputation of a limb is a stressful event for the patient, involving a major life change (see Chapter 7). Reactions will depend upon the patient's personality, cultural and life experience, and also the significance of the limb loss. A patient who may have suffered with a painful, immobile limb for many weeks or months may be able to adjust to the reality of amputation and the relief it will bring. A major responsibility of the nurse is to help the patient develop coping strategies. The loss of a limb takes away the patient's freedom and they feel their mobility is restricted and their independence lost. It is vital to provide complementary care and stress the importance of an increased awareness of the psychosocial and existential consequences of losing a limb (Norlyk et al, 2013). Special attention should be given to the postoperative patient's mental status, which should include potential need for psychiatric evaluation and care (Adams & Lakra, 2018).

Assessment may reveal a very positive attitude in some patients who have a supportive family, whereas another patient may have less family support and may feel very isolated and negative about the future. A preoperative visit to the local limb-fitting centre and a visit from another amputee patient may also offer some positive support.

Patients must be fully informed about what to expect after the operation as well as what to expect regarding their rehabilitation, both physically and emotionally. Allowing patients to make an informed choice is critical in helping them accept the need for amputation. A preoperative environmental visit to the patient's home by the occupational therapist is recommended if time allows, to aid discharge planning at an early stage.

Physiological preparation

Pain control

Pain management is often very complicated in surgical amputees due to the presence of polypharmacy and severe comorbidities, which include ischaemic heart disease and renal compromise. These patients remain a high-risk patient group with a 22% 30-day mortality from emergency surgery (Neil, 2016). Failure to optimize acute pain control can lead to detrimental pathophysiological stress response for the patient, functional recovery and predisposes to chronic stump and phantom pain (Neil, 2016). Opioid analgesics should be administered by regular oral, epidural or patient-controlled analgesia. Phantom limb pain and sensations should be discussed with patients preoperatively, reassuring them that this is normal following amputation. These feelings may vary from tingling sensations to a more unpleasant sensation resembling the pain felt in the limb prior to amputation.

If no regional anaesthesia is available, the stump pain should be managed by strong opioids as baseline pain management. Due to sedative side-effects of opioids, sometimes adjuvant analgesics such as intravenous ketamine are used to control the pain (Neil, 2016). Normally, the acute stump pain resolves in the first few weeks after amputation; however, approximately 10% of patients experience persistent stump pain requiring pain management through a multidisciplinary team approach (Neil, 2016).

Nutritional status and pressure ulcer risk

Nutritional status and pressure ulcer risk should be reassessed due to the patient's reduced mobility and pain. High-protein drinks should be encouraged, and a review of blood glucose control should be undertaken in diabetes.

Physiological care following amputation

- Blood pressure, pulse and respiratory rate must be regularly monitored on return from theatre for early detection of haemorrhage or respiratory complications.
- Oxygen therapy is administered overnight, and saturation levels monitored.
- Intravenous fluids are administered to prevent dehydration until the patient is able to drink adequately. Frail, elderly patients may need an infusion over a longer time period if they are unable to drink adequate amounts orally to maintain hydration over the first few days.
- Urine output is monitored to ensure the patient is adequately hydrated. A urinary catheter may be *in situ* until the patient is more mobile and able to use a bed pan or commode/toilet.
- The dietitian may need to see the patient, as malnutrition can prevent wound healing and development of pressure ulcers.
- Blood glucose control in people with diabetes is essential to aid stump healing.
- Deep breathing exercises should be encouraged hourly to prevent chest infection, and thromboprophylaxis with low-molecular-weight heparin is given to prevent DVT or pulmonary embolism.
- Postoperative pain will need reassessing and appropriate analgesics administered regularly. Epidural or patient-controlled analgesia should continue until regular oral morphine is tolerated.
- 80% of amputees feel phantom limb pain and at least 75% of patients develop phantom pain within the first week after amputation (Neil, 2016). Uncontrolled phantom limb pain or sensation may cause the patient some distress. It is typically felt in the distal extremity of the absent limb and patients often describe it as cramping, burning or even shooting in nature. These sensations of the limb still being present are often so vivid that the patient may even attempt to walk on the missing limb. Reassurance will need to be given that these are normal sensations which will decrease or disappear; however, this may take time (Neil, 2016).
- Non-analgesic medication can also be used in conjunction with conventional analgesics such as

morphine to help reduce phantom limb pain and sensation. The most common medications used in acute management of phantom limb pain are tricyclic antidepressants, gabapentin, salmon calcitonin, clonidine, and NMDA antagonists (ketamine, memantine), but the approach to these patients' pain management should be multidisciplinary/multimodal (Neil, 2016).

Care of the stump

- The stump dressing should be observed for signs of haemorrhage on return from theatre and should ideally be left undisturbed for a minimum of 3 days. Severe pain or pyrexia may necessitate earlier wound inspection for signs of infection or stump ischaemia.
- Staples, sutures or Steri-Strips or a combination of these are used for wound closure and are removed 14–21 days postoperatively.
- To facilitate fitting of the prosthesis, the ideal stump shape should be conical. Incorrect stump bandaging performed by an inexperienced nurse will lead to poor stump shape and delays in limb fitting. Tight bandages must not be used, as patients with vascular disease are especially at risk from stump ischaemia, and a poorly applied stump bandage will contribute to this. Therefore, the application of a light tubular support bandage in theatre, e.g. Tubifast, applied double over a sterile wound dressing, is recommended instead of bandaging, as this will reduce oedema and promote healing.
- A bed-cradle will help prevent bed clothes resting directly on the stump wound.
- Vacuum drains are removed 24–48 hours postoperatively.
- Prophylactic antibiotics are given to prevent wound infection.
- When the stump has healed, a Juzo stump sock can be applied by the patient to give support and reduce oedema 2–3 weeks postoperatively.
- Longer-term stump care includes daily bathing of the stump and application of a moisturizing cream. Stump socks should be changed daily, and the patient should not wear the prosthesis if an ulcer develops and should contact their limb-fitting centre as soon as possible.

Mobility and rehabilitation

Rehabilitation will commence on the first postoperative day to enable patients to feel more independent and self-confident at an early stage if their general condition allows. Patients are encouraged to provide as much self-care as possible to maintain their independence in daily living activities. Help and assistance with toilet or commode transfers will be required, ensuring the patient's privacy is maintained until they can transfer independently. Patients should also be encouraged to wear comfortable day clothes as soon as possible after the operation, which will help them regain their self-esteem.

Dynamic stump exercises will be taught by the physiotherapist. Patients who have had a below-knee amputation should be encouraged to exercise and completely extend the knee hourly on the first postoperative day, to help prevent a flexion contracture developing. Full hip extension exercises are also taught and encouraged, to prevent hip contracture, as the risk of muscle contracture is increased in patients who spend long periods of time lying or sitting postoperatively.

A wheelchair should be provided on the first or second postoperative day to promote independence. The patient is taught how to safely transfer to and from the wheelchair, and a slide board and other mobility devices may be required. The physiotherapist and occupational therapist will assess sitting and standing balance and teach arm/leg strengthening exercises and wheelchair mobility. It is important to take patients to the gym as soon as possible following surgery, to help them regain their confidence. Walking training in the parallel bars is practiced daily to regain balance. Hopping with crutches is not recommended for new amputees, as this can be both unsafe and tiring for the patient. This practice can also prevent reduction of stump oedema and may also cause an abnormal gait.

It is important for the physiotherapist and occupational therapist to establish at an early stage whether the patient will be able to cope safely with mobilizing on an artificial limb, as this will require strength, free joint movement and an efficient cardiopulmonary system. This decision should be made after ascertaining what the patient's expectations of rehabilitation are and if limb fitting is a realistic option. In some vascular patients with arthritis, eyesight problems or cardiopulmonary insufficiency, aiming for wheelchair independence is often a more realistic rehabilitation choice.

Mobilization with an early walking aid, known as a pneumatic post-amputation mobility aid (Fig. 22.10) (or similar mobility aid), should commence after 7 days, and a temporary limb prosthesis can be fitted within 3–4 weeks.

The occupational therapist will assess and teach the patient how to regain independence with everyday activities, e.g. washing and dressing practice, bathing, kitchen activities, hobbies and work skills.

Limb-fitting referral

An appointment will be made with the local limb-fitting centre for prosthetic limb fitting if appropriate. The initial assessment will be made when the stump has healed,

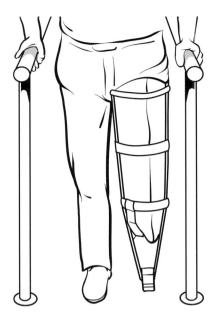

Figure 22.10 Pneumatic post-amputation mobility aid.

sutures have been removed and swelling has reduced, and when the patient is competent using an early walking aid. The design, construction and fitting techniques of prostheses have become very sophisticated over the last few years. The prosthesis is selected to meet the individual's requirements and can be dressed in accordance with the amputee's taste of shoes, socks or stockings, so as to look cosmetically attractive. A referral can also be made for a cosmetic prosthesis if the amputee is unsuitable for a walking prosthesis.

A patient will often experience initial discomfort with their prosthesis, and regular visits to the prosthetist at the centre will be required until the limb fits correctly. If they are able to manage at home in a wheelchair, arrangements can be made for the patient to continue walking training on an outpatient basis, until they achieve independence with the prosthesis.

Psychological support

Ongoing psychosocial support for the amputee and their family is required for many months following amputation. The patient may continue to express grief over the loss of their leg and will have alteration in their body image. All patients must be given adequate counselling, and this is particularly important for patients who have undergone an emergency amputation. The nurse has an important role to play and can assist the patient to adjust to this loss by encouraging open communication with the patient, relatives and health professionals. Some denial and anger may be shown by the patient towards the nurses, physiotherapist and relatives. Postoperatively, the patient may initially wish to hide the stump under bedclothes until they feel able to cope with looking at and touching their stump. The nurse should allow the amputee opportunity to express their feelings and concerns. Praise of the positive accomplishments achieved by the patient will also help them feel more positive about the future, bearing in mind that full acceptance of such a major alteration of their body image will require time.

Discharge planning

Discharge planning will ideally have commenced prior to surgery. A home environment assessment will be carried out by the social worker and occupational therapist. Plans can be made for discharge when the patient is wheelchair-independent or safely using their prosthesis. Home adaptations, rehousing or even consideration for residential or nursing care may be necessary for some patients. Weekend leave or a day out at home, prior to discharge, may help the patient and their family adapt to the reality of leaving the protective hospital environment.

Some patients may want to return to work if appropriate and will need to discuss this with their GP and employer. All patients, particularly those with diabetes, should also be given advice on care of their remaining limb and may require podiatry or specialist foot clinic follow-up.

Advice and support for smoking cessation and medication concordance to reduce risk factors for further complications should be reiterated. If patients wish to continue driving, their doctor will tell them when they are able to do so again. They will also need to inform the Driver and Vehicle Licensing Agency (DVLA) of their disability, who will advise them of how to adapt the car to a satisfactory standard.

Management of the patient with an abdominal aortic aneurysm

An aneurysm is an abnormal dilatation of an artery. *True aneurysms* may be saccular in shape, or fusiform, where the entire circumference of the affected aorta is dilated (see Fig. 22.1). An aneurysm may affect any large or medium-sized blood vessel. They occur more commonly in the aorta, below the origin of the renal arteries (infrarenal), and often extend to the common iliac vessels. Aneurysms can also occur commonly in the thoracic, femoral and popliteal arteries. An abdominal aortic aneurysm (AAA) occurs once the abdominal aorta just below the renal arteries expands to 3 cm or more.

The weakening of the aortic wall can lead to progressive dilatation and, in some cases, rupture; a ruptured aorta is life-threatening and causes 2% of all male deaths in the UK (PHE, 2015). If immediate medical care is not given to these patients, approximately 80% of patients will die of sudden cardiovascular collapse (Smith-Burgess, 2017) and ruptured AAAs account for 6000 deaths per year in the UK (PHE, 2015). AAAs are 4–6 times more common in men than in women and several risk factors play a role in the development of AAAs, including patients being more than 65 years old, smoking, hypertension, cerebral vascular disease and family history (Smith-Burgess, 2017).

Aetiology

In addition to the modifiable and genetic risk factors, AAA pathogenesis includes inflammation of the arterial wall, smooth muscle cell apoptosis, extracellular matrix degradation of connective tissue and oxidative stress (Kuivaniemi et al, 2015).

The chronic inflammatory process on the aortic wall has been identified but is of unclear etiology. Other risk factors including cystic medial wall necrosis, dissection of the vessel wall, syphilis, HIV, Marfan's syndrome and Ehlers–Danlos syndrome have been identified. The constant pressure on the aortic wall follows the Law of Laplace (wall stress is proportional to the radius of the aneurysm) and presence of hypertension increases the risk (Shaw et al, 2019).

AAAs normally occur due to the failure of the structural proteins of the aorta. The cause of these proteins to fail is still unknown but it results in the gradual weakening of the aortic wall. The main composition of the aortic wall is collagen lamellar units, but in AAAs there is a huge decrease in collagen and elastin which leads to higher incidence of aneurysmal formation (Shaw et al, 2019).

Elderly white men have the highest risk of developing AAAs and they are uncommon in Asian, African American and Hispanic individuals (Zommorodi et al, 2018).

Screening

The NHS Abdominal Aortic Aneurysm Screening Programme (NAAASP) was started by Public Health England (PHE) to reduce aneurysm-related mortality through early detection, appropriate monitoring and treatment. This scheme invites men for ultrasound screening during the year they turn 65, while men over 65 who have not previously been screened can self-refer (PHE, 2016). Healthcare professionals should consider an aortic ultrasound for women aged 70 and over if AAA has not already been excluded on abdominal imaging with any co-morbidities (NICE, 2018b).

Asymptomatic AAA patients with abdominal aorta diameter of 5.5 cm or larger should be referred to the specialist unit and they should be seen within 2 weeks of diagnosis. Patients with abdominal aorta diameter of 3−5.5 cm should be seen within 12 weeks of diagnosis (NICE, 2018b). Symptomatic patients should be seen immediately in the regional vascular service.

Clinical features

As most patients with an abdominal aortic aneurysm will have no symptoms, diagnosis may occur when they or their doctor detect a pulsatile mass, or incidentally while having routine investigations. Other patients may complain of vague abdominal and/or lumbar pain, which is more common in patients with inflammatory aneurysms.

Diagnosis

Palpation of the abdomen is insufficient for routinely diagnosing an aneurysm. It is usually confirmed by ultrasound, which gives an accurate size and position of the aneurysm. More accurate confirmation of its position in relation to the renal arteries can be obtained by a CT scan or MRA.

Emergency surgery for ruptured abdominal aortic aneurysm

The patient presenting with a ruptured aneurysm will usually arrive clinically shocked, with severe abdominal and lower back pain, in the Emergency Department. A rupture may also occur in a patient who has already been admitted to a vascular ward and is awaiting surgery. Without emergency surgery there is 100% fatality. On diagnosis, the patient will be taken immediately for surgery. The nurse will need to provide reassurance and emotional support for the patient and their family, at the same time recognizing that this situation is a dire emergency. Only minimal physical preparation may be possible, and this should be performed calmly and competently, as the patient will be very frightened by the need for major surgical intervention. The patient will be hypovolaemic and may be semiconscious. The main priority of care will be to maintain the patient's airway, breathing and circulation, to optimize oxygen delivery and tissue perfusion. Immediate resuscitation with prescribed IV fluids if blood is not available, using a pressure infuser, will be continued during transfer of the patient to theatre.

Indications and treatment options

Patients with smaller aneurysms can usually be treated by actively reducing risk factors and carrying out regular ultrasound scans to detect any increase in size. Patients with unruptured abdominal aortic aneurysm, if it is symptomatic, asymptomatic and 5.5 cm or larger, or asymptomatic, larger than 4 cm and has grown by more than 1 cm in a year, should have a surgical repair unless there are anaesthetic or medical contraindications (NICE, 2018b). Ruptured aneurysm should be treated either via endovascular or open surgical repair.

Conventional repair of aneurysms requires a major open surgical procedure to replace the aneurysm with a prosthetic graft, whilst endovascular repair is a less invasive treatment option now commonly used in patients with a suitable anatomy.

The decision to perform elective surgery depends on balancing the risk of aneurysm rupture against the risks of operative morbidity and mortality for the patient concerned. Patients needing aneurysm repair require preoperative day care admission for more detailed investigations and assessment. Patients and their relatives will then be advised of treatment options and the increased risk of rupture if surgery is not performed.

Endovascular repair of abdominal aortic aneurysm

The aim of this treatment is to isolate the aneurysm from the circulation, preventing further expansion, rather than replacing it. A prosthetic stent graft is introduced usually through bilateral groin incisions into the common femoral artery and positioned up into the aorta and iliac arteries under X-ray guidance, to exclude the aneurysm from the circulation to prevent rupture (Fig. 22.11).

Endovascular abdominal aortic aneurysm repair (EVAR) has improved surgical treatment outcomes especially for women and for men over the age of 70 (NICE, 2018b). EVAR should not be offered to people with an unruptured infrarenal AAA. This technique has advantages over conventional surgery, in that it is minimally invasive, requires a postoperative hospital stay of only 2−3 days and is associated with minimal discomfort. Endovascular repair is now being undertaken in some large vascular units for patients with ruptured abdominal aortic aneurysm.

Depending on the patient's general condition, the procedure can be performed under local or general anaesthesia. A high-dependency bed may be required, depending on the patient's fitness, or the patient can be closely monitored by experienced nurses on a dedicated vascular surgery ward.

Blood pressure, pulse, urine output and oxygen saturations are closely monitored overnight using NEWS2. The intravenous infusion is removed the following day, as there is no restriction on oral intake. The urinary catheter and any wound drains are also removed the next day and the patient encouraged to mobilize early. Patients are normally fit for discharge 2−3 days after the procedure and instructions given for removal of sutures after 10 days. A duplex ultrasound is usually undertaken prior to discharge to check for an endoleak, and a CT scan arranged 4 weeks postoperatively with a 6-week outpatient appointment.

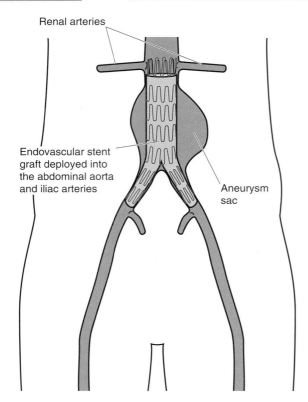

Figure 22.11 Endovascular aneurysm repair (EVAR) with bifurcated stent graft.

Renal arteries

Endovascular stent graft deployed into the abdominal aorta and iliac arteries

Aneurysm sac

Current studies demonstrate that patients treated with endovascular repair show better outcomes than open repair in the USA, England and other parts of the world (Mayer et al, 2012; Mani et al, 2009; Karthikesalingam et al, 2014).

Conventional open repair of abdominal aortic aneurysm

The surgical procedure involves replacing the abdominal aneurysm with a straight synthetic (PTFE) tube graft or with an aorto-bifemoral graft if the aneurysm extends to the common iliac arteries. Care requirements are significantly more complex than those for endovascular repair, as this is a major surgical procedure.

Preparation of patients for elective surgical aneurysm repair

- The patient will have been assessed both physically and psychologically in a pre-admission clinic prior to surgery. This allows the patient and their family time to be fully informed of the proposed operation, length of stay, associated risks of surgery and the care involved. It also allows time to discuss any concerns with an anaesthetist regarding any special preoperative investigations which may be needed.
- Pre-existing cardiac disease is a significant risk factor for patients undergoing surgery; therefore, a full cardiorespiratory and renal assessment is undertaken. Relevant investigations discussed under the assessment section earlier in the chapter will be needed before the patient is assessed by the anaesthetist.
- The patient may then be admitted the day prior to surgery to become familiar with the ward environment and members of the multidisciplinary team.
- Infection prophylaxis is essential to minimize risk of infection of the prosthetic graft, which could pose a catastrophic risk to the patient. A routine screen for MRSA and MSSA should be taken in the pre-admission clinic and the patient admitted into a side room. Antiseptic showers are recommended prior to theatre to help reduce skin microbes, and prophylactic antibiotics will be commenced in theatre according to local antimicrobial policy (NICE, 2016).
- Written consent will be obtained from the patient following several prior discussions with the vascular surgeon of the risks and benefits of the operation.
- DVT prophylaxis with low-molecular-weight heparin is prescribed and administered in the evening to avoid the risk of dural haematoma if epidural anaesthesia is used.
- The patient and their family should be informed of the need for close monitoring on the high dependency or intensive care unit immediately following surgery.
- Anti-embolism stockings may only be worn if there is no evidence of arterial insufficiency of the lower limbs.

Postoperative care

- Immediate nursing care will be given in the high dependency or intensive care unit for continuous monitoring following prolonged anaesthesia. Most patients are extubated following surgery and will only require high dependency care for 24–48 hours. Patients requiring longer intubation/ventilation will remain in intensive care.
- The patient will be transferred back to a ward with nurses experienced in managing vascular patients when their cardiac, respiratory and renal functions are considered stable.
- A profiling bed assists with maintaining the patient sitting upright to aid lung expansion. A pressure-relief mattress and heel protection will be required until mobility increases, as epidural analgesics will increase the risk of pressure ulcer development if the patient is unable to feel discomfort to vulnerable areas.

- NEWS2 should be commenced on the patient's return from the unit, with support from the critical care outreach team if the score increases.
- Vital signs and oxygenation should be closely monitored, initially 1/4-hourly and then 1/2-hourly to hourly. Humidified oxygen can be given via a facemask until the targeted oxygen saturation is achieved (most patients 94–98%).
- Respiratory rate, SpO2 is monitored hourly and is a good indicator of the onset of chest complications. Deep breathing exercises must be encouraged to ensure lung expansion, and regular physiotherapy is given.
- Blood pressure should be monitored, and normal BP should be maintained as hypertension can cause bleeding at the graft anastomosis and hypotension can result in multiorgan failure.
- Hourly urine output and central venous pressure observations will be required to assess hydration.
- Pain control is essential to allow adequate chest expansion, which will reduce the risk of chest infection. Epidural analgesia is recommended for 2–3 days, until the patient is able to tolerate oral analgesics.
- Limb observations should initially be undertaken 1–2-hourly to assess for warmth, colour, sensation and movement, with Doppler assessment of pedal pulses. Distal embolization ('trash foot') can occur following aortic surgery. Caution is therefore needed if anti-embolism stockings are *in situ*, as full examination of the limb can be hindered, and onset of limb ischaemia can go unnoticed or be compounded by the stockings. Assessment of limb movement is important, as the rare complication of paraplegia following this type of surgery may be missed in acutely unwell patients or those with epidural analgesia.
- Nutritional status will be regularly assessed, as it will take several days for normal gut peristalsis to be established due to handling of the bowel during surgery. A nasogastric tube will be *in situ* and aspirated regularly, and the patient allowed to drink small amounts of water immediately postoperatively. This can be increased as bowel sounds return, and nasogastric aspirate lessens. High-calorie/high-protein sip feed supplements should be introduced when nasogastric tube aspirate lessens, and the tube is then removed. Diet can be recommended when free fluids are tolerated, and high-protein drinks continued until appetite returns. Total parenteral nutrition will need considering if prolonged paralytic ileus occurs.
- Mobility should be encouraged at an early stage, with the patient sitting out of bed for short periods and gradually increasing walking distance.
- Patients often experience diarrhoea following aortic aneurysm repair and a stool specimen should be sent to exclude *Clostridium difficile*. If diarrhoea persists and the patient's abdomen becomes distended and tender, further investigation will be required, as bowel necrosis can occur due to the lengthy clamping of the mesenteric artery during surgery.

Health promotion and discharge advice

- Temporary loss of appetite and excessive tiredness often occur following abdominal aortic aneurysm repair. The patient should be warned of this and advised to eat regular small nourishing meals and take regular naps initially. Full recovery will take at least 3–6 months.
- Patients should be advised not to lift anything heavy for the first 4 weeks but should be encouraged to lead an active life, gradually increasing their activity level, and taking daily walks. Stair practice should be undertaken with the physiotherapist prior to discharge.
- Moderate exercise does not cause rupture. Patients should be doing exercise as part of their rehabilitation programme.
- Driving should not be resumed until the patient is reviewed in the outpatient clinic.
- The patient should be advised about the best way to achieve and maintain a healthy lifestyle in relation to diet and taking regular exercise. Smoking must not be resumed in patients who have smoked previously, and ongoing specialist support will be required.
- Discharge drugs will probably include aspirin, antiplatelet and statin therapy, and the importance of taking this, as well as any other prescribed medications, should be explained. The patient should also be instructed to have regular blood pressure checks and to continue taking any required antihypertensive medications.
- Patients should also inform any dentist or doctor they may consult that they have an artificial graft in their aorta, as they may require prophylactic antibiotics before any procedure is undertaken.
- A follow-up appointment is required 4 weeks after discharge. The patient should be given an information leaflet with a contact phone number in case any problems are encountered following discharge.

Management of the patient requiring carotid endarterectomy

A stroke can leave a patient with severe physical and mental disability, making them highly dependent on family and society. Public Health England (PHE) data from 2016 show that 57,000 people had a first-time stroke and it is estimated that around 30% of people who have had a stroke will go on to experience another stroke. There are around 32,000 stroke-related deaths in England each year. Deaths related to stroke have declined by 49% in the past 15 years due to the combination of better prevention, earlier treatment and more advanced medical treatment. Awareness is crucial because 1.9 million nerve cells in the brain are lost every minute that a stroke which is left untreated, which can result in slurred speech and paralysis (PHE, 2018).

Most strokes (80%) are ischaemic, and 10% of strokes are secondary to extracranial carotid atherosclerosis. In carotid disease, atheromatous plaques occur at the origin of the internal carotid artery in the neck. Classic symptoms of carotid disease are a sudden loss of focal cerebral function such as difficulty or loss of speech, weakness/numbness of one or both contralateral limbs, or transient ipsilateral blindness. Transient monocular blindness (*amaurosis fugax*) is described as like a blind being drawn down or across one eye. Symptoms of carotid artery disease are rarely global, such as general dizziness, unsteady gait or coma.

Sudden loss of focal cerebral function lasting less than 24 hours is referred to as a *transient ischaemic attack* (TIA). Symptoms which last for more than 24 hours are called a stroke. All suspected patients should be treated and admitted in the specialist acute stroke unit within 24 hours of referral, whether from the community, the emergency department or from outpatient clinics (NICE, 2019).

The current guidelines recommend that triage of patients on the basis of the risk of stroke should be assessed by the ABCD (age, blood pressure, clinical findings, duration of symptoms and presence or absence of diabetes) score (Lovett et al, 2003; Amarenco et al, 2016). These scores range from 0 to 7, with higher scores indicating the greater risk of stroke. Previous stroke studies indicated that the risk of stroke after minor stroke/TIA was 12−20%. However, the TIAregistry.org project concluded that they observed a lower rate of stoke (5.1%) or cardiovascular events (6.2%) after TIA/minor stroke due to faster implementation of secondary stroke prevention strategies (e.g. immediate initiation of antiplatelet agents, oral anticoagulation in the event of atrial fibrillation, urgent revascularization for critical carotid stenosis and anti-hypertensive/statin drugs) (Amarenco et al, 2016).

Interestingly, NICE (2019) suggests that health professionals should use validated tools such as FAST (Face, Arm, Speech Test) outside the hospital and ROSIER (Recognition of Stroke in the Emergency Room) in A&E and not use the ABCD2 scoring system to assess the risk of subsequent stroke or to inform the urgency of referral for people who have had a suspected or confirmed TIA; they should be treated as soon as possible.

The decision to perform carotid endarterectomy therefore depends on balancing the risk of stroke occurring if surgery is not performed against the risk of perioperative or postoperative stroke occurring. These risks and benefits will need to be carefully discussed at a multidisciplinary neurovascular meeting, and with the patient and their family in order for them to make an informed decision about the proposed operation.

Management of patients with asymptomatic carotid stenosis

The first line of treatment for these patients should be medical therapy unless they are identified as having a high risk of stroke and should have surgical intervention (Paraskevas et al, 2016). The intense medical therapy should include lifestyle modification, smoking cessation, a Mediterranean diet, antiplatelet drugs, lipid-lowering drugs, blood pressure control and vitamin B to lower homocysteine. The main aim for these asymptomatic patients should be treating the arteries rather than treating the risk factors (Spence et al, 2016).

Investigations

All patients presenting for investigation of a TIA or a stroke should have an urgent duplex ultrasound scan to identify disease and accurately measure the degree of stenosis. MRA may also be needed to confirm the extent of stenosis; however, duplex ultrasound has now become the gold standard investigation and is repeated immediately before surgery (NICE, 2019). Computed tomographic angiography, carotid imaging, and MRI scan should be considered according to the severity of the stenosis and should be carried out on the same day as the assessment. Patients with stable neurological symptoms from acute non-disabling stroke or TIA who have symptomatic carotid stenosis of 50−99% according to the North American Symptomatic Carotid Endarterectomy Trial (NASCET) criteria should be referred urgently for carotid endarterectomy following current national standards and best medical treatment (NICE, 2019).

Carotid endarterectomy is one of the most common surgical interventions to prevent stroke in symptomatic and asymptomatic patients with significant carotid artery stenosis. The NASCET Trial and the Asymptomatic Carotid Atherosclerosis study found class 1 evidence of superior outcomes with surgery compared with medical therapy in the prevention of stroke (Garzon-Muvdi et al, 2016). In addition, the morbidity and mortality associated with surgery are very low, which makes this a safe intervention for patients with severe stenosis (Babu et al, 2013).

Health promotion and risk factor management

Even if surgery is not required, assessment of risk factors and 'best medical therapy' includes smoking cessation support, well-controlled blood pressure and cholesterol, and weight and diabetes control, to prevent disease progression. Antiplatelet therapy, comprising aspirin, clopidogrel or a combination of aspirin and dipyridamole, is recommended for all patients with stenosis, unless otherwise indicated (Garzon-Muvdi et al, 2016).

Multiple factors can contribute to restenosis after surgery and one of the main factors is family history of stroke. It is important to have a close clinical surveillance and frequent vascular imaging studies, and a multidisciplinary management approach may also be valuable in ensuring correction of modifiable factors to prevent restenosis after surgery (Garzon-Muvdi et al, 2016).

Preoperative preparation of the patient undergoing carotid endarterectomy

- Depending on the urgency for surgery, the patient will be assessed in the pre-admission clinic the week before surgery. This allows time for the patient and their relatives to discuss any further anxieties and to reconfirm the indication for surgery. The clinic nurse should carefully explain the care pathway requirements and proposed discharge day to the patient and relatives to help allay anxiety.
- Routine blood screening and screening for MRSA will be undertaken, and a full cardiorespiratory and renal assessment performed. Investigations will include a chest X-ray, ECG and possibly an echocardiogram. A cardiology opinion may also be required for patients with cardiac symptoms.
- A review of the antiplatelet therapy with the vascular consultant surgeon or neurologist should be undertaken at this stage, as patients having combination therapy with aspirin and clopidogrel may need to have the clopidogrel stopped several days before the operation owing to reports of excessive bleeding during surgery.
- The patient is usually admitted the afternoon prior to surgery into an area of the ward where there is a low risk of contamination from MRSA.
- Due to the increased risk and complications of haematoma formation during and after surgery, DVT prophylaxis with low-molecular-weight heparin is omitted in many centres and only anti-embolism stockings provided unless contraindicated. Patients undergoing carotid endarterectomy are mobilized quickly, which decreases the risk of DVT in comparison to the risk of severe haemorrhage.
- A full neurological examination is normally performed by the neurologist to identify and document any pre-existing deficit. The anaesthetist will review the patient and discuss the type of anaesthetic

required, as local anaesthesia is an option for suitable patients.
- Informed written consent is obtained and the risks of a stroke occurring during or after surgery will be again explained to the patient and relatives by the surgeon. Other risks of surgery — e.g. heart attack, minor haemorrhage, temporary numbness of the face/neck, tongue and mouth weakness — are also explained, which will inevitably heighten anxiety. A vein patch may be required and will be obtained from the patient's neck or leg veins, or a prosthetic patch can be used. This patch is anastomosed onto the carotid artery to widen the vessel, preventing narrowing at the incision site. The patient needs to be informed that this may occur.
- An antiseptic shower immediately prior to operation is recommended, to help reduce skin microbes.
- Medications for risk factors will need to be given on the morning of surgery and these will include aspirin and antihypertensive drugs. Due to the risk of stroke immediately prior to surgery, antiplatelet therapy, including clopidogrel, should not be stopped unless specific written instructions are given to do so by the senior surgeon.
- Monitoring of the patient's cerebral function during the operation can be undertaken in an 'awake' patient having local anaesthesia, by asking the patient simple questions and testing their grip power on the contralateral hand. Transcranial Doppler (TCD) monitoring is now more commonly used for both local and general anaesthesia, to assess cerebral blood flow.

Postoperative care

- The patient will require either an extended recovery or brief high dependency stay if they are considered a high-risk patient prior to return to the vascular surgery ward for monitoring by experienced nurses.
- National Early Warning Score 2 should be commenced on the patient's return to the ward.
- Close monitoring of vital signs, oxygenation, and for recovery of consciousness, speech, facial weakness and limb function are required for early detection of any neurological deficit.
- Blood pressure should be carefully monitored. The parameters and necessary treatment to stabilize blood pressure must be clearly documented in the medical notes or care pathway by the anaesthetist or surgeon before the patient leaves the recovery ward.
- Oxygen is given as prescribed for up to 24 hours and saturations recorded 1—2 hourly initially, to maintain >95%.

- Blood pressure, pulse and respiratory observations are undertaken:
  - 1/4-hourly for 1 hour
  - 1/2-hourly for 6 hours
  - hourly for 12 hours, then 4 hourly if stable.
- The patient is observed for stridor or other signs of respiratory distress, which should be immediately reported to the surgeons.
- Urine output is carefully monitored and recorded on the output chart. IV fluids are administered for approximately 24 hours and removed when the patient is drinking adequately by oral.
- Blood glucose monitoring is required for known diabetes patients and treatment should be undertaken according to the local diabetes management policy. A systematic literature review and meta-analysis of randomized controlled trials to evaluate the effectiveness of the Regular Insulin Sliding Scale (RISS) concluded that the use of RISS alone or even with antidiabetic medications did not provide any benefits in blood glucose control. So, the use of sliding scale insulin should be discontinued in hospitals (Lee et al, 2015). Normal diet can be resumed as desired when the patient is awake.
- The wound dressing, situated behind the angle of the jaw, should be observed for haemorrhage or haematoma formation. Staples are removed 5 days following surgery.
- A vacuum drain is usually inserted and removed on the first postoperative day.
- Deep breathing and leg exercises are encouraged.
- Analgesics are administered as necessary, as patients usually experience only minor discomfort following surgery.
- The patient may mobilize the following morning once normotensive and may be discharged on the first or second postoperative day.

Follow-up advice

- Slight numbness to the face or some tongue weakness, due to trauma of the nerves during the operation, is not uncommon following surgery. Patients need to be informed that this is quite normal and may take some weeks to disappear.
- Modification of risk factors must be re-emphasized to the patient and relatives, especially in relation to smoking, blood pressure and diet.
- Patients need to be reminded of the importance of taking their prescribed antiplatelet therapy and other medications and should continue to have their blood pressure monitored regularly.
- A follow-up outpatient appointment is normally arranged for 6 weeks after discharge.

Management of the patient with varicose veins

Varicose veins and chronic venous insufficiency are a very common conditions affecting almost one-third of the adult population, with a substantial negative impact on healthcare cost and on the patient's health-related quality of life (Molnar et al, 2019). It is estimated that approximately 10–15% of male subjects and around 20–25% of female subjects are affected by the varicose veins but it varies across the geographic locations (Molnar et al, 2019). Malfunctioning valves in the veins anastomosing the deep and superficial veins, called perforators, cause an increase in pressure, which leads to tortuous and dilated superficial varicose veins.

Most varicose veins are *primary* where the exact cause is unknown, but is possibly a congenital defect giving rise to valvular incompetence and weakness in the vein wall. Only a minority are *secondary* to conditions following DVT, pregnancy or pelvic tumours. The valves become damaged by increased pressure, causing back flow from the deep to the superficial veins.

Structural changes in the vein wall contribute to pathological weakening and resultant dilation. Overproduction of collagen type 1, decreased synthesis of collagen type III and disruption of the arrangement of smooth muscle cells and elastin fibers have been observed in histological studies of varicose venous segments. Increased levels of transforming growth factors β1 and fibroblast growth factor β have also been seen in the walls of varicose veins and may contribute to structural degradation of the vessel wall (Piazza, 2014).

There are three types of superficial varicose veins:
- true or trunk varicose veins are widened, tortuous and bulging
- reticular veins are normal but more visually prominent superficial veins which do not usually become widened
- spider or thread veins (telangiectases).

Risk factors

Risk factors for varicose veins can be categorized as hormonal, lifestyle, acquired and inherited (Piazza, 2014).
- Hormonal:
  - Female due to high oestrogen state.
  - Prolonged standing or sitting due to venous hypertension.
- Lifestyle:
  - Smoking due to venous endothelial injury but modifiable risk factor.
  - Obesity due to venous hypertension.
  - Pregnancy due to high oestrogen and venous hypertension.

- Acquired:
  - Deep vein thrombosis due to venous valvular incompetence.
  - Age due to venous valvular incompetence.
  - Family history due to venous valvular incompetence.
- Inherited:
  - Tall height due to venous hypertension.
  - Congenital syndromes due to incompetence valve, hypertension and deep venous obstruction.

Symptoms

Symptoms that commonly occur are tiredness, swelling, aching, itching, throbbing, post-thrombotic syndrome and restless legs. These are made worse by standing for long periods and hot weather and are relieved by walking. Many patients have no symptoms but will present with varicose veins because they are worried about the cosmetic appearance. Dilated, tortuous, lumpy veins can cause considerable disfigurement and give rise to cosmetic concern.

Complications of varicose veins

Complications include superficial inflammation (phlebitis) and superficial thrombosis (thrombophlebitis). Haemorrhage from a ruptured vein through the skin may result from trauma, and spontaneous rupture can also occur, particularly in elderly people with thin overlying skin. Some severe cases will have dermatitis, lipodermatosclerosis, atrophy, itching in the lower legs, congestion, irritation, local hyperthermia, skin hyper-/hypopigmentation, leg oedema, or swelling with serous ooze (Molnar et al, 2019).

Investigations

Duplex ultrasound scanning

This procedure is a non-invasive scan to accurately assess sites of valve incompetence in the deep and superficial venous systems and is considered the gold standard method of investigation (NICE, 2013).

Trendelenburg test

This test can confirm the source of venous incompetence. A tourniquet is placed around the upper thigh after raising the leg. Veins that fill slowly when the patient stands, but fill rapidly on releasing the tourniquet, have incompetent saphenofemoral valves. The test can be used with the tourniquet placed below the knee to assess the short saphenous vein.

Doppler ultrasound

Doppler ultrasound can be used to determine the presence of venous reflux in the veins behind the knee.

Treatment

The symptoms of varicose veins can be managed by wearing compression stockings. If compression stocking does not relieve the symptoms, surgical treatment can be considered. It is one of the most common forms of surgery. These varicose veins are closed off using several different techniques such as vein stripping, phlebectomy, radiofrequency ablation, endovascular laser ablation and transilluminated powered phlebectomy. This will not disturb the normal blood supply in the legs because the blood will be re-directed into other healthy veins. The common side-effects of surgery are pain, bleeding, swelling, scarring and discoloration of the skin. The rare complications are infection, thrombosis and nerve damage.

Compression hosiery

Support hosiery will help relieve symptoms by aiding venous return and will conceal varicosities. They require correct fitting to achieve results and aid concordance. Significant arterial disease should be excluded before applying compression hosiery. The patient should also be advised to moisturize their skin well to avoid dryness. Other measures, such as staying active, reducing weight, and elevating legs when resting, can help reduce symptoms.

Sclerotherapy

Ultrasound-guided foam sclerotherapy involves injecting a chemical agent (a sclerosant) to induce blood vessel scarring and closure of the vessel. It has a combination of air and the chemical agent which creates a foam, which fills the vein, causing the vein to spasm and scar. It has a good success rate with 80—90% of veins remaining closed after 3 years of injection (Weiss et al, 2014; Mwipatayi et al, 2016). It has a good minor below-knee reticular veins and thread veins are frequently treated with this method for cosmetic reasons. Compression bandaging is initially applied, and compression hosiery supplied, which should be worn for 2—3 weeks following sclerotherapy treatment.

Another variation of sclerosing agent (3% sodium tetradecyl/sulphate) is injected into the lumen of the prominent veins. This agent eliminates the varicosity by creating inflammation of the lumen walls, which become adherent when immediate local pressure is applied with pads. Prior to injection treatment for cosmetic reasons, the patient should be informed that there is a risk of developing bruising, skin pigmentation and some rare complications such as nerve damage, skin and soft tissue necrosis. Almost 10 out of 100 people develop phlebitis after they have had a sclerotherapy (Mwipatayi et al, 2016).

Phlebectomy

Small skin incisions (a few millimetres) are made along the surface of the vein's anatomical area. A small hook is inserted through these skin incisions and the vein is pulled out from its original place as far as possible and then it is cut and removed in several small sections. This technique is used only for small veins which branches off from the main vein and it produces small scars rather than a massive scar.

Radiofrequency ablation

This technique uses heat generated by electromagnetic waves to close off the veins by inserting the radiofrequency ablation probe into the vein through a small skin incision. This probe catheter heats the vein until it is closed off on either end.

Transilluminated powered phlebectomy

This procedure involves a tiny rotating blade inserted into the vein to cut it and then the cut vein tissue is removed by using suction. The surgeon visualizes the vein through the skin by an illuminated light and this approach is only carried out for the great saphenous vein varicosity.

Endovascular laser therapy (EVLT)

EVLT is a minimally invasive alternative to surgical stripping of the long saphenous vein, which can be performed under local anaesthetic in a suitable outpatient clinic or day surgery unit equipped for laser use. Under ultrasound guidance, a catheter is placed into the long saphenous vein. A laser fibre is then introduced and the fibre is slowly withdrawn while the laser is repeatedly applied in short pulses along the entire vein to destroy it.

Ligation and stripping of varicose veins
During surgery, the long or short saphenous veins are stripped out distally with a wire stripper. Several small incisions may be made if it is not possible to remove the entire vein through one incision. The vessel will be ligated where it meets the perforators at the saphenofemoral junction.

Preoperative preparation
- The surgeon will mark the skin over the vein to be stripped, and the nurse should ensure that these markings are not removed prior to surgery.
- Many patients are concerned with the cosmetic appearances after surgery and may have unrealistic expectations. It is therefore important for the surgeon to explain that the small incisions made at operation will leave small scars.

- Women taking a combined oral contraceptive should stop taking it 4 weeks before surgery and use an alternative method.

Aftercare
- The wound dressings should be observed for bleeding. Compression bandages will have been applied from toes to thigh. Bedrest is usually only required for 2–3 hours after day care surgery or maybe longer, depending on the extent of the surgery.
- Patients are at risk of DVT and should be encouraged to mobilize when there is no further risk of haemorrhage. DVT prophylaxis is usually prescribed for patients if an overnight stay is required, as their mobility may be limited if they are more elderly or have had bilateral surgery.

Discharge advice
- The patient is advised to remove the bandaging after 48 hours. Either medium-strength (Class II) elastic support stockings or anti-embolism stockings should then be worn for 10 days following surgery, but can be removed at night.
- The patient is advised to keep the wounds as dry as possible. Soluble sutures are normally used for groin incisions, with Steri-Strips over the multiple avulsions, which can be peeled off after 48 hours.
- Bruising to the legs and discomfort are not uncommon. The patient should be forewarned of this, and the small possibility of numbness due to nerve damage, when consent is obtained prior to surgery.
- Walking exercise should be encouraged following surgery, and the patient's legs should be elevated while sitting, to prevent swelling. To avoid recurrence of varicosities, patients should avoid standing still for long periods of time, as gravity can cause pooling of blood in the legs. Weight gain should also be avoided, as excess adipose tissue gives poor support to the venous system.

SUMMARY OF KEY POINTS

- Patients with peripheral vascular disorders (PVD) may require hospitalization for treatment by either radiological or surgical intervention.
- Care of patients with PVD, both in primary and acute settings, is challenging, requiring early detection, risk factor reduction and vigilant monitoring to prevent onset of limb-threatening disease.
- Community screening for abdominal aortic aneurysm is essential to prevent death from rupture.

(Continued)

(cont'd)

- Caring for vascular patients within acute care environments requires a broad range of skills and expertise to encompass critical care, wound and tissue viability, nutritional, pain and diabetes management, as well as palliative care.
- Nurses must be aware of the importance of correct assessment, diagnosis and treatment of venous and arterial leg ulceration.
- Active control of risk factors and education is a key component of care, requiring a team approach to enable vascular patients to increase control over and improve their own health.

REFLECTIVE LEARNING POINTS

Having read this chapter, think about what you now know and what you still need to find out about. These questions may help:

- Describe the nurse's role in patient education and smoking cessation
- Specifically, what are the key areas the nurse needs to address preoperatively with the patient (and, if appropriate, their family) with regards to lower limb amputation?
- Discuss the strategies required to help alleviate preoperative anxiety prior to surgery for peripheral vascular disease.

References

Editor's Choice – 2017 European Society of Cardiology Guidelines on the Diagnosis and Treatment of Peripheral Arterial Diseases, in collaboration with the European Society for Vascular Surgery. In V. Aboyans, J. B. Ricco, M. L. Bartelink, M. Bjorck, M. Brodmann, T. Cohnert, et al. (Eds.), *European Journal of Vascular Endovascular Surgery* (55, pp. 305–368). .

Adams, C.T., & Lakra, A. (2018). Below knee amputation (BKA). *StatPearls* (internet). Treasure Island (FL): StatPearls Publishing. Available from: <www.ncbi.nlm.nih.gov/books/NBK534773>

Ahmad, N., Thomas, G. N., Gill, P., Chan, C., & Torella, F. (2014). Lower limb amputation in England: prevalence, regional variation and relationship with revascularisation, deprivation and risk factors. A retrospective review of hospital data. *Journal of Royal Society of Medicine, 107*(12), 483–489.

Ahmad, N., Thomas, G. N., Gill, P., & Torella, F. (2016). The prevalence of major lower limb amputation in the diabetic and non-diabetic population of England 2003–2013. *Diabetes and Vascular Disease Research, 13*(5), 348–353.

Alshehri, A. M. (2010). Metabolic syndrome and cardiovascular risk. *Journal of Family Community Medicine, 17*(2), 73–78.

Amarenco, P., Lavallee, P. C., Labreuche, J., Albers, G. W., Bornstein, N. M., Canhao, P., et al. (2016). One-year risk of stroke after transient ischemic attack or minor stroke. *The New England Journal of Medicine, 374*, 1533–1542.

American Diabetes Association. (2003). Peripheral arterial disease in people with diabetes. *Diabetes Care, 26*, 3333–3341.

Anderson, J. L., Antman, E. M., Harold, J. G., Jessup, M., O'Gara, P. T., Pinto, F. J., et al. (2014). Clinical practice guidelines on perioperative cardiovascular evaluation: collaborative efforts among the ACC, AHA, and ESC. *Circulation, 130*, 2213–2214.

Appleton, N. D., Bosanquet, D., Morris-Stiff, G., Ahmed, H., Sanjay, P., & Lewis, M. H. (2010). *Annals of Royal College of Surgeons England, 92*(6), 499–502.

Arya, S., Binney, Z., Khakharia, A., Brewster, L. P., Goodney, P., Patzer, R., et al. (2018). Race and Socioeconomic Status Independently Affect Risk of Major Amputation in Peripheral Artery Disease. *Journal of American Heart Association, 7*, e007425.

Babu, M. A., Meissner, I., & Meyer, F. B. (2013). The durability of carotid endarterectomy: long-term results for restenosis and stroke. *Neurosurgery, 72*, 835–838.

Bailey, M. A., Griffin, K. J., & Scott, D. J. A. (2014). Clinical assessment of patients with peripheral arterial disease. *Seminars in Interventional Radiology, 31*(4), 292–299.

Baszczuk, A., & Kopczynski, Z. (2014). Hyperhomocysteinemia in patients with cardiovascular disease (Abstract). *Postepy Hig Med Dosw (online), 68*, 579.

Berger, J. S., Hochman, J., Lobach, I., Adelman, M. A., Riles, T. S., &

Rockman, C. B. (2013). Modifiable risk factor burden and the prevalence of peripheral artery disease in different vascular territories. *Journal of Vascular Surgery, 58*(3), 673–681.el.

Brearley, S. (2013). Acute leg ischaemia. *British Medical Journal, 346*, f2681.

Brodmann, M., Werner, M., Brinton, T. J., Illindala, U., Lansky, A., Jaff, M. R., et al. (2017). Safety and performance of lithoplasty for treatment of calcified peripheral artery lesions. *Journal of American College of Cardiology, 70*(7), 908–910.

Callum, K., & Bradbury, A. (2000). ABC of arterial and venous disease: Acute limb ischemia. *British Medical Journal, 320* (7237), 764–767.

Conte, S. M., & Vale, P. R. (2018). Peripheral arterial disease. *Heart, Lung and Circulation, 27*, 427–432.

Cote, M. C., Ligeti, R., Cutler, B. C., & Nelson, P. R. (2003). Management of hyperlipidaemia in patients with vascular disease. *Journal of Vascular Nursing, 21*(2), 63–67.

Crismaru, I., & Diaconu, C. C. (2015). European Society of Cardiology article on the lipid-lowering therapy with peripheral artery disease. *E-journal of Cardiology Practice, 1*, 31.

Dake, M. D., Ansel, G. M., Jaff, M. R., Ohki, T., Saxon, R. R., Smouse, H. B., et al. (2016). Durable clinical effectiveness with paclitaxel-eluting stents in the femoropopliteal artery: 5-year results of the Zilver PTX randomized trial. *Circulation, 133*, 1472–1483.

Delewi, R., Yang, H., & Kastelein, J. (2013). Atherosclerosis. *Textbook of Cardiology, 369*(7), 676–677. Available at: <www.textbookofcardiology.org/wiki/atherosclerosis>.

Dormandy, J. (2000). Management of peripheral arterial disease. TASC working group. Transatlantic Inter-Society Consensus (TASC). *Journal of Vascular Surgery, 31*, 1.

Earnshaw, J. J., Gaines, P. A., & Beard, J. D. (2001). Management of acute lower leg ischaemia. In J. D. Beard, & P. A. Gaines (Eds.), *Vascular and endovascular surgery* (2nd ed.). London: W.B. Saunders.

Erb, W. (1911). Klinische beitrage zur pathologie des intermittierenden hinkens. *Munch Med Wochenschr, 2*, 2487.

European Working Group. (1991). Second european consensus document on critical leg ischaemia. *Circulation, 84* (4 Suppl.), IV–1IV–26.

Ewles, L., & Simnett, I. (2017). *Promoting health: A practical guide* (7th ed.). Elsevier Ltd.

Fowkes, F. G., Rudan, D., Rudan, I., Aboyans, V., Denenberg, J. O., McDermott, M. M., et al. (2013). Comparison of global estimates of prevalence and risks factors for peripheral artery disease in 2000 and 2010: a systematic review and analysis. *Lancet, 382*, 1329–1340.

Ganguly, P., & Alam, F. S. (2015). Role of homocysteine in the development of cardiovascular disease. *Nutrition Journal, 14*, 6.

Garg, A., Gupta, A. K., & Khandelwal, N. (2018). *Diagnostic radiology: Chest and cardiovascular imaging* (4th ed., p. 515) Jaypee Brothers Medical Publishers (P) Ltd.

Garzon-Muvdi, T., Yang, W., Rong, X., Caplan, J. M., Ye, X., Colby, G. P., et al. (2016). Restenosis after carotid endarterectomy: Insight into risk factors and modification of postoperative management. *World Neurosurgery, 89*, 159–167.

Global Burden of Disease (GBD) 2013. (2015). Mortality and causes of death collaborators. global, regional, and national age-sex specific all-cause and cause-specific mortality for 240 causes of death, 1990-2013: a systematic analysis for the Global Burden of Disease Study 2013. *Lancet, 385*(9963), 117–171.

Greenhalgh, R. (1990). *The cause and management of aneurysms*. London: W.B. Saunders.

Grone, E., Uceyler, N., Abahji, T., Fleckenstein, J., Mussack, T., Hoffmann, U., et al. (2014). Reduced intraepidermal nerve fiber density in patients with chronic ischemic pain in peripheral arterial disease. *Pain, 155* (9), 1784–1792.

Guy, J. B., Bertoletti, L., Magne, N., Rancoule, C., Mahe, L., Font, C., et al. (2017). Venous thromboembolism in radiation therapy cancer patients: Findings from the RIETE registry. *Critical Review Oncology Hematology, 113*, 83–89.

Heart Protection Study Collaborative Group. (2007). Randomised trial of the effects of cholesterol-lowering with simvastatin on peripheral vascular and other major vascular outcomes in 20,536 people with peripheral arterial disease and other high-risk conditions. *Journal of Vascular Surgery, 45*(4), 645–654.

Hiramoto, J. S., Katz, R., Weisman, S., & Conte, M. (2014). Gender-specific risk factors for peripheral artery disease in a voluntary screening population. *Journal of American Heart Association, 3*(2), e000651.

Hordacre, B., Birks, V., Quinn, S., Barr, C., Patritti, B. L., & Crotty, M. (2012). Physiotherapy rehabilitation for individuals with lower limb amputation: A 15-year clinical series. *Physiotherapy Research International Journal, 18*(2), 70–80.

Hu, Y. Y., Arriaga, A. F., Peyre, S. E., Corso, K. A., Roth, E. M., & Greenberg, C. C. (2012). Deconstructing intraoperative communication failures. *Journal of Surgical Research, 177*(1), 37–42.

Hwang, J. Y. (2017). Doppler ultrasonography of the lower extremity arteries: anatomy and scanning guidelines. *Ultrasonography, 36*, 111–119.

Indes, J. E., Pfaff, M. J., Farrokhyar, F., Brown, H., Hashim, P., Cheung, K., et al. (2013). Clinical outcomes of 5358 patients undergoing direct open bypass or endovascular treatment for aortoiliac occlusive disease: a systematic review and meta-analysis. *Journal of Endovascular Therapy, 20*, 443–455.

Kannel, W. B., Skinner, J. J., Jr, & Schwartz, M. J. (1970). Intermittent claudication: incidence in the Framingham study. *Circulation, 41*, 875–883.

Karthikesalingam, A., Holt, P. J., Vidal-Diez, A., Ozedemir, B. A., Poloniecki, J. D., Hinchliffe, R. J., et al. (2014). Mortality from ruptured abdominal aortic aneurysms: clinical lessons from a comparison of outcomes in England and the USA. *Lancet, 383*, 963–969.

Kiel, J., Kaiser, K. (2019). Tibial anterior compartment syndrome. *StatPearls* [Internet]. Treasure Island (FL): StatPearls Publishing. Available at: <www.ncbi.nlm.nih.gov/books/NBK518970/>

Klinkert, P., Post, P. N., Breslau, P. J., & van Bockel, J. H. (2004). Saphenous vein versus PTFE for above-knee femoropopliteal bypass. A review of the literature. *European Journal of Vascular Endovascular Surgery, 27*, 357–362.

Kuivaniemi, H., Ryer, E. J., Elmore, J. R., & Tromp, G. (2015). Understanding the pathogenesis of abdominal aortic aneurysms. *Expert Review Cardiovascular Therapy, 13*(9), 975–987.

Langer, V. (2014). Compression therapy for leg ulcers. *Indian Dermatology Online Journal, 5*(4), 533–534.

Lassila, R., & Lepantalo, M. (1988). Cigarette smoking and the outcome after lower limb arterial surgery. *Acta Chirurgica Scandinavica, 154*, 635–640.

Lee, Y. Y., Lin, Y. M., Leu, W. J., Wu, M. Y., Tseng, J. H., Hsu, M. T., et al. (2015). Sliding-scale insulin used for blood glucose control: a meta-analysis of randomized controlled trials. *Metabolism, 64*(9), 1183–1192.

Li, Y., Huang, T., Zheng, Y., Muka, T., Troup, J., & Hu, F. B. (2016). Folic acid supplementation and the risk of cardiovascular diseases: a meta-analysis of randomized controlled trials. *Journal of American Heart Association, 5*(8), e003768.

Lingard, L., Espin, S., Whyte, S., Regehr, G., Baker, G. R., Reznick, R., et al. (2004). Communication failures in the operating room: An observational classification of recurrent types and effects. *Quality and Safety Health Care, 13*(5), 330–334.

Livingston, E. H. (2010). Solutions for improving patient safety. *JAMA, 303*, 159–161.

Lovett, J. K., Dennis, M. S., Sandercock, P. A., Bamford, J., Warlow, C. P., & Rothwell, P. M. (2003). Very early risk of stroke after a first transient ischemic attack. *Stroke, 34*(8), e138–140.

Lu, L., Mackay, D. F., & Pell, J. P. (2014). Meta-analysis of the association between cigarette smoking and peripheral arterial disease. *Heart, 100*(5), 414.

Mani, K., Bjorck, M., Lundkvist, J., & Wanhainen, A. (2009). Improved long-term survival after abdominal aortic aneurysm repair. *Circulation, 120*(3), 201–211.

Mayer, D., Aeschbacher, S., Pfammatter, T., et al. (2012). Complete replacement of open repair for ruptured abdominal aortic aneurysms by endovascular aneurysm repair: a two-center 14-year experience. *Annals of Surgery, 256,* 688—695.

McCallum, J. C., Besley, R. P., Darling, J. D., Hamdan, A. D., Wyers, M. C., Hile, C., et al. (2017). Open surgical revision provides a more durable repair than endovascular treatment for unfavorable vein graft lesions. *Journal of Vascular Surgery, 63*(1), 142—147.

McDermott, M. M., Ferrucci, L., Liu, K., Guralnik, J. M., Tian, L., Kibbe, M., et al. (2011). Women with peripheral arterial disease experience faster functional decline than men with peripheral arterial disease. *Journal of American College of Cardiology, 57,* 707—714.

Molnar, C., Opincariu, D., Benedek, T., Toma, M., & Nicolescu, C. (2019). Association between varicose veins anatomical pattern and procedural complications following endovascular laser photothermolysis for chronic venous insufficiency. *Brazilian Journal of Medical and Biological Research, 52* (4), e8330.

Muir, R. L. (2009). Peripheral arterial disease: Pathophysiology, risk factors, diagnosis, treatment and prevention. *Journal of Vascular Nursing, 27*(2), 26—30.

Mwipatayi, B. P., Western, C. E., Wong, J., & Angel, D. (2016). Atypical leg ulcers after sclerotherapy for treatment of varicose veins: Case reports and literature review. *International Journal of Surgery Case Reports, 25,* 161—164.

Nagpal, K., Vats, A., Lamb, B., Ashrafian, H., Sevadalis, N., Vincent, C., et al. (2010). Information transfer and communication in surgery: a systematic review. *Annals of Surgery, 252,* 225—239.

National Confidential Enquiry into Patient Outcomes and Death (NCEPOD). (2014). Lower Limb Amputation: Working Together. Available at: <www.ncepod.org.uk/2014report2/downloads/WorkingTogetherFullReport.pdf>

National Institute for Health and Care Excellence (NICE). (2012). *Lower limb peripheral arterial disease: diagnosis and management.* NICE guideline [CG147]. Available at: <guidance.nice.org.uk/CG147>.

National Institute of Health and Care Excellence (NICE). (2013). *Varicose veins in the legs: the diagnosis and management of varicose veins.* NICE Clinical Guidelines, No. 168. London: National Institute for Health and

Care Excellence (UK). Available at: <www.ncbi.nlm.nih.gov/books/NBK328012/>

National Institute of Health and Care Excellence (NICE). (2014a). *Peripheral arterial disease.* NICE clinical guideline 147. Available at: <www.nice.org.uk/guidance/CG147>

National Institute for Health and Care Excellence (NICE). (2014b). *The prevention and management of pressure ulcers in primary and secondary care.* National Clinical Guideline Centre (UK), No.179. Available at: <www.nice.org.uk/guidance/CG179>

National Institute of Health and Care Excellence (NICE). (2015). *Diabetic foot problems: prevention and management.* NICE guidelines [NG19]. Available at: <www.nice.org.uk/guidance/ng19>

National Institute of Health and Care Excellence (NICE). (2016). *Surgical site infection.* NICE clinical guideline QS49. Available at: <www.nice.org.uk/guidance/QS49>.

National Institute for Health and Care Excellence (NICE). (2018a). *Decision-making and mental capacity.* NICE guidelines (NG108). Available at: <www.nice.org.uk/guidance/ng108>

National Institute for Health and Care Excellence (NICE). (2018b). *Peripheral arterial disease: Diagnosis and management.* NICE guideline [CG147]. Available at: <www.nice.org.uk/guidance/cg147/evidence/evidence-review-a-determining-diagnosis-and-severity-of-peripheral-arterial-disease-in-people-with-diabetes-pdf-4776839533>.

National Institute for Health and Care Excellence (NICE). (2019). *Stroke and transient ischaemic attack in over 16s: diagnosis and initial management.* NICE guideline [NG128]. Available at: www.nice.org.uk/guidance/ng128

Neil, M. J. E. (2016). Pain after amputation. *British Journal of Academic Education, 16*(3), 107—112.

NHS England. (2018). The Atlas of Shared Learning, Case study: Improving venous leg ulcer healing in the community. Available at: <www.england.nhs.uk/atlas_case_study/improving-venous-leg-ulcer-healing-in-the-community>

Norlyk, A., Martinsen, B., & Kjaer-Petersen, K. (2013). Living with clipped wings-patients' experience of losing a leg. *International Journal of Qualitative Studies on Health and Well-being, 8,* 21891.

Nursing and Midwifery Council (NMC). (2018). *The code. Professional standards*

of practice and behaviour for nurses, midwives and nursing associates. Available at: <www.nmc.org.uk/standards/code>

O'Donnell, M. E., Reid, J. A., Lau, L. L., Hannon, R. J., & Lee, B. (2011). Optimal management of peripheral arterial disease for the non-specialist. *Ulster Medical Journal, 80*(1), 33—41.

Ousey, K., Stephenson, J., Barrett, S., King, B., Morton, N., Fenwick, K., et al. (2013). Wound Care in five English NHS Trusts: Results of a Survey. *Wound UK, 9*(4), 20—28.

Pande, R. L., & Creager, M. A. (2014). Socioeconomic inequality and peripheral artery disease prevalence in US adults. *Cardiovascular Quality and Outcomes, 7*(4), 532—539.

Paraskevas, K. L., Mikhailidis, D. P., Veith, F. J., & Spence, J. D. (2016). Definition of best medical treatment in asymptomatic and symptomatic carotid artery stenosis. *Angiology, 67*(5), 411—419.

Patel, M. R., Conte, M. S., Cutlip, D. E., Dib, N., Geraghty, P., Gray, W., et al. (2015). Evaluation and treatment of patients with lower extremity peripheral artery disease: consensus definitions from Peripheral Academic Research Consortium (PARC). *Journal of the American College of Cardiology, 65* (9), 931—941.

Peach, G., Griffin, M., Jones, K. G., Thompson, M. M., & Hinchliffe, R. J. (2012). Diagnosis and management of peripheral arterial disease. *British Medical Journal, 345,* e-5208.

Piazza, G. (2014). Varicose veins. *Circulation, 130*(7), 582—587.

Public Health England (PHE). (2015). *Abdominal aortic aneurysm screening: programme overview.* Available at: <www.gov.uk/guidance/abdominal-aortic-aneurysm-screening-programme-overview>

Public Health England (PHE). (2016). Abdominal aortic aneurysm screening programme: standards. Version 1.3. Available at: <www.gov.uk/government/publications/aaa-screening-quality-standards-and-service-objectives>

Public Health England (PHE). (2018). *New figures show larger proportion of strokes in the middle aged.* Available at: <www.gov.uk/government/news/new-figures-show-larger-proportion-of-strokes-in-the-middle-aged>

Ramot, Y., Nyska, A., & Spectre, G. (2013). Drug-induced thrombosis: an update. *Drug Safety, 36*(8), 585—603.

481

Robertson, L., Ghouri, M. A., & Kovacs, F. (2012). Antiplatelet and anticoagulant drugs for prevention of restenosis/reocclusion following peripheral endovascular treatment. *Cochrane Systematic Review Intervention, 8*, CD002071.

Rooke, T. W., Hirsch, A. T., & Misra, S. (2011). ACCF/AHA Focused Update of the Guideline for the Management of Patients With Peripheral Arterial Disease (updating the 2005 guideline): a report of the American College of Cardiology Foundation/American Heart Association Task Force on Practice Guidelines. *Circulation, 124* (18), 2020–2024.

Roper, N., Logan, W., & Tierney, A. (1981). *Learning to Use the Process of Nursing.* Edinburgh: Churchill Livingstone.

Royal College of Physicians. (2017). *National Early Warning Score (NEWS) 2: Standardising the assessment of acute-illness severity in the NHS. Updated report of a working party.* London: RCP.

Schwindt, A. G., Bennett, J. G., Crowder, W. H., Dohad, S., Janzer, S. F., George, J. C., et al. (2017). Lower extremity revascularization using optical coherence tomography-guided directional atherectomy: final results of the EValuatIon of the PantheriS OptIcal COherence Tomography ImagiNg Atherectomy System for Use in the Peripheral Vasculature (VISION) Study. *Journal of Endovascular Therapy, 24*(3), 355–366.

Scottish Intercollegiate Guidelines Network. Management of chronic venous leg ulcers.Edinburgh: SIGN;2010. (SIGN guideline No.120). (cited Available from http://www.sign.ac.uk/assets/sign120.pdf)

Sebelius, K. (2010). *How tobacco smoke causes disease: The Biology and behavioral basis for smoking-attributable disease: A report of the surgeon general.* Cardiovascular disease. Centers for Disease Control and Prevention (US); National Center for Chronic Disease Prevention and Health Promotion (US); Office on Smoking and Health (US). Chapter 6, Available at: <www.ncbi.nlm.nih.gov/books/NBK53012/>.

Selvin, E., & Erlinger, T. P. (2004). Prevalence of and risk factors for peripheral arterial disease in the United States: results from the National Health and Nutrition Examination Survey, 1999-2000. *Circulation, 110*, 738–743.

Seretny, M., & Colvin, L. A. (2016). Pain management in patients with vascular disease. *British Journal of Anaesthesia, 117*(2), ii95–ii106.

Shaw, P.M., Loree, J., & Gibbons, R.C. (2019). Abdominal Aortic Aneurysm (AAA). *StatPearls* [Internet]. Treasure Island (FL): StatPearls Publishing. Available at: <www.ncbi.nlm.nih.gov/books/NBK470237>

Shearman, A., Shearman, C. (2012). Failure to diagnose acute limb ischaemia (ALI); an avoidable cause of limb loss. *Association of Surgeons of Great Britain and Ireland, 2012 International Surgical Congress.*

Shepperd, S., Lannin, N. A., Clemson, L. M., McCluskey, A., Cameron, I. D., & Barras, S. L. (2013). Discharge planning from hospital to home. *Cochrane Database Systematic Review, 31*(1), CD000313.

Smeili, L. A. A., & Lotufo, P. A. (2015). Incidence and predictors of cardiovascular complications and death after vascular surgery. *Arquivos Brasileiros De Cardiologia, 105*(5), 510–518.

Smith, B. H., Macfarlane, G. J., & Torrance, N. (2007). Epidemiology of chronic pain, from the laboratory to the bus stop: time to add understanding of biological mechanisms to the study of risk factors in population-based research? *Pain, 127*, 5–10.

Smith-Burgess, L. (2017). Early identification and detection of abdominal aortic aneurysms. *Nursing Times [online], 113* (3), 36–39.

Spence, J. D., Song, H., & Cheng, G. (2016). Appropriate management of asymptomatic carotid stenosis. *Stroke and Vascular Neurology, 1*(2), 64–70.

Thomas, C. (2018). Intrinsic and extrinsic sources and prevention of infection (in surgery). *Infection Surgery, 37*, 1.

Topfer, L.A., Spry, C. (2018). New technologies for the treatment of peripheral artery disease. Canadian Agency for Drugs and Technologies in Health: *Issues in Emerging Health Technologies,* 172. Available at: <www.ncbi.nlm.nih.gov/books/NBK519606>

Valentijn, T. M., & Stolker, R. J. (2012). Lessons from the REACH Registry in Europe. *Current Vascular Pharmacology, 10*, 725–727.

Walker, W. F. (1988). *A colour atlas of peripheral vascular disease.* London: Wolfe Medical Publications.

Wariyapola, C., Littlehales, E., Abayasekara, K., Fall, D., Parker, V., & Hatton, G. (2016). Improving the quality of vascular surgical discharge planning in a hub centre. *Annals of Royal College of Surgery England, 98*(4), 275–279.

Watson, L., Ellis, B., & Leng, G. C. (2008). Exercise for intermittent claudication. *Cochrane Database Systematic Review, 4*, CD000990.

Weiss, M. A., Hsu, J. T., Neuhaus, I., Sadick, N. S., & Duffy, D. M. (2014). Consensus for sclerotherapy. *Dermatology Surgery, 40*, 1309–1318.

Weledji, E. P., & Fokam, P. (2014). Treatment of the diabetes foot – to amputate or not? *BioMed Central Surgery, 14*, 83.

Willigendael, E. M., Teijink, J. A., & Bartelink, M. L. (2004). Influence of smoking on incidence and prevalence of peripheral arterial disease. *Journal of Vascular Surgery, 40*, 1158–1165.

Wilson, D. G., Harris, S. K., Peck, H., Hart, K., Jung, E., Azarbal, A. F., et al. (2017). Patterns of care in hospitalized vascular surgery patients at end of life. *JAMA Surgery, 152*(2), 183–190.

Wise, J., White, A., Stinner, D. J., & Fergason, J. R. (2017). *Advanced Wound Care, 6*(8), 253–260.

Wood, A.M., Kaptoge, S., Butterworth, A.S., et al., for the Emerging Risk Factors Collaboration/EPIC-CVD/UK Biobank Alcohol Study Group. (2018). Risk thresholds for alcohol consumption: combined analysis of individual-participant data for 599 912 current drinkers in 83 prospective studies. *Lancet, 391*(101129), 1513–1523.

Yahagi, K., Kolodgie, F. D., Lutter, C., Mori, H., Romero, M. E., Finn, A. V., et al. (2017). Pathology of human coronary and carotid artery atherosclerosis and vascular calicification in diabetes mellitus. *Atherosclerosis, Thrombosis and Vascular Biology, 37*(2), 191–204.

Yau, W. J., Teoh, H., & Verma, S. (2015). Endothelial cell control of thrombosis. *BioMed Central Cardiovascular Disorder, 15*, 130.

Zommorodi, S., Leander, K., Roy, J., Steuer, J., & Hultgren, R. (2018). Understanding abdominal aortic aneurysm epidemiology: socioeconomic position affects outcome. *Journal Epidemiology Community Health, 72*(10), 904–910.

Further reading

Engstrom, B., & Van de Ven, C. (1999). *Therapy for amputees*. London: Churchill Livingstone.

Hands, L., & Thompson, M. (2015). Vascular surgery *(Oxford Specialist Handbooks in surgery)* (2nd ed.). Oxford: Oxford University Press.

Loftus, I., & Hinchliffe, R. J. (2018). *Vascular and endovascular surgery: A companion to specialist surgical practice* (6th ed.). Elsevier.

MacVittie, B. (1998). *Vascular surgery: Mosby's perioperative nursing series.* London: Mosby.

Mangus, J. A. (2019). *LIMB LOSS LIFE: The first few days, weeks, months and years as a new amputee.* Independently published.

McMonagle, M., & Stephenson, M. (2014). *Vascular and endovascular surgery at a glance.* Chichester: Wiley-Blackwell.

Murray, S. (2001). *Vascular disease: nursing and management.* London: Whurr Publishers.

Sidawy, A. N., & Perler, B. A. (2018). (9th ed.). *Rutherford's vascular and endovascular therapy,* (2-volume set. 9e). Elsevier.

Smith, L. (2016). *Cardiac vascular nursing: review and resource manual* (4th ed.). Silver Spring, MD: American Nurses Association.

Zollinger, R., & Ellison, E. (2016). *Zollinger's atlas of surgical operations* (10th ed.). New York: McGraw Hill.

Chapter | **23** |

Patients requiring orthopaedic surgery

Giles Farrington

KEY OBJECTIVES OF THE CHAPTER

At the end of this chapter the reader should be able to:

- describe the structure and function of the musculoskeletal system
- classify bones according to their structure
- classify joints according to their structure and degree of movement
- discuss specific orthopaedic investigations and common orthopaedic conditions
- discuss the importance of pre-assessment and education in preparing the orthopaedic patient for their surgery
- demonstrate knowledge of the nursing care of patients requiring surgery to the hip, knee, foot, shoulder, forearm, hand and spine
- discuss the process of bone healing
- discuss types of fracture and how they are managed
- discuss the relevance of neurovascular observations in detecting compromise and the actions to be taken if detected
- discuss specific issues in planning a patient's discharge and the importance of patient education in rehabilitation.

Areas to think about before reading the chapter

How do bones heal?

- Compare and contrast the role and function of the nurse and physiotherapist.
- What do you understand by the multidisciplinary team?

Introduction

The term 'orthopaedics' is applied to all conditions affecting the musculoskeletal system. The scope of orthopaedic nursing includes the treatment, management and rehabilitation of patients with musculoskeletal conditions through either conservative or surgical methods. A fully functioning musculoskeletal system is essential for optimal health in the human being, and disease or injury involving this system can significantly affect the individual's quality of life.

There are two types of orthopaedic surgery: trauma (emergency) and elective surgery. Trauma surgery is carried out on patients who require urgent surgery, such as following an accident. Elective orthopaedic surgery is for patients waiting for planned orthopaedic procedures such as joint replacements for progressive osteoarthritis.

The field of orthopaedics and orthopaedic nursing has become extremely diverse and is changing at an unprecedented rate. Advances in surgical techniques, and developments within nursing and within healthcare provision are all contributing to the advancement within the specialty of orthopaedics.

One change that has affected orthopaedic nursing is the reduced time a patient now spends in hospital. Many patients now have surgery as a day case admission, instead of remaining in hospital overnight or for several days. Innovations such as preoperative assessment clinics and early discharge schemes, where patients are cared for in their own home, also significantly reduce the length of time a patient spends in hospital.

In the context of change, orthopaedic nurses must continue to promote healing, maximize independence within the individual's capability and promote optimal rehabilitation.

This chapter will describe some of the more common disorders of the musculoskeletal system that are caused by disease and trauma and will explain orthopaedic surgical procedures and the relevant nursing care.

The musculoskeletal system

Most of the body's mass is made up of the musculoskeletal system. It comprises bones, joints, ligaments, muscles and cartilage. The musculoskeletal system performs and enables several essential functions (Bulstrode, 2017; Tortora & Derrickson, 2017):

- the maintenance of body shape
- the support and protection of soft tissue structures such as internal organs
- movement
- breathing
- the manufacture of red blood cells, white blood cells and platelets in the bone marrow
- the storage and main supply of reserve phosphate and calcium in bone.

Bone

Bones are classified by their shape and fall into five categories:

- *Long bones*: these are greater in length than width. Pulled by contracting muscles, they act as levers for body movement. Long bones include the femur, tibia, fibula, radius, ulna and humerus.
- *Short bones*: these measure approximately the same in length and width and are irregular in shape. They are found where only limited movement is necessary, such as the carpal and tarsal bones.

- *Flat bones*: these are generally curved or thin. They have a protective function and facilitate muscle attachment. Flat bones include the ribs, sternum, scapulae and bones of the cranium.
- *Sesamoid bones*: these small bones are found where tendons pass over the joint of a long bone. Their key role is protection, such as the patella bone of the knee joint.
- *Irregular bones*: these do not fit neatly into any of the other categories. The facial bones and the vertebrae are examples of irregular bones.

Anatomy of a long bone

A typical long bone consists of the following parts:
- *Diaphysis* – the shaft or long part of the bone.
- *Epiphysis* – a proximal and distal epiphysis can be found at opposite ends of the bone.
- *Metaphysis* – separates the diaphysis from the epiphysis at either end of the bone. It is made up of the adjacent trabeculae of spongy bone.
- *Medullary cavity* – contains fatty yellow marrow and can be found within the diaphysis.
- *Endosteum* – the membrane that lines the internal cavities of bone.
- *Articular cartilage* – the layer of hyaline cartilage which covers the epiphysis and allows a joint to function more effectively by reducing friction.
- *Periosteum* – the fibrous membrane that covers the outer surface of bone that has not been covered by articular cartilage. It contains nerves, capillaries and lymphatic vessels and is essential for bone nutrition, growth and repair.

Bone tissue

Bone tissue comprises cells embedded in a matrix of ground substance, collagenous fibres and inorganic salts. The salts harden the bone, whereas the ground substance and collagenous fibres provide flexibility and strength.

The two main types of bone tissue are cancellous bone and compact bone.

Cancellous bone

- Cancellous bone consists of thin plates of bone tissue called trabeculae and is also known as spongy bone because of its lattice-like appearance.
- Red marrow fills the spaces between the trabeculae, and within the trabeculae lie lacunae, which store osteocytes. The osteocytes are nourished through the marrow cavities from circulating blood.
- Cancellous bone stores some red and yellow marrow, and its main function is support.

Compact bone

- Compact bone is hard and contains cylinders of calcified bone known as osteons or Haversian systems. These systems are surrounded by calcified intercellular rings called lamellae.
- Centrally within the Haversian systems are Haversian canals, which contain nerves, blood vessels and lymphatic vessels. Haversian canals are longitudinal channels which generally branch into perforating canals called Volkmann's canals. The Volkmann's canals extend the vessels and nerves inward to the endosteum and outwards to the periosteum.
- Spaces called lacunae, which store osteocytes, can be found between the lamellae, and radiating from the lacunae are tiny canaliculi, which transport waste and nutrients into and out of blood vessels in the Haversian canals.
- Compact bone lies over cancellous bone and its main functions are support and protection.

Bone cells

Bone tissue contains four types of cell.
- *Osteogenic cells* – found in the periosteum, endosteum and the Haversian and Volkmann's canals. They can be transformed into osteoblasts or osteoclasts during the healing process or at stressful times, e.g. following trauma.
- *Osteoblasts* – found in the growing parts of bones and the periosteum. They secrete some of the organic components and mineral salts involved in bone formation, and their main function is bone building.
- *Osteocytes* – the main cells of bone tissue. They derive from osteoblasts that have deposited bone tissue around themselves. Osteocytes keep the matrix healthy and help maintain homeostasis by assisting in the release of calcium into the blood.
- *Osteoclasts* – giant multinuclear cells found around bone surfaces, which do exactly the opposite of osteoblasts. Their main function is in resorption (dissolved and assimilated), which is essential in bone development, growth, maintenance and repair.

Bone ossification

Bones develop through a process known as ossification (osteogenesis). This process begins during the sixth week of embryonic life.

There are two types of ossification:
- *intramembranous ossification*, when bone is formed by mesenchymal tissue (embryonic connective tissue cells)
- *endochondral ossification*, when bone develops by replacing a cartilage model.

The primary ossification centre of a long bone is in the diaphysis. As a result of cartilage degeneration, cavities merge, forming the marrow cavity, and osteoblasts lay down bone. Ossification then occurs in the epiphyses but not for the epiphyseal plate.

Homeostasis

Bone assists homeostasis (a state of inner balance and stability) by the storage and release of minerals and calcium, as required in the blood and tissues to maintain appropriate levels. Normal bone growth depends on calcium and phosphorus, and adequate levels of vitamins A, C and D are essential for bone growth and maintenance.

Effects of hormones on bone

Bones have an effect on hormone secretion and several hormones have an effect on bones. The parathyroid hormone assists in osteoclast production, increasing bone remodelling, whereas calcitonin (a hormone released by the thyroid gland) reduces the calcium level in the blood and reduces bone resorption. Other hormones such as thyroxine, growth hormone, the sex hormones from the gonads and vitamins A, C and D are significantly involved in bone maturation, with thyroxine and the growth hormones stimulating endochondral ossification.

Effects of ageing on bone

The ageing process affects bone in two key ways:
1. The loss of calcium from bone starts in females at around 30 years of age and this loss increases as oestrogen levels decrease in the early 40s. By the age of 70, as much as 30% of the calcium in bone is lost; however, in the male, calcium loss does not generally start until over 60 years of age (Tortora & Derrickson, 2017).
2. There is a decrease in protein formation, which results in a decreased ability to produce the organic part of the bone matrix. This leads to osteoporotic bones in the elderly and an increased risk of fractures (Cheung et al, 2016).

Cartilage

Cartilage is a tough, avascular, flexible connective tissue which assists with the support systems of the body. There are three types of cartilage.
- *Hyaline cartilage* is firm and smooth and is found on the articulating surfaces of synovial joints.
- *Fibrocartilage* is tough, flexible and tension-resistant, and is found between the intervertebral discs.
- *Elastic cartilage* retains its strength while stretched, as it has more elastic fibres, and is found in the epiglottis and external ear.

487

Joints

A joint is the site at which two or more bones are united. A joint provides the mechanism that allows body movement. Based on the structure or type of tissue that connects the bones, joints are classified into three major groups: fibrous, cartilaginous and synovial.

Fibrous joints

The bones are united by fibrous connective tissue and allow very minimal movement, e.g. sutures between the bones of the skull.

Cartilaginous joints

The bones are united by a plate of hyaline cartilage (primary cartilaginous) or fibrocartilage (secondary cartilaginous), and will allow slight movement, e.g. the pubic symphysis or between the bodies of the vertebrae.

Synovial joints

Synovial joints contain a synovial (joint) cavity, articular capsule, synovial membrane and synovial fluid.

A synovial (joint) cavity is the space between two articulating bones. Articular cartilage covers the surfaces of the articulating bones but does not hold the bones together. Synovial joints are surrounded by an articular capsule, and the inner lining of the capsule is called the synovial membrane. The synovial membrane secretes synovial fluid to lubricate the joint and provides nourishment for the articular cartilage.

An extensive range of movement is possible with this type of joint. Based on the shape of the articulating surfaces and the range of movements possible, there are several different types of synovial joint, e.g. the ball and socket joint of the hip and shoulder, and the hinge joint of the knee.

Common orthopaedic disorders

Rheumatoid arthritis

Rheumatoid arthritis is the commonest chronic inflammatory disease of joints and affects 3% of women and 1% of men (Bulstrode, 2017). The cause is unknown, but the inflammation is the result of an abnormality of both cellular and humoral immunity with environmental and genetic factors involved (Elias-Jones et al, 2018; Bulstrode, 2017). As it is a systemic disease, unlike osteoarthritis, rheumatoid arthritis affects structures all over the body.

Pathophysiology

The target for this disease is the synovium. In the early stages of the disease the synovial membrane is affected and the joints become warm, swollen and tender, and range of movement is reduced. This disease generally presents in the small peripheral joints, usually of the hands and feet, with the wrists, knees and elbows also being susceptible. Unlike osteoarthritis it nearly always affects several joints at the same time (Bulstrode, 2017). The affected synovium contains plasma cells and lymphocytes, a reflection of the autoimmune nature of the disease, and, left untreated, the inflammatory reaction affects the neighbouring structures. As the disease progresses, there is joint cartilage, capsule and ligament destruction, leading to joint instability, subluxation and deformity (Solomon et al, 2014).

Although rheumatoid arthritis is mainly treated by rheumatologists, it does involve orthopaedic surgeons when conservative treatments have proved to be unsuccessful. Orthopaedic surgeons are involved when joints and ligaments require stabilization or reconstruction.

Osteoarthritis

Osteoarthritis is a degenerative 'wear and tear' process occurring in joints that are impaired by congenital defect, vascular insufficiency or previous disease or injury. It is by far the commonest variety of arthritis (Bulstrode, 2017), affecting up to 85% of the population at some time in their lives (Elias-Jones et al, 2018).

Osteoarthritis is defined as primary or secondary.

- *Primary osteoarthritis* has no obvious cause (Solomon et al, 2014), is most common in white females during their 50s and 60s and affects several joints (Bulstrode, 2017).
- *Secondary osteoarthritis* has many causes and follows a demonstrable abnormality of which the commonest are obesity, malunited fractures, joint instability, genetic or developmental abnormalities, metabolic or endocrine disease, inflammatory diseases, osteonecrosis and neuropathies (Bulstrode, 2017; White et al, 2015).

Pain, limited mobility and a decrease in functional ability are the main clinical features. X-ray or imaging is undertaken to confirm the diagnosis of osteoarthritis (Jester, 2014; Bulstrode, 2017).

Pathophysiology

In osteoarthritis the articular cartilage is slowly worn away, resulting in the exposure of underlying bone. The subchondral bone becomes hard and glossy (eburnated), and bone at the margins of the joint forms protruding ridges and spurs known as osteophytes. These spurs can break off, causing further restriction of movement and additional pain. It is the pain, stiffness and often deformity that force the patient to seek treatment.

Treatment of rheumatoid arthritis and osteoarthritis

Treatment can be conservative or operative. Orthopaedic surgery should not be recommended until all conservative measures have been considered.

Conservative treatment

- *Weight reduction*: if overweight, the patient is encouraged to reduce weight, so that less weight is forced on to the joint. The patient needs to be informed of the problems caused by excess weight and understand that, by reducing their weight, they will assist in reducing their level of pain. This may be difficult for the patient, owing to the nature of the disease. It is therefore important to set small achievable targets and offer praise and encouragement as they achieve satisfactory weight loss.
- *Physiotherapy*: passive and active exercises can assist the range of joint movement, prevent contractures and improve coordination or balance. Heat therapy can often produce relief from pain.
- *Hydrotherapy*: the warmth and buoyancy of the water allows the patient active, pain-free movement and relieves muscle spasm.
- *Use of a walking stick*: the patient is encouraged to use the walking stick correctly, holding it in the opposite hand to the affected hip/knee.
- *Aids and appliances*: these can help the patient with activities of living, e.g. a helping hand to pick up dropped articles or an aid to assist with putting shoes and socks on.
- *A shoe raise*: application of a shoe raise to the shorter limb can correct the apparent shortening, relieving strain on the lumbar spine and opposite hip.
- *Drug therapy*: simple analgesics such as paracetamol or dihydrocodeine can be effective in reducing the pain caused by raw bone rubbing on bone; however, they are not useful in reducing the sinusitis of osteoarthritis. Non-steroidal anti-inflammatory drugs (NSAIDs) reduce the inflammatory response and many people find them useful before physical activity or at night. Disease-modifying anti-rheumatic drugs, corticosteroids and immunosuppressive drugs may be used for patients with rheumatoid arthritis.
- *Intra-articular therapy*: local injection of hydrocortisone into the joint may help to restore comfort and mobility.

Operative treatment

All patients need to be carefully assessed before a decision to undertake surgery is made, because some patients will benefit from surgery more than others, according to their physical, psychological and social circumstances. Only when conservative treatments have failed should operative treatment be considered.

The following criteria are often used to decide on the need for surgery:
- pain
- radiological changes
- joint stability
- loss of function
- immobility.

The most common surgical procedures for patients with osteoarthritis and rheumatoid arthritis are synovectomy, osteotomy, arthrodesis and arthroplasty.
- *Synovectomy* involves excision of diseased synovial membrane and is performed more frequently for the patient with rheumatoid arthritis.
- *Osteotomy* involves surgically cutting across the bone. It is used to correct bone deformity or to relieve joint pain.
- *Arthrodesis* is carried out to surgically fuse a joint. It is used to stabilize a joint, or for pain relief in a joint severely damaged or diseased.
- *Arthroplasty* is replacement of the joint by an artificial component and one of the most successful operations in orthopaedic surgery (Bulstrode, 2017).

Nursing assessment of the orthopaedic patient

When assessing orthopaedic patients, it is important to first establish what their normal functional abilities were and then to see how their presenting complaint is decreasing this functional ability. A thorough nursing assessment is required to obtain essential information from patients about the physical, psychological, socio-cultural, environmental and politico-economic factors affecting their activities of living and how they cope with these problems. Once the patient's problems have been identified, the nurse can set goals, take nursing action and evaluate any subsequent care. The Roper, Logan and Tierney model of nursing (Roper et al, 1996) is one example of a model used in the nursing management of an orthopaedic patient and an example of this can be seen in Table 23.1.

Every patient is a unique individual and the nursing assessment should be tailored to address these individual needs. The

Table 23.1 Postoperative care plan for a patient following a total hip replacement, using the Roper, Logan and Tierney model of nursing

Assessment/usual routine	Patients problem	Goal	Nursing action	Evaluation
Maintaining a safe environment				
Uncemented hip prosthesis in correct position following anterior approach on return from operating theatre	Potential risk of dislocation of hip prosthesis	To prevent hip dislocation	Ensure Louise has a copy of the dos and don'ts on how not to dislocate her hip Reinforce the information at regular intervals Ensure Louise does not flex the hip to an angle of 90 degrees or more Ensure Louise uses a high toilet seat on the ward and at home for 3 months	Louise's hip prosthesis did not dislocate
Louise's skin is healthy and intact	Pre- and postoperative skin checks to identify existing or new skin ulcers/ pressure sores Potential wound infection or haematoma following surgery	To prevent wound infection and haematoma	Administer prophylactic antibiotics as prescribed Observe the wound for bleeding, swelling and excessive drainage Use aseptic technique when dealing with dressings and drains Record temperature {1/2}—1 hourly initially, then 2—4-hourly for a 24-hour period	Louise remained apyrexial and the wound healed with no sign of infection
	Potential risk of pressure ulcers as her mobility is reduced	Assess pressure ulcer risk using Waterlow score and use appropriate mattress if indicated	Encourage mobilization on day 1	Louise's pressure areas remained intact TED stockings fitted to reduce chance of embolism formation, to remain in place until patient is fully mobile
Louise's temperature was normal, 37.1°C, on admission to hospital	On return to the ward Louise's temperature was 35°C	To assist body temperature back to normal limits	Place a Bair Hugger next to Louise's body and apply extra bed linen Record Louise's temperature at regular intervals until it has returned to within normal limits	Within 2 hours Louise's temperature had risen to 36.2°C and the Bair Hugger was removed Louise's temperature remained above 36.2°C and below 37.5°C

(Continued)

Table 23.1 Postoperative care plan for a patient following a total hip replacement, using the Roper, Logan and Tierney model of nursing—cont'd

Assessment/usual routine	Patients problem	Goal	Nursing action	Evaluation
Mobilization				
Louise's mobilization and distance she could walk without pain prior to surgery was approximately 300 yards	Postoperatively, Louise had lack of confidence mobilizing, but her pain was under control	Louise to regain confidence mobilizing	Give explanations and reassurance prior to and when mobilizing Observe for signs of dislocation On day 1 begin mobilizing Louise with the aid of a physiotherapist, starting with transfers from bed to chair, learning the correct way to sit in a chair and progressing on to how to use the sticks safely to avoid dislocation Louise will need to mobilize partial weight-bearing on the operated leg for 6 weeks	Louise can safely mobilize and transfer from bed to chair and bed to toilet with confidence
Work and play				
Louise works as a part-time secretary for a small local firm The firm is having some financial problems and there have been some redundancies	Louise is warned she may lose her job due to her sick leave She likes to get out and does not wish to retire	To return to work as soon as she is able	Encourage Louise to express her fears Refer to a social worker	The surgeon wrote a supportive letter to her employer, who was very sympathetic and supportive
Louise is a keen gardener	Louise is concerned that she will not be able to return to her hobby of gardening, although she admits that she has been unable to do any gardening during the 6 months prior to surgery	For Louise to return to light gardening activities	Refer Louise to the physiotherapist for advice on safe movement while gardening	As yet, Louise has not returned to gardening but looks forward to doing so She has learnt what she can do safely and accepts this
Expressing sexuality				
Louise and her husband have been married for 32 years and still enjoy a	Fear of dislocating hip during sexual relations	Louise to return to sexual relations with	Give Louise advice and reassurance that she can resume sexual intercourse in the passive role at approximately 6 weeks	Louise has yet to resume sexual intercourse but feels

(Continued)

Table 23.1 Postoperative care plan for a patient following a total hip replacement, using the Roper, Logan and Tierney model of nursing—cont'd

Assessment/usual routine	Patients problem	Goal	Nursing action	Evaluation
sexual relationship. This has been affected by pain in recent months, and Louise confided that her husband had offered to sleep in the spare room to give her more room and to prevent her dislocating her hip when she got home		her husband without dislocating her hip	Give Louise helpline number and email address of Outsiders, the organisation that aids the sexual and personal relationships of people with a disability, and provide a leaflet on positions postoperatively	she knows how not to dislocate the hip

following points, however, are often discussed and assessed in an orthopaedic nursing assessment (Jester, 2014).

- Mobility
  - Is movement restricted, and, if so, how restricted is the movement?
  - Is the range of movement limited?
  - Is active range of movement less than passive?
  - Does mobility improve throughout the day?
  - What is the condition of the patient's musculoskeletal system?
  - What is the neurological status of the affected limb?
  - Does the patient require aids to assist mobility?
- Pain
  - Where is the maximum site of pain?
  - Does the pain radiate away from the site of injury?
  - Does the pain change during the course of the day?
  - How would the pain be described?
  - Is there swelling or deformity?
- Sleep
  - Is sleep affected by pain?
- Sexuality
  - Has a limp, limb-shortening or a deformity altered the patient's body image?
  - Has the patient had surgery that is affecting their sexual relationship?
- Psychological well-being
  - Is the patient anxious or depressed?
  - Does the patient have dementia or a poor attention span?
- Hygiene
  - Can the patient manage with their own personal cleansing and dressing?
  - Does the patient require assistance or special aids/appliances to assist with hygiene care?

- Breathing
  - Does the patient smoke?
  - Does the patient have a history of cardiovascular problems?
  - Does the patient have any sort of curvature of the spine that is affecting their respiratory system?
- Working and playing
  - Has the problem affected the patient's work and/or social activities?
  - Does the patient require assistance for household activities?

The main aim of the orthopaedic nursing assessment and subsequent care that is planned is to assist the patient to be as independent as is realistically possible.

Orthopaedic investigations and tests

Standard X-rays

Standard X-rays assist in the diagnosis and confirmation of the injury or disease, e.g. fractures, loss of joint space in osteoarthritis. Usually, no specific preparation is required.

Computerized axial tomography

A computerized axial tomography (CAT or CT) scan combines X-rays with computer technology to show cross-sectional views (tomograms) of internal body structures. The patient is intravenously injected with a low-level radioactive tracer and lies on a table slowly passing through a circular tunnel in the scanner, where rotation of a low-intensity X-ray beam across the width of the body takes place. Detectors opposite the X-ray beam record the degree to which the X-ray is absorbed by various body tissues and convert the modified beams into electronic signals that are fed into the computer. Changes in the X-ray beams are then analysed by the computer, and high-resolution images are shown on a monitor. These images are kept on film and examined one section at a time. This investigation is particularly useful in the diagnosis of spinal and skull disorders.

Magnetic resonance imaging

Magnetic resonance imaging (MRI) is a non-invasive investigation of the body's deep structures. The patient is required to lie on a non-magnetic stretcher and is passed into a scanner where the body is exposed to a strong magnetic field. This magnetic field causes the body's protons to line upright in rows parallel to the field. The patient's body is then exposed to radiofrequency waves, which cause the protons to fall out of line. When the radiofrequency waves are stopped, the protons return to their previous position. Images of this movement are taken and visually displaced. MRI is particularly useful to show changes in the vascularity of bone following trauma, and degenerative changes in the ligaments and intervertebral discs (Bulstrode, 2017).

Many patients who undergo an MRI scan experience anxiety or panic attacks and nurses should therefore help reduce stress by maintaining verbal contact.

Radioisotope bone scan

The patient is given an intravenous injection of radioisotope substance, which is taken up in the bone. The amount of uptake reflects the bone turnover and is of value in the early detection of tumour invasion, bone death and repair.

Dual-energy X-ray absorptiometry (DXA) or bone densitometry

This technique is carried out to measure bone mineral density in patients with metabolic bone disease and may be required for the whole of the patient's body or an identified area. This measurement assists the clinician to make an informed opinion on the most appropriate treatment for the patient.

Arthroscopy

Arthroscopy is an invasive procedure which involves the introduction of an instrument called an arthroscope into a joint, under general anaesthetic. Arthroscopy enables inspection of the interior of the joint with and without joint movement and allows manipulation of individual structures with a probe or hook. It can also be used to aspirate fluid and wash out a joint.

Nerve conduction studies (NCS)

Nerve conduction studies measure how fast an electrical impulse moves through your nerve. NCS can identify nerve damage and be used to plan treatment for various conditions, NCS are the gold standard test for carpal tunnel syndrome. Electromyography (EMG) is normally carried out at the same time. An EMG measures electrical activity in response to a nerve's stimulation of the muscle. The test is used to help detect neuromuscular abnormalities. During the test small needles are inserted through the skin into the muscle and electrical activity is measured resting the muscle and contracting the muscle. Both of these tests are outpatient procedures and the whole test takes approximately 60–90 minutes.

Lower limb orthopaedic surgery

The hip

Total hip replacement (arthroplasty)

Total hip replacement (arthroplasty) is the most popular operation for osteoarthritis of the hip (Bulstrode, 2017). In a total hip replacement, the worn acetabulum and femoral head are removed and replaced with artificial components, which can be either cemented or uncemented.

- *Cemented*: this involves the use of a dense cup, usually polyethylene, and a metal or metal alloy femoral component. Each of these parts is secured by the compound methylmethacrylate, which has properties resembling bone. A disadvantage of the cemented prostheses is the potential bone destruction caused if the prosthesis becomes loose.
- *Uncemented*: where cement would have been placed, more cortical bone is preserved. This allows younger patients to have total hip replacement surgery with increased choice for revision surgery in the future.

Minimally invasive hip replacement
Minimally invasive hip (MIH) surgery involves the insertion of the prostheses via one or two incisions, each less than 10 cm, compared with a traditional incision of 20–30 cm (Eskelinen, 2017). While appealing to patients, when MIH is compared with traditional-incision total hip replacement surgery there is yet a lack of large-scale long-term robust clinical trials on its success (Lloyd et al, 2012).

Preoperative assessment and care

It is recommended that patients undergoing total hip replacement attend the preoperative assessment clinic and education classes 2–3 weeks prior to surgery.

Preoperative assessment enables the multidisciplinary team to ensure that the patient is as medically fit as is possible, in order that they are not cancelled because of medical problems when admitted to hospital. This allows effective use of resources such as theatre time and hospital beds and avoids patient disappointment when their surgery is cancelled (Flynn & Lucas 2014).

Depending on whether preoperative education classes are available, the preoperative assessment clinic may be run by a nurse practitioner alone or by a variety of members of the multidisciplinary team. The preoperative assessment will consist of:

- routine blood tests for a full blood count, urea and electrolytes, group and save and crossmatching, and any other indicated tests, e.g. glucose, sickle cell screen
- vital signs monitoring, including blood pressure, pulse, temperature, respirations and oxygen saturation levels
- neurovascular assessment to provide a baseline for postoperative monitoring
- electrocardiograph, if indicated
- X-rays of the hip and chest, if indicated
- a comprehensive health history and physical examination.

Preoperative education class. Many patients now have the opportunity to attend a preoperative education class, which is run by the multidisciplinary team alongside the patient's visit to the preassessment clinic. If education classes are not available, the multidisciplinary team will provide information at the preassessment clinic. The patient is given a detailed explanation about what the operation will involve and what they should expect postoperatively.

- Patients are often anxious about the postoperative pain they may experience. Explanations are given about the use of analgesia, spinal and regional anaesthesia, and distraction techniques such as deep breathing and guided imagery to control their pain (Carpenter et al, 2017).
- Patients are informed that they will receive prophylactic antibiotics to prevent infection, and prophylaxis against deep venous thrombosis, such as anti-embolism stockings, sequential compression devices and anticoagulant therapy.
- Patients are made aware of the risks of their surgery, such as dislocation of the hip, and will be taught how to prevent this during the class. A list of 'dos and don'ts' following surgery is given to the patient (Fig. 23.1).
- The physiotherapist will assess patients' gait and range of movement and will teach patients their postoperative exercises during the class so that they can practise them prior to their admission.
- The occupational therapist will carry out a daily living assessment to see what activities the patient is having difficulty with. The patient is taught how to preserve energy and adapt daily living as required. Those

DOs and DON'Ts after a total hip replacement

DOs

Do the exercises you have been taught twice a day, if possible

Do continue to lie flat on your back, for a short period daily (half an hour twice a day) for a couple of weeks after leaving hospital

Do use your stick(s), especially outside the house. It is advisable to use one stick for 6 weeks

Do be critical of your own posture in sitting, standing and walking

Do sleep on the side of your new hip, if you want to, and put a pillow between your legs for comfort

Do use equipment you have been given for putting on socks or stockings or shoes

Do ask advice if in doubt about any activity

DON'Ts

After Hip Replacement Surgery, surrounding muscles and other tissues take time to heal and strengthen. During this time your new hip is at risk of dislocating. To minimize this risk you must take the following precautions for at least 6 weeks following your operation

Don't cross your legs

Don't sit on a low chair or toilet

Don't sleep on your unaffected side for 2 months

Don't squat or bend down to pick up things from the floor

Don't try to bend the affected leg up to your chest

Don't attempt getting in or out of the bath for 6 weeks after the operation

Don't drive until 6 weeks after the operation

Figure 23.1 Dos and don'ts following a total hip replacement.

scheduled for surgery are shown aids that may be required, e.g. raised toilet seats, and those that may help patients with their activities of living, e.g. sock aids, long-handled sponges and helping hands.

- The discharge coordinator or care manager will work with all members of the multidisciplinary team, to ensure that the patient has a safe home environment to be discharged to.

Information is reinforced in the form of written documentation, which the patient can take away with them.

Postoperative care

Following total hip replacement, the patient may return to the ward with an intravenous infusion, unless they are already taking oral fluids. To prevent neurovascular compromise, neurovascular observations of the toes and foot will be carried out and recorded at 30-minute intervals initially, progressing to 4-hourly for up to 24 hours (Fig. 23.2). Each digit of the affected limb is examined for temperature, colour, sensation and mobility. One of the patient's pedal pulses is palpated and compared with the pulse on the unaffected foot, and any abnormalities are reported immediately. A pain score is also recorded.

The patient will initially return to the ward with a pressure dressing *in situ*, which is usually taken down after 24 hours to leave the primary dressing exposed. A transparent vapour-permeable film is recommended as a primary dressing so that the wound can be inspected without the dressing being removed, thus reducing the risk of infection. The wound is closed with either sutures or staples, which are removed between 7 and 10 days postoperatively.

Postoperative care plan. The care plan given in Table 23.1 illustrates the care of Louise, a 62-year-old woman who requires a total hip replacement.

Potential postoperative complications

Deep venous thrombosis (DVT). Patients are at risk of developing a DVT following surgery. To prevent this, patients receive a variety of prophylactic measures, including administration of low-molecular-weight heparin injections, oral anticoagulants, anti-embolism stockings and intermittent pressure devices, as well as being taught to dorsi- and plantarflex their ankles and deep breathe.

Infection. Patients are at risk of bacterial infection to both bone and wound. Prophylactic intravenous antibiotics are administered and strict wound asepsis is carried out. Deep prosthetic bacterial infection after total hip arthroplasty is one of the most devastating complications in hip surgery. Patients are initially treated with targeted antibiotic therapy following culture and sensitivity (Bulstrode, 2017), as well as serial surgical washouts of the infection site. Infection may result in removal of the prosthesis and insertion of a temporary spacer, resulting in an unstable joint with revision in the future.

Dislocation of the hip. Dislocation following total hip replacement is an unfortunate complication that is either patient- or technique-related (Cunningham et al, 2017). The patient is given written and verbal information on how to prevent dislocation.

The knee

Total knee replacement (arthroplasty)

Total knee replacement (arthroplasty) is generally performed to relieve patients' pain, and improve mobility and stability which have been impaired by conditions such as osteoarthritis. Excellent and durable results are now being achieved in over 80% of patients, with only 3.37% needing revising at the 10-year point (Sugand & Gupte, 2018).

Arthroplasty of the knee can be unicondylar (partial) or total (Fig. 23.3). Unicondylar knee arthroplasty is only suitable for early disease or disease of one compartment only. Total knee replacement is far more common.

Total knee arthroplasty involves the worn femoral and tibial surfaces being removed and replaced with metal and polyethylene components, respectively, providing gliding articular surfaces.

Preoperative care

The preoperative care for a patient undergoing a total knee replacement is much the same as for a patient undergoing a total hip replacement, with a few exceptions. At preoperative assessment, the physiotherapist teaches the patient specific leg exercises, such as static quadriceps, straight leg raising and knee bending, to help strengthen the quadriceps muscles. The patient is informed that postoperatively it is likely the leg will be painful, swollen and bruised.

- *Static quadriceps exercises*: the patient is instructed to place their hand behind the affected knee, then press their knee on to their hand and then to relax. Some patients such as those with rheumatoid arthritis of the hands have great difficulty with this, but they can generally manage to press their knee downwards into the bed.
- *Straight leg raising exercises*: the patient is instructed to tighten the thigh muscles of the affected leg, and then raise the leg as high as they can.

Teaching and carrying out physiotherapy exercises preoperatively has a direct beneficial effect on a patient's functional ability postoperatively (Flynn & Lucas, 2014).

Postoperative care

Following total knee replacement, the patient will return to the ward with an intravenous infusion, if they are not taking oral fluids yet, and a pressure dressing of wool and crepe from ankle to thigh. To prevent neurovascular compromise, neurovascular observations of the toes and foot will be carried out as per post hip replacement (Clarke &

NAME	WARD	PROCEDURE/INJURY:
CONSULTANT	NUMBER	AREA TO BE OBSERVED:
DATE OF ADMISSION		FREQUENCY OF OBSERVATIONS:

DATE										
TIME										
PAIN SCORE (0–5)										

VASCULAR	COLOUR	Normal									
		Pale									
		Cyanotic									
		Mottled									
	WARMTH	Hot									
		Warm									
		Cold									
		Cool									
	SWELLING	Nil									
		Moderate									
		Marked									
	CAPILLARY REFILL <2 SECONDS										
	PULSE	Strong									
		Weak									
		Absent									
MOVEMENT	ANKLE DORSI-FLEXION	No active contraction detected									
		Active movement no pain									
		Active movement with pain									
		Passive movement no pain									
	ANKLE PLANTAR-FLEXION	No active contraction detected									
		Active movement no pain									
		Active movement with pain									
		Passive movement no pain									

Figure 23.2 Neurovascular chart.

MOVEMENT	TOE EXTENSION	No active contraction detected											
		Active movement no pain											
		Active movement with pain											
		Passive movement no pain											
	TOE FLEXION	No active contraction detected											
		Active movement no pain											
		Active movement with pain											
		Passive movement no pain											
SENSATION	DORSAL WEB SPACE 1st & 2nd TOE	No sensation											
		Tingling/ numbness											
		Full sensation											
	WEB SPACE 3rd & 4th TOE	No sensation											
		Tingling/ numbness											
		Full sensation											
	SOLE OF FOOT/ TOES	No sensation											
		Tingling/ numbness											
		Full sensation											
	MEDIAL ARCH OF FOOT	No sensation											
		Tingling/ numbness											
		Full sensation											
INITIALS													

Always compare with unaffected limb.
If both limbs are affected use a separate chart for each limb.
If abnormalities occur, report to the nurse-in-charge or the medical team immediately.
Document all actions taken.

Figure 23.2 (Continued).

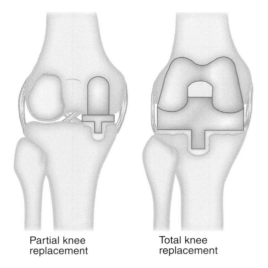

Partial knee
replacement

Total knee
replacement

Figure 23.3 Knee arthroplasty.

Santy-Tomlinson, 2014). The wound is closed with either sutures or staples, which are removed between 7 and 10 days postoperatively.

Potential complications are similar to those for total hip replacement, e.g. DVT and infection. It is important that the patient undergoing a total knee replacement continues to flex and extend the knee in order that a range of movement is achieved and maintained, and joint contracture does not occur. For this reason, pillows must not be placed under the knee, particularly at night, leaving the knee in a fixed flexion position.

The care plan in Table 23.2 illustrates the care of Daljit, a 74-year-old man who requires a total knee replacement.

Discharge planning following total knee replacement

All members of the multidisciplinary team must be satisfied that the patient has achieved the defined functional milestones:

- independently mobile with an appropriate aid
- able to climb stairs (if appropriate)
- full understanding of exercises and precautions
- independent with transfers
- active knee flexion of 70–90 degrees
- wound has healed
- is medically fit.

The patient is reviewed in the outpatient department 4–6 weeks following discharge.

Knee injuries

Tears of the menisci

Tears of the menisci are common sports injuries, and are frequently found in individuals with occupations involving kneeling and crouching, such as electricians and miners, or in professional footballers with a history of repeated knee injuries (White et al, 2015).

Meniscus tears fall into three categories (Fig. 23.4).

- *Bucket handle tear*: complete tearing practically divides the meniscus in two, and the inner part flips over like the action of a bucket handle to create this most common tear.
- *Posterior or anterior tear*: these may only affect the posterior or anterior horns.
- *Parrot beak tear*: this is a horizontal cleavage tear that produces a flap between the condyles, which resembles a parrot's beak.

These patients tend to be young males with a history of twisting a flexed knee with the weight on that leg. They experience pain and feel something tear. The knee may lock so that they cannot extend their leg; however, manipulation of the knee will cause it to unlock. There may be swelling, tenderness over the meniscus and loss of full extension. However, as the menisci are avascular and have no nerve supply on their inner two-thirds, there may be no pain or swelling (Bulstrode 2017; Sugand & Gupte, 2018).

The knee is usually treated initially with pressure bandaging, e.g. a wool and crepe bandage from ankle to thigh, and the symptoms should gradually settle down.

When diagnosis is reached, the loose fragment should be removed and as much of the healthy meniscal tissue should be left as is possible. This procedure is commonly done arthroscopically as a day case because it allows a more precise diagnosis and careful excision.

Following arthroscopic day surgery, the patient is prescribed analgesics and mobilized weight-bearing as pain allows with crutches, given an exercise plan by the physiotherapist and advised to do light work 1 week after surgery and heavy work 2 weeks after surgery.

Ligament injuries

The knee depends heavily on the anterior and posterior cruciate ligaments for stability. Ruptures of the cruciate ligaments are commonly found in the young adult involved in contact sports (Sugand & Gupte, 2018).

Anterior cruciate rupture

The patient feels and hears a 'pop' and cannot continue the activity they were doing. The knee swells, and a haemarthrosis (blood in the joint space) is present. The presence of a haemarthrosis generally indicates a substantial injury to the joint and will cause the patient great pain (Sugand & Gupte, 2018). In the acute stage, investigations to test the stability of ligaments are difficult to carry out because of the swelling; thus, the haemarthrosis should be aspirated first.

Table 23.2 Postoperative care plan for a patient following a total knee replacement, using the Roper, Logan and Tierney model of nursing

Assessment/usual routine	Patients problem	Goal	Nursing action	Evaluation
Eliminating				
Daljit occasionally has difficulty passing urine. He is concerned he may not be able to pass urine while on bedrest	Potential risk of urinary retention	To prevent urinary retention	Reassure Daljit and try to allay anxiety Encourage at least 2 L of fluids in 24 hours Position Daljit comfortably in the upright position in bed Sit out on commode and encourage Daljit to mobilize out to the toilet as soon as possible Pass a catheter if indicated	All nursing action failed Daljit had urinary retention Daljit was catheterized and passed 400 mL On removal of catheter, Daljit had no further problems passing urine
Daljit opens his bowels daily	At risk of constipation while on bedrest	To prevent constipation	Encourage fluids, fruit and high-fibre diet Monitor bowel action and record daily	Daljit opened his bowels on the 2nd postoperative day
Mobilizing				
Daljit's knee is stiff and painful and his muscles are weak	Potential risk of stiff new knee prosthesis with limited function	To achieve maximum result from knee replacement Aim for 70–90-degree flexion prior to discharge from hospital	Assess Daljit's pain and administer prescribed analgesics Reassure Daljit Encourage quadriceps and straight leg raising exercises Aim for 70–90-degree flexion by discharge Daljit achieved 90-degree flexion by discharge	He was discharged on day 2, mobilizing fully weight-bearing with two sticks
Maintaining a safe environment				
Daljit is concerned he may not be able to do his shopping or heavy household chores when discharged	Daljit is concerned he will not be able to do his own shopping or heavy housework for up to 3 months	Ensure Daljit has assistance with shopping and housework when discharged from hospital	Refer Daljit to social services for assistance with shopping and housework when discharged	Daljit was discharged with Meals on Wheels for 2 weeks and has a home help once a week for shopping and housework until he can manage himself

The initial treatment is to provide the patient with analgesics and aspirate the joint to relieve pressure within the capsule. Many surgeons carry out an emergency arthroscopy to wash out the haemarthrosis. When the blood has been removed, physiotherapy is commenced to build up the muscles. Treatment does depend on age; younger patients who are active and playing contact sports will benefit more from surgical repair, whereas the older more sedentary patient may benefit from physiotherapy and activity modification only (Sugand & Gupte, 2018; Bulstrode, 2017).

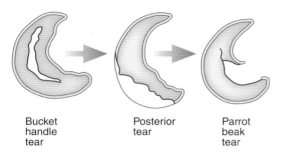

Bucket handle tear **Posterior tear** **Parrot beak tear**

Figure 23.4 Types of menisci tears.

Surgical treatment. Reconstruction involves the anterior cruciate ligament being replaced with natural tissue such as the medial third of the patellar tendon or the hamstring. This complex surgery requires 3–6 months of physiotherapy and 6–12 months away from sport. Satisfactory outcomes are achieved in a majority of patients, but only 50% achieve normal stability and only 60–70% of patients return to a pre-surgery level of sport (Bulstrode, 2017).

Posterior cruciate rupture

This ligament is injured less frequently than the anterior cruciate ligament, and most patients make an excellent recovery without treatment (Sugand & Gupte, 2018). Conservative treatment consists of joint aspiration or arthroscopy followed by quadriceps exercises. Surgery is only carried out if there is ongoing instability and a failure to heal (Sugand & Gupte, 2018).

The foot

Hallux valgus

With hallux valgus, the first metatarsal deviates medially and the great toe deviates laterally. A bunion develops over an exostosis on the first metatarsal head, and this can become inflamed and infected (White et al, 2015).

This condition may start late in childhood or in early adult life and is more common in females.

Conservative treatment such as chiropody, padding the bunion to relieve pressure, steroid injections and special footwear helps make the patient more comfortable but it does not correct the deformity. Pain and deformity are the main reasons why patients have surgical treatment.

Surgical treatment

There are several surgical techniques have been introduced for correction of hallux valgus, from soft tissue procedures to a number of osteotomies (Bulstrode, 2017). The majority of corrective foot surgery is carried out as a day procedure under general anaesthesia. The most common surgical procedures are as follows.

- *Bunionectomy*: the exostosis is trimmed and the bunion removed.
- *Distal metatarsal osteotomy*: a cut is made through the neck of the first metatarsal head, and the head is inwardly displaced and left to unite, e.g. Mitchell's osteotomy or Chevron osteotomy .
- *Arthroplasty*: the most common arthroplasty is the Keller's arthroplasty. This involves excision of the proximal half of the great toe first phalanx, creating a flail joint. The position of the second toe is often affected, and this can be corrected with a Kirschner wire.
- *Arthrodesis of the metatarsophalangeal joint*: the joint is fused in slight valgus, and the great toe continues to take part in weight-bearing.

Hallux rigidus

Osteoarthritis of the first metatarsophalangeal joint is often referred to as hallux rigidus (Bulstrode, 2017). The joint becomes painful when walking, stiffens, and the toe becomes rigid (White et al, 2015).

Conservative treatment includes the use of NSAIDs and orthoses which aim to reduce the movement that produces pain (Kunnasegaran & Thevendran, 2015).

Surgical treatment is by arthrodesis of the joint, as it is the most reliable procedure to give lasting pain relief, although this limits the height of a shoe heel that a woman can wear.

Mallet toe

Mallet toe is a congenital abnormality of the distal interphalangeal joint and is usually genetic. The shoe rubs against the toe, and blisters may develop. Conservative treatment such as wearing wider-fitting shoes, having regular chiropody and padding the tip of the toe to stop it rubbing against the shoe can help. Surgical treatment is by arthrodesis, or amputation of the terminal phalanx, which may be necessary if there is excessive pressure on the tip of the toe.

Hammer toe

A hammer toe consists of fixed flexion at the proximal interphalangeal joint, with hyperextension at the distal interphalangeal joint. This deformity generally involves the second toe, and a painful corn develops over the prominent head of the proximal phalanx.

Conservative treatment is by padding the corn to relieve pressure, or by strapping the toe and carrying out gentle stretching. However, this is effective in mild cases only. Surgical treatment is by arthrodesis of the joint in an extended position.

Nursing care for patients undergoing foot surgery

The majority of surgical procedures carried out on the foot are carried out as day surgery procedures under general anaesthesia with local anaesthetic administered for postoperative pain.

Preoperative care

The condition of the patient's foot is assessed for any circulatory disorders, infection or corns, and the surgeon is notified if there are any lesions or cuts. The pedal pulses should be recorded to give a baseline for postoperative monitoring, and any skin discoloration should be noted. A full explanation regarding the surgery and the type of footwear to be worn postoperatively should be given to the patient.

Postoperative care

Upon return from surgery, the patient's foot will be in either a below-knee cast or a pressure dressing; both should be closely observed for oozing or bleeding. Neurovascular observations should be recorded and the bed end should be elevated to prevent the foot swelling and aid venous return, particularly following a Keller's arthroplasty where a metal Kirschner wire extends through the dressing and is covered with a pin protector. Patients will experience severe pain in the early stages and will require regular analgesics when they start mobilizing. Patients are taught to walk on their heels supported by a walking aid, e.g. frame or crutches.

Discharge planning

Patients are discharged when they can safely mobilize, usually with a walking aid and often wearing a special sandal if they are not in a cast. Analgesics are also given to the patient to take home. Kirschner wires are removed after 4–6 weeks at the outpatient appointment.

Upper limb orthopaedic surgery

The shoulder

Total shoulder replacement (arthroplasty)

Following the success of hip and knee arthroplasty, shoulder arthroplasty is now carried out, although it is not as common. A total shoulder arthroplasty is indicated when there is severe destruction of the joint from trauma or a disease process such as rheumatoid arthritis (Bulstrode, 2017). The total shoulder arthroplasty replaces the humeral head with a metallic component and resurfaces the glenoid cavity (Sugand & Gupte, 2018). Total shoulder replacements are carried out under general anaesthesia and as an inpatient procedure, requiring a 2–3 day stay in hospital.

Preoperative care

- Preoperative tests and investigations for a patient undergoing a total shoulder arthroplasty are similar to those carried out for hip or knee arthroplasty.
- It is useful to encourage the patient to begin to use their non-dominant arm and hand if the dominant arm is being operated on.
- The neurovascular status of both arms should be recorded and used as baseline observations in the postoperative period.
- Full explanations regarding the surgery, postoperative care and recovery period should be given to the patient.
- Patients should be taught deep breathing exercises and be made aware that these may be restricted because their arm will be in an immobilizer, which may slightly restrict chest movement (Fig. 23.5).

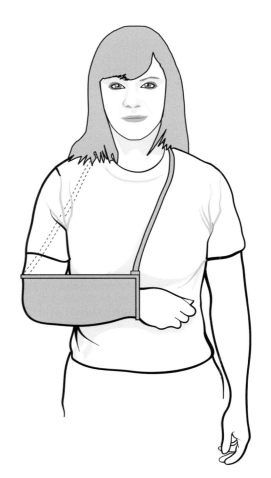

Figure 23.5 A shoulder immobilizer.

Postoperative care

- The patient's temperature, pulse, respirations and blood pressure should be recorded half-hourly until stable, then gradually built up to 4-hourly observations for a 24-hour period.
- Neurovascular observations of the affected limb should be carried out and recorded.
- An intravenous infusion may be running and a vacuum drain *in situ*, which require monitoring and output record.
- When the patient has tolerated adequate oral fluids and is hydrated, the intravenous infusion may be discontinued and a normal diet commenced. The patient will need assistance with cutting up food.
- The patient's pain is controlled with either a PCA pump or regional anaesthesia and its efficacy evaluated.
- Prophylactic antibiotics are administered to prevent infection.
- Sutures are generally removed 7–10 days postoperatively, unless they are self-dissolving.
- The physiotherapist will encourage the patient to do finger, wrist and hand movements and static exercises of the deltoid muscle in the early postoperative period.
- Following X-ray to confirm implant position on day 2, the patient will be encouraged to use the affected shoulder, assisted by the unaffected shoulder. Arm exercises such as walking the fingers up a wall and circulating the arm outwards and inwards (known as pendulum exercises) are encouraged.
- The patient will require assistance with hygiene care and dressing but should be encouraged to actively participate as a mode of rehabilitation.

Discharge planning

Following shoulder arthroplasty, it may take up to 6 months before the patient feels the full benefit of the surgery. For this reason, many patients require some social service assistance, e.g. help with cleaning and shopping.

The patient needs to be advised on how not to dislocate the shoulder arthroplasty, and have a full understanding of their individual exercise regimen and its importance. Exercise regimens are tailored to individual needs, but usually include movement of the shoulder using the unaffected arm, finger-walking up a wall, grasping of a gymnastic ball and pendulum exercises.

The patient is reviewed in the outpatient department 2–3 weeks following discharge.

Recurrent dislocation of the shoulder

Dislocation of the shoulder is a common injury, usually as a result of falling onto the hand or arm in the elderly population, or as a result of a sporting injury in the young. The dislocation more often than not occurs anteriorly. The patient presents with a painful immobile shoulder that is flattened in appearance, producing a drop in the shoulder line. If this injury recurs, then surgery can be considered. Arthroscopic repair under general anaesthesia as a day patient is the most common surgical treatment (Bulstrode, 2017).

Postoperative care

- The arm is positioned in a shoulder immobilizer. When and how quickly the patient's shoulder is mobilized is dependent on the surgeon. The shoulder immobilizer remains *in situ* under clothing for 3 weeks.
- Physiotherapy starts with gentle assisted exercises only and progresses to more active exercises following the 3-week follow-up appointment.

Discharge

The patient is discharged with an individual exercise regimen and analgesics, and is made fully aware that it will take several months before maximum use of the shoulder is possible. The patient is followed up in the outpatient department at 3 and 6 weeks.

The elbow

Total elbow replacement (arthroplasty)

An arthroplasty of the elbow is less common than that of the hip or knee; however, it is regarded as a well-established surgical procedure. It is increasingly being carried out to relieve pain in patients with a severely painful elbow and joint destruction caused by rheumatoid arthritis and to restore stability and improve mobility of the elbow joint.

Preoperative care

The preoperative care is similar to that for a patient undergoing shoulder arthroplasty and is carried out under general anaesthesia with an inpatient stay of 2–3 days.

Specific postoperative care

- A plaster backslab may be used over the dressings to immobilize the elbow joint for the first few days.
- The arm will be elevated in a sling. An intravenous infusion will be *in situ*, and, depending on surgeon preference, a vacuum drain, which will usually be removed at 24 hours.
- The nurse should carefully monitor and record the neurovascular observations of the affected arm, looking for signs of ulnar nerve decompression due to elbow oedema, e.g. altered sensation in the little and ring fingers, and report any changes immediately.

- Most exercises are focused on the activities of living, such as flexion of the elbow to brush the hair or to feed self.

Discharge

Recovery can take months, and the patient may require assistance with activities of living and social service support for several weeks.

The hand

Dupuytren's contracture

This condition occurs as a result of a thickening of the palmar fascia. The cause is unknown but it is associated with family history, liver disease, alcoholism and epilepsy (BSSH, 2016a). Dupuytren's contracture is more common in men than in women and often both hands are affected (BSSH, 2016a). There is a slow-progressing flexion contracture of one or more of the fingers, which are pulled into the palm of the hand. The thickened palmar fascia tends to pucker the outlying skin (Fig. 23.6).

Surgery is the only effective treatment and involves the excision of the thickened fascia. Surgery is carried out as a day surgery procedure under local or regional anaesthesia.

Postoperative care

- The hand is elevated in a Bradford sling to prevent oedema.
- Neurovascular observations need to be monitored and recorded, as there is a high risk of bleeding and swelling owing to the vascular nature of the palm of the hand.
- The wound needs careful observation, as haematomas are not uncommon.

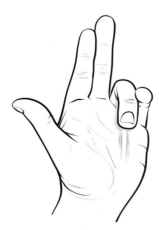

Figure 23.6 Dupuytren's contracture.

- Some surgeons use a resting hand splint, whereas others prefer to leave the hand alone.
- Gentle massage of the scar helps to decrease swelling and helps to stimulate the circulation and improve healing.

Discharge

It can take months for the hand to return to full use. Patients are sent home with a gentle exercise regimen, analgesics, oils, and, in some cases, with silicone for hand baths.

Carpal tunnel syndrome

In this condition there is compression of the median nerve as it passes beneath the flexor retinaculum in the carpal tunnel. There may be altered sensation in half of the ring, middle and index fingers and thumb. This often affects the patient's sleep and is particularly common in young to middle-aged and pregnant women (BSSH, 2016b; Sugand & Gupte, 2018). Conditions such as rheumatoid arthritis or Colles' fractures, which cause synovial thickening, can also cause carpal tunnel syndrome (BSSH, 2016b; Sugand & Gupte, 2018).

Conservative treatments are generally tried initially, but the majority of patients require surgery in the long term. Conservative treatments include the use of rest, night splints with the wrist held in the neutral position to reduce compression within the tunnel, injection of hydrocortisone into the carpal tunnel to relieve pain, and the use of anti-inflammatory drugs to reduce inflammation.

Surgery is the only effective treatment, and involves the division of the flexor retinaculum and median nerve decompression. This surgery is generally a day case procedure and carried out under local anaesthesia.

Postoperative care

- The arm is elevated in a Bradford sling. It is important that exercises are carried out at least 4-hourly. This involves the wrist, fingers, elbow and shoulder, ensuring a full range of movement.
- Neurovascular observations require careful monitoring, recording and reporting when indicated.
- The wound needs to be observed for bleeding, and the dressing is reduced 24 hours postoperatively, with sutures removed at 7–10 days.
- Advice is given to the patient regarding the importance of keeping the hand elevated while at rest.

Discharge

The patient is advised not to get their hands wet, and instructed to use plastic bags in the shower to prevent this occurring. The importance of keeping the hand elevated while at rest and the continuation of exercises is reinforced, and the patient is advised to avoid heavy lifting for several weeks.

Orthopaedic surgery of the spine

Back pain is a common complaint. Up to 84% of adults have had back pain at some time in their lives. The majority of patients treated within primary care have a non-specific back pain which clears up within 4 weeks, with a small minority of patients developing chronic back pain lasting longer than 12 weeks (Oliveira et al, 2018). Backstrain is generally the result of incorrect lifting, and nurses have many opportunities in the workplace to advise patients and their families how to avoid backstrain.

On its own, back pain is not an orthopaedic problem and is best treated conservatively (Sugand & Gupte, 2018). The majority of patients with back pain are managed conservatively with analgesics to reduce pain and anti-inflammatory drugs to reduce inflammation, physiotherapy to improve range of movement and posture. Exercise to improve flexibility, which will help ease pain, and for stabilization by building up core muscles. Braces are also available and they can reduce pain and lessen the chance of further injury.

Attention to weight, avoiding heavy lifting where possible, and instruction in back care, e.g. back strengthening exercises and sleeping posture, are all helpful. Surgery is only considered when conservative methods have been unsuccessful, and it may be undertaken in an orthopaedic or neurosciences unit.

The criteria used to determine surgery relate to CT/MRI findings and the following:

- when conservative treatment has failed to relieve the pain
- when general health is deteriorating because of disturbed sleep caused by sciatic nerve pain
- when there is neurological disturbance, e.g. disruption of bowel and bladder control.

A variety of surgical options are available, all carried out under general anaesthesia as inpatients; the length of stay is defined by the surgical procedure and patient recovery:

- *microsurgery*: the carrying out of surgery using a microscope and miniature instruments
- *discectomy*: surgical removal of the protruding disc
- *laminectomy*: surgical removal of the protruding disc and one or more of the laminae
- *spinal fusion*: fusion of the spinal vertebrae to stabilize the vertebral column.

Specific postoperative care for patients following spinal surgery

- The patient is nursed flat on a firm bed with one pillow.
- Temperature, pulse, respirations, blood pressure and neurovascular observations are monitored {1/2}-hourly initially and gradually progressed to 4-hourly.

- The patient is log-rolled for pressure area care and observation of the wound.
- A small drain may be *in situ* for 24 hours, and this should be monitored and blood loss recorded.
- Sutures/staples are removed at days 7–10.
- Analgesics should be administered if the patient is in pain.
- An intravenous infusion requires monitoring and may be removed when the patient has tolerated adequate amounts of oral fluids.
- Urinary output should be monitored and recorded, as the patient is at risk of urinary retention due to their position in bed.
- Diet may be commenced when the patient is tolerating oral fluids, and a high-fibre diet will help prevent constipation, a complication which many back surgery patients experience.
- Deep breathing exercises, foot exercises and back strengthening exercises are encouraged.
- Following discectomy and laminectomy, a patient may be mobilized 24 hours postoperatively if pain allows by the nursing staff under direction from the surgeon and physiotherapists. Following spinal fusion, patients tend to require more time in bed, but mobility is encouraged as soon as pain allows.
- Some surgeons prefer a corset to be worn for a specified period of time.
- Patients are instructed how to safely sit, bend and stand, and given written information tailored to their individual needs to support this.

Discharge

Advice on the importance of physiotherapy exercises, avoiding heavy lifting and good posture is reinforced and supported with written information. If the patient has been supplied with a corset, they need to be taught how to apply and care for it. The patient is reviewed in the outpatient department 2 weeks after discharge. Return to work is dependent on the type of spinal surgery and the patient's recovery and can be anything from a couple of weeks following discectomy or laminectomy to several months following spinal fusion.

Fractures

A fracture can be defined as a loss or break in the continuity of a bone (Clarke & Santy-Tomlinson, 2014). Fractures are classified according to the type, complexity and location of the break (Table 23.3). The stages of bone healing are illustrated in Fig. 23.7.

Table 23.3 Classification of fractures

Type	Definition
Complete	The bone is fractured completely into two or more pieces
Partial (incomplete)	The bone does not fracture completely
Open (compound)	The bone is fractured and breaks through the skin
Closed (simple)	The bone is fractured but does not break through the skin
Greenstick	The bone is fractured on one side and bent on the other. It is a common fracture in children
Comminuted	The bone is splintered and crushed into smaller fragments
Oblique	The bone is fractured at a 45-degree angle to the long bone axis
Spiral	The bone is twisted apart
Transverse	The bone is fractured at right angles to the long bone axis
Impacted	A fracture where one part of the bone is forcefully driven into another
Pathological	A fracture due to bone weakening caused by diseases such as osteoporosis or neoplasia

Fracture management

Early management is directed towards converting any contaminated wounds to clean wounds. The main aims of fracture treatment are then:
- *reduction*: to restore normal alignment of the bone
- *immobilization*: to ensure the reduced position is maintained until bone union has taken place
- *rehabilitation*: either to restore normal function or to assist the patient to cope with disability.

Reduction

Reduction may be achieved by either closed manipulation, or open reduction.
- *Closed* – involves the pulling of displaced bone fragments into their normal anatomical position, restoring alignment.
- *Open* – this is achieved through a surgical incision. It is indicated when closed reduction has been unsuccessful or where it is desirable to avoid external splintage of the part, e.g. in elderly patients with fractures of the neck of femur where early immobilization is necessary.

Immobilization

Immobilization may be achieved by external or internal splintage, which comes in many forms. External splintage can be achieved either conservatively or surgically and includes non-rigid methods of support, e.g. slings, cast immobilization, skin or skeletal traction, or external fixator frames.

Cast immobilization
- *Plaster of Paris* is most commonly used for patients who have just sustained their injuries, because it allows for swelling (Szostakowski et al, 2017). It is less expensive than synthetic casts but a disadvantage is that it is heavy and takes 48 hours before it is completely dry.
- *Synthetic casts* allow early weight-bearing, as they dry within 20 minutes, and are ideal for those elderly patients where early mobilization is necessary. However, they are more expensive than plaster of Paris and do not allow for swelling; therefore they should not be used on patients who have just received their injuries.
- *Cast braces* can be used for fractures of the upper or lower limb. They are moulded closely to the shape of the limb and fitted with hinges to allow joint movement.

Specific care for a patient in a cast
- Limbs encased in casts should be elevated to prevent oedema and aid venous return.
- The cast should not be rested on a hard or sharp surface and must be handled using the palms of the hands to avoid denting, as this could result in pressure to the underlying skin. The signs of pressure ulcer formation include a burning pain, offensive odour and cast discoloration. A window can be cut in the cast to permit treatment, but it must always be replaced so as to avoid further swelling into the space.
- The colour, sensation, temperature and mobility of all individual digits should be checked to ensure that circulation and nerve conduction are not impaired. In

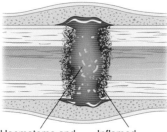

Haematoma and bone fragments   Inflamed area

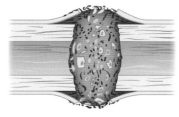

Phagocytosis of clot and debris.
Growth of granulation tissue begins

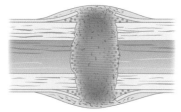

Osteoblasts begin to form new bone

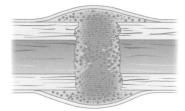

Gradual spread of new bone to bridge gap

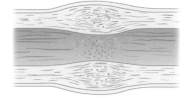

Bone healed. Osteoblasts reshape and canalize new bone

Figure 23.7 Stages of bone healing. (Reproduced from Wilson, 2018.)

addition, a pain assessment should be undertaken and the cast checked for tightness at the proximal and distal regions. A digit that is cold, blanched or blue, painful and oedematous has impaired circulation (Jester et al, 2011).

- If signs and symptoms of neurovascular impairment are evident, the cast should be split down both sides (bivalved) immediately, the padding cut and a medical opinion sought. A tight cast can cause ischaemia of muscle compartments, which can lead to irreversible damage (Szostakowski et al, 2017).

Many patients go home wearing casts, and it is essential that they are given clear verbal instructions and written information on how to care for their specific cast. The Nursing and Midwifery Council (NMC) (2018) make it clear in *The Code* that the nurse is required to provide the patient with information that can help to enhance their health and well-being and this is just as important when providing information in the orthopaedic setting. Information must be provided in such a way as the patient can understand it; there may be a need to provide information in various forms, for example, in large type or Braille.

Traction

Traction is the application of a pulling force to a body part, with a counter-traction force applied in the opposite direction. Traction falls into two main categories:

- *Fixed traction*: the Thomas splint is the best example of fixed traction, with the counter force being applied to the ischial tuberosity. Thomas splints are now rarely used, with the exception of paediatrics and during transfers.
- *Balanced or sliding traction*: balanced traction involves the use of weights on a limb, and counter-traction is achieved when the foot of the bed is elevated.

Traction can be exerted by applying skin traction in the form of strapping to the patient's affected limb (Fig. 23.8). This strapping can be adhesive or non-adhesive; however, due to the increased risk of skin deterioration, non-adhesive strapping is advised. The second method of applying traction is skeletal traction, which involves the insertion of a metal pin through a bone, allowing heavier weights to be applied (Sugand & Gupte, 2018; Jester et al, 2011) (Fig. 23.9).

Specific care for a patient in traction

- Traction equipment should be checked at every handover to ensure traction and counter-traction is maintained.
- Traction cords should be taut at all times and should only be untied when traction or counter-traction is applied, e.g. manually.
- A bed-cradle can be used to prevent the bedclothes interfering with the traction.
- Skin traction should be removed at least daily, for limb washing and skin inspection.

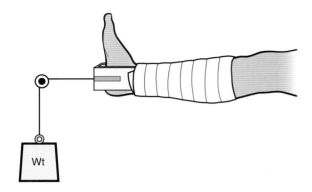

Figure 23.8 Skin traction.

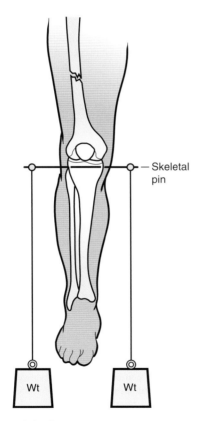

- Skeletal
pin

Figure 23.9 Skeletal traction.

- Patients with skeletal traction should be advised not to touch the pin or pin sites, and pin covers should be used to cover sharp pin ends to prevent the patient from injuring themselves.

- Skeletal pin sites should be checked regularly for signs of infection, such as redness, warmth or oozing, and should be cleaned weekly with minimal disturbance.
- The colour, sensation, temperature and movement of the extremities, and signs of pain or swelling should be observed and recorded.
- Two-hourly pressure area care is essential. The heels should rest over a Leonard's pad, and, where slings are used, areas under the edges of the slings should be observed for signs of pressure.
- Pulleys should run freely, and traction cords should run on straight lines. Weights should hang freely and not rest on the floor or chair, and should be the correct weight. Cords should be checked for fraying.

The patient will also require general nursing care and physiotherapy to prevent deep venous thrombosis, chest infection, muscle wasting or foot drop (Jester et al, 2011).

External fixation

Fractures that cannot be held reduced in a cast or on traction need to be fixed externally or internally. External fixation tends to be used in fractures where there is significant bone loss or extensive soft tissue damage (McNally & Catagni, 2011). This involves the holding of bone and bone fragments by metal pins attached to an external frame (Fig. 23.10).

Specific care for a patient with an external fixator

- Observe for altered neurovascular status, as previously discussed.
- Give patients a full explanation and support in managing the external fixator, ensuring they are aware of benefits such as early-assisted mobilization.
- Concordance to treatment is essential in the use of an external fixator. Patients will require a lot of reassurance and support to help them accept the unsightly external fixator frame, which may significantly alter their body image.
- The patient with an external fixator is at a high risk of developing a pin-site infection. This may be superficial and treated with simple antibiotics; however, if not treated, the infection can progress along the pin tract to the bone, which can then have devastating effects.
- Pin-site care should be carried out weekly with minimal disturbance to crust and scab formation. Patients should be encouraged, where possible, to undertake this themselves to help with acceptance of the fixator.

Internal fixation

There are many types of internal fixation devices, such as intramedullary nails, compression nails, plates and screws (Fig. 23.11). Internal fixation is used in the following situations:

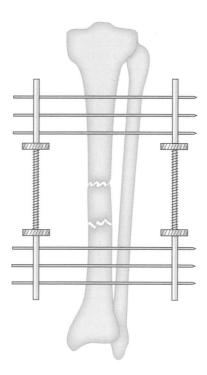

Figure 23.10 External fixation used in treatment of tibial fractures.

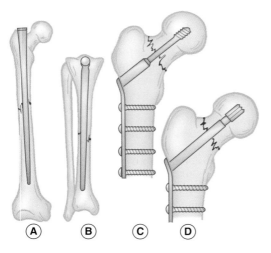

Figure 23.11 Types of internal fixation: (A, B) intramedullary nails; (C) compression nail for fixation of the femoral neck; (D) sliding nail fixation of the femoral neck.

- to allow early limb or joint movement, or to avoid a long period of immobilization in bed, e.g. the elderly patient with a fractured neck of femur (Solomon et al, 2014)
- when sufficient reduction cannot be maintained by external fixation, e.g. fractures involving joint surfaces
- in multiple fractures where internal fixation of one or more of the fractures may assist in making the treatment of other injuries more simple
- in certain pathological fractures where the patient's life expectancy may be short, e.g. malignancy, or where union may be uncertain.

Complications of fractures

Patients with fractures are at risk of complications, which are described in terms of immediate, early or late complications (Table 23.4). The nurse should be observant for these complications and take preventative measures.

Compartment syndrome

One particular complication of concern to the orthopaedic nurse following a fracture or orthopaedic surgery is that of compartment syndrome. There is a progressive build-up of pressure in a confined space (muscle compartment), which compromises circulation, diminishes oxygen supply and, thus, jeopardizes function of tissues within that space.

The onset of the symptoms can vary, and should be treated as a medical emergency. If pressure is not relieved in the compartment, irreversible nerve and tissue damage will result in contractures, paralysis and loss of sensation, and, in some cases, amputation. If pressure is not relieved in sufficient time, a fasciotomy will be performed in which the muscle compartments are incised to relieve the pressure. The fasciotomy wounds are left open and the patient is taken back to theatre to have the ischaemic muscle debrided and, in some cases, the wounds skin-grafted (Bulstrode, 2017).

The orthopaedic nurse plays a vital role in detecting compartment syndrome through the assessment of the 'five Ps' of the limb: pain, pale, pulseless, paralysed and paraesthetic (Schinco & Hassid, 2018). These should be assessed and recorded on a neurovascular observation chart (see Fig. 23.2), and any changes reported immediately.

General discharge planning and advice

Discharge planning commences for elective orthopaedic patients at the pre-assessment clinic prior to admission, or

Table 23.4 Complications of fractures

Immediate	Early	Late
Soft tissue damage	Infection	Malunion
Nerve injury	Neurovascular compromise	Delayed union
Haemorrhage	Fat embolism	Non-union
	Pulmonary embolism	Osteoarthritis
	Deep venous thrombosis	Avascular necrosis
	Pressure ulcers	
	Chest infection	
	Exacerbation of generalized illness	

from the first day of admission for trauma patients. Many patients are discharged home to early discharge schemes where they are cared for in their own homes.

Each patient requires a systematic but individualized documented discharge plan, as the needs of orthopaedic patients vary greatly because of the wide variety of orthopaedic conditions and ages of the patients.

Patients should be actively involved in their discharge planning, and it is paramount that every member of the multidisciplinary team ensures that, through a thorough assessment, the patient is fit for a safe discharge home.

In many cases patients require aids, appliances or adaptations to their home, such as stair rails, to assist them with their activities of living, or social services support and assistance by a community nurse. Some patients may require transportation to take them home and to return for follow-up.

Verbal and written information in the form of booklets or pamphlets should be given to the patient, with a list of contact numbers should the patient require further advice, support or information while at home.

Most patients will require a follow-up appointment with the orthopaedic surgeon, and the time period from discharge to appointment will vary depending on the patient's condition.

Conclusion

This chapter has outlined some of the fundamental principles of nursing the trauma and elective orthopaedic patient, discussing some of the more common orthopaedic conditions and surgical procedures. Orthopaedics is changing at an unprecedented rate and this chapter has introduced some of the developments in orthopaedic techniques and the specialty of orthopaedic nursing.

SUMMARY OF KEY POINTS

- Orthopaedic surgery is carried out for patients with disease or injury to the musculoskeletal system. Elective orthopaedic surgery is planned surgery for patients with disease to the musculoskeletal system, such as osteoarthritis. Trauma surgery is performed as an emergency, such as following a fracture.
- It is paramount that the orthopaedic practitioner considers the physical, psychological, social and cultural needs of all elective and trauma orthopaedic patients.
- Where possible, all orthopaedic patients should be offered advice, support, and verbal and written information regarding their condition prior to admission. Where admission is as an emergency, this should be addressed as soon after admission as is possible and continued until discharge.
- Nursing care of the orthopaedic patient aims to promote healing, prevent further injury or complications, maximize independence and promote optimal rehabilitation.

REFLECTIVE LEARNING POINTS

Having read this chapter, think about what you now know and what you still need to find out about. These questions may help:

- How might surgical preparation for the person undergoing elective and emergency orthopaedic surgery differ?
- What are the key legal, physical and psychological issues the nurse must consider for the person undergoing orthopaedic surgery?
- How can the nurse ensure that those who have undergone orthopaedic surgery are discharged in a safe and appropriate manner?

Useful addresses

Versus Arthritis
Copeman House
St Mary's Court
St Mary's Gate
Chesterfield
Derbyshire S41 7TD
Disabled Living Foundation
Unit 1, 34 Chatfield Road
Wandsworth
London SW11 3SE

Royal Osteoporosis Society
Manor Farm
Skinners Hill
Camerton
Bath BA2 0PJ
RCN Society of Orthopaedic and Trauma Nurses
20 Cavendish Square
Marylebone
London W1G 0RN

References

British Society for Surgery of the Hand (BSSH). (2016a). *Dupuytren's contracture* [Online]. Available at: <www.bssh.ac.uk/patients/conditions/25/dupuytrens_disease>

British Society for Surgery of the Hand (BSSH). (2016b). *Carpal tunnel syndrome* [Online]. Available at: <www.BSSH.ac.uk/patients/commonhandconditions/carpaltunnelsyndrome>

Bulstrode, C. (2017). *Oxford textbook of trauma and orthopaedics* (2nd ed.). New York: Oxford University Press.

Carpenter, J., Hines, S., & Lan, V. (2017). Guided imagery for pain management in postoperative orthopedic patients: an integrative literature review. *Journal of Holistic Nursing, 35*(4), 342–351.

Cheung, W., Miclau, T., Chow, S., Yang, F., & Alt, V. (2016). Fracture healing in osteoporotic bone. *Injury, 47,* S21–S26.

Clarke, S., & Santy-Tomlinson, J. (2014). *Orthopaedic and trauma nursing.* Chichester, West Sussex: Wiley Blackwell.

Cunningham, R., Beck, D., & Peterson, C. (2017). Dislocation following total hip arthroplasty. *JBJS Journal of Orthopaedics for Physician Assistants, 5*(1), e8.

Elias-Jones, D., Aitken, M., Gibson, A., & Perry, M. (2018). *Crash course rheumatology and orthopaedics* (4th ed.). Amsterdam: Elsevier.

Eskelinen, A. (2017). Minimally invasive THA. *Journal of Bone and Joint Surgery, 99*(20), e109.

Flynn, S., & Lucas, B. (2014). The team approach and nursing roles in orthopaedic and musculoskeletal trauma care. In S. Clarke, & J. Santy-Tomlinson (Eds.), *Orthopaedic and trauma nursing* (pp. 48–58). Chichester: Wiley Blackwell.

Jester, R. (2014). Clinical assessment of the orthopaedic and trauma patient. In S. Clarke, & J. Santy-Tomlinson (Eds.), *Orthopaedic and trauma nursing* (pp. 69–79). Chichester: Wiley Blackwell.

Jester, R., Santy, J., & Rogers, J. (2011). *Oxford handbook of orthopaedic and trauma nursing* (pp. 355–385). Oxford: Oxford University Press.

Kunnasegaran, R., & Thevendran, G. (2015). Hallux rigidus. *Foot and Ankle Clinics, 20*(3), 401–412.

Lloyd, J., Wainwright, T., & Middleton, R. (2012). What is the role of minimally invasive surgery in a fast track hip and knee replacement pathway? *Annals of The Royal College of Surgeons of England, 94*(3), 148–151.

McNally, M., & Catagni, M. (2011). Principles of circular external fixation in trauma. In C. Bulstrode (Ed.), *Oxford textbook of trauma and orthopaedics* (2nd ed.). Oxford: Oxford University Press.

Oliveira, C., Maher, C., Pinto, R., Traeger, R., Lin, C., Chenot, J., et al. (2018). Clinical practice guidelines for the management of non-specific low back pain in primary care: an updated overview. *European Spine Journal, 27*(11), 2791–2803.

Roper, N., Logan, W., & Tierney, A. (1996). *The elements of nursing* (4th ed.). Edinburgh: Churchill Livingstone.

Schinco, M., & Hassid, V. (2018). Compartment syndrome of extremities – symptoms, diagnosis and treatment. *BMJ Best Practice.* Available at: <bestpractice.bmj.com/topics/en-gb/502>.

Solomon, L., Warwick, D., & Nayagam, S. (2014). *Apley's concise system of orthopaedics and trauma* (4th ed.). Boca Raton: CRC Press.

Sugand, K., & Gupte, C. (2018). *ABC of orthopaedics and trauma* (1st ed.). Chichester: Wiley-Blackwell.

Szostakowski, B., Smitham, P., & Khan, W. (2017). Plaster of Paris – short history of casting and injured limb immobilization. *The Open Orthopaedics Journal, 11*(1), 291–296.

The Nursing and Midwifery Council (NMC). (2018). *The Code. Professional standards of practice and behaviour for nurses, midwives and nursing associates.* Available at: <www.nmc.org.uk/globalassets/sitedocuments/nmc-publications/nmc-code.pdf>

Tortora, G., & Derrickson, B. (2017). Principles of anatomy and pysiology (15th ed.). New York: Wiley.

White, T., Mackenzie, S., & Gray, A. (2015). *McRae's orthopaedic trauma and emergency fracture management* (3rd ed.). Amsterdam: Elsevier.

Relevant websites

British Orthopaedic Association: www.boa.ac.uk

Hip and Knee Institute: www.hipsand-knees.com

National Association of Orthopaedic Nurses: www.orthonurse.org

National Joint Registry: www.njrcentre.org.uk/njrcentre/default.aspx

Orthopaedic Terminology: orthopaedics.org.uk

Versus Arthritis (formerly Arthritis Care and Arthritis Research UK): www.versusarthritis.org

Chapter | 24 |

Patients requiring plastic surgery

Jane Holden

KEY OBJECTIVES IN THE CHAPTER

By the end of the chapter the reader will be able to:

- understand the relevance that key plastic surgery procedures have across all surgical specialties
- understand what a skin graft is and have knowledge about nursing skills needed to manage skin grafts and their donor sites
- understand what a flap is and differentiate between various types of flap reconstruction
- identify nursing principles of care for patients with a microvascular flap and how to assess the vascular status of a flap
- identify the roles of the nurses is assisting patients in adapting to changes following plastic surgery.

Areas to think about before reading the chapter

- Describe the differences between reconstructive surgery and cosmetic (also called aesthetic) surgery
- Some people's emotions have a very big effect on how they think they look; how might the nurse offer support to people when these emotions are having a negative impact on a person's health and well-being?

Introduction

Plastic surgery, derived from the Greek word *plastikos* meaning to mould or to shape (Mazzola & Mazzola, 2018; Thorne, 2014), is surgery that involves the 'moulding' of any part of the human body. The specialty focuses on surgical procedures as opposed to anatomical sites (Thorne, 2014), which have relevance from the newborn to patients in their very senior years. Despite the evolution of plastic surgery in terms of 'life-saving, changing and enhancing surgeries' (Asbery, 2017), there remains an association by the public with predominantly cosmetic procedures. Although these are important, they represent only one aspect of an extensive and exciting area of surgery that involves congenital, gender-related, traumatic and cancer-related challenges.

Fundamental techniques associated with the specialty include skin grafting and reconstruction with flaps. Although previously these procedures were undertaken primarily by plastic surgeons, the fact that the techniques are not restricted to an organ has led to their application by many surgeons throughout the surgical spectrum (Thorne, 2014). Consequently, nursing people having plastic surgery in specialized units (Asbery, 2018) is fast becoming a thing of the past. Instead, patients in any surgical specialty, cared for on a ward or in the community, may have undergone these procedures. This highlights the relevance to all surgical nurses to develop knowledge and skills to competently manage these patients. This chapter's focus is on the two most common techniques in plastic surgery, being skin grafts and flaps. It aims to provide practical tips that link the theory to practice in achieving optimum outcomes. Acting as a basic introduction, the author hopes that readers will be encouraged to access the numerous articles and books published on the topic with relevance to their area of practice. The author assumes the reader acknowledges the relevance of the chapters in Section 1 of this book in managing patients having plastic surgery at different points of the patient's pathway.

Surgical procedures associated with plastic surgery

Decision-making in wound closure has historically been considered in terms of the reconstruction ladder. This arranges closure techniques in order of complexity, moving from the simpler approaches on the bottom rungs to the more technically challenging on the higher rungs (Black & Black, 2012; Hsieh, 2015). The evolution of new wound closure techniques has resulted in modifications (Fig. 24.1) and an acceptance that surgeons will select the most appropriate methods, and not just select the simplest option and then move up the steps in succession for every case (Janis et al, 2011). Consequently, more complex procedures may be more suited to the issue in question and selected accordingly to ensure the best outcomes in terms of both function and aesthetics.

Skin grafts

A skin graft is a segment of dermis and epidermis that is removed in a sheet from its own blood supply, the donor site, and placed onto another area of the body to provide skin cover over a defect, the recipient site (McGregor & McGregor, 2000). Skin grafts are categorized as split or full thickness, with the thickness of the skin graft being dictated by the thickness of the dermis included in the skin graft. A full-thickness skin graft (FTSG) contains all the epidermis and dermis and is only applied as a sheet. In contrast, a split-thickness skin graft (STSG/SSG) contains all the epidermis and varying degrees of the dermis, hence the dermis is split. It can be applied in one piece with no holes (referred to as a sheet), with holes inserted to permit exudate to pass through it (referred to as fenestrated), or put through an electrical apparatus that insets much larger holes (referred to as meshed). Meshing an STSG permits stretching of the graft to cover a larger surface area and facilitates exudate drainage (Beldon, 2007). Initially the meshed graft resembles the appearance of a 'string vest', with raw areas in between. The larger the mesh, the larger the holes. These areas heal

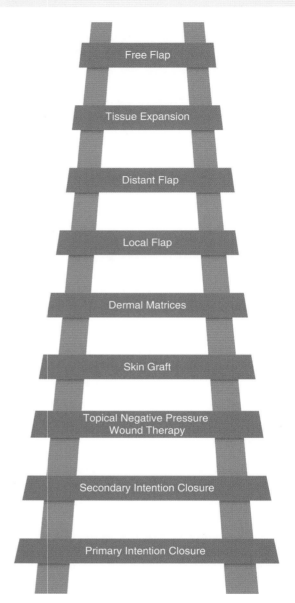

Figure 24.1 Reconstructive ladder.

as re-epithelialization occurs. The final scar will retain the meshed appearance, making it a less-pleasing aesthetic result and therefore less favourable in areas on constant view such as the face or head (McGregor & McGregor, 2000). Table 24.1 outlines the differences between the STSG and FTSG.

Indications for skin grafting are to resurface a vascularized surface, including:

- removal of skin lesions
- skin cover for a free muscle flap
- replacing skin loss due to trauma such as degloving injuries or surgical debridement
- closure of fasciotomy sites
- closure of a chronic wounds, e.g. venous leg ulcer
- temporary reconstruction for preservation before more complex reconstruction can occur
- correction of deformities such as scar contractures and release of webbed fingers, knowns as syndactyly.

The success of a skin graft is assessed and articulated as the degree of 'take', which refers to the adherence of the skin graft to the recipient bed and uptake of a new blood supply from that area. The process of 'take' has been divided into three phases, known as serum imbibition, revascularization and maturation (Scherer-Pietramaggiori et al, 2018).

Phase 1: serum imbibition occurs in the first few days when the newly applied skin graft is nourished by oxygen and nutrients that diffuse through the plasma between the graft and recipient site. The conversion of fibrinogen to fibrin fixes the graft to the recipient site.

Phase 2: revascularization is essential for the long-term survival of a skin graft. It involves anastomosis, neovascularization and endothelial cell ingrowth.

- Anastomosis involves the reconnection of existing blood vessels in the recipient site to vessel ends in the skin graft.
- Neovascularization involves new vessel ingrowth between the recipient site and the skin graft.

Table 24.1 Differences between FTSGs and STSGs

Variation	Full-thickness skin graft (FTSG)	Split-thickness skin graft (STSG or SSG)
Layers	All the epidermis and dermis down to but not including the subcutaneous tissue.	All the epidermis and various levels of the dermis but not all of the dermis.
Harvesting	Cut with a scalpel.	Cut with a Humby knife or dermatome.
Size	Size limited by the need to directly close the donor site so areas are relatively small.	Can be extensive. Meshing allows an increase of 2–3 times the surface area of the skin originally harvested.
Application	In one piece, no holes in the graft.	In one piece as a sheet; fenestrated with small holes or meshed with larger holes.
Blood supply	Both are separated from their own blood supply and once applied are completely dependent on the recipient site to develop a new blood supply.	
Contraction	Less contraction during maturation.	The thinner the graft, the greater the contraction during maturation.
Sensation	More sensory innervation due to transfer of nerves but end result variable.	Partial sensation regained from nerves on the wound bed but less than FTSG and also variable.
Aesthetics	Better aesthetic result due to less contraction. The closer the donor site is to the recipient site, the better matched the skin colour.	Sheet grafts have a better aesthetic result than fenestrated or meshed. The more fenestrations and larger the mesh, the less aesthetically pleasing. Skin colour mismatch at site of graft.
Resilience	More robust although still susceptible to trauma.	More vulnerable to trauma.
Donor site	No epidermal elements left after harvesting so direct closure required, healing by primary intention. Taken from sites with laxity to accommodate direct closure, e.g. pre-/postauricular, antecubital fossa, supraclavicular region, groin.	Remnant epidermal apparatus such as glands and hair follicles remain so re-epithelialization occurs, healing by secondary intention. Common sites are thigh and buttocks but can be anywhere depending on the amount of skin required to cover the defect.

From McGregor & McGregor (2000); Beldon (2007).

- Endothelial cell ingrowth involves the proliferation of endothelial cells in the recipient site.

Phase 3: maturation refers to the period when the skin graft is completely integrated in the recipient site. All of the tissue begins to remodel and contract, mirroring the final phase of wound healing.

Successful 'take' is dependent on the recipient site being infection free, having a good blood supply, and for close continuous contact between the skin graft and recipient site until the new blood supply has been established. Studies suggest variations in timing of this process, which begins within hours and lasts several days depending on the thickness of the skin graft (Scherer-Pietramaggiori et al, 2018). Accepted time frames are 5–7 days for an STSG and 7–10 days for an FTSG (McGregor & McGregor, 2000). Prior planning before skin grafting is essential to ensure the recipient site has an adequate blood supply to support the skin graft, and is infection free. Vascular issues in the recipient site can be due to:

- a poorly prepared recipient site where there is non-viable tissue and inadequate debridement.
- application of skin grafts over poorly vascularized areas such as bone without periosteum, tendon without paratenon, cartilage and fat. It is possible for a skin graft to 'take' over exposed bone and tendon through the phenomenon described as 'bridging'. This is when the blood supply develops successfully in the skin graft around and is adequate to support the viability of the graft area over these structures. However, this can only occur over very small areas (McGregor & McGregor, 2000). In general, skin grafts applied over structures, no matter how small, with no or limited blood supply are likely to fail.
- in areas where the blood supply is affected by underlying disease processes including vascular disease and previous radiotherapy sites.

Absence of infection in the area is essential prior to skin graft application. Specific organisms that challenge successful take include *Streptococcus pyogenes* and *Pseudomonas aeruginosa*. Confirmation of absence of these organisms is recommended prior to undertaking the procedure (McGregor & McGregor, 2000).

Skin grafting can occur using a local or general anaesthetic, being influenced by the area being grafted and patient assessment. An FTSG will be cut to the precise shape of the defect and then secured in place (Fig. 24.2), in contrast to the STSG, which is often applied to the defect with some overlap at the edges (Fig. 24.3).

The surgeon uses a variety of securing methods such as glue, dissolving and non-dissolving sutures or staples. Once applied, it is essential for the skin graft to stay in close continuous contact with the recipient bed. Failure to achieve this can result from inadequate splinting or

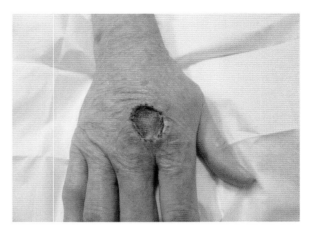

Figure 24.2 Full-thickness skin graft cut to size of defect.

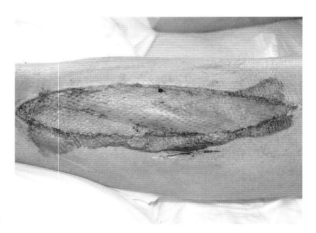

Figure 24.3 Split-thickness skin graft (meshed) with overlapped skin.

immobilization resulting in friction or shearing between the skin graft and the recipient site. Seroma or haematoma collection under the graft will also prevent the process of imbibition and anastomosis but may sometimes not be evident until the first postoperative skin graft dressing. Pressure application to ensure sustained close, continuous contact is achieved by the primary dressing fixation and in any secondary fixation required. The method used depends on the site and area grafted. Common primary fixation methods are outlined in Table 24.2.

Table 24.2 Skin graft primary fixation

Body part	Common primary fixation	Comments
Head; face; ears	Bolster of foam; gauze or cotton stitched or stapled to the skin graft and surrounding skin. Alternatively, the bolster may be stitched to skin graft and threads of stitch material tied over the dressing – known as a 'tie-over' dressing.	Secures the dressing well without the need for additional fixation. Excellent in awkward areas such as the face and fingers. Can be awkward to remove if: • area has bled and the dressing is stuck – needs soaking to soften and remove • stitches/staples are tight and difficult to cut – may need to cut around the stitches to remove dressing and expose stitch material for removal • the colour of the stitches used in the tie-over dressing are difficult to see against the dressing material – use good lighting.
Trunk	Paraffin gauze dressings with gauze and adhesive. Topical negative pressure (TNP) wound therapy.	Primary dressing of paraffin gauze may adhere to skin graft so requires careful removal with soaking and use of gloved finger to support skin graft while easing dressing away. TNP provides an excellent splint (Yin et al, 2018). Difficulties with TNP include: • can delay discharge planning if equipment is not transferable to community setting • if the negative pressure seal is lost it needs to be removed as close, continuous contact is no longer being maintained.
Limbs	As outlined in trunk areas but requires secondary fixation with bandages. May also have a plaster of Paris/thermoplastic splint to immobilize.	Bandages should be joint to joint to provide good limb support and prevent swelling at either end. In the leg it is advisable to bandage from the toes to prevent foot swelling distal to the bandage end. Mobility of the limb will be reduced, and elevation is important to reduce oedema. Preoperative advice not to drive is essential.
Hands, fingers, foot and toes	Bolster dressings as above. Paraffin gauze dressings with gauze and adhesive. May also have a plaster of Paris/thermoplastic splint to immobilize.	The balance is between keeping a joint mobile and allowing immobilization long enough for the skin graft to take. Dressing can stick in these areas so copious soaking and gentle removal is essential. Following any period of immobility the patient will need to be shown how to exercise all joints to regain full function.

Specific preoperative advice is essential and dependent on the areas being grafted. The balance is between keeping the patient moving while not compromising the skin graft. The author's experience highlights the need to explicitly advise on activity and driving. The nurse should not assume patients will realize the modifications needed in the initial postoperative period in order to optimize the outcome. Ongoing advice can be provided at subsequent follow-up dressings.

Skin graft first dressing

The first inspection of a newly applied skin graft can occur in any clinical setting (Holden, 2015) and at any time with the understanding that the earlier the timing of this, the more fragile the graft is. The more fragile the graft, the greater the risk of separating it from the newly forming vasculature. In line with the physiological process of 'take', it is logical to try to leave the initial skin graft dressing in place for at least 5 days providing the dressing is adequately securing the skin graft and there are no clinical indications to inspect sooner. Clinical indications for early inspection will be signs of infection or bleeding under the skin graft, both of which will result in skin graft failure if not addressed. The thicker the skin graft, the longer the process of revascularization. In practice it is accepted that skin grafts will be inspected any time from 5–10 days following application.

Advice for the first skin graft dressing

Reading operative notes will direct the nurse to the location of the skin graft and associated donor site; the type of fixation of the skin graft, the type of dressing and any directions for aftercare such as stitch removal, ongoing use of a splint or mobility restrictions. It is essential to prepare the patient for the graft appearance and the degree of success of the procedure (Holden, 2015). Analgesia prior to the event and explanation about the mixture of colours that will differ from the surrounding skin and varying contours is essential (see Fig. 24.2). Tie-over packs or negative

pressure dressings may indicate the size to expect but this still does not prepare the patient for what they are about to see. Establishing whether the patient wants to see or hear about the progress of the wound at this time should underpin how the nurse conducts this aspect of care.

The aim of this first inspection is to ensure that removal of the skin graft dressing does not pull and lift the skin graft, highlighting the importance of a gentle approach to the procedure. This can be achieved by removing layer by layer, soaking any adhered dressing with copious amounts of normal saline and applying a gloved finger under the dressing to support the skin graft so that removal does not pull at the skin or traumatize the skin graft.

Once the dressing has been removed, the nurse completes a systematic wound assessment. Assessment models such as TIMES (Wounds UK, 2016) provide such an approach and can be applied as illustrated in Table 24.3. Specific to the skin graft is an estimation of what percentage of the skin graft has 'taken' and how stable the adherence is. Although subjective, this is widely adopted terminology in skin graft assessment (Holden, 2015). To make this assessment the nurse needs to consider out of 100% how much of the wound has a skin graft in place — this gives the percentage. Then, wearing a sterile glove, gentle palpation of the graft indicates how much of that percentage is adhered and stable.

Table 24.3 TIMES Framework to assess at first skin graft dressing

Category	Action
Tissue type and how to manage it. A skin graft is epithelial tissue.	Comment on: • appearance of graft and % that has adhered • % of the adhered skin graft that is stable • % of area of the skin graft that may lift in areas over fat, fascia or bone if suspected • % of any other tissue present • any fluid collection under the skin graft such as a seroma or haematoma.
Infection or inflammation	Comment if erythema/inflammation is infection or inflammation from another source such as tight stitches, exudate or friction from the dressing. If infection suspected take a swab and document action taken.
Moisture imbalance	Document if odour present and consistency of the fluid, both can indicate infection. The larger the holes or mesh, the more fluid is expected. Assess presence of oedema in the area and consider management, e.g. lower limb may require assessment for compression.
Edges and epithelial advancement	Document % of take and any raw areas at the edges of the skin graft. Document overlapped skin (Fig. 24.3) and action taken.
Surrounding skin	Comment on any inflammation. Comment on dryness and fragility with consideration of management.

Throughout the first inspection, the impact on first seeing the skin graft needs to be considered for the patient and their adaptation to an altered body image. No amount of explanation can ever mirror the image when the patient first looks, but reassurance that this will change over time and opportunities to answer questions can contribute to a more positive experience.

In theory, at the time of the first dressing any suture or staples securing the skin graft will have served their purpose and should be removed (Beldon, 2007). This is good practice at five days onwards for stable grafts, together with trimming of excess skin that overlaps intact skin at the edges of the graft. However, if the graft is less stable, there are concerns about the fragility or the patient's experience of the first dressing is difficult to tolerate, then this can be delayed until future dressing changes. Unstable grafts may not 'take' but can remain in place to act as a biological dressing, although all sutures, staples and non-viable skin should be removed by 7—10 days (Holden, 2015).

Selection of the primary dressing is based on assessment of graft 'take' and type of tissue where the graft has not 'taken'. If there is 100% take and stability in an area that is not subject to mechanical stress, the area can be left exposed and the patient can commence moisturizing and massaging the skin graft (Holden, 2015) However, the author's experience is that this is rare and applies to very small areas around the nose and eyes in patients who feel able to immediately adapt to the new appearance. In the majority of situations, a new dressing will need selecting in line with systemic assessment, aims of care, impact of the product on the skin graft, local policy and associated dressing formularies. The impact some types of dressings may have on new skin grafts are outlined in Table 24.4.

Secondary dressings and fixation options to secure a new skin graft

The aim of the secondary dressing is to add absorption or further secure the primary dressing against the skin graft. In skin grafts where there are dips and crevices, the primary dressing selected needs to be moulded along the contours and then gauze can be opened out and

Table 24.4 Potential impact of primary dressings on new skin grafts (5—10 days)

Category	Advantage	Disadvantage
Paraffin gauze	If >90% take, the area continues re-epithelializing so this can be useful over large areas or in difficult areas.	Dries after 24—48 hours so requires frequent dressing changes.
Iodine and silver-based products	Can reduce bioburden if required.	Should not be used routinely if there is no concern over bioburden or infection risk.
Silicone	Low adherence and can stay intact for several days.	Can cause fluid collection underneath leading to maceration or dried scabs.
Foams	Useful if cut to the size as they apply pressure to splint and support indented grafts.	Do not conform well over joints and curves so can cause friction on the new skin graft if not firmly fixed.
Hydrocolloid	Can help to secure and moisturize very stable skin grafts in difficult areas such as the scalp, face and ears.	Can lift grafts that are not stable so should be avoided in fragile grafts.
Alginates and hydrofibre	If the majority of skin graft has failed and the wound is wet, these can help with exudate management.	The products are gel-forming, having the potential to cause maceration to the newly adhering skin.
Hydrogels	Only for use in areas with complete skin graft failure.	The products will cause maceration to newly adhered skin and should be avoided in the initial dressing.
Topical negative pressure	Excellent splint for a skin graft when first applied but should not be reapplied unless skin graft failure.	Due to the potential for maceration it should not be reapplied after the initial dressing.

scrunched or fluffed into balls that can be positioned into crevices, holding the primary dressing firmly against the skin graft. Selection of foam cut to the size of the grafted area if it is deep can have further support applied with a second piece of foam over the top. Careful positioning of gauze to support the primary dressings is recommended over indiscriminate application.

Fixation needs to be secure and will vary in line with the body part being dressed. Where tape is indicated, firm tapes such as Hypafix (Smith & Nephew) or Mefix (Mölnlycke Health Care) can be useful but should not be used where surrounding skin is fragile.

In all new skin grafts on limbs, joint to joint fixation is recommended with a liner, then wool bandage to shape and protect the limb followed by crepe type support bandages. Further support can be provided by an elastic tubular bandage such as Tubigrip, providing there is no vascular contraindication. The author recommends assessing patients with lower leg grafts who have oedematous limbs or signs of venous hypertension for compression suitability where possible preoperatively. Alternatively, after the first inspection, use of compression where indicated and appropriate should be considered to facilitate healing.

Ongoing nursing management of a skin graft

Subsequent dressing changes will see the skin graft becoming more robust over time and, where the graft did not initially take, re-epithelialization will occur as healing continues. Hence, reference to the 'take' of a skin graft is only relevant at the first dressing inspection. Subsequent assessments should be stated in terms of how much of the wound has healed and should employ the principles of all wound assessment and management (Lucas & King, 2010). The new graft is newly formed epithelial tissue and the absence of self-moisturizing glands highlights the importance of patient education and advice on massage, moisturizing and protection from trauma and UV sunlight (Holden, 2015).

Skin graft donor sites

The FTSG skin graft donor site is directly closed at the time of the harvesting and therefore heals by primary intention, being managed in the same way as any stitch line. STSGs, however, heal by secondary intention, where the initial nursing priorities are pain and exudate management (Beldon, 2003). This wound may be more problematic for the patient compared to the actual skin graft as pain levels will be at their greatest over the first few days, followed by itching as the donor site heals. Patients need to be warned about this and advised about taking adequate pain control. If the pain does not settle after 3–5 days despite appropriate analgesia and good fixation, the donor site should be inspected in case of infection.

In the initial few days the STSG donor site will produce large amounts of fluid; the larger the donor site, the more fluid produced. This is then followed by a later period of the wound drying out and the potential for the primary dressing adhering to newly forming epithelium. Although healing time of the STSG donor site mirrors the depth of the wound together with patient factors affecting healing, on average the healing trajectory should be 7–21 days (McGregor & McGregor, 2000; Beldon, 2003).

Studies exploring dressings for donor site management indicate there is no ideal dressing and systematic reviews highlight the need for quality research on the topic (Voineskos et al, 2009). Facilitating moist wound healing is frequently documented, with popularity currently remaining with alginate, hydrofibre and foam dressings due to their ability to manage exudate in the early days (Higgins et al, 2012). Alternatively, the practice of using an adhesive tape, such as Hypafix (Smith & Nephew) or Mefix (Mölnlycke Health Care), directly to the wound is supported by authors who have demonstrated positive patient outcomes, including the benefit of being able to shower throughout the healing process (Hormbrey et al, 2003). The author's experience with this practice is mixed and suggests the adoption of this practice by surgeons should be selective. Examples of the postoperative dressings the nurse may encounter are outlined in Table 24.5.

In some circumstances, such as in the elderly or where harvesting of the skin is in excess of what is applied, donor sites are overgrafted where the skin is re-applied over the donor site (Keilani et al, 2017). The author recommends treating the wound as a donor site, as the primary issues will still be the open raw areas that need to have exudate managed. Irrespective of the dressing selection, the nursing care must focus on optimizing the local environment to facilitate healing. This will include secure fixation to help reduce pain and discomfort by reducing friction between the newly healing wound and the primary dressing. Thighs do not lend themselves to bandaging, which should be avoided in preference for fixation with secure tapes. Failure to manage exudate and trauma caused by dressing movement may result in an infected donor site and delayed healing. *Pseudomonas aeruginosa* can become established in a donor site, presenting as a bright green exudate with odour. Management of this may simply be a case of changing the dressing more regularly or selecting a topical antimicrobial product (Wounds UK, 2013a). Extended periods of inflammation resulting from increased infection and trauma may result in over-granulation and this needs prompt management with a topical steroid (Holden, 2015). Non-healing or recurrent breakdown of a donor site may indicate a high

Table 24.5 Donor site dressings

Dressing	Postoperative	Ongoing dressing management
Alginate/hydrofibre with gauze and Hypafix (Smith & Nephew) or Mefix (Mölnlycke Health Care) as a secondary dressing	Allows some vapour permeability and initial 'strike through' of exudate to top layer of dressing can be re-padded. Assess extent of wetness of the dressing and redress if requiring more than one re-padding. Adhesive tape is essential to fix in place on places like the thigh or buttock where bandaging will slip and therefore should be avoided.	If exudate comes to the outer layers within 24 hours, re-padding is acceptable but after this each dressing layer that is wet needs removal to assess if complete redressing is required. Careful removal of the layers down to the wettest one prevents bulky dressings that can pull on the wound. If the alginate is wet, it has reached its full absorbency capacity and can no longer manage the exudate. Wet dressings can damage surrounding skin and become a harbour for bacteria to then increase the risk of infection (Wounds UK, 2013b). As soon as alginate or hydrofibre dries out it can have a secondary dressing of semipermeable film to hydrate and lift the primary dressing from the newly formed epithelial tissue.
Alginate/hydrofibre with a polyurethane film as a secondary dressing	Only appropriate on very small STSG donor site. If exudate too much for this to manage, redress with an alternative.	Move to this regime once the alginate is dry and exudate is more manageable.
Foam	Change as exudate indicates (Terrill et al, 2007).	Types of foam dressings can absorb fluid and limit adhesion to wound bed so can be a useful dressing (Beldon, 2003).
Adhesive tapes	Single sheet applied and then gauze padding and more tape on top – this can be changed each time exudate comes to the outer layers. Once dry it can remain in place and patients can shower (Hormbrey et al, 2003).	Only re-apply new gauze when the tape is wet. Trim edges as they start lifting. If fluid collects under the tape or there are signs of infection, remove the tape and use alternative following assessment.
Semi-permeable films	Should not be used in initial postoperative dressing as exudate too high.	Can be used only as a secondary dressing with alginates or hydrofibre dressings when exudate is not too heavy. Useful in hydrating dry alginate/hydrofibre that then separate spontaneously from the newly formed epithelial tissue.
Hydrocolloid	Not used in initial postoperative dressing as exudate too high.	Useful for superficial raw areas in healing STSG donor site.
Paraffin gauze	The paraffin dries and the gauze adheres to the donor site causing trauma on removal (McGregor & McGregor, 2000; Beldon, 2003). **This should always be avoided in donor sites**.	Only to be used as a medication carrier if topical steroids are used for the management of over-granulation.

bioburden that needs managing. The author recommends referring patients with delayed donor site healing for specialist advice.

Newly healed donor sites are fragile and may need an extended period of protection. Avoiding dressing fabric that will rub and damage the skin is advisable. For some patients, extra time with a protective dressing may be required. The nurse needs to consider this in the assessment. Patient education about managing the healed donor site mirrors that of any maturing wound that requires moisturizing, massage and protection against trauma and the sun.

Flaps

A flap is a mass of tissue with a blood supply that is transferred from a donor site to a recipient site (Levine, 2014). Therefore, although flaps and skin grafts are procedures involving the transfer of tissue, the inherent difference is that the flap brings with it a blood supply while the skin graft does not (Del Rosario & Barkley, 2017). In essence, the flap can be described as a tongue of tissue comprising tissue of various types containing its own independent circulation. This circulation may result from the vascular supply remaining intact during tissue transfer, or as a result of complete detachment and then re-attachment by surgically joining vessels together at the recipient site. Although principles of flap reconstructions and similarities in anatomy will exist, no two flaps will be the same as they are uniquely specific to the patient and the surgeon undertaking the reconstruction. Essentially there will be the primary site to which the flap has been applied and a flap donor site from where it has come. The only exception to this is when a digit is replanted following traumatic amputation. Flap surgery is adopted across all surgical specialties in a huge range of reconstruction situations, including:

- for primary defects following tumour excision from any part of the body, or a defect resulting from trauma, that require vascularized tissue
- for a defect with inadequate vascularization to support a skin graft, such as exposed bone or areas that have undergone radiotherapy (Levine, 2014)
- in an area of wear and tear, such as repair of a defect resulting from a pressure ulcer (Black & Black, 2012)
- in areas where other tissue is required, such as intra-oral repair (Wax, 2013) or nerve innervation
- replantation of anatomical parts detached as a result of traumatic amputation (Spiers, 2018).

Various flap classification systems exist (Levine, 2014), but the terms used can be confusing, as elements of a flap can overlap and fit into more than one category. To understand the surgery and implications for nursing the flap, the author recommends the nurse considers flaps in terms of type of tissue transferred, proximity between the donor and recipient sites, sphere of transfer and blood supply, as outlined in Table 24.6.

Access to the internet and search engines facilitates swift access to clarification and illustration with images if the terms used are not familiar to the nurse. Understanding the operation will enable the nurse to appreciate the structures involved and relevance to nursing care with specific reference to the initial monitoring of a flap if required. Additionally, it underpins explanations to patients where unexpected incision wounds may be explained if additional

Table 24.6 Categories of flaps

Category	Flap classification	Nursing considerations
Type of tissue	Cutaneous — skin and superficial fascia. Fasciocutaneous — skin and deep fascia (Fig. 24.4). Myocutaneous — skin and muscle. Osteomyocutaneous — skin, muscle and bone. Muscle used, e.g. latissimus dorsi, deltopectoral, gastrocnemius. Muscle and other tissues, e.g. transverse rectus abdominis myocutaneous (TRAM) — indicates the muscle taken and overlying cutaneous tissue.	The viability of any flap with a cutaneous portion can be assessed by capillary refill and should resemble the donor site. A combination of tissue may be selected to fill large defects that exceed the volume provided by one tissue type or where multiple tissue types are required to achieve the desired outcome (Levine, 2014).
Proximity	Local is where the donor site is next to the recipient site. Distant is where the donor site is some distance from the recipient site.	Positioning will be affected by both where the flap is and the associated donor site.

(Continued)

Table 24.6 Categories of flaps—cont'd

Category	Flap classification	Nursing considerations
Sphere of transfer	Rotation — the tissue is turned locally on an axis or pivot and is usually semi-circular in design. Transposition — the tissue is moved immediately adjacent and tends to be square or rectangular in shape. Island — skin is transferred under the skin still attached to a blood vessel. Advancement — not moved on a pivot but moved directly forward. Free flap — the tissue is completely detached from the arterial and venous circulation and the vessels re-anastomosed once inset into the recipient site. Pedicle — the tissue remains attached to its blood supply via a pedicle and will be limited by arc of rotation (Levine, 2014).	Avoiding kinking and pressure on the pedicle is essential. Knowledge of the location of the anastomosis is essential to avoid pressure on the area and for monitoring.
Blood supply	Random pattern — non-specified circulation supporting the tissue transferred, flap length ratio to width is critical for survival. Axial pattern — based on an identified anatomical vascular supply positioned longitudinally in the flap. Perforator flaps — name of blood vessel on which survival of the flap depends, e.g. deep inferior epigastric perforator (DIEP); superficial inferior epigastric artery (SIEA); thoracodorsal artery perforator (TAP); superior or inferior gluteal artery perforator (SGAP/IGAP). Free and pedicle as indicated above.	Random flaps are restricted in terms of size of the defect. Knowledge of the blood supply and anastomosis is essential for safe care.

Table 24.7 Flap planning considerations

Defect for reconstruction (recipient site)	Donor site
• Area and location • Quality of surrounding tissue • Reasons for surgery including desired end result • Method to be adopted to bring donor and defect together	• Tissue match • Size of amount of tissue required to close the defect including volume and thickness • Associated blood supply of the donor site to meet the defect requirements • Morbidities associated with the donor site (Hsieh, 2015)

procedures were required, such as vein grafts to stabilize circulation.

Selection of the flap will be planned by the surgeon who considers both the defect to be reconstructed and the attributes of the donor site from which the flap will come (Table 24.7). The success of any technical expertise will be dependent on thorough planning before the surgery (Salgado et al, 2010).

Preoperative imaging methods are variable but are recommended in selecting appropriate donor sites to harvest where the viability of vessels can be confirmed before the surgery (Thimmappa et al, 2019). A delayed flap refers

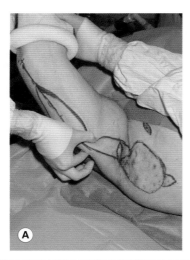

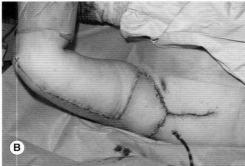

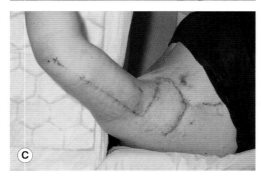

Figure 24.4 Fasciocutaneous local pedicle flap. (A) Planning of a posterior arm flap. (B) Inset at operation. (C) One week later.

to a situation where procedures are employed to increase the success of a viable blood supply on transfer. It may involve raising the flap but not transferring it at the same time or using techniques such as tissue expansion prior to transfer (Levine, 2014). Additional influencing factors include whether it is an emergency or elective procedure,

the patient's condition and associated morbidities. Factors such as tobacco use, diabetes and malnutrition need to be managed to optimize a patient's condition where possible (Salgado et al, 2010; Hsieh, 2015).

Preoperative discussions with the patient are essential to ensure informed consent and will include:

- donor site or potential donor sites as the extent of a resection or debris removal may be unknown and flexibility has to accommodate intraoperative discoveries (Butler & Adelman, 2014)
- potential for partial or full flap failure and associated monitoring regime expected after the surgery, including plans for a period in intensive care
- postoperative care involving intravenous fluid, drains, indwelling urinary catheter, restricted mobility and possible use of leech therapy
- potential complications associated with any type of surgery including bleeding, haematoma, infection and pain
- estimated recovery period and impact on daily activities
- subsequent surgical procedures anticipated, such as excision of a paddle of skin used for monitoring or division of a pedicle as in the forehead flap
- specific scarring anticipated in both the reconstructed and donor sites (Fig. 24.5).

Nursing care

Many small, local flaps will be managed as day cases with little input from the nursing team until the first postoperative review in clinic. However, where monitoring is required, skilled and experienced nursing care is critical in the early detection of clinical problems (McGregor & McGregor, 2000; Nahabedian & Nahabedian, 2016; Del Rosario & Barkley, 2017; Wax, 2013). Examples of more complex flaps requiring observation include local flaps such as a pedicled nipple in a breast reduction or a fasciocutaneous flap in the leg, as well as distant pedicle flaps such as the forehead flap or the sophisticated microvascular free flaps that can involve any part of the body. Ideally, management of complex microvascular flap surgery should occur in specialized units with experienced and knowledgeable nurses (Broyles et al, 2016), as the complexity and skill needed in accurate assessment should not be underestimated (Khan et al, 2010). Nursing care must be based on systematic patient assessment with identification of actual and potential problems. A variety of nursing models can be employed by the nurse, who will be influenced by their own experience and the practice in the clinical area within which the patient is nursed. The author has based the outline of potential problems in line with the activities of living (AL) (Roper et al, 2000) (Box 24.1). The emphasis, however, in the immediate

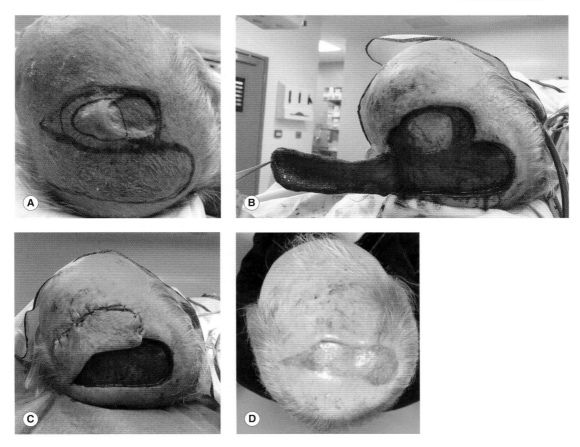

Figure 24.5 Scarring — the flap, the split-thickness skin graft used on the flap donor site and the split-thickness skin graft donor site. (A) Defect for reconstruction. (B) Raising of flap to cover bone. (C) Flap inset and flap donor site required a split-thickness skin graft. (D) Healed flap and flap donor site.

postoperative management focuses on facilitating a safe recovery and maintaining a sustainable circulation to ensure flap success.

Maintaining a safe environment (AL 1)

This includes safe recovery of the patient after the surgery, as discussed in Chapter 2. Specific to flap surgery is the importance of systemic support to maintain adequate blood flow through the anastomosis, which is dependent on good fluid balance, prevention and management of abnormalities in blood pressure, and maintaining a warm environment to prevent hypothermia resulting in circulatory shut down (Chao & Lamp, 2014). Good pain control, discussed in Chapter 4, is fundamental to prevent sympathetic nervous system activity that has the potential

to reduce blood flow to the flap (Del Rosario & Barkley, 2017). Comfortable positioning can also reduce pain but needs to be balanced with the position required for the vascular supply and drainage from the flap. Surgeon's instructions about the impact of positioning on the anastomosis or pedicle are important, as certain flaps, such as in the head and neck, have been shown to depend heavily of positioning in the initial postoperative period (Wax, 2013).

Regular physical examination of the flap means any subtle changes in vascularity that suggest compromise can be swiftly reported and acted on (Nahabedian & Nahabedian, 2016). This increases the potential for flap salvage to 75% in those that are struggling (Hsieh, 2015). Duration of intense monitoring is specific to the flap location and specifications of the surgeon but is usually a minimum of hourly for the first 24 hours (Salgado et al,

2010; Chao & Lamp, 2014). This need for intensive nursing intervention, together with the extended operation times required for complex reconstruction, underpins the reason some patients may be nursed in high dependency or intensive care units for 24−48 hours.

Safe recovery is dependent on understanding operation notes and clarification of details about the anastomosis and positioning of the pedicle, if present. Full patient and procedural handover is essential with clarification of any details that are not clear. Requested monitoring parameters help direct the staff about when to call for medical review (Salgado et al, 2010). Additionally, knowledge of any intraoperative problems with vessels either in the pedicle or at the site of a microvascular anastomosis can alert the nurse to the elevated potential for postoperative circulation problems (Wax, 2013).

Acute problems with the blood supply to the flap may necessitate a return to the operating theatre to explore and rectify the problem (Del Rosario & Barkley, 2017), so preparation for safe return may be part of the postoperative nursing care. Accurate documentation is an essential element of nursing care (NMC, 2018) and use of charts and local protocols may exist to provide guidelines on how to monitor flaps (Khan et al, 2010). An example of a flap monitoring chart with descriptive explanations currently used in a London teaching hospital is illustrated in Fig. 24.6. It is recommended that, in the initial 24−72 hours, each nurse taking over the responsibility of the flap observations do their first set alongside a practitioner who has previously monitored the flap (Chao & Lamp, 2014). This will provide the baseline and promote consistency in accurate reporting.

Vascular complications

Detecting blood flow involves using equipment to detect the flow through the flap and assessing the flap for colour, capillary refill, temperature and texture. Flaps that are buried without any visible portion cannot be monitored, but knowledge of blood supply is needed to prevent inappropriate positioning or pressure on the vascular pedicle or anastomosis (Salgado et al, 2010). Where possible, if a flap is buried, exposing a small paddle of the cutaneous portion of the flap, e.g. in a transverse rectus abdominis myocutaneous (TRAM) or deep inferior epigastric perforator (DIEP) in skin-sparing mastectomy, facilitates monitoring. For accessible flaps with a visible portion that can be monitored or for replanted digits, the blood flow is commonly assessed using a hand-held external Doppler with a suture inserted on the skin or muscle where the perforator signal should be detected (Salgado et al, 2010; Butler & Adelman, 2014; Wax, 2013). Marking the site to assess is important to avoid confusion in picking up signals from adjacent vessels (Salgado et al, 2010). Developments in technology have seen the introduction of implantable methods and laser Doppler flowmetry (Del Rosario & Barkley, 2017). Flaps that experience vascular problems intraoperatively have been shown to be at a higher risk of having subsequent vascular problems in the head and neck area. Consequently, recommendations exist to use implantable intraoperative Doppler to detect vascular problems intraoperatively, with the added advantage that subsequent postoperative blood flow can continue in the first few days after surgery (Wax, 2013). However, irrespective of the postoperative monitoring technology used, it needs to occur alongside the clinical examination of the flap, which remains the gold standard in assessing flap viability (Butler & Adelman, 2014; Chao & Lamp, 2014; Hsieh, 2015).

The new in-growth for venous drainage in a flap develops gradually over several days and can be less easy to accomplish then the arterial anastomosis (Spear, 2016). Both can be affected by thrombus with a need for antithrombotic treatment. The use of antithrombotic prophylaxis or active treatment is controversial (Salgado et al, 2010; Hsieh, 2015), and the absence of robust evidence has resulted in a variety of regimes directed by the surgeon's experiences and patient-specific issues (Del Rosario & Barkley, 2017). Even in the absence of thrombus formation, efficient venous circulation is gradual. Hence, venous compromise is the more common circulation issue where outflow does not match arterial inflow resulting in venous congestion (Wax, 2013). Factors that can contribute to the congestion include kinking of the flap pedicle; positioning of the body part to which the flap has been transferred; constricting dressings or support garment, e.g. bra post breast reconstruction; rigid bandages or splinting; tight stitches or non-functioning vacuum drains. Hence, assessment of these potential causes and relief of obstructions should occur in the first instance (Chao & Lamp, 2014). The need for regular inspection and pressure relief may result in flaps being left dressing-free and exposed, thus challenging the nurses' skills in managing infection control if there is leaking around the flap and in preventing

Name of operation:			**Please complete or affix label:**												
			Forename:												
			Surname:												
			DOB:												
			Hospital Number:												
Medical team name and contact numbers:															
Operative instructions:															
State light source used:															
Date															
Time															
Assessor's initial															
Colour: Red flesh (RF); Pink (P); Cream (C); White (W); Blue (Blu); Mauve (M); Black (Bla)															
Temp	Cold														
	Cool														
	Warm														
	Hot														
Capillary refill (not for non-cutaneous flaps)	No blanch														
	> 3 seconds														
	3 seconds														
	< 3 seconds														
	No refill / fixed staining														
Texture	Soft														
	Spongy														
	Firm														
	Hard														
Doppler	Audible														
	Faint														
	No sound														
Comments															

Figure 24.6 Flap/digit monitoring chart.

Observation explanation - The first set of observations to be recorded by the surgeon with the nurse.	
Name of operation	Ensure you understand type of tissue transferred, blood supply, sphere of transfer. Ensure you understand where the anastomosis/pedicle is.
Medical team and contact numbers	Get the contact numbers and names of the operating team so that problems detected with the flap can be reported promptly to increase the chances of flap salvage and survival. Put on chart name / number of who to contact – it will be in the notes.
Postoperative instructions	Read ALL instructions. Be aware of: ○ special positioning that may affect the blood supply; ○ the position of the anastomosis or pedicle to avoid jeopardizing this; ○ recording observations as specifically directed by the surgeon or ½-hourly for four hours; 1-hourly for 48 hours; reducing as surgeon instructs and according to flap condition; ○ using the same light source to inspect the flap; ○ handing over observations between different nurses to confirm the baseline; ○ flap changes often occur over a period of time so report subtle changes.
Colour	Perfusion is monitored through the colour of a flap. Report changing colour to the team as soon as it is noted. The early diagnosis of a failing flap is crucial. Muscle flaps with split-thickness skin cover should appear bright red and resemble fresh meat or red flesh (RF) if healthy. Flaps with cutaneous cover may vary in colours but should always be compared to the skin colour in the donor area. Intra-oral flaps appear a little pale when compared to normal oral mucosa. The baseline colour from the surgeon will provide the guide against which to measure changes. Pale flaps suggest arterial insufficiency and a white (W) flap indicates arterial occlusion. Varying shades of blue (Blu) or mauve (M), suggest venous obstruction. This is the most frequent cause of flap failure. Black (Bla) flaps indicate necrosis.
Temperature	Keep patients warm to facilitate vasodilation and optimum blood flow through the flap. Avoid drafts around the flap and prolonged exposure. Warm fluid for cleansing. The flap should be of a similar temperature to that of the surrounding normal tissue. Test by putting one gloved finger on the flap and one on the surrounding tissue. Cold flaps suggest a failed blood supply, which may be arterial and/or venous. Cool flaps are suggestive of deterioration of the vascularity of a flap and should be acted on promptly. Warm flaps are suggestive of a perfused flap.
Capillary refill	This indicates perfusion but can only be assessed in flaps with a cutaneous component. 3–5 seconds for refill can be considered normal Less than 3 seconds may highlight the venous congestion. More than 3 seconds may show arterial sluggishness No refill indicates an arterial occlusion.
Texture	A flap should feel soft to the touch. A spongy flap with reduced tissue turgor may indicate arterial insufficiency. A firm flap may indicate venous congestion and can be caused by oedema within the flap and/or kinking of the pedicle/anastomosis. A firm/hard texture is a sign of impending flap failure that needs immediate attention.
Doppler	Unless otherwise stated a Doppler probe should be placed to assess the flap. The position of the anastomosis may be marked with a stitch or pen. If no arterial Doppler signal is audible then call the team immediately.

Figure 24.6 (Continued).

overexposure with cooling of the flap. In addition, issues relating to the altered body image and impact of the appearance of the exposed flap on the patient need to be assessed and addressed.

Flap colour. The colour should be comparable to the donor site. Hence, any flap with a cutaneous component should match the cutaneous area from where it has come (Hsieh, 2015). Changes in this colour vary depending on the underlying vascular problem. Paler flaps, when compared to their donor site, indicate a reduced arterial inflow (Wax, 2013). Colour changes due to venous outflow vary according to the degree of congestion and may include pinkish hues to varying shades of purple/blue (Hsieh, 2015). Darker pigmented skin can be more difficult to assess. Salgado et al (2010) recommends photographing the flap, against which future assessments can be compared. Muscle flaps should appear as red vascular tissue. Colour changes can be very subtle and are less specific to the type of vascular problem, but darker red shades through to mauve indicate a failing flap (Storch & Rice, 2005). An STSG may be meshed and used to cover the muscle flap. In the absence of infection, failure of STSG 'take' can be an indication that the blood supply in the muscle flap is failing (Hsieh, 2015).

Temperature. The theory that a warm flap is perfused underpins the reason to assess temperature (Hsieh, 2015). A cool flap assessed using a gloved finger in line with body temperature suggests problems with arterial supply (Wax, 2013). However, the subjective nature of this assessment methodology needs to be recognized. Furthermore, intraoral flaps can be difficult to assess as their temperature is also influenced by the cooling effect of any secretions that surround the flap (Wax, 2013). Where temperature is monitored, comparisons must be made to the temperature of the surrounding tissue and considerations about the impact of prolonged exposure of a flap must be appreciated as this may be the cause of a cool flap as opposed to a circulatory failure.

Capillary refill. Flaps with a cutaneous portion can be assessed by applying pressure with the gloved finger to cause blanching and assessing the speed the colour returns on pressure removal. Normal capillary refill times may vary although quoted timings range from 2 to 5 seconds (Hsieh, 2015; Wax, 2013). Challenges in observing this can occur with the position of the flap and variations in lighting. Capillary refill that lasts longer or starts to extend in time may suggest a reduction in arterial inflow with absence of refill indicating a definite arterial problem. Alternatively, a quicker refill time implies venous congestion. Wax (2013) recommends that surgeons undertake a 'pin prick' to assess the rate and type of bleeding that occurs in flaps where the capillary refill time is of concern. This can be assessed using a needle to prick the flap; providing the pin prick is adequate, prompt bleeding will indicate good arterial inflow, with

absence of bleeding indicating arterial occlusion (Hsieh, 2015). A dark red colouring suggests venous outflow obstruction (Hsieh, 2015).

Texture or turgor. Using a gloved finger and gently palpating the flap will inform the assessor of flap turgor (rigidity). The thicker and boggier a flap is, the more fluid within it, which can imply venous outflow problems. However, this finding must not be seen in isolation to the other observations (Wax, 2013), as other causes may be positioning and non-functioning vacuum drains. A spongy or visually collapsed flap with reducing firmness or wrinkles in the skin may indicate reduced arterial inflow (Chao & Lamp, 2014; Spiers, 2018).

The diligence of the nurse in assessment and reporting any concerns that arise cannot be understated as this informs the surgeon of the need to return to theatre to explore the flap. Butler and Adelman (2014) suggest the surgeon should have a low threshold for this in a flap that is developing clinical signs that it is failing. Flaps with arterial failure will always need operative exploration if salvage is considered to be possible. However, in situations where a cutaneous flap or a replanted digit starts to show signs of venous congestion, there is the option of using leeches to aid decongestion until the newly developing venous drainage becomes more robust and efficient.

Use of leeches in reconstructive surgery

The medicinal leech, *Hirudo medicinalis*, is an essential adjunct to the salvage of the venous congested flap with a cutaneous component and replanted digits (Spear, 2016; Spiers, 2018). The therapy creates an exit point for accumulating blood in the flap until such time as a competent venous circulation is established (Welshhans & Hom, 2016; Spear, 2016; Biopharm, 2019). Leeches must never be used in the arterially compromised flap (Del Rosario & Barkley, 2017), but if this occurs due to venous congestion, relief of the congestion may resolve the pressure on the arterial anastomosis. The patient can be reassured that attachment is painless due to a local anaesthetic released by the leech at the bite site. Once attached, the leech releases powerful anticoagulants, including hirudin, enabling blood to flow from the site (Welshhans & Hom, 2016). It is estimated that the leech has the potential to remove 5−20 mL directly but ongoing bleeding from the site will continue for hours (Fig. 24.7). This is the most important therapeutic aspect of leeching (Spear, 2016).

The decision of when to start or stop the therapy is largely empirical, being based on physical assessment of the flap (Spear, 2016). Although their use has been shown as fundamental in salvaging a venous congested flap, there is an increased risk of infection from *Aeromonas hydrophila* bacteria in the leeches' gut (Biopharm, 2019). This necessitates commencement of antibiotic therapy prior to and throughout their use. Blood loss needs to be monitored and

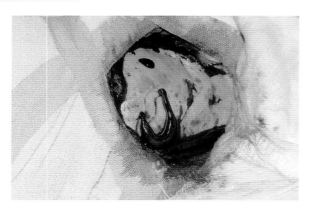

Figure 24.7 Sucking leech and ongoing bleeding points in venous congestion.

haemoglobin assessed throughout the treatment period (Sig et al, 2017). In addition, leeching poses psychological challenges for the patient and staff (Spiers, 2018; Welshhans & Hom, 2016). Clear explanation of benefits, how they will be managed, and a professional approach are essential. Following consent, application can be challenging (Spear, 2016), so needs to be undertaken by someone familiar with the process. Nurses are in an ideal position to implement this therapy but can have difficulties with the sight, handling and destruction of the leech after use (Reynolds & OBoyle, 2016). The author accepts the difficulties posed but would encourage nurses to overcome visual displays of such emotions in front of patients who are already psychologically burdened by their situation. Application instructions are available via the Biopharm website (Biopharm, 2019) and nurses should consult local standard operating procedures in areas using this therapy.

Non-salvageable flaps

In flaps where salvage is not possible, or only partial loss has occurred, approaches to their management thereafter may vary. Immediate removal of non-salvageable flaps has been recommended (Butler & Adelman, 2014), however management in such situations will vary between patients and surgeons. Hence wound care principles and debridement approaches will be adopted. The dynamic nature of wound healing means that once the circulatory success has declared itself, attention will move from the monitoring of the flap to the total healing of all the associated tissues.

Communication (AL 2)

Excellent communication applies to the preoperative preparation of the patient, the reading and understanding of operative notes, the postoperative support with adapting to an altered body image, and ongoing patient education throughout the trajectory. Psychological support and discussion about the altered body image is essential. This can be challenged further with flap reconstruction in the head and neck, where verbal communication may be reduced or absent. The decision not to look at the reconstruction will be challenged by the need for intensive and repeated observations to be carried out. Timing of patient discussions and education is dependent on the reason for surgery and timing. However, patient education regarding reconstructive procedures needs to be introduced at the soonest possible opportunity and reinforced throughout the entire period of recovery (Lucas & King, 2010; Del Rosario & Barkley, 2017). Involvement in care empowers the patient and assists in concordance. As the goals of care change, explanation of these to the patient is essential to avoid frustration with the process of recovery (Lucas & King, 2010).

Adapting to a change in body image is discussed in more detail in Chapter 7 and may also be assisted by external support agencies, examples of which include:

- **Let's Face It** — a charity providing an international support network for people and families affected by facial cancer and disfigurement: www.lets-face-it.org.uk
- **Changing Faces** — a charity providing advice, support and psychosocial services to children, young people and adults: www.changingfaces.org.uk
- **Saving Faces** — The Facial Surgery Research Foundation charity solely dedicated to the worldwide reduction of facial injuries and diseases: www.savingfaces.co.uk
- **British Association of Skin Camouflage** (BSAC) — an independent association using the application of specialized camouflage products to reduce psychological, physical and social effects resulting from an altered image: www.skin-camouflage.net. The use of products by people wanting to conceal scars or skin blemishes has been shown to have advantages for self-esteem (Kornhaber et al, 2018), but also disadvantages as it can be time-consuming and sometimes noticeable (Pasterfield et al, 2019), so patient selection and referral needs consideration.

Breathing (AL 3)

Reduced mobility enforced in the early stages has implication for breathing and the potential for chest infection. It is not unusual to perform a tracheostomy in patients undergoing head and neck reconstruction (Salgado et al, 2010), and careful positioning of ties is important in preventing flap constriction. Tobacco negatively impacts on the cardiovascular system, angiogenesis and skin capillary perfusion (Rau et al, 2017), hence lifelong cessation needs to be encouraged.

Eating and drinking (AL 4)

Good nutritional intake is essential for recovery and wound healing, as outlined in Chapter 6. However, resuming normal fluid and diet intake may be delayed if return to theatre in the first 24 hours is anticipated. Intravenous fluids will be ongoing until oral intake is safe and adequate. Flaps of the head and neck may necessitate nasogastric or enteral feeding. Previous recommendations to avoid caffeine-containing food and drink have subsequently been challenged with a call for more robust investigation of the impact on flap perfusion (Zelken & Berli, 2015).

Elimination (AL 5)

The extended operation time and need to balance fluid following surgery necessitates the use of a urinary indwelling catheter to monitor output. Monitoring urine output will indicate potential fluid balance issues and knowing accepted parameters will guide the nurse to report readings that are marginal or low. This can be addressed with increasing fluid input to maintain good systemic perfusion and therefore flap circulation (Chao & Lamp, 2014). Once close monitoring is no longer required this can be removed, although in genitourinary reconstructions the catheter may have to remain for longer periods. The impact of opioids and reduced mobility on bowel function needs assessment and management (Chao & Lamp, 2014). Elimination issues can be further challenged in patients with perianal reconstruction where the need to avoid pressure on the flap negates the possibility of the patient being able to sit on a bedpan or toilet to open their bowels.

Washing and dressing (AL 6)

Restrictions from drains, intravenous drips, catheter, enforced immobility, and specific positioning will need to be considered in meeting general hygiene care.

Controlling temperature (AL 7)

Maintenance of a warm environment is common practice in the first few days following surgery to maintain peripheral vasodilation, perfusion and flap circulation (Chao & Lamp, 2014). This may be achieved with the use of convective temperature management systems (Madrid et al, 2016), such as a heating blanket, e.g. 3 M Bair Hugger. This is usually only required for the first 24−48 hours and can be very uncomfortable for the patient. Additional actions include preventing drafts to the flap and reducing exposure time of the flap.

Mobilization (AL 8)

Restriction of mobility and positioning will be specific to the flap alongside any other condition, such as a bone injury, but it is expected that there will be a 24-hour period of enforced bedrest (Salgado et al, 2010).

Irrespective of the flap the need to ensure pressure relief is a key requirement to prevent arterial occlusion (Chao & Lamp, 2014). In addition, the impact of movement and position on the flap donor site also needs to be considered when planning care.

- In lower limb trauma the patient will have to keep the affected limb elevated for 24 hours a day until the flap is stable enough to commence 'dangling'. Dangling is the process of letting the limb dangle and assessing the impact on the gravitational change to the circulation in the limb. As the vascular circulation becomes more established, so the period of time for dangling can be extended. This will be directed by the surgical team and is patient-specific. Initially this process will last only 5 minutes and it is important to watch the impact on the flap regarding colouring and any changes that suggest vascular compromise in the flap. Mobility will also need to consider any bone injury and directions provided by the orthopaedic team regarding weight-bearing status and splinting.
- Head and neck flaps need the patient to be positioned upright to reduce swelling, and close airway monitoring is essential. Bed rest may only be required for a short period of time although restrictions on bending over and head movement may need enforcing.
- In the breast, after the initial period of bedrest and once the flap is stable, mobility will be encouraged. However, if the flap donor site is the abdomen, care is required to avoid overstretching and putting pressure on the abdominal scar. Relief of this can be facilitated by having bent legs in bed supported by pillows and rolling onto the side and gradually sitting up when getting out of bed.
- Reconstruction to the sacral area demands complete pressure relief necessitating side to side or prone positioning. Return to seating will be over a graduated extension of sitting time with assessment of the impact on the area. This progress is patient-specific and, in some cases, can extend for several weeks.
- Hand reconstruction, including replantation of digits, will require elevation but within the limits of those directed by the surgeon. Although elevation will reduce oedema, the reality that if the elevation is too high it may compromise the arterial inflow highlights the importance of following surgical instructions or enquiring on each basis if this is not clear.

Working and playing (AL 9)

Resuming normal activities will be dependent on a patient's recovery, how the wounds progress, weight-bearing restrictions from other injuries (Chao & Lamp, 2014), the nature of the work and how the person would travel to it. For example, a patient with a pedicled forehead flap who works from a computer at home may feel able to return to a level of work sooner than someone who has to travel to work. In general, activities will be altered for a minimum of 3 months with graduated return in line with the nature of the surgery. Flap reconstruction of the lower limb is susceptible to long-term swelling. Long-term management may require compression once the surgeon is satisfied this will not compromise the flap.

Sleeping (AL 10)

Although essential for recovery in the first 24 hours after surgery, repeated disturbance for flap monitoring can result in sleep deprivation (Storch & Rice, 2005). This too will impact on the ability of the patient to rest and recover from the surgery. Therefore, where possible, planning to undertake nursing interventions collectively should occur.

Flap donor sites

The nature of the donor site and nursing care issues will depend on the type of flap that has been lifted. It may be directly closed, as in the case of latissimus dorsi or gastrocnemius muscle flaps. However, where direct closure is not possible the area may need to have an STSG graft applied, as in the case of a local, pedicled fasciocutaneous flap on the leg (Fig. 24.8).

The type and origin of tissue used in the flap may have functional consequences, such as muscle taken from the abdomen where a mesh may be used to provide abdominal support and prevent an abdominal hernia occurring. In addition, complications may relate to the nature and place of the donor site or the amount of tension it is

under. Alterations in strength and impact on exercise may occur as a result of muscle removal. For example, use of the latissimus dorsi will reduce muscular strength in the back and impact on activities that depend on that muscle function. Potential problems include bleeding, seroma formation, delayed healing and further scarring.

Bleeding is part of the postoperative monitoring and specifically includes watching for swelling in the donor site that might suggest haematoma formation and checking the drainage in the vacuum drains. Seroma formation is a collection of serous fluid in the dead space resulting from the movement of tissue used for the flap reconstruction. Recommended management varies in the literature due to paucity of evidence to support one approach over another (Massey et al, 2018). Management options for small seromas include using fitted support garments such as compression pants, to apply pressure to the area, or waiting for spontaneous resolution as the new scar tissue forms and obliterates the space for the fluid to collect. However, large seromas may necessitate serial aspiration with the possibility of injecting sclerosing agents to prevent re-accumulation (Daoud et al, 2018). In some cases, chronic seromas may require surgical intervention for resolution (Sadeghi & Malata, 2013). Delayed wound healing can occur where pressure is applied on the wound edges from seroma formation as a result of infection or because removing the tissue for the flap results in tight closure. These wounds should be managed in line with the principles of wound management outlined in Chapter 5. The additional scarring may result in altered sensation and impacts further on the body image challenges facing patients undergoing this surgery.

Conclusion

Plastic surgery is based on techniques that repair and reconstruct any part of the body, which are being increasingly used by surgeons across the full spectrum of surgery. In both skin grafting and flap surgery there will be at least two wounds, a recipient and donor site. The complexity of the reconstruction varies considerably, and nursing care is dependent on the nurse understanding the surgery undertaken, following operative instructions, and applying management to the patient-specific situation. The wounds should be managed by understanding the physiology associated with them and applying the principles of wound assessment and management. All reconstruction results in a wound and subsequent scar, so assisting patients with an altered body image underpins all aspects of this surgical specialty. Referral to support agencies can assist in this, although the importance of the nurse managing these patients in the early days of exposure to an altered body image must not be underestimated.

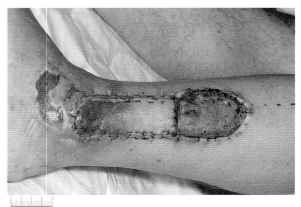

cmD750 105mm 1m

Figure 24.8 Fasciocutaneous local flap rotated with a vascular pedicle and a skin-grafted flap donor site.

SUMMARY OF KEY POINTS

- Skin grafts are at their most vulnerable in the first 5–10 days and inspection demands a careful approach.
- Split-thickness skin graft donor sites need exudate and pain management and extended healing times should be referred for specialist advice.
- Nurses need to understand terminology and associated surgery when dealing with flaps.
- Complex flaps require intense monitoring where visual observation remains the gold standard.
- The impact of surgery on body image remains a key nursing consideration throughout the entire patient trajectory when undergoing any plastic surgery procedure.

REFLECTIVE LEARNING POINTS

Having read this chapter, think about what you now know and what you still need to find out about. These questions may help:

- What is the role of plastic surgery with regards to burns?
- Describe the role and function of the nurse with regards to the post-surgical care of patients undergoing reconstructive surgery to the head and neck.
- List and discuss four congenital conditions that are treated with reconstructive surgery.

References

Asbery, J. (2017). The development of plastic and reconstructive surgery nursing (Part 1). *The Dissector*, *45*(2), 12–14.

Asbery, J. (2018). The development of plastic and reconstructive surgery nursing (Part 2). *The Dissector*, *46*(1), 32–34.

Beldon, P. (2003). Skin grafts 2: management of donor site wounds in the community. *British Journal of Community Nursing*, *8*(9), S6, S8, S10, S12.

Beldon, P. (2007). What you need to know about skin grafts and donor site wounds. *Wound Essentials*, *2*, 149–155.

Biopharm. (2019). *Biopharm leeches*. [Online] Available at: <www.bio-pharm-leeches.com/applying1.html>

Black, J. M., & Black, S. B. (2012). Reconstructive surgery. In R. A. Bryant, & D. P. Nix (Eds.), *Acute and chronic wounds current management concepts* (4th ed.). St Louis: Elsevier Mosby.

Broyles, J. M., Smith, M., Coon, D., & Bonawitz, S. C. (2016). Assessment of nursing deficiencies in the postoperative care of microsurgical patients. *Journal of Reconstructive Microsurgery*, *32*(8), 615–624.

Butler, C. E., & Adelman, D. M. (2014). Principles of microsurgery. In C. H. Thorne (Ed.), *Grabb and Smith's plastic surgery* (7th ed.). London: Lippincott Wiiliams and Wilkins.

Chao, A., & Lamp, S. (2014). Current approaches to free flap monitoring. *Plastic Surgical Nursing*, *34*(2), 52–56.

Daoud, F. A., Thayer, A., Daswani, G. S., Maraqa, T., Perinjelil., & Mercer, L. (2018). Management of chronic abdominal wall seroma with Doxycycline sclerotherapy using a negative pressure wound therapy system. *International Journal of Surgical Case Reports*, *51*, 25–28.

Del Rosario, C., & Barkley, T. W. (2017). Postoperative graft and flap care: what clinical nurses need to know. *Medsurg Nursing*, *26*(3), 180–192.

Higgins, L., Wasiak, J., Spinks, A., & Cleland, H. (2012). Split thickness skin graft donor site management: a randomized controlled trial comparing polyurethane with calcium alginate dressings. *International Wound Journal*, *9*(2), 126–131.

Holden, J. (2015). Top tips for skin graft and donor site management. *Wound Essentials*, *10*(2), 7–13.

Hormbrey, E., Pandya, A., & Giele, H. (2003). Adhesive retention dressings are more comfortable than alginate dressings on split-skin-graft donor sites. *The British Association of Plastic Surgeons*, *56*(5), 498–503.

Hsieh, S.T. (2015). *Free tissue transfer flaps*. [Online] Available at: <emedicine.medscape.com/article/1284841-overview>

Janis, J. E., Kwon, R. K., & Attinger, C. E. (2011). The new reconstructive ladder; modifications to a traditional model. *Plastic and Reconstructive Surgery*, *127*, 205S–212S.

Keilani, C., Duhoux, D., Lakhel, A., Giraud, O., Brachet, M., Duhamel, P., et al. (2017). Grafting both acute wound site and adjacent donor site with the same graft: an easy and safe procedure to improve healing and minimize pain in the elderly and bed-ridden patients. *Annals of Burns and Fire Disasters*, *30*(1), 52–56.

Khan, M., Mohan, A., Ahmed, W., & Rayatt, S. (2010). Nursing monitoring and management of free and pedicled flaps outcomes of teaching sessions on flap care. *Plastic Surgical Nursing*, *30*(4), 213–216.

Kornhaber, R., Visentin, D., Thapa, D. K., West, S., McKittrick, A., Haik, J., et al. (2018). Cosmetic camouflage improves quality of life among patients with skin disfigurement: a systematic review. *Body Image*, *27*, 98–108.

Levine, P. L. (2014). Muscle flaps and their blood supply. In C. H. Thorne (Ed.), *Grabb and Smith's plastic surgery* (7th ed.). London: Lippincott Williams and Wilkins.

Lucas, V. S., & King, A. W. (2010). Wound care for the plastic surgery nurse. *Plastic Surgical Nursing*, *30*(3), 158–169.

Madrid, E., Urrútia, G., Roqué, I., Figuls, M., Pardo-Hernandez, H., Campos, J., et al. (2016). Active body surface warming systems for preventing complications caused by inadvertent perioperative hypothermia in adults. *Cochrane Database of Systematic Reviews*, *4*, CD009016. Available at: <www.cochrane.org/CD009016/ANAESTH_body-warming-people-undergoing-surgery-avoid-complications-and-increase-comfort-after-surgery>.

Massey, L. H., Pathak, A., Bhargava, A., Smart, N. J., & Daniels, I. R. (2018). The use of adjuncts to reduce seroma in open incisional hernia repair: a systematic review. *Hernia, 22,* 273–283.

Mazzola, R. F., & Mazzola, I. C. (2018). History of reconstructive and aesthetic surgery. In G. C. Gurtner, & P. C. Neligan (Eds.), *Plastic surgery* (4th ed.). St Louis: Elsevier.

McGregor, I. A., & McGregor, A. D. (2000). *Fundamental techniques of plastic surgery* (10th ed.). Edinburgh: Churchill Livingstone.

Nahabedian, M. Y., & Nahabedian, A. G. (2016). Autologous microvascular breast reconstruction: Postoperative strategies to improve outcomes. *Nursing, 46*(12), 26–34.

Nursing and Midwifery Council (NMC). (2018). *The Code: Professional standards of practice and behaviour for nurses, midwives and nursing associates.* Available at: <www.nmc.org.uk/standards/code/read-the-code-online>

Pasterfield, M., Thompson, A. R., & Clarke, S. A. (2019). A qualitative examination of the experience of skin camouflage by people living with visible skin conditions. *The British Journal of Dermatology, 180*(6), 1531–1532.

Rau, A. S., Viktorja, R., Schmidt, E. P., Taraseviciene-Stewart, L., & Deleyiannis, F. W. (2017). Electronic cigarettes are as tonic to skin flap survival as tobacco cigarettes. *Annals of Plastic Surgery, 79*(1), 86–91.

Reynolds, A., & OBoyle, C. (2016). Nurses' experiences of leech therapy in plastic and reconstructive surgery. *British Journal of Nursing, 25*(13), 629–733.

Roper, N., Logan, W. W., & Tierney, A. J. (2000). *The Roper-Logan-Tierny model for nursing based on activities of living.* Edinburgh: Churchill Livingstone.

Sadeghi, A., & Malata, C. (2013). Case report persistent seromas in abdominal free flap donor sites after postmastectomy breast reconstruction surgery: case reports and literature review. *Eplasty, 13,* e24. Available at: <www.ncbi.nlm.nih.gov/pmc/articles/PMC3676264>.

Salgado, C. J., Chim, H., Schoenoff, S., & Mardini, S. (2010). Postoperative care and monitoring of the reconstructed head and neck patient. *Seminars in Plastic Surgery, 24*(3), 281–287.

Scherer-Pietramaggiori, S. S., Pietramaggiori, G., & Orgil, D. P. (2018). Skin graft. In G. C. Gurtner, & P. C. Neligan (Eds.), *Plastic surgery* (4th ed.). St Louis: Elsevier.

Sig, A. K., Guney, M., Guclu, A. U., & Ozmen, E. (2017). Medicinal leech therapy – an overall perspective. *Integrative Medicine Research, 6*(4), 337–343. Available at: <www.sciencedirect.com/science/article/pii/S221342201730104X>.

Spear, M. (2016). Medicinal leech therapy: friend or foe. *Plastic Surgical Nursing, 36*(3), 121–125.

Spiers, E. (2018). Managing vascular compromise of hand and digit replantation following traumatic amputation. *British Journal of Nursing, 27*(20), S50–S56.

Storch, J. E., & Rice, J. (2005). *Reconstructive plastic surgical nursing.* Oxford: Blackwell Publishing.

Terrill, P. J., Goh, R. C. W., & Bailey, M. J. (2007). Split thickness skin graft donor sites: a comparative study of two absorbent dressings. *Journal of Wound Care, 16*(10), 433–438.

Thimmappa, N. D., Vasile, J. V., Ahn, C. Y., Levine, J. L., & Prince, M. R. (2019). MRA of the skin: mapping for advanced breast reconstructive surgery. *Clinical Radiology, 74*(1), 13–28.

Thorne, C. H. (2014). Techniques and principles in plastic surgery. In C. H. Thorne (Ed.), *Grabb and Smith's plastic surgery* (7th ed.). London: Lippincott Wiiliams and Wilkins.

Voineskos, S. H., Ayeni, O. A., McKnight, L., & Thoma, A. (2009). Systematic review of skin graft donor site dressings. *Plastic and Reconstructive Surgery, 124*(1), 298–306.

Wax, M. ,K. (2013). The role of the implantable Doppler probe in free flap surgery. *Laryngoscope, 124,* S1–S12.

Welshhans, J. L., & Hom, D. B. (2016). Are leeches effective in local/regional skin flap salvage? *Laryngoscope, 126,* 1271–1272.

Wounds UK. (2013a). *Best practice statement: The use of topical antimicrobial agents in wound management* [Online]. Available at: <www.wounds-uk.com/resources/details/best-practice-statement-use-topical-antimicrobial-agents-wound-management>

Wounds UK. (2013b). *Best practice statement: Effective exudate management* [Online]. Available at: <www.wounds-uk.com/resources/details/best-practice-statement-effective-exudate-management>

Wounds UK. (2016). *Best practice statement: holistic management of venous leg ulceration* [Online]. Available at: <www.wounds-uk.com/resources/details/best-practice-statement-holistic-management-of-venous-leg-ulceration>

Yin, Y., Zhang, R., Li, S., Guo, J., Hou, Z., & Zhang, Y. (2018). Negative-pressure therapy versus conventional therapy on split-thickness skin graft: A systematic review and meta-analysis. *International Journal of Surgery, 50,* 43–48.

Zelken, J. A., & Berli, J. U. (2015). Coffee, tea, and chocolate after microsurgery why not? *Annals of Plastic Surgery, 74*(2), 139.

Index

Index